Angioplasty and Stenting Procedures

Angioplasty and Stenting Procedures

Editor: Casey Judd

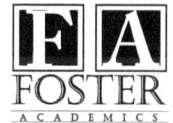

FOSTER
ACADEMICS

www.fosteracademics.com

www.fosteracademics.com

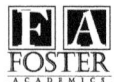
FOSTER
ACADEMICS

Cataloging-in-Publication Data

Angioplasty and stenting procedures / edited by Casey Judd.
    p. cm.
Includes bibliographical references and index.
ISBN 978-1-63242-476-1
1. Angioplasty. 2. Stents (Surgery). 3. Blood-vessels--Surgery. 4. Coronary heart disease--Treatment.
I. Judd, Casey.
RD598.35.A53 A54 2017
617413--dc23

Foster Academics,
118-35 Queens Blvd., Suite 400,
Forest Hills, NY 11375, USA

ISBN 978-1-63242-476-1 (Hardback)

Contents

Preface

The purpose of the book is to provide a glimpse into the dynamics and to present opinions and studies of some of the scientists engaged in the development of new ideas in the field from very different standpoints. This book will prove useful to students and researchers owing to its high content quality.

Angioplasty is defined as a medical procedure that widens obstructed arteries and veins in the human body. This book on angioplasty discusses techniques and methods followed during the surgical procedure. This book elucidates the concepts and innovative models around prospective developments with respect to angioplasty. While understanding the long-term perspective of the topics, the book makes an effort in highlighting their impacts as a modern tool for the growth of the discipline. This book on angioplasty will be useful to students, experts and professionals in the field of vascular surgery, cardiology and medical imaging.

At the end, I would like to appreciate all the efforts made by the authors in completing their chapters professionally. I express my deepest gratitude to all of them for contributing to this book by sharing their valuable works. A special thanks to my family and friends for their constant support in this journey.

Editor

Treatment for Stable Coronary Artery Disease: A Network Meta-Analysis of Cost-Effectiveness Studies

Thibaut Caruba[1]***, Sandrine Katsahian**[2,3]**, Catherine Schramm**[2]**, Anaïs Charles Nelson**[2]**, Pierre Durieux**[3,4]**,
Dominique Bégué[5]**, Yves Juillière**[6]**, Olivier Dubourg**[7,8]**, Nicolas Danchin**[9,10⑨]**, Brigitte Sabatier**[1,3⑨]

1 Pharmacie, Hôpital Européen Georges Pompidou, APHP, Paris, France, 2 URC Hôpital Henri Mondor, APHP, Créteil, France, 3 Equipe 22, Centre de Recherche des Cordeliers, UMRS 762 INSERM, Paris, France, 4 Département de Santé Publique et Informatique, Hôpital Européen Georges Pompidou, APHP, Paris, France, 5 Faculté de Pharmacie, Université René Descartes, Paris, France, 6 Cardiologie, Institut Lorrain du Cœur et des Vaisseaux Louis Mathieu, Nancy, France, 7 Cardiologie, Hôpital Ambroise Paré, APHP, Boulogne Billancourt, France, 8 Université de Versailles-Saint Quentin, Montigny-Le-Bretonneux, France, 9 Cardiologie, Hôpital Européen Georges Pompidou, APHP, Paris, France, 10 Faculté de Médecine, Université René Descartes, Paris, France

Abstract

Introduction and Objectives: Numerous studies have assessed cost-effectiveness of different treatment modalities for stable angina. Direct comparisons, however, are uncommon. We therefore set out to compare the efficacy and mean cost per patient after 1 and 3 years of follow-up, of the following treatments as assessed in randomized controlled trials (RCT): medical therapy (MT), percutaneous coronary intervention (PCI) without stent (PTCA), with bare-metal stent (BMS), with drug-eluting stent (DES), and elective coronary artery bypass graft (CABG).

Methods: RCT comparing at least two of the five treatments and reporting clinical and cost data were identified by a systematic search. Clinical end-points were mortality and myocardial infarction (MI). The costs described in the different trials were standardized and expressed in US $ 2008, based on purchasing power parity. A network meta-analysis was used to compare costs.

Results: Fifteen RCT were selected. Mortality and MI rates were similar in the five treatment groups both for 1-year and 3-year follow-up. Weighted cost per patient however differed markedly for the five treatment modalities, at both one year and three years (P<0.0001). MT was the least expensive treatment modality: US $3069 and 13 864 after one and three years of follow-up, while CABG was the most costly: US $27 003 and 28 670 after one and three years. PCI, whether with plain balloon, BMS or DES came in between, but was closer to the costs of CABG.

Conclusions: Appreciable savings in health expenditures can be achieved by using MT in the management of patients with stable angina.

Editor: Yu-Kang Tu, National Taiwan University, Taiwan

Funding: The authors have no support or funding to report.

Competing Interests: The authors have read the journal's policy. Three co-authors have the following conflicts: 1) Pr Dubourg: consultancy: Bracco Altam Pharma; and grant: Sorin France and Medtronic. 2) Pr Juillière: consultancy: Abbott vascular, AstraZeneca, Bayer, Bristol-Myers-Squibb, MSD-Schering, Novartis, Sanofi Aventis and Servier; and grant: AstraZeneca. 3) Pr Danchin: board membership: AstraZeneca, Bayer, Daiichi-Sankyo, Eli-Lilly, Novo-nordisk and Servier; consultancy: GSK and Sanofi Aventis; and grant: MSD, AstraZeneca, Daiichi-Sankyo, Eli-Lilly, GSK, Novartis and Sanofi Aventis.

* E-mail: thibaut.caruba@egp.aphp.fr

⑨ These authors contributed equally to this work.

Introduction

Expenses related to the management of coronary artery disease represent a considerable burden for healthcare systems. The estimated direct and indirect cost of heart disease in 2010 in the USA was $177.13 billion [1]. The recent increase in expenditure can be explained by the rising number of invasive procedures, and by higher costs for percutaneous coronary intervention (PCI) due to the widespread use of drug-eluting stents (DES). In the USA, coronary revascularization is one of the most common major medical interventions provided by the healthcare system; between 2001 and 2008, the number of coronary revascularization procedures rose by 6% with over 1 million performed in 2006

[2]. In the same year, in the USA, over 70% of PCI were performed with DES [3]. Although DES do reduce the risk of repeat procedures as compared to bare-metal stents (BMS), widespread use of this technique has not led to the anticipated reduction in the total number of procedures performed [4].

Clinical data have failed to demonstrate clear superiority of any of the treatment modalities available (medical therapy alone, PCI or coronary artery bypass graft [CABG]) for stable coronary artery disease in terms of hard clinical events [5–7] for non-specific populations [8] (i.e., patients with diabetes, peripheral arterial disease, etc). Comparing the costs of these different management strategies therefore appears warranted and numerous studies have previously assessed the cost-effectiveness of the different pairwise therapeutic options [9–14].

In order to clarify this important public healthcare issue, we set out to compare, through a network meta-analysis, the efficacy and mean cost per patient (after one and three years of follow-up) of the following treatments as assessed in randomized controlled trials (RCT): MT, percutaneous coronary intervention without stent (PTCA), with BMS, with -DES, and elective CABG.

Methods

Search strategy

Our strategy involved searching Medline via PubMed, Embase and the Cochrane library and relevant websites (www.theheart. org, www.pcronline.com, www.tctmd.com, www. clinicaltrialresults.org, www.crtonline.org and stent manufacturer web pages). The search was also extended to proceedings of the American Heart Association, the American College of Cardiology, the British Cardiac Society and the European Society of Cardiology.

Keywords (used as free text words) for the PubMed search were "coronary artery disease", "myocardial revascularization" and "costs". We selected the following filters: "humans", "clinical trial" (for the type of study) and "English" for the language. The same keywords were used to search in the Cochrane Library. For the Embase search, two keywords were combined: "ischemic heart disease" and "cost". The search was filtered on the term "humans", and limited to RCT. Lastly, to avoid duplication, we excluded the PubMed database that is accessible via Embase (figure S1).

The search was restricted to the period between January 1, 1980 and June 1, 2012.

Two authors (TC and BS) independently reviewed titles, abstract, and the full text as required to determine whether the studies met our inclusion criteria. Any conflict between reviewers was resolved by re-review and discussion.

Inclusion and exclusion criteria

We conducted our analysis on adult patients with stable or stabilized unstable angina (stabilization was defined by symptoms older than 48 hours) or documented silent myocardial ischemia. All patients were assessed, regardless of whether they had single or multivessel coronary artery disease. Indeed, for these clinical situations, all three treatment modalities (MT only, PCI, CABG) are considered possible alternatives by learned societies, based on the results of RCT and the related meta-analyses [5–7,15,16]. We did not include RCT where patients had acute coronary syndromes (ACS), non-stabilized unstable angina (symptoms within 48 hours of randomization) or myocardial infarction in the previous 48 hours (MI), because revascularisation is usually considered the preferred therapeutic option for such patients [17,18]. We also excluded studies performed in patients with in-stent restenosis because revascularization is the standard approach in these situations [19–21].

We selected all published randomized controlled trials that documented at least two of the five treatment modalities: MT, PTCA without stent, PCI with BMS or DES and elective CABG with cardiopulmonary bypass. Time periods with at least one event in any group were included in the analyses.

Studies were included in the clinical review if they reported 1) rates of death and MI, and 2) direct costs due to medical expenses for the management of the disease over a follow-up period of one year and/or three years. Indeed, costs relating to treatment of stable coronary artery disease are related to hospitalization due to complications such as subsequent revascularisation, MI and death.

We excluded all studies focusing on specific patient profiles, such as those with as diabetes mellitus, all studies with data based on economic models, and studies on non-conventional treatment modalities such as off-pump coronary artery bypass grafting, complete vessel treatment with PCI, etc. Lastly, all studies comprising clinical data alone were also excluded.

Data extraction and cost conversions

We recorded information from each trial about the publication (first author, journal, and year of publication); patient demographics (mean age, proportion of men, prior revascularization, prior MI, diabetic participants, and patients with multivessel disease); the type of treatments that were compared and the number of patients assigned to each group; years of patient enrolment; whether the trial was blinded; and follow-up duration.

We recorded death and MI rates in each arm of the studies. To study the economical outcome we sought the direct costs related to treatment in each study. We extracted the direct medical-care costs for the management of the disease. Costs were recorded with the currency and year of calculation.

A cascading adjustment was made to generate costs for the patient that would be comparable across the different countries. We used a comparison adjustment by purchasing power parity (PPP). The costs recorded ineach study were converted into US $ 2008 and then: 1) costs were collected in the original currency used in the study; 2) if necessary, costs were converted into the currency of the country where the economic study was conducted; 3) between the year the costs were calculated and 2008, we applied the consumer price index of the country where the economic study was conducted; 4) costs were converted to US $ 2008 using the PPP in 2008 (available on the Organisation for Economic Co-operation and Development website [15]). The currency conversion rate expresses the purchasing power of different currencies in one common unit (i.e. US $); it incorporates not only the exchange rates between currencies, but also the amount of currency needed to buy the same basket of goods and services in different countries. This method has been used previously in several studies [16–18].

Additionally, for each RCT, we recorded the source of the costs studied. Direct costs of treatment for stable coronary artery disease were related to hospitalisation (for an initial revascularization procedure or for management of complications), to outpatient care (medical visit, radiological and biological examinations, etc), and to outpatient drug prescriptions (antiplatelet drugs, antianginal drugs, etc).

Assessment of methodological quality

Quality was evaluated using two checklists. Relevance of clinical data was assessed using methods put forward by the Heart Collaborative Review Group [19]. The 4 criteria considered are: the randomization process, the allocation concealment process, the potential for selection bias after allocation and the adequacy of masking. For each criterion, three or four answers are possible, "A" being the best. The "Drummond checklist" was used to measure the methodological quality of full economic evaluations conducted alongside single effectiveness studies [20]. This checklist evaluates 35 criteria grouped into three themes: study design, data collection, and analysis and interpretation of results. These checklists are presented in the figures S2 and S3.

Statistical analysis

We performed a network meta-analysis to compare MT *versus* PTCA *versus* PCI with BMS *versus* PCI and with DES *versus* CABG, separately all with regard to rates for death and MI.

Initially, Bayesian random effects models were used for multiple treatment comparisons; this approach preserves the within-trial randomised treatment comparison of each analysis. We compared the five treatments after one year of follow-up and then after three years of follow-up. Then, we used an extension of this model to compare the five treatment approaches throughout the whole follow-up period [21–24]. We used a random walk model based on piece-wise constant hazards to account for varying follow-up times [25]. In a random walk model, log hazard at time t depends on the log hazard at previous times. The model included random effects of the trials, adjacent time periods, interaction between trials and periods and treatment comparisons, and was fitted to the three pre-specified time periods (years 1 to 3).

Lastly, a sensitivity analysis was conducted to verify the robustness of the results. This focused only on studies that included outpatient costs (outpatient care and/or outpatient drugs) in addition to hospital costs.

Hazard ratios (HR) and cumulative incidences were estimated from the median of the posterior distribution. A HR lower than 1 indicates a benefit from the treatment. All results are given with 95% credibility intervals (CI) from the 2.5^{th} and 97.5^{th} percentiles of the posterior distribution. A result was considered significant when the CI of the HR did not contain 1. We also calculated the probability that each treatment was the best.

All results are based on 130 000 simulations with 30 000 burn-in. In all analyses, MT was considered as the reference treatment.

Mean costs, weighted by the number of patients in each study for each treatment, were calculated and compared by an ANOVA after 1 and 3 years of follow-up.

All analyses were carried out with WinBUGS version 1.4 and R version 2.12.

Results

We screened the titles and abstracts of 246 potentially eligible reports and examined the full text of 70 articles. We identified 15 RCT with 18 articles and two oral communications presented at major medical congresses that met our inclusion criteria (Figure 1): ACME [26] (*The Veterans Affairs Cooperative Study: Angioplasty Compared to Medicine*), ARTS [27,28] (*Arterial Revascularization Therapy Study*), BENESTENT II [29] (*Randomised comparison of implantation of heparin-coated stents with balloon angioplasty in selected patients with coronary artery disease*), COURAGE [14] (*Optimal Medical Therapy with or without PCI for Stable Coronary Disease*), EAST [30] (*Emory Angioplasty Versus Surgery Trial*), ENDEAVOR II [12,31–33] (*Randomized Controlled Trial to Evaluate the Safety and Efficacy of the Medtronic AVE ABT-578 Eluting Driver Coronary Stent in De Novo Native Coronary Artery Lesions*), ERACI [34,35] (*Argentine Randomized Trial of Percutaneous Transluminal Coronary Angioplasty Versus Coronary Artery Bypass Surgery in Multivessel Disease*), MASS II [36] (*The Medicine, Angioplasty, or Surgery Study II*), RAVEL [37] (*randomised study with the sirolimus eluting Bx Velocity balloon expandable stent in the treatment of patients with de novo native coronary artery lesions*), RITA 2 [38] (*The second Randomised Intervention Treatment of Angina*), SIRIUS [11] (*Sirolimus-Eluting Stent in De-Novo Native Coronary Lesions*), SoS [10] (*the Stent or Surgery trial*), STRESS [39] (*Stent Restenosis Study*), SYNTAX [40] (*Synergy between PCI with Taxus and Cardiac Surgery*) and TAXUS IV [41] (*A polymer-based, paclitaxel-eluting stent in patients with coronary artery disease*). The table S4 entitled "List of excluded and selected studies" presents the main reasons for exclusion.

The characteristics of included RCT are presented in table 1. Six of these trials involved patients with multivessel disease: ARTS [27,28], COURAGE [14], EAST [30], ERACI [34,35], MASS II [36] and SoS [10]. The other clinical trials included patients with single vessel disease. For eight trials, the duration of follow-up was one year: BENESTENT II [29], MASS II [36], RAVEL [37], SIRIUS [11], SoS [10], STRESS [39], SYNTAX [40] and TAXUS IV [41]. For four trials, 3-year follow-up was available: ACME [26], COURAGE [14], EAST [30] and RITA 2 [38]. Two trials included both 1 and 3-year follow-up data: ARTS [27,28] and ERACI [34,35]. Lastly, in ENDEAVOR II [12,31–33], duration of follow-up was 1, 2, 3 and 4 years.

Figure 2 shows the comparators and the duration of patient follow-up for each RCT. The BENESTENT II [29] trial was a comparison of a heparin-coated stent *versus* PTCA. We considered this particular stent as a bare-metal stent because drug-eluting stent referred to stents with antiproliferative coating. Only one trial compared three treatment modalities: MT, BMS and CABG: MASS II [36].

According to the recommendations put forward by the Heart Collaborative Review Group, eleven trials described appropriate methods of randomization: ARTS [27,28], BENESTENT II [29], COURAGE [14], ENDEAVOR II, MASS II [36], RAVEL [37], SIRIUS [11], SoS [10], STRESS [39], SYNTAX [40] and TAXUS IV [41]. The methods used to conceal treatment allocation were considered adequate in ten trials: ARTS [27,28], BENESTENT II [29], COURAGE [14], MASS II [36], RAVEL [37], SIRIUS [11], SoS [10], STRESS [39], SYNTAX [40] and TAXUS IV [41]. Four of the sixteen trials were double blind: ENDEAVOR II, RAVEL [37], SIRIUS [11] and TAXUS IV [41]. Quality assessment of the clinical methodology is reported in the table S1.

According to the Drummond checklist, one trial did not specify the method used for estimating quantities and unit cost (checklist item 17): ERACI [34,35]. Three of the eight trials with a 3-year follow-up did not apply the discount rate as recommended (checklist item 23): ARTS [27,28], EAST [30] and ERACI [34,35]. For eight trials, there was no approach to sensitivity analysis (checklist item 27): ARTS [27,28], BENESTENT II [29], EAST [30], ENDEAVOR II [12,31–33], ERACI [34,35], MASS II [36], SoS [10] and STRESS [39]. Results of quality assessment of economical methodology are displayed in the table S2.

Clinical analysis

In all, the 15 trials included had enrolled 9 565 patients followed for one year and 6 443 patients for three years. The percentages of men or diabetic patients were similarly distributed among the treatment arms, regardless of duration of follow-up (P = 0.22 for the percentage of men and 0.23 for the percentage of diabetes mellitus).

After one year of follow-up, 202 patients died: three of the 203 patients on MT (1.5%), 60 of the 2 221 patients with CABG (2.7%), nine of the 578 patients with PTCA (1.6%), 60 of the 3 693 patients with BMS (1.6%) and 70 of the 2 796 patients with DES (2.5%). After three years of follow-up, 345 patients had died: 111 of the 1 759 patients on MT (6.3%), 43 of the 863 patients with CABG (5.0%), 39 of the 870 patients with PTCA (4.5%), 133 of the 2 336 patients with BMS (5.7%) and 19 of the 584 patients with DES (3.2%).

After one year of follow-up, 394 patients had a MI: eight of the 203 patients on MT (3.9%), 96 of the 2 221 patients with CABG (4.3%), 33 of the 578 patients with PTCA (5.7%), 171 of the 3 693 patients with BMS (4.6%) and 86 of the 2 769 patients with DES (3.1%). After three years of follow-up, 530 patients had a MI: 147 of the 1 759 patients on MT (8.3%), 80 of the 841 patients with CABG (9.5%), 67 of the 845 patients with PTCA (7.9%), 212 of the 2 336 patients with BMS (9.1%) and 19 of the 584 patients with DES (3.3%).

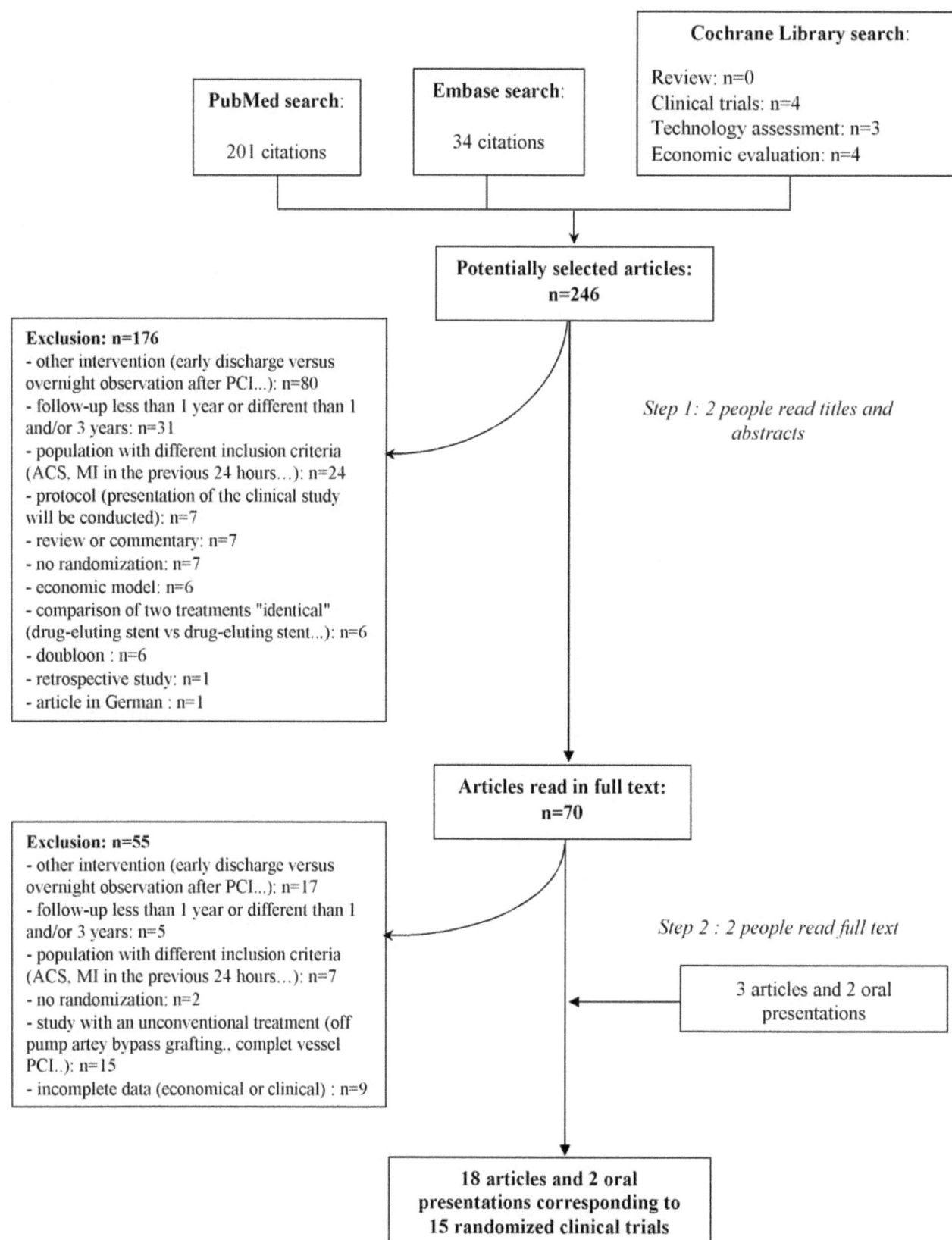

Figure 1. Flow diagram of the screening process.

Table 1. Baseline characteristics of patients in the studies selected.

Study	Inclusion	Inclusion criteria	Blinded	Single- or multi-vessel disease	Number of centres	Number of patients	Mean age (years)	Diabetes mellitus (%)	Sex (% men)	Previous MI (%)	Previous revascularisation (%)	Follow-up (years)
PTCA versus MT												
ACME [26]	1987–1990	stable angina pectoris, a strikingly positive exercise tolerance test or an MI within the past 3 months	no	single	8	200	62	18	100	30	0	3
RITA 2 [38]	1992–1996	angiographically-documented coronary artery disease	no	single	20	1 018	58	9	82	47	0	3
PTCA versus CABG												
ERACI [34,35]	1988–1990	severe stenosis >70% in ≥1 major epicardial coronary artery, severely limiting stable angina or refractory resting unstable angina despite optimal medical therapy, no or minimal symptoms but with a large area of myocardium at risk identified by exercise testing	no	multi	1	127	57	11	85	50	NA	1 and 3
EAST [30]	1987–1990	stable or unstable angina or objective signs of ischemia	no	multi	1	392	61	23	74	41	0	3
CABG versus MT												
MASS II [36]	1995–2000	symptomatic multivessel coronary disease (2 or more epicardial coronary arteries with ≥70% narrowing),	no	multi	1	611	60	14	85	22	0	1
CABG versus PCI with BMS												
MASS II [36]	1995–2000	symptomatic multivessel coronary disease (≥2 epicardial coronary arteries with ≥70% narrowing),	no	multi	1	611	60	14	85	22	0	1
SoS [10]	1996–1999	symptomatic patients with multivessel coronary artery disease	no	multi	53	988	61	14	79	45	0	1
ARTS [27,28]	1997–1998	stable angina pectoris or unstable angina pectoris or silent myocardial ischemia	no	multi	67	1 205	61	17	76	43	0	1 and 3

Table 1. Cont.

Study	Inclu sion	Inclusion criteria	Blinded	Single- or multi-vessel disease	Number of centres	Number of patients	Mean age (years)	Diabetes mellitus (%)	Sex (% men)	Previous MI (%)	Previous revascularisation (%)	Follow-up (years)
CABG versus PCI with DES												
SYNTAX [40]	2005–2007	stable or unstable angina pectoris with ischemia; or patients with atypical chest pain or asymptomatic with demonstrated myocardial ischemia	no	multi	85	1 740	65	28	78	32	0	1
PCI with BMS versus PCI with DES												
SIRIUS [11]	2001	history of stable or unstable angina and signs of myocardial ischemia.	double	single	53	1 058	62	26	71	31	NA	1
TAXUS IV [41]	2002	stable or unstable angina or inducible ischemia	double	single	73	1 314	63	24	72	30	NA	1
RAVEL [37]	2000–2001	stable or unstable angina or silent ischemia	double	single	19	238	61	19	76	36	NA	1
ENDEA VOR II [12,31–33]	2003–2004	patients with clinical evidence of ischemia or a positive functional test	double	single	72	1 197	62	20	76	41	20	1, 2 and 3
PCI with BMS versus PTCA												
STRESS [39]	1991–1993	symptomatic ischemic heart disease	no	single	8	207	61	14	72	35	6	1
MT versus PCI with BMS												
MASS II [36]	1995–2000	symptomatic multivessel coronary disease	no	multi	1	611	60	14	85	22	0	1
COURAGE [14]	1999–2004	chronic angina pectoris CCS I-III, stable post-MI patients, and asymptomatic patients with objective evidence of myocardial ischemia.	no	multi	50	2 287	62	33	85	38	25	3
CABG versus PCI with DES												
BENE STENT II [29]	1995–1996	stable angina or unstable angina	no	single	50	823	54	12	78	26	9	1

MT: medical therapy, PTCA: percutaneous coronary angioplasty, CABG: coronary artery bypass graft, DES: drug-eluting stent, BMS: bare-metal stent, NA: not available.

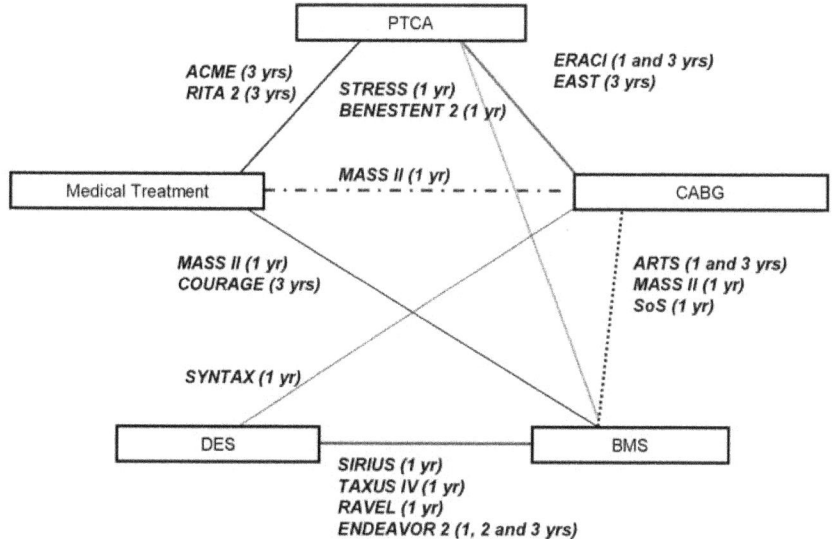

Figure 2. Comparators and duration of patient follow-up for the trials selected.

After one and three years of follow-up there was no statistically significant difference between the death and MI rates of the five treatments. Because of non-significant results, the rating of treatment efficacy is not informative (Table 2 and figure 3).

Economic analysis

Table 3 and figure 4 present the evaluation of cost per patient for each RCT: cost published in the article (year of publication and currency used) and cost per patient adjusted in US $ 2008. Figure 5 presents the mean cost per patient for each treatment. After one year of follow-up, the mean weighted cost per patient in US $ 2008 was: $3069 with MT, $27 003 with CABG, $12 483 with PTCA, $15 228 with BMS, and $23 973 with DES. After three years of follow-up, the mean weighted cost was: $13 864 with MT, $28 670 with CABG, $14 277 with PTCA, $25 513 with BMS, and $20 536 with DES. There was a statistically significant difference of weighted cost per patient for the comparison of the five treatments: P value was <0.0001 after one year and after three years. Between one and three years of follow-up, the greatest increase in average weighted cost per patient was observed with MT (+ $10 795, +352% compared with the cost per patient after one year). During this period, weighted cost with treatment by CABG was stable (+ $1667, +6% compared with cost per patient after one year). We performed a comparison of the weighted cost of each treatment in at least two clinical studies. For all these comparisons, at one and three years of follow-up, the differences observed were significant (P<0.0001): CABG versus PTCA after one year, CABG versus BMS after one year, CABG versus DES after one year, etc.

Table 2. Comparison of the rates of death and myocardial infarction between the 5 treatments (MT *versus* CABG *versus* PTCA *versus* BMS *versus* DES).

		Events				
		MT*	CABG	PTCA	BMS	DES
death within the first year of follow-up	HR (95% CI)	1	2.61 (0.63; 12.55)	3.78 (0.66; 25.28)	3.10 (0.76; 15.18)	4.01 (0.95; 21.12)
	probability treatment is the best	0.87	0.06	0.05	0.02	0.00
death within the first three years of follow-up	HR (95% CI)	1	1.01 (0.41; 2.25)	1.24 (0.57; 2.61)	0.83 (0.41; 1.46)	0.79 (0.23; 2.56)
	probability treatment is the best	0.11	0.15	0.05	0.24	0.49
MI within the first year of follow-up	HR (95% CI)	1	1.07 (0.37; 2.89)	1.67 (0.47; 5.47)	1.70 (0.59; 4.57)	1.14 (0.33; 3.25)
	probability treatment is the best	0.51	0.27	0.04	0.00	0.18
MI within the first three years of follow-up	HR (95% CI)	1	1.48 (0.52; 5.20)	1.36 (0.57; 3.97)	1.76 (0.72; 3.45)	1.03 (0.23; 6.11)
	probability treatment is the best	0.37	0.07	0.09	0.02	0.45

HR: hazard ratio, MI: myocardial infarction, MT: medical therapy, PTCA: percutaneous coronary angioplasty, CABG: coronary artery bypass graft, DES: drug-eluting stent, BMS: bare-metal stent, CI: confidence interval.
* medical therapy was the reference treatment.

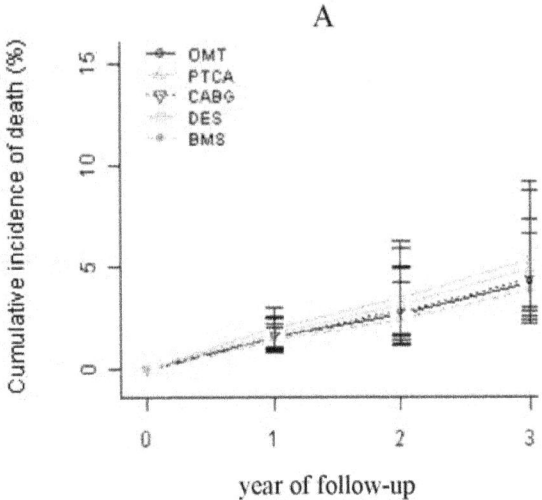
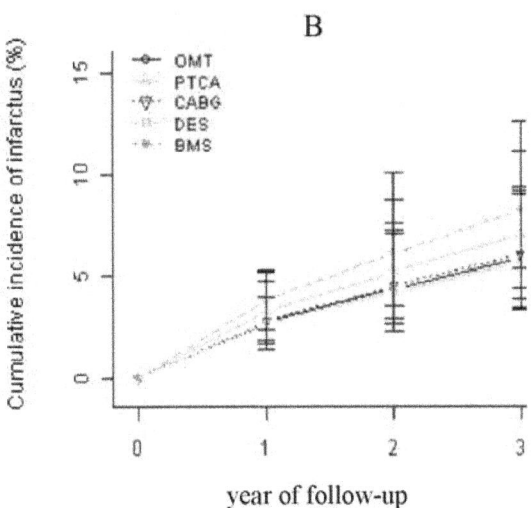

Figure 3. Cumulative incidences of death and MI.

For five trials, only hospital costs were assessed: BENESTENT II [29], ENDEAVOR II [12,31–33], EAST [30], ERACI [34,35] and STRESS [39]. For ARTS [27,28], costs related to outpatient medical visits were studied in addition to hospital costs. In four studies, the costs assessed were related to hospitalization and outpatient drugs: MASS II [36], RAVEL [37] TAXUS IV [41] and SoS [10]. In five studies, costs assessed were related to hospitalization, outpatient care (medical visit and/or cardiovascular testing) and outpatient drugs: ACME [26], COURAGE [14], RITA 2 [38], SIRIUS [11] and SYNTAX [40].

Sensitivity analysis

In this analysis, we excluded trials reporting only hospital costs: BENESTENT II [29], ENDEAVOR II [12,31–33], EAST [30], ERACI [34,35] and STRESS [39]. Consequently, not all treatment modalities could be compared at one year and three years of patient follow-up: at one year, data on PTCA alone were not available for the sensitivity analysis; likewise, data on DES after three years of follow-up could not be used in the sensitivity analysis.

After one year of follow-up, results of the sensitivity analysis were consistent with the main results. MT remained the least expensive, followed by BMS, then DES and lastly CABG (P< 0.0001). After 3 years however, the results were different. Treatment with PTCA appeared to be the least expensive and CABG was still the most costly strategy (P<0.0001). Table S3.

Discussion

The present network meta-analysis confirms the absence of a statistically significant difference between medical therapy, angioplasty without stent, angioplasty with BMS, angioplasty with DES and coronary artery bypass graft on mortality and myocardial infarction rates at one and three years of follow-up. These results concord with those reported in recent meta-analyses and therefore justify the cost-comparison of the different treatment strategies [5–7,42].

Our economic analysis demonstrates a significant difference of weighted costs per patient between the five treatment options. Medical therapy is the least expensive with a weighted cost per patient of US $3069 after one year of follow-up and US $13 864

after three years of follow-up. Coronary artery bypass grafting is the most costly treatment modality: US $27 003 and US $28 670 at one and three years respectively. Between one and three years of follow-up, however, the largest increase in average weighted cost per patient was observed with MT (+ $10 795, +352% compared with the cost after one year), followed by BMS (+ $10 285, +67%), then PTCA (+ $1794, +14%) and CABG (+ $1667, +6%). This significant increase in expenditures, particularly for the MT group, can probably be explained by the need for (additional) revascularization during mid-term follow-up. The sensitivity analysis, performed on the 10 studies that followed, in addition to hospital costs, outpatient costs (outpatient care and/or outpatient drugs), yielded results that are consistent with those of the primary analysis after one year of follow-up. At three years, balloon PTCA and MT had comparable low costs, while there was little difference in the costs of BMS and CABG.

The apparent decrease in cost from one year to three years with DES is artefactual, and due to the fact that only one trial (ENDEAVOR II [12,31–33]) reported 3-year results, whereas several trials were pooled to derive one-year costs. When considering change in costs from one to three years in ENDEAVOR II, an 18% increase was observed, which is consistent with the reduced need for additional revascularization with DES, compared with BMS [12]. The cost increase in ENDEAVOR II is in line with that found in ENDEAVOR III, a clinical trial comparing two different DES: +23% for the sirolimus-eluting stent and +24% for the zotarolimus-eluting stent [43]. In addition, after three years of follow-up we observed a lower cost per patient for the treatment with PTCA compared with treatment with BMS. This surprising observation can probably be explained by the different proportion of patients with SVD: 70% of patients treated by PTCA versus 25% in the BMS group after three years of follow-up.

Overall, the increased initial cost related to initial performance of myocardial revascularization was not counterbalanced by equivalent savings during the three subsequent years of follow-up, although the difference at one year was notably attenuated at three years. A cost advantage for MT compared with myocardial revascularisation was also observed in BARI 2D after four years of follow-up [44]. In this study, which only included patients with type 2 diabetes mellitus, medical costs per patient were higher for

Table 3. Cost per patient for each treatment.

	Trial	FU (year)	Cost per patient as published (currency, year, country)	Cost followed	multi or single vessel disease	Cost per patient adjusted (US $ 2008)
MT	MASS II	1	2 285 (US $, 1998, Netherlands)	H+D	MVD	3 069
	ACME	3	6 311 (Aus $, 1994, Australia)	H+C+D	SVD	6 299
	RITA 2	3	3 613 (£, 1999, UK)	H+C+D	SVD	6 633
	COURAGE	3	15 653 (US $, 2004, USA)	H+C+D	MVD	17 842
CABG	ARTS	1	13 638 (US $, 1998, Netherlands)	H+C	MVD	19 100
	ERACI	1	12 938 (US $, 1991, Argentina)	H	MVD	23 733
	MASS II	1	11 794 (US $, 1998, Netherlands)	H+D	MVD	15 846
	SoS	1	8 905 (£2000, UK)	H+D	MVD	16 222
	SYNTAX	1	39 581 (US $, 2007, USA)	H+C+D	MVD	41 101
	ARTS	3	16 100 (€, 1998, Netherlands)	H+C	MVD	23 596
	EAST	3	25 310 (US $, 1997, USA)	H	MVD	46 083
	ERACI	3	13 000 (US $, 1991, Argentina)	H	MVD	23 847
PTCA	BENESTENT II	1	16 727 (Dfl, 1996, Netherlands)	H	SVD	11 596
	STRESS	1	10 865 (US $, 1994, USA)	H	SVD	15 782
	ERACI	1	6 952 (US $, 1991, Argentina)	H	MVD	12 753
	ACME	3	6 790 (Aus $, 1994, Australia)	H+C+D	SVD	6 777
	RITA 2	3	6 299 (£1999, UK)	H+C+D	SVD	11 565
	ERACI	3	7 523 (US $, 1991, Argentina)	H	MVD	13 800
	EAST	3	23 734 (US $, 1997, USA)	H	MVD	25 310
BMS	BENESTENT II	1	18 812 (Dfl, 1996, Netherlands)	H	SVD	13 041
	ENDEAVOR II	1	16 641 (US $, 2008, USA)	H	SVD	16 641
	RAVEL	1	9 915 (€, 2001, Netherlands)	H+D	SVD	13 339
	SIRIUS	1	16 504 (US $, 2002, USA)	H+C+D	SVD	19 755
	STRESS	1	11 656 (US $, 1994, USA)	H	SVD	16 931
	TAXUS IV	1	14 011 (US $, 2004, USA)	H+D	SVD	15 971
	ARTS	1	10 665 (US $, 1998, Netherlands)	H+C	MVD	14 936
	MASS II	1	8 676 (US $, 1998, Netherlands)	H+D	MVD	11 656
	SoS	1	6 296 (£2000, UK)	H+D	MVD	11 469
	ENDEAVOR II	3	20 348 (US $, 2008, USA)	H	SVD	20 348
	ARTS	3	14 302 (€, 1998, Netherlands)	H+C	MVD	20 961
	COURAGE	3	26 847 (US $, 2004, USA)	H+C+D	MVD	30 602
DES	ENDEAVOR II	1	17 422 (US $, 2008, USA)	H	SVD	17 422
	RAVEL	1	9 969 (€, 2001, Netherlands)	H+D	SVD	13 412
	SIRIUS	1	16 813 (US $, 2002, USA)	H+C+D	SVD	20 124
	TAXUS IV	1	15 447 (US $, 2004, USA)	H+D	SVD	16 624
	SYNTAX	1	35 991 (US $, 2007, USA)	H+C+D	MVD	37 373
	ENDEAVOR II	3	20 536 (US $, 2008, USA)	H	SVD	20 536

FU: follow-up, MT: medical therapy, PTCA: percutaneous coronary angioplasty, CABG: coronary artery bypass graft, DES: drug-eluting stent, BMS: bare-metal stent, SVD: single vessel disease, MVD: multi vessel disease, H: hospital cost, C: costs related to outpatient care, D: costs related to outpatient drugs.

CABG or PCI than for MT. Costs (in US$ 2007) were 80 900, 73 400 and 65 600 respectively after four years of follow-up.

Because of the relatively small number of studies in the meta-analysis, and as we did not use individual data, we were unable to perform separate analyses for patients with single-vessel disease versus multivessel disease. It is possible that the benefit of MT in terms of costs might be more limited in patients with multi-vessel coronary artery disease who are more likely to need subsequent myocardial revascularization.

Nowadays, plain balloon angioplasty (PTCA) is only used in very rare instances. We did keep these studies in our analysis, however, in order to provide additional data on the treatment

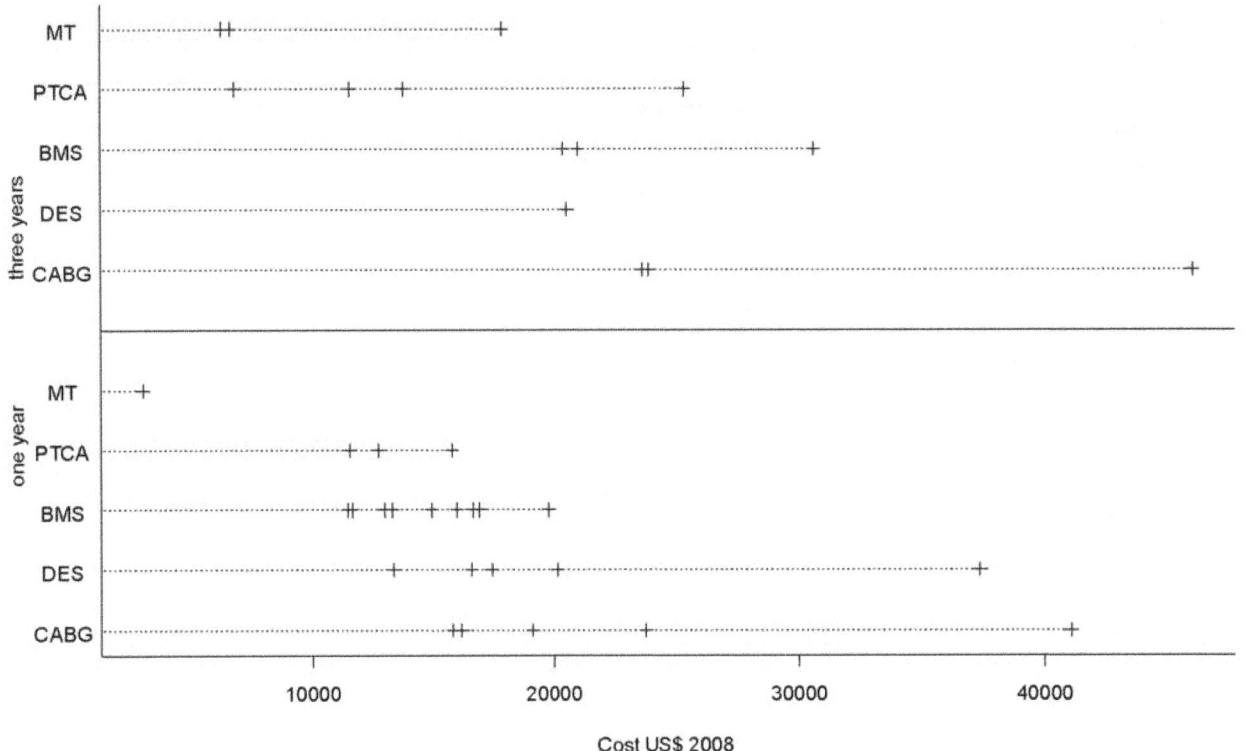

Figure 4. Cost per patient adjusted in US $ 2008 after 1 and 3 years of follow-up (each mark represents a clinical study).

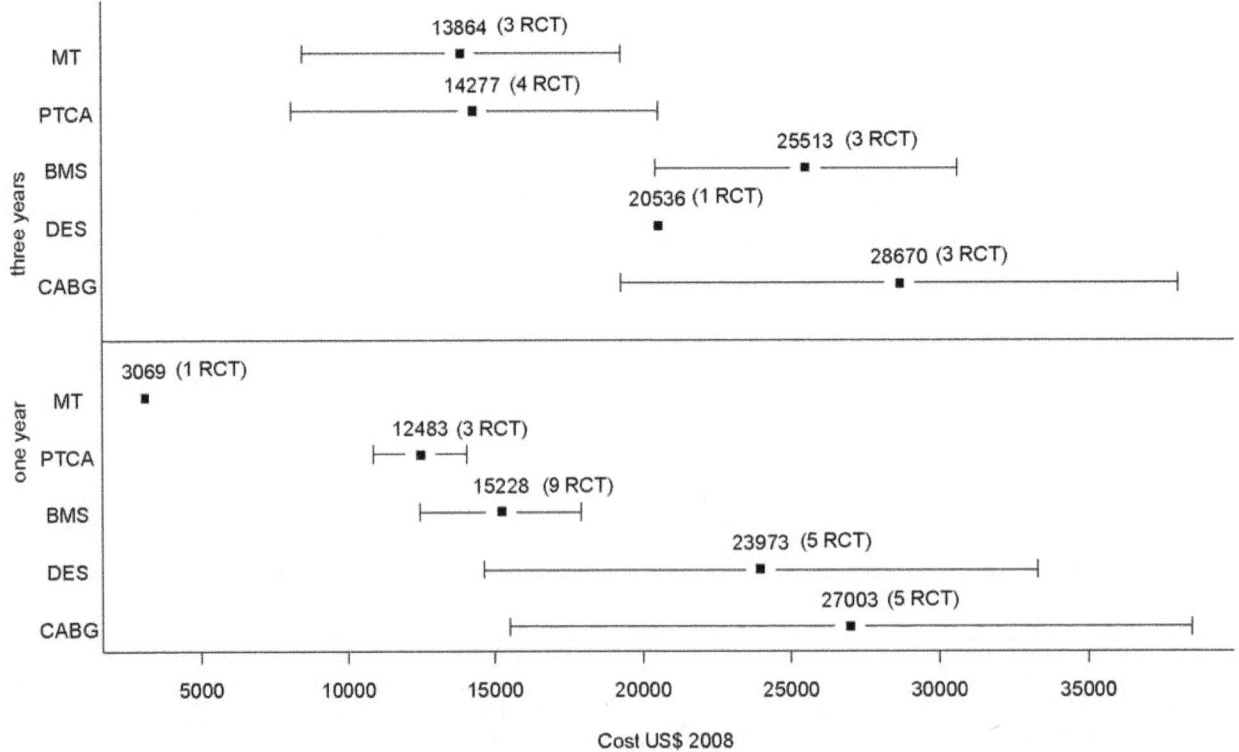

Figure 5. Mean weighted cost per patient in US $ 2008 and standard deviation (number of RCT available).

modalities studied in the non-PTCA arms of the trials (CABG or medical treatment); indeed, excluding the six studies using balloon angioplasty would have resulted in also excluding two studies with medical treatment (ACME and RITA 2), two studies with CABG (ERACI and EAST) and two studies with BMS (BENESTENT 2 and STRESS), thereby much decreasing the statistical power of our analyses.

We also adopted the approach to consider BMS and DES studies separately. In fact, although DES are increasingly used, a substantial proportion of procedures still use BMS, with wide between-country variations; the proportion of DES in published studies varied from 23% (Sweden, 2007, Gudnason et al.), 45% (France, 2004-2008, Puymirat et al.), 61% (Spain, 2009, Diaz J et al.) and 70% (USA, 2011, Dehmer GJ et al.) [45-48].

Critical appraisal of costing methods

We must emphasize that the definition of costs in each study varies. In the management of coronary artery disease, direct costs correspond to three items of expenditure: hospitalization (for invasive treatment and/or care of complications of the disease), outpatient care (medical visits, radiological and biological tests, home visits by nurses, etc.) and outpatient medications (anti-platelet drugs, anti-anginal drugs, etc). All 15 studies included in our economical analysis assessed hospitalization-related costs. Among the 15 RCT, 10 measured both hospital and ambulatory costs (assessment of ambulatory care and /or medication costs). For seven of these 10 RCT, separate hospital and ambulatory cost analyses were available. After one year, ambulatory costs represented an average of 8% of the total cost (from 2.9% in TAXUS-IV to 15% in SoS); after three years, only one study (RITA-2) provided a detailed analysis of the respective proportion of hospital and ambulatory costs; as expected, the percentage of the total cost related to ambulatory care was higher than that observed at one year. Furthermore, a number of the studies analysed the cost of all cardiovascular drugs (ARTS, SYNTAX, RITA 2 etc), whereas the SIRIUS trial analysed the cost of thienopyridines only.

Moreover, the methods used to calculate the cost per patient vary in the studies analyzed. In practice, as published by Reed et al. [49], the calculation of the average cost depends on two parameters. The first is the approach used in the clinical trial to estimate the resource consumed. Indeed, resource-use can be based on data from patients in all countries participating in the clinical trial or from patients belonging to one center or one country. The second is the costing approach; again, the unit cost applied for the whole trial population can be derived from individual countries, from a single country, or from one center. According to these two parameters, studies can be classified into six groups: fully pooled with multi-country costing, fully pooled with one-country costing, partially split with multi-country costing, partially split with one-country costing, fully split with multi-country costing and fully split with one-country costing. The 15 trials we analyzed belong to two of these six groups. Eight trials are classified as "fully pooled with one-country costing": ARTS [27,28], BENES-TENT II [29], COURAGE [14],, ENDEAVOR II [12,31–33], RAVEL [37], RITA 2 [38], SoS [10] and SYNTAX [40]. The seven other studies are classified as "fully split with one-country costing": ACME [26], EAST [30], ERACI [34,35], MASS II [36], SIRIUS [11], STRESS [39] and TAXUS IV [41]. Our conclusions may therefore be limited by the methodological variability of the 16 trials we analyzed,

although the results were fairly consistent regardless of the costing methods used.

Limitations

Our meta-analysis included trials that were conducted at a time when the technique of PCI used would be considered completely obsolete in today's terms. In such earlier studies, the rates of subsequent revascularisation following PCI were definitely higher than those that would currently be observed, leading to higher follow-up costs than would be found nowadays.

Also, as some trials planned angiographic follow-up for all patients, including those who were asymptomatic, the rates of repeat revascularization may have been higher that those that would have been observed in a real-life situation, because of the "oculostenotic reflex" that mandatory coronary angiography during follow-up may have induced. In fact, only six studies did not include routine angiographic follow-up: ARTS [27,28], COURAGE [14], ERACI [34,35], RITA 2 [38], SoS [10] and SYNTAX [40]. Studies in which angiographic follow-up was planned, tended to have higher treatment costs.

Another limitation of our analysis is that the period over which we selected the studies expands over two decades, with the oldest trial (EAST) recruiting patients from 1987 to 1990, and the most recent (SYNTAX) between 2005 and 2007. During this period, the cost of BMS and DES has decreased substantially. Among the trials selected, five reported the unit cost of stents (RAVEL, SIRIUS, TAXUS IV, SYNTAX et ENDEAVOR II): the cost of BMS remained relatively stable (US $900 to 700) while the absolute price decrease for DES was greater (from US $2900 to 2100). The differential cost between BMS and DES remained stable ($\approx$ US $2000), except for the two most recent trials (SYNTAX, 2007 and ENDEAV-OR II, 2008), where the difference was smaller. Although we lacked the power to fully take these changes into consideration, they should be kept in mind when analysing our results.

In addition, it must be emphasized that the nature of costs varied across the 15 RCT. All measured hospital costs, while 10 also assessed ambulatory costs. A specific sensitivity analysis, however, was performed to take this variability into account.

Lastly, we used data from one single randomized clinical trial in two situations: medical therapy with one year follow-up (MASS II [36]) and treatment with DES with three years of follow-up (ENDEAVOR II [12,31–33]). As mentioned above, this may have led to inconsistencies, such as the seemingly lower costs from one to three years in patients with DES.

Conclusions

This network meta-analysis documents considerable differences in treatment costs at 3-year follow-up, when comparing five treatment modalities that provided similar clinical results, in terms of death and risk of myocardial infarction. Medical therapy in patients without acute coronary syndromes therefore appears to be the most cost-effective option, which may achieve appreciable savings in healthcare expenditures. Our findings, however, may be limited by methodological considerations pertaining to the way costs are evaluated in long-term random-ized trials, and by the fact that we did not take into account potential differences between treatment modalities in terms of symptoms.

Author Contributions

Conceived and designed the experiments: TC BS PD DB ND. Performed the experiments: TC BS PD ND. Analyzed the data: SK CS ACN. Wrote the paper: TC BS SK PD OD YJ ND.

References

1. Fihn SD, Gardin JM, Abrams J, Berra K, Blankenship JC, et al. (2012) 2012 ACCF/AHA/ACP/AATS/PCNA/SCAI/STS Guideline for the diagnosis and management of patients with stable ischemic heart disease: a report of the American College of Cardiology Foundation/American Heart Association Task Force on Practice Guidelines, and the American College of Physicians, American Association for Thoracic Surgery, Preventive Cardiovascular Nurses Association, Society for Cardiovascular Angiography and Interventions, and Society of Thoracic Surgeons. J Am Coll Cardiol 60: e44–e164. doi:10.1016/j.jacc.2012.07.013.

2. Epstein AJ, Polsky D, Yang F, Yang L, Groeneveld PW (2011) Coronary revascularization trends in the United States, 2001-2008. JAMA J Am Med Assoc 305: 1769–1776. doi:10.1001/jama.2011.551.

3. Eisenberg MJ (2006) Drug-eluting stents: the price is not right. Circulation 114: 1745–1754; discussion 1754. doi:10.1161/CIRCULATIONAHA.106.646190.

4. Kirtane AJ, Gupta A, Iyengar S, Moses JW, Leon MB, et al. (2009) Safety and efficacy of drug-eluting and bare metal stents: comprehensive meta-analysis of randomized trials and observational studies. Circulation 119: 3198–3206. doi:10.1161/CIRCULATIONAHA.108.826479.

5. Pursnani S, Korley F, Gopaul R, Kanade P, Chandra N, et al. (2012) Percutaneous coronary intervention versus optimal medical therapy in stable coronary artery disease: a systematic review and meta-analysis of randomized clinical trials. Circ Cardiovasc Interv 5: 476–490. doi:10.1161/CIRCINTER-VENTIONS.112.970954.

6. Hlatky MA, Boothroyd DB, Bravata DM, Boersma E, Booth J, et al. (2009) Coronary artery bypass surgery compared with percutaneous coronary interventions for multivessel disease: a collaborative analysis of individual patient data from ten randomised trials. Lancet 373: 1190–1197. doi:10.1016/S0140-6736(09)60552-3.

7. Stergiopoulos K, Brown DL (2012) Initial coronary stent implantation with medical therapy vs medical therapy alone for stable coronary artery disease: meta-analysis of randomized controlled trials. Arch Intern Med 172: 312–319. doi:10.1001/archinternmed.2011.1484.

8. Hlatky MA, Boothroyd DB, Baker L, Kazi DS, Solomon MD, et al. (2013) Comparative effectiveness of multivessel coronary bypass surgery and multivessel percutaneous coronary intervention: a cohort study. Ann Intern Med 158: 727–734. doi:10.7326/0003-4819-158-10-201305210-00639.

9. Hill RA, Boland A, Dickson R, Dündar Y, Haycox A, et al. (2007) Drug-eluting stents: a systematic review and economic evaluation. Health Technol Assess Winch Engl 11: iii, xi–221.

10. Weintraub WS, Mahoney EM, Zhang Z, Chu H, Hutton J, et al. (2004) One year comparison of costs of coronary surgery versus percutaneous coronary intervention in the stent or surgery trial. Heart Br Card Soc 90: 782–788. doi:10.1136/hrt.2003.015057.

11. Cohen DJ, Bakhai A, Shi C, Githiora L, Lavelle T, et al. (2004) Cost-effectiveness of sirolimus-eluting stents for treatment of complex coronary stenoses: results from the Sirolimus-Eluting Balloon Expandable Stent in the Treatment of Patients With De Novo Native Coronary Artery Lesions (SIRIUS) trial. Circulation 110: 508–514. doi:10.1161/01.CIR.0000136821.99814.43.

12. Eisenstein EL, Wijns W, Fajadet J, Mauri L, Edwards R, et al. (2009) Long-term clinical and economic analysis of the Endeavor drug-eluting stent versus the Driver bare-metal stent: 4-year results from the ENDEAVOR II trial (Randomized Controlled Trial to Evaluate the Safety and Efficacy of the Medtronic AVE ABT-578 Eluting Driver Coronary Stent in De Novo Native Coronary Artery Lesions). JACC Cardiovasc Interv 2: 1178–1187. doi:10.1016/j.jcin.2009.10.011.

13. Hlatky MA, Rogers WJ, Johnstone I, Boothroyd D, Brooks MM, et al. (1997) Medical care costs and quality of life after randomization to coronary angioplasty or coronary bypass surgery. Bypass Angioplasty Revascularization Investigation (BARI) Investigators. N Engl J Med 336: 92–99. doi:10.1056/NEJM199701093360203.

14. Weintraub WS, Boden WE, Zhang Z, Kolm P, Zhang Z, et al. (2008) Cost-effectiveness of percutaneous coronary intervention in optimally treated stable coronary patients. Circ Cardiovasc Qual Outcomes 1: 12–20. doi:10.1161/CIRCOUTCOMES.108.798462.

15. OED website. Available: http://www.oecd.org/std/prices-ppp/ (n.d.).

16. Bertoldi EG, Rohde LE, Zimerman LI, Pimentel M, Polanczyk CA (2011) Cost-effectiveness of cardiac resynchronization therapy in patients with heart failure: The perspective of a middle-income country's public health system. Int J Cardiol. doi:10.1016/j.ijcard.2011.06.046.

17. Kühr EM, Ribeiro RA, Rohde LEP, Polanczyk CA (2011) Cost-effectiveness of supervised exercise therapy in heart failure patients. Value Health J Int Soc Pharmacoeconomics Outcomes Res 14: S100–107. doi:10.1016/j.jval.2011.05.006.

18. Antioch KM, Jennings G, Botti M, Chapman R, Wulfsohn V (2002) Integrating cost-effectiveness evidence into clinical practice guidelines in Australia for acute myocardial infarction. Eur J Health Econ HEPAC Health Econ Prev Care 3: 26–39. doi:10.1007/s10198-001-0088-z.

19. Villanueva EV, Wasiak J, Petherick ES (2003) Percutaneous transluminal rotational atherectomy for coronary artery disease. Cochrane Database Syst Rev Online: CD003334. doi:10.1002/14651858.CD003334.

20. Evers S, Goossens M, de Vet H, van Tulder M, Ament A (2005) Criteria list for assessment of methodological quality of economic evaluations: Consensus on Health Economic Criteria. Int J Technol Assess Health Care 21: 240–245.

21. Woods BS, Hawkins N, Scott DA (2010) Network meta-analysis on the log-hazard scale, combining count and hazard ratio statistics accounting for multi-arm trials: a tutorial. BMC Med Res Methodol 10: 54. doi:10.1186/1471-2288-10-54.

22. Lu G, Ades AE (2004) Combination of direct and indirect evidence in mixed treatment comparisons. Stat Med 23: 3105–3124. doi:10.1002/sim.1875.

23. Higgins JP, Whitehead A (1996) Borrowing strength from external trials in a meta-analysis. Stat Med 15: 2733–2749. doi:10.1002/(SICI)1097-0258(19961230)15:24<2733::AID-SIM562>3.0.CO;2-0.

24. Smith TC, Spiegelhalter DJ, Thomas A (1995) Bayesian approaches to random-effects meta-analysis: a comparative study. Stat Med 14: 2685–2699.

25. Lu G, Ades AE, Sutton AJ, Cooper NJ, Briggs AH, et al. (2007) Meta-analysis of mixed treatment comparisons at multiple follow-up times. Stat Med 26: 3681–3699. doi:10.1002/sim.2831.

26. Kinlay S (1996) Cost-effectiveness of coronary angioplasty versus medical treatment: the impact of cost-shifting. Aust N Z J Med 26: 20–26.

27. Serruys PW, Unger F, Sousa JE, Jatene A, Bonnier HJ, et al. (2001) Comparison of coronary-artery bypass surgery and stenting for the treatment of multivessel disease. N Engl J Med 344: 1117–1124. doi:10.1056/NEJM200104123441502.

28. Legrand VMG, Serruys PW, Unger F, van Hout BA, Vrolix MCM, et al. (2004) Three-year outcome after coronary stenting versus bypass surgery for the treatment of multivessel disease. Circulation 109: 1114–1120. doi:10.1161/01.CIR.0000118504.61212.4B.

29. Serruys PW, van Hout B, Bonnier H, Legrand V, Garcia E, et al. (1998) Randomised comparison of implantation of heparin-coated stents with balloon angioplasty in selected patients with coronary artery disease (Benestent II). Lancet 352: 673–681.

30. Weintraub WS, Mauldin PD, Becker E, Kosinski AS, King SB 3rd (1995) A comparison of the costs of and quality of life after coronary angioplasty or coronary surgery for multivessel coronary artery disease. Results from the Emory Angioplasty Versus Surgery Trial (EAST). Circulation 92: 2831–2840.

31. Meredith I (n.d.) Trial updates & long term follow-up - ENDEAVOR I: 3-year, ENDEAVOR II: 2-year clinical results. May 16-19 2006 Eur Paris 2006.

32. Meredith I, Wijns W (n.d.) Clinical Trial Update. ENDEAVOR I & II clinical program: long term follow-up. 4 Sept 2005 ESC Stockh 2005.

33. Zeiher A (n.d.) ENDEAVOR clinical Program Update. ENDEAVOR I: 4-year clinical follow-up. ENDEAVOR II: 3-year clinical follow-up. May 22 2007 Eur Barc 2007.

34. Rodriguez A, Boullon F, Perez-Baliño N, Paviotti C, Liprandi MI, et al. (1993) Argentine randomized trial of percutaneous transluminal coronary angioplasty versus coronary artery bypass surgery in multivessel disease (ERACI): in-hospital results and 1-year follow-up. ERACI Group. J Am Coll Cardiol 22: 1060–1067.

35. Rodriguez A, Mele E, Peyregne E, Bullon F, Perez-Baliño N, et al. (1996) Three-year follow-up of the Argentine Randomized Trial of Percutaneous Transluminal Coronary Angioplasty Versus Coronary Artery Bypass Surgery in Multivessel Disease (ERACI). J Am Coll Cardiol 27: 1178–1184.

36. Favarato D, Hueb W, Gersh BJ, Soares PR, Cesar LAM, et al. (2003) Relative cost comparison of treatments for coronary artery disease: the First Year Follow-Up of MASS II Study. Circulation 108 Suppl 1: II21–23. doi:10.1161/01.cir.0000087381.98299.7b.

37. Van Hout BA, Serruys PW, Lemos PA, van den Brand MJBM, van Es G-A, et al. (2005) One year cost effectiveness of sirolimus eluting stents compared with bare metal stents in the treatment of single native de novo coronary lesions: an analysis from the RAVEL trial. Heart Br Card Soc 91: 507–512. doi:10.1136/hrt.2004.034454.

38. Sculpher M, Smith D, Clayton T, Henderson R, Buxton M, et al. (2002) Coronary angioplasty versus medical therapy for angina. Health service costs based on the second Randomized Intervention Treatment of Angina (RITA-2) trial. Eur Heart J 23: 1291–1300.

39. Cohen DJ, Krumholz HM, Sukin CA, Ho KK, Siegrist RB, et al. (1995) In-hospital and one-year economic outcomes after coronary stenting or balloon angioplasty. Results from a randomized clinical trial. Stent Restenosis Study Investigators. Circulation 92: 2480–2487.

40. Cohen DJ, Lavelle TA, Van Hout B, Li H, Lei Y, et al. (2012) Economic outcomes of percutaneous coronary intervention with drug-eluting stents versus bypass surgery for patients with left main or three-vessel coronary artery disease: one-year results from the SYNTAX trial. Catheter Cardiovasc Interv Off J Soc Card Angiogr Interv 79: 198–209. doi:10.1002/ccd.23147.

41. Bakhai A, Stone GW, Mahoney E, Lavelle TA, Shi C, et al. (2006) Cost effectiveness of paclitaxel-eluting stents for patients undergoing percutaneous coronary revascularization: results from the TAXUS-IV Trial. J Am Coll Cardiol 48: 253–261. doi:10.1016/j.jacc.2006.02.063.

42. Schömig A, Mehilli J, de Waha A, Seyfarth M, Pache J, et al. (2008) A meta-analysis of 17 randomized trials of a percutaneous coronary intervention-based strategy in patients with stable coronary artery disease. J Am Coll Cardiol 52: 894–904. doi:10.1016/j.jacc.2008.05.051.

43. Eisenstein EL, Leon MB, Kandzari DE, Mauri L, Edwards R, et al. (2009) Long-term clinical and economic analysis of the Endeavor zotarolimus-eluting stent versus the cypher sirolimus-eluting stent: 3-year results from the ENDEAVOR III trial (Randomized Controlled Trial of the Medtronic Endeavor Drug [ABT-578] Eluting Coronary Stent System Versus the Cypher Sirolimus-Eluting Coronary Stent System in De Novo Native Coronary Artery Lesions). JACC Cardiovasc Interv 2: 1199–1207. doi:10.1016/j.jcin.2009.10.009.

44. Hlatky MA, Boothroyd DB, Melsop KA, Kennedy L, Rihal C, et al. (2009) Economic outcomes of treatment strategies for type 2 diabetes mellitus and coronary artery disease in the Bypass Angioplasty Revascularization Investigation 2 Diabetes trial. Circulation 120: 2550–2558. doi:10.1161/CIRCULATIONAHA.109.912709.

45. Gudnason T, Gudnadottir GS, Lagerqvist B, Eyjolfsson K, Nilsson T, et al. (2013) Comparison of interventional cardiology in two European countries: a nationwide internet based registry study. Int J Cardiol 168: 1237–1242. doi:10.1016/j.ijcard.2012.11.054.

46. Puymirat E, Blanchard D, Perier M-C, Piadonataccio M, Gilard M, et al. (2013) Study Design and Baseline Characteristics of the National Observational Study of Diagnostic and Interventional Cardiac Catheterization by the French Society of Cardiology. Am J Cardiol. doi:10.1016/j.amjcard.2013.03.030.

47. Díaz JF, de La Torre JM, Sabaté M, Goicolea J (2012) Spanish Cardiac Catheterization and Coronary Intervention Registry. 21st official report of the Spanish Society of Cardiology Working Group on Cardiac Catheterization and Interventional Cardiology (1990-2011). Rev Esp Cardiol Engl Ed 65: 1106–1116. doi:10.1016/j.recesp.2012.07.021.

48. Dehmer GJ, Weaver D, Roe MT, Milford-Beland S, Fitzgerald S, et al. (2012) A contemporary view of diagnostic cardiac catheterization and percutaneous coronary intervention in the United States: a report from the CathPCI Registry of the National Cardiovascular Data Registry, 2010 through June 2011. J Am Coll Cardiol 60: 2017–2031. doi:10.1016/j.jacc.2012.08.966.

49. Reed SD, Anstrom KJ, Bakhai A, Briggs AH, Califf RM, et al. (2005) Conducting economic evaluations alongside multinational clinical trials: toward a research consensus. Am Heart J 149: 434–443. doi:10.1016/j.ahj.2004.11.001.

2

Incidence, Risk Factors, Treatment and Prognosis of Popliteal Artery Embolization in the Superficial Femoral Artery Interventions

Weiwei Wu[1,2¶], Surong Hua[1¶], Yongjun Li[1], Wei Ye[1], Bao Liu[1], Yuehong Zheng[1], Xiaojun Song[1], Changwei Liu[1]*

1 Department of Vascular Surgery, Peking Union Medical College Hospital, Chinese Academy of Medical Science, Beijing, China, 2 Department of Vascular Surgery, Beijing Tsinghua Changgung Hospital, Beijing Tsinghua University, Beijing, China

Abstract

Objective: Percutaneous transluminal angioplasty and stenting (PTA + stent) has gained acceptance as a primary treatment modality for the superficial femoral artery (SFA) diseases. Popliteal artery embolization (PAE) is a severe complication in SFA interventions. The purpose of this study was to evaluate the incidence, risk factors, treatment and prognosis of PAE in primary SFA PTA + stent.

Methods: Chronic SFA arteriosclerosis cases that underwent primary PTA + stent were reviewed from a retrospectively maintained database. Runoff vessels were evaluated in all cases before and after the interventions for PAE detection. The primary patency, secondary patency and limb salvage rates were calculated using Kaplan-Meier analysis and compared using log-rank analysis. Cox multivariate regression was performed to evaluate predictors of patency and limb salvage rates.

Results: There were 436 lesions treated in 388 patients with 10 PAE events (2.3%) in total. PAE rate was significantly higher in Transatlantic Inter-Society Consensus (TASC) C/D group compared with TASC A/B group (OR = 8.91, $P = .002$), in chronic total occlusion (CTO) lesions compared with stenotic lesions ($P < .0001$), and in group with history of cerebral ischemic stroke (OR = 6.11, $P = .007$). PAE rates were not significantly affected by age, sex, smoking, hypertension, diabetes, hyperlipidemia and runoff status. The binary logistic regression showed that only the TASC C/D was an independent predictor of PAE ($P = .031$). The 12-month and 24-month primary patency, secondary patency and limb salvage rates in PAE group showed no significant differences comparing with non-PAE group.

Conclusions: PAE is a rare event in primary SFA PTA + stent. TASC C/D lesion, CTO and cerebral ischemic stroke history are risk factors for PAE. PAE is typically reversible by comprehensive techniques. If the popliteal flow is restored in time, PAE has no significant effect on long-term patency and limb salvage rates.

Editor: Hiroyoshi Ariga, Hokkaido University, Japan

Funding: The authors have no support or funding to report.

Competing Interests: The authors have declared that no competing interests exist.

* Email: liucw@vip.sina.com

¶ These authors are co-first authors on this work.

Introduction

Distal embolization (DE) of thromboembolic material generated during lower extremity endovascular intervention is a known complication following potential severe ischemic consequences [1]. The reported incidence of DE, detected angiographically or clinically, ranges from 1% to 5% [2]. DE may necessitate additional intervention, including thrombectomy or thrombolysis, resulting in longer procedure time, more contrast used, and greater radiation exposure [3]. The concern for DE in lower extremity interventions has led to a debate [4]. Some recommend the use of a variety of embolic protection devices (EPDs) [5,6,7], while other evidence suggested that EPDs may be unnecessary [2,8]. Clinical data have shown that the application of EPDs in lower extremity is generally safe [4]. More trial data may be necessary to find the balance between the increase in cost, complexity, risks and the potential benefit [9]. DE rate can differ a lot in different lesion types and treatment methods. It was reported that reintervention may have a higher rate of DE, and the use of newer atherectomy devices may be more emboligenic than angioplasty with or without stenting [2]. However, it is still not quite sure to tell which type of lesion or treatment methods could benefit from EPDs. More retrospective or prospective studies need to be done to identify the incidence and prognosis of DE in each subgroup.

The superficial femoral artery (SFA) is one of the most common affected target vessels in the atherosclerotic occlusive disease of the lower extremities. For most doctors, endovascular therapy, especially percutaneous transluminal angioplasty and stenting (PTA + stent), has become the primary choice for SFA occlusion. However, DE remains a concern in SFA interventions. Popliteal artery embolization (PAE) is the most severe type of DE. The acute occlusion before popliteal trifurcation in SFA interventions may cause sudden pain, worsening ischemia or later limb loss, which will be a nightmare for both patient and operator.

It is reported that DE has no effects on patency rates and limb salvage for all kinds of lower extremity interventions [2]. But this previous research did not separate PAE from other runoff vessel embolization, nor PTA + stent from other interventions. So far there have been no literatures clearly demonstrating the rate, treatment and prognosis of PAE in primary SFA PTA + stent. This study was aim to evaluate the incidence, risk factors, treatment and prognosis of PAE in chronic SFA arteriosclerosis cases underwent primary PTA + stent.

Methods

Patient Selection

All patients treated percutaneously for chronic lower extremity ischemia with atherosclerotic occlusive disease in a single center were identified in a retrospectively maintained database. All SFA cases that underwent primary PTA + stent from November 2008 to December 2012 were reviewed. Indications for intervention were peripheral arterial disease greater than Rutherford's category 2, including moderate to severe claudication or critical limb ischemia, defined as rest pain, tissue loss, or non-healing ulceration. All patients suffered from lower extremity ischemia for at least 3 months, and all procedures were performed by 4 experienced vascular surgeons. The medication included: routine antiplatelet therapy (at least one week of aspirin 100 mg daily prior and indefinitely after the procedure, and clopidogrel 75 mg daily for three months after the procedure) and intensive lipid-lowering therapy (mostly atorvastatin). Patients with acute or subacute limb ischemia less than 3 months were excluded. The study protocol was reviewed and approved by the Ethics Committee of Peking Union Medical College Hospital. Written informed consents for both the procedure and the use in anonymous observational research were collected from all patients.

Treatments and Technique

PTA + stent was carried out in all cases. Most procedures were performed under local anesthesia. A crossover approach from the contralateral side was established and a long sheath was placed for the proximal SFA lesions, while an antegrade transfemoral access was selected for the ipsilateral middle or distal SFA lesions. Retrograde or transbrachial approaches were not used in this group. Anticoagulation included 80–100 unit/kg of unfractionated heparin given intravenously at the beginning of the procedure and another 500–1000 unit/h during the procedure to maintain an activated clotting time between 250 and 300 seconds (maximum total dose of heparin 10,000 units). Angiography of the total SFA and distal runoff was performed in all cases. The 0.035 inch hydrophilic guide wires were used to cross the stenosis lesions, and appropriated sized self-expanding bared stents (often 6 or 7 mm in diameter) were deployed overlapping the lesions. The 0.018 inch or 0.014 inch guide wires supported by a noncompliant balloon (often 2.5 or 3.0 mm in diameter) were usually chosen to cross the

occluded lesions with either an intraluminal or subintimal technique. After the wires got back into the distal true lumen, the supported balloons were inflated to its nominal pressure to predilate the occluded lesions, in order to facilitate the subsequent delivery of the self-expanding bare stents. Post-dilation was then performed with noncompliant balloons (often 1 mm less than the stent in diameter) within the stents. Completion angiography with evaluation of the distal runoff was performed after all interventions.

In case of PAE, the salvage intraluminal techniques including aspiration with guiding catheters, local thrombolysis with urokinase, and/or angioplasty with small sized noncompliant balloons would be used at once. If all of the above did not open the popliteal artery occlusion, popliteal artery embolectomy through a below-knee medial longitudinal incision would be performed as quickly as possible under general anesthesia.

Data Collection and Follow-up

Operative reports and angiograms were examined by two separate reviewers to determine lesion type and Transatlantic Inter-Society Consensus (TASC) II classification [10]. The lesion with angiography proved blood flow interruption at SFA segment was defined as chronic total occlusion (CTO) lesion, otherwise was defined as stenotic lesion. Runoff vessel evaluation (including the popliteal, anterior tibial, posterior tibial and peroneal artery) was performed in all cases before and after intervention for PAE detection. PAE was defined as new onset of angiographic contrast filling defect in the popliteal artery with all below-knee runoff vessels blocked at any time during the procedure, other than vasospasm and dissection. Patients were followed up at 1, 3, 6, and 12 months after the interventions, and annually thereafter. Physical examination (ankle-brachial index and pulse examination) and duplex ultrasonography (DUS) were performed on each follow-up visit. Follow-up angiography was indicated when the findings on DUS suggested restenosis over 50 percent. Loss of primary or secondary patency was defined as the presence of over 50% stenosis during angiography after the primary or secondary intervention. Loss of limb salvage was defined as any amputation above the level of the ankle joint.

Statistical Analysis

Chi-square analysis or Fisher's exact test were used to assess significance based on $P < .05$ for categorical data. Odds ratio (OR) and 95% confidence intervals (CI) were also calculated when $P < .05$. The primary patency, secondary patency and limb salvage rates were calculated using Kaplan-Meier analysis and compared using log-rank analysis. Cox multivariate regression was performed to evaluate whether PAE and other factors were predictor of decreased patency and limb salvage rates. All analysis was done with SPSS 19.0 software (SPSS Inc, Chicago).

Results

There were 436 lesions treated in 388 patients. Demographic data and comorbidities are outlined in Table 1. Two hundred and ninety two patients (75.3%) were men and 96 patients (24.7%) were women. The average age was 68.9±8.5 years (range from 44 to 87 years). Lesion types and characteristics are listed in Table 2. One hundred and ninety one lesions (43.8%) were in Transatlantic Inter-Society Consensus (TASC) II A group, while 105 (24.1%), 51 (11.7%) and 89 (20.4%) lesions were in TASC B, C and D group, respectively.

There were 15 DE events (3.4%) in the popliteal, tibial or peroneal artery, ten of which were PAE. The other 5 DE events

Table 1. Patient demographics and comorbidities.

Variable	
Total patients	388 (100.0%)
Age (years)	68.9±8.5
Male	292 (75.3%)
Smokers (current and former)	184 (47.4%)
Hypertension	281 (72.4%)
Diabetes mellitus	208 (53.6%)
Hyperlipidemia	153 (39.4%)
Coronary artery disease	108 (27.8%)
Cerebral ischemic stroke	81 (20.9%)
Chronic renal insufficiency	8 (2.1%)
Other peripheral artery diseases	70 (18.0%)
Rutherford's category	
2	35 (9.0%)
3	207 (53.4%)
4	72 (18.6%)
5	58 (14.9%)
6	16 (4.1%)

Continuous data are presented as means ± standard deviation; categorical data are given as counts (percentages).

located in the tibial or peroneal artery with the popliteal artery and at least one other runoff vessel patent showed no symptoms, thus, no specific treatments were carried out. Table 3 summarizes and compares the rates of PAE in different groups. There were 10 PAE events (2.3%) in total, of which 2 happened in TASC B group, 2 in C group and 6 in D group. The PAE rate was significantly higher in TASC C/D group compared with TASC A/B group (OR = 8.91, 95% CI: 1.87–42.53, P = .002), in CTO lesions

Table 2. Lesion types and characteristics.

Variable	
Total lesions	436
Lesion type	
Stenosis	278 (63.8)
Chronic total occlusion	158 (36.2)
TASC II classification	
A	191 (43.8)
B	105 (24.1)
C	51 (11.7)
D	89 (20.4)
A/B (low TASC grade)	296 (67.9)
C/D (high TASC grade)	140 (32.1)
Preoperative runoff vessels	1.82±0.81
Preoperative runoff	
0	9 (2.1)
1	160 (36.7)
2	166 (38.1)
3	101 (23.2)
0/1 (insufficient runoff)	169 (38.8)
2/3 (sufficient runoff)	267 (61.2)

Continuous data are presented as means ± standard deviation; categorical data are given as counts (percentages).
TASC, Transatlantic Inter-Society Consensus.

compared with stenotic lesions ($P<.0001$), and in group with history of cerebral ischemic stroke (OR = 6.11, 95% CI: 1.69–22.13, $P = .007$). The mean age was 67.0±4.6 years in PAE group compared with 68.6±8.6 years in non-PAE group ($P = .553$). PAE rates were not significantly affected by age, sex, smoking, hypertension, diabetes, hyperlipidemia and runoff status. The binary logistic regression showed that only the TASC C/D was an independent predictor of PAE ($P = .031$), while others were not. We noticed that all 10 PAE events happened in male patients and CTO lesions. Within the CTO group, PAE rates in the intraluminal (5.38%, 5/93) and subintimal subgroup (7.69%, 5/65) were not significantly different ($P = .915$).

Patency of the popliteal artery and at least one runoff vessel was restored at the completion of the procedure in all cases of PAE. Aspiration and local thrombolysis were not working in any case. Angioplasty with noncompliant balloons (3.0 or 3.5 mm in diameter) had opened the PAE and restored the flow of at least one below-knee runoff vessel in 6 cases. Embolectomy was performed immediately in the rest 4 cases that were not salvaged by the intraluminal techniques. Pathology exams showed that all emboli were atheromatous plaque rather than thrombus. Kaplan-

Meier curves and log-rank test analysis results of the primary patency, secondary patency and limb salvage rates in the PAE and non-PAE group are shown in Figs. 1, 2 and 3. The median follow-up time of the PAE group is 29.5 months (7–50 months), while that of the non-PAE group is 20 months (1–56 months). The dropout percentage of follow-up is 7.8% (34/436). The overall primary patency ($P = .475$), secondary patency ($P = .736$) and limb salvage rates ($P = .298$) between the PAE and non-PAE group show no significant differences. At 12 months, the two groups (PAE vs. non-PAE) were equivalent in terms of primary patency (PAE: 80.0%, non-PAE: 80.1%, $P = 1.000$), secondary patency (PAE: 90%, non-PAE: 89.6%, $P = 1.000$), and limb salvage (PAE: 90%, non-PAE: 96.7%, $P = .298$). There were also no significant differences between the two groups at 24 months or 36 months in primary patency, secondary patency, or limb salvage ($P>.05$, Table 4). Cox multivariate regression model showed that PAE was not an independent predictor of risk in primary patency, secondary patency or limb salvage ($P>.05$, Table 5). Diabetes mellitus and hyperlipidemia were independent predictors of risk for primary patency, while hyperlipidemia and CTO were independent predictors for poor secondary patency. However, we found that

Table 3. PAE rates in different subgroups.

Subgroup	Lesions		PAE		P value
	Total No.		No. (%)		
Male	320		10 (3.1%)		.069
Female	116		0 (0%)		
Smokers (current and former)	210		4 (1.9%)		.753
Non-smokers	226		6 (2.7%)		
Hypertension	312		6 (1.9%)		.480
Without hypertension	124		4 (3.2%)		
Diabetes mellitus	235		4 (1.7%)		.524
Without diabetes mellitus	201		6 (3.0%)		
Hyperlipidemia	175		4 (2.3%)		1.000
Without hyperlipidemia	261		6 (2.3%)		
Coronary artery disease	109		4 (3.7%)		.276
Without coronary artery disease	327		6 (1.8%)		
Cerebral ischemic stroke	90		6 (6.7%)		**.007**[a]
Without cerebral ischemic stroke	346		4 (1.6%)		
Chronic renal insufficiency	8		0 (0%)		1.000
Without chronic renal insufficiency	428		10 (2.3%)		
Lesion type					
Chronic total occlusion	158		10 (6.3%)		**<.0001**
Stenosis	278		0 (0%)		
TASC II classification					
C/D (high TASC grade)	140		8 (5.7%)		**.002**[b]
A/B (low TASC grade)	296		2 (0.7%)		
Preoperative runoff					
2/3 (sufficient runoff)	267		8 (3.0%)		.329
0/1 (insufficient runoff)	169		2 (1.2%)		

Categorical data are given as counts (percentages).
PAE, Popliteal artery embolization; TASC, Transatlantic Inter-Society Consensus.
P values of <.05 are in bold.
[a]Odds ratio (OR) = 6.11, 95% confidence interval (CI): 1.69–22.13.
[b]OR = 8.91, 95% CI: 1.87–42.53.

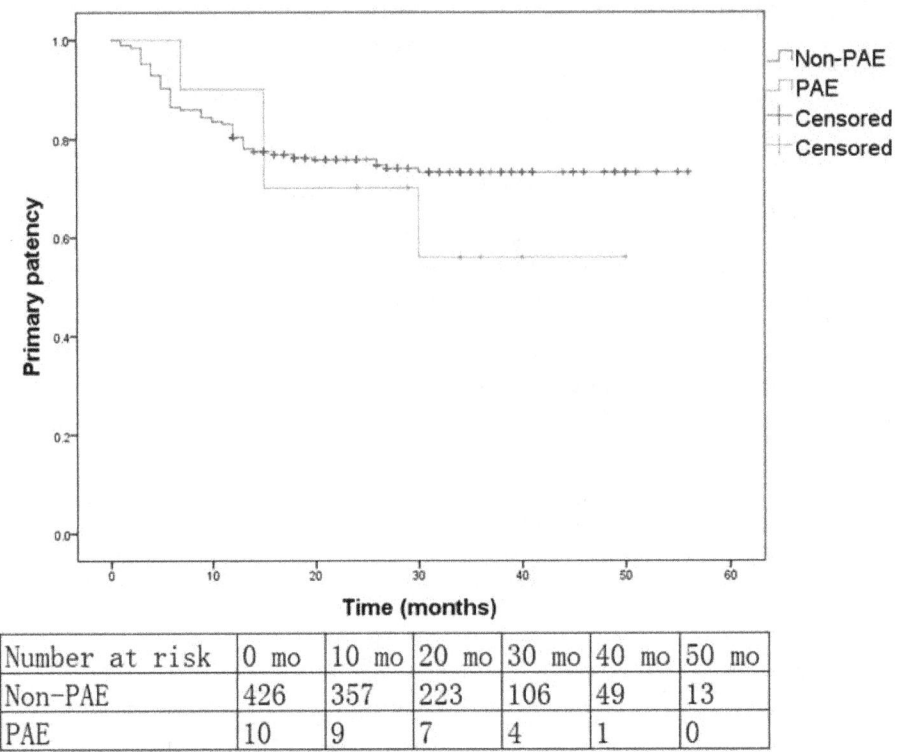

Number at risk	0 mo	10 mo	20 mo	30 mo	40 mo	50 mo
Non-PAE	426	357	223	106	49	13
PAE	10	9	7	4	1	0

Figure 1. Kaplan-Meier curves for primary patency between the popliteal artery embolization (PAE) group and the non-PAE group (Log rank test: $P = .475$**).**

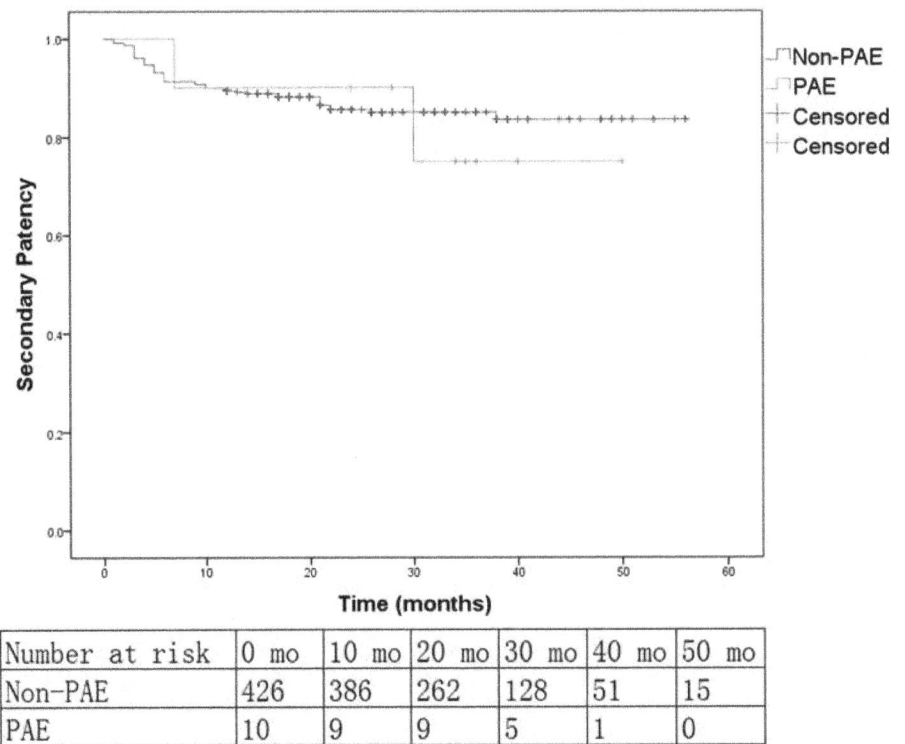

Number at risk	0 mo	10 mo	20 mo	30 mo	40 mo	50 mo
Non-PAE	426	386	262	128	51	15
PAE	10	9	9	5	1	0

Figure 2. Kaplan-Meier curves for secondary patency between the popliteal artery embolization (PAE) group and the non-PAE group (Log rank test: $P = .736$**).**

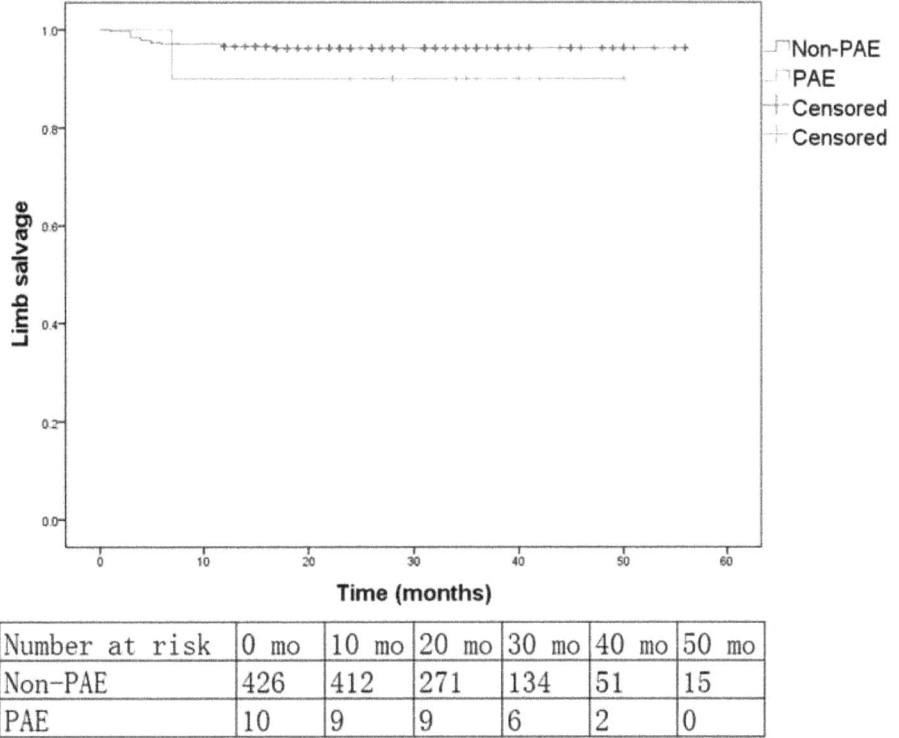

Number at risk	0 mo	10 mo	20 mo	30 mo	40 mo	50 mo
Non-PAE	426	412	271	134	51	15
PAE	10	9	9	6	2	0

Figure 3. Kaplan-Meier curves for limb salvage between the popliteal artery embolization (PAE) group and the non-PAE group (Log rank test: *P* = .298).

hypertension was associated with decreased risk in primary patency.

Discussion

Contemporary studies have demonstrated a higher rate of DE in the filter of EPDs (20–58%) [3,7,11], or detected by Doppler ultrasound (100%) [8,12], than angiographically (1%–5%) [1,2].

The reported incidence of limb-threatening DE during routine lower extremity intervention is 1–2% [1,13]. Most of the limb-threatening DE are PAE according to our experience. The incidence of PAE was seldom discussed in literature, and our data suggests that PAE rate (2.3%) is similar to limb-threatening DE rate. Published research reported that DE rate was significantly higher in CTO lesions compared with stenotic lesions, and in TASC C/D group compared with TASC A/B group [2]. We

Table 4. Comparison of patency and limb salvage rates.

Patency rate	12 months	24 months	36 months
	value ± SE	value ± SE	value ± SE
Primary patency			
Non-PAE	80.1±1.9%	75.4±2.1%	72.5±2.4%
PAE	80.0±12.6%	70.0±14.5%	56.0±17.1%
P value	1.000	.714	.474
Secondary patency			
Non-PAE	89.6±1.5%	85.9±1.8%	84.8±1.9%
PAE	90.0±9.5%	90.0±9.5%	75.0±15.8%
P value	1.000	1.000	.656
Limb salvage			
Non-PAE	96.7±0.9%	96.4±0.9%	96.4±0.9%
PAE	90.0±9.5%	90.0±9.5%	90.0±9.5%
P value	.298	.315	.315

PAE, Popliteal artery embolization; SE, Standard error.

Table 5. Cox multivariate analysis of risk factors.

Variable	HR (95% CI)	*P* value
Primary patency		
PAE	1.60 (0.54–4.79)	.401
Diabetes mellitus	2.14 (1.39–3.28)	.001
Hypertension	0.63 (0.41–0.97)	.035
Hyperlipidemia	1.67 (1.12–2.50)	.013
Secondary patency		
PAE	0.92 (0.20–4.22)	.912
Hyperlipidemia	2.51 (1.43–4.40)	.001
Chronic total occlusion	1.93 (1.07–3.47)	.028
Limb salvage		
PAE	4.35 (0.36–52.16)	.246

CI, Confidence interval; HR, hazard ratio; PAE, Popliteal artery embolization.

found the results were consistent with PAE. TASC C/D lesion, CTO lesion and history of cerebral ischemic stroke are risk factors for PAE. Aspiration and local thrombolysis were not working in all PAE cases, and all emboli retrieved from embolectomy were atheromatous plaques, suggesting that the embolic debris was mainly made of atheromatous plaque, not thrombus. The possible mechanism for PAE may be that debris is more likely to drop or release from unstable plaque in TASC C/D or CTO lesions during the intervention, in course of which the guide wire or other devices are often used to pass the occlusion by force. Once the occluded lesion is open, the debris will be flushed to the distal vessels by chance. There is little clinical evidence about cerebral ischemic stroke increases DE rate in peripheral intervention as far as we know. But basic research showed that several genes were associated with altered macrophage activity or endothelial function, resulting in increased stroke incidence and unstable plaque in cerebrovascular diseases [14,15]. It is reasonable to presume that in patients with history of cerebral ischemic stroke in this study might be inclined to form unstable plaque in the SFA lesions, resulting in increased PAE risk during interventions. Further research should be done to verify the hypothesis and the mechanism. Another interesting finding was that hypertension was an independent protective predictor of primary patency. We noticed that there were no similar reports in the literatures. The mechanism need to be studied in the future.

The treatments of PAE include aspiration, local thrombolysis, angioplasty with balloons and embolectomy. Keeping in mind that PAE is an acute limb ischemia that could lead to limb loss, and prompt restoration of the popliteal flow is urged. Angioplasty with balloons should be carried out in time if aspiration or local thrombolysis were not working. The possible mechanism of balloon angioplasty is that it may help those emboli made of soft atheromatous plaque to break into tiny particles and be flushed into distal vessels, or crush the emboli into a distal vessel from the popliteal artery. If the endovascular techniques do not work, embolectomy under general anesthesia should be carried out to open popliteal artery without delay. At least one runoff vessel flow should be restored before the procedure can be terminated after a PAE event. Our experience suggests that PAE is typically reversible by comprehensive techniques.

The concern for DE has led to a debate on the use of EPDs during lower extremity intervention. Published reports have evaluated the use of several kinds of EPDs and confirmed of the

presence of debris [6,11]. However, since these studies did not involve any control groups to confirm the short term or long term clinical efficacy of EPDs, so far it can only demonstrate that certain EPDs are safe and efficient in collecting debris during the procedure. In the Preventing Lower Extremity Distal Embolization Using Embolic Filter Protection (PROTECT) study recruiting 56 lesions treated in 40 patients all with EPDs, a side branch embolization occurred in one patient, and a no-flow phenomenon occurred in another as a result of an overfilled filter [3]. The potential benefit of EPDs must therefore be balanced against the associated complications. A study by Shrikhande and colleagues indicates that DE is typically reversible with endovascular techniques and is not associated with unfavorable clinical outcomes in a 24-month follow up, suggesting that EPDs may be unnecessary for lower extremity intervention [2]. On the other hand, the use of distal protection to prevent DE during intervention in carotid angioplasty and stenting is well established [16,17,18]. It is reasonable to believe that EPDs might be beneficial for some certain lesion types and treatment methods in lower extremity interventions. This study focus on chronic SFA arteriosclerosis cases underwent primary PTA + stent. Our data suggests that PAE events are not associated with significant lower long-term primary patency, secondary patency or limb salvage rates in both Kaplan-Meier analysis and Cox multivariate regression, if the popliteal flow is restored in time. This is similar to some previous research that complete resolution of macro-embolization may not affect long-term patency and limb salvage [2]. The results do not support routine application of EPDs. However, these results must be viewed with caution.

This study has some limitations that require attention. First, we only focus on chronic SFA arteriosclerosis cases underwent primary PTA + stent, other lesion types treated by other methods are not included in this study. Reinterventions and some new atherectomy devices are associated with higher DE rate [19,20], thus more likely to benefit from EPDs, but not discussed here. Second, the PAE rate is so low that the sheer event number is small. Thus the power to detect differences in outcome may be insufficient. Third, patency rates and limb salvage can only present a part of the clinical outcome. Distal neuromuscular function was not compared, the assessment of other collateral runoff vessels in the foot was not routinely performed neither. In addition, the mean age was less than 70 years old, which means this is a young cohort for arteriosclerosis patients who can somehow compensate from the ischemia. Therefore we don't know if EPDs could improve long-term distal neuromuscular function in patients with more advanced age.

Conclusions

PAE is a rare event that occurs in primary SFA PTA + stent. TASC C/D lesion, CTO and history of cerebral ischemic stroke are risk factors for PAE. PAE is typically reversible by comprehensive techniques. If the popliteal flow is restored in time, PAE has no significant effect on SFA patency and limb salvage rates.

Author Contributions

Conceived and designed the experiments: WW SH CL. Performed the experiments: WW YL WY BL YZ XS. Analyzed the data: WW SH. Contributed reagents/materials/analysis tools: WW SH CL. Wrote the paper: WW SH CL.

References

1. Davies MG, Bismuth J, Saad WE, Naoum JJ, Mohiuddin IT, et al. (2010) Implications of in situ thrombosis and distal embolization during superficial femoral artery endoluminal intervention. Ann Vasc Surg 24: 14–22.
2. Shrikhande GV, Khan SZ, Hussain HG, Dayal R, McKinsey JF, et al. (2011) Lesion types and device characteristics that predict distal embolization during percutaneous lower extremity interventions. J Vasc Surg 53: 347–352.
3. Shammas NW, Dippel EJ, Coiner D, Shammas GA, Jerin M, et al. (2008) Preventing lower extremity distal embolization using embolic filter protection: results of the PROTECT registry. J Endovasc Ther 15: 270–276.
4. Muller-Hulsbeck S, Schafer PJ, Humme TH, Charalambous N, Elhoft H, et al. (2009) Embolic protection devices for peripheral application: wasteful or useful? J Endovasc Ther 16 Suppl 1: I163–I169.
5. Zeller T, Schmidt A, Rastan A, Noory E, Sixt S, et al. (2012) Initial Experience With the 5×300-mm Proteus Embolic Capture Angioplasty Balloon in the Treatment of Peripheral Vascular Disease. J Endovasc Ther 19: 826–833.
6. Hadidi OF, Mohammad A, Zankar A, Brilakis ES, Banerjee S (2012) Embolic capture angioplasty in peripheral artery interventions. J Endovasc Ther 19: 611–616.
7. Karnabatidis D, Katsanos K, Kagadis GC, Ravazoula P, Diamantopoulos A, et al. (2006) Distal embolism during percutaneous revascularization of infra-aortic arterial occlusive disease: an underestimated phenomenon. J Endovasc Ther 13: 269–280.
8. Lam RC, Shah S, Faries PL, McKinsey JF, Kent KC, et al. (2007) Incidence and clinical significance of distal embolization during percutaneous interventions involving the superficial femoral artery. J Vasc Surg 46: 1155–1159.
9. Lookstein RA, Lewis S (2010) Distal embolic protection for infrainguinal interventions: how to and when? Tech Vasc Interv Radiol 13: 54–58.
10. Norgren L, Hiatt WR, Dormandy JA, Nehler MR, Harris KA, et al. (2007) Inter-Society Consensus for the Management of Peripheral Arterial Disease (TASC II). J Vasc Surg 45 Suppl S: S5–S67.
11. Shammas NW, Coiner D, Shammas GA, Christensen L, Dippel EJ, et al. (2009) Distal embolic event protection using excimer laser ablation in peripheral vascular interventions: results of the DEEP EMBOLI registry. J Endovasc Ther 16: 197–202.
12. Banerjee S, Iqbal A, Sun S, Master R, Brilakis ES (2011) Peripheral embolic events during endovascular treatment of infra-inguinal chronic total occlusion. Cardiovasc Revasc Med 12: 134–137.
13. Matsi PJ, Manninen HI (1998) Complications of lower-limb percutaneous transluminal angioplasty: a prospective analysis of 410 procedures on 295 consecutive patients. Cardiovasc Intervent Radiol 21: 361–366.
14. Schlittenhardt D, Schober A, Strelau J, Bonaterra GA, Schmiedt W, et al. (2004) Involvement of growth differentiation factor-15/macrophage inhibitory cytokine-1 (GDF-15/MIC-1) in oxLDL-induced apoptosis of human macrophages in vitro and in arteriosclerotic lesions. Cell Tissue Res 318: 325–333.
15. Fatini C, Sofi F, Gensini F, Sticchi E, Lari B, et al. (2004) Influence of eNOS gene polymorphisms on carotid atherosclerosis. Eur J Vasc Endovasc Surg 27: 540–544.
16. Bosiers M, Deloose K, Verbist J, Peeters P (2008) The impact of embolic protection device and stent design on the outcome of CAS. Perspect Vasc Surg Endovasc Ther 20: 272–279.
17. Goodney PP, Schermerhorn ML, Powell RJ (2006) Current status of carotid artery stenting. J Vasc Surg 43: 406–411.
18. Cohen SN (2007) Incidence of new brain lesions after carotid stenting with and without cerebral protection. Stroke 38: e18, e19–e20.
19. Shammas NW, Coiner D, Shammas GA, Dippel EJ, Christensen L, et al. (2011) Percutaneous lower-extremity arterial interventions with primary balloon angioplasty versus Silverhawk atherectomy and adjunctive balloon angioplasty: randomized trial. J Vasc Interv Radiol 22: 1223–1228.
20. Suri R, Wholey MH, Postoak D, Hagino RT, Toursarkissian B (2006) Distal embolic protection during femoropopliteal atherectomy. Catheter Cardiovasc Interv 67: 417–422.

3

Safety and Efficacy of Biodegradable Drug-Eluting vs. Bare Metal Stents

Yangguang Yin[1][9], **Yao Zhang**[2][9], **Xiaohui Zhao**[1]*

1 Cardiovascular Disease Research Center, Xinqiao Hospital, Third Military Medical University, Chongqing, China, **2** The Evidence Based Medicine and Clinic Epidemiology Center, Third Military Medical University, Chongqing, China

Abstract

Background: Biodegradable polymeric coatings have been proposed as a promising strategy to enhance biocompatibility and improve the delayed healing in the vessel. However, the efficacy and safety of biodegradable polymer drug-eluting stents (BP-DES) vs. bare metal stents (BMS) are unknown. The aim of this study was to perform a meta-analysis of randomized controlled trials (RCTs) comparing the outcomes of BP-DES vs. BMS.

Methods and Results: PubMed, Embase, and Cochrane Central Register of Controlled Trials (CENTRAL) were searched for randomized clinical trials, until December 2013, that compared any of approved BP-DES and BMS. Efficacy endpoints were target-vessel revascularization (TVR), target-lesion revascularization (TLR) and in-stent late loss (ISLL). Safety endpoints were death, myocardial infarction (MI), definite stent thrombosis (DST). The meta-analysis included 7 RCTs with 2,409 patients. As compared with BMS, there was a significantly reduced TVR (OR [95% CI] = 0.37 [0.28–0.50]), ISLL (OR [95% CI] = −0.41 [−0.48–0.34]) and TLR (OR [95% CI] = 0.38 [0.27–0.52]) in BP-DES patients. However, there were no difference for safety outcomes between BP-DES and BMS.

Conclusions: BP-DES is more effective in reducing ISLL, TVR and TLR, as safe as standard BMS with regard to death, ST and MI. Further large RCTs with long-term follow-up are warranted to better define the relative merits of BP-DES.

Editor: Claudio Moretti, S.G. Battista Hospital, Italy

Funding: This study was supported by grants from National Natural Science Foundation of China (81070168 and 81370213) and Third Military Medical University (2010XLC28). The funders had no role in study design, data collection and analysis, decision to publish, or preparation of the manuscript.

Competing Interests: The authors have declared that no competing interests exist.

* Email: zxhwn@tmmu.edu.cn

[9] These authors contributed equally to this work.

Introduction

The development of bare-metal stents (BMS) represents a considerable advance over balloon angioplasty in preventing restenosis by attenuating early arterial recoil and contraction. However, 15% to 20% of patients required ≥1 repeat revascularization procedure within the 6 to 12 months after BMS implantation [1]. Polymer based drug-eluting stents (DES) are currently widely used to reduce restenosis and the need for repeat revascularization, representing a major advance for percutaneous coronary intervention (PCI). [2] However, well publicized concerns raises with the long-term safety of stent thrombosis (ST) [3].

At present, great efforts have been prompted to develop alternative stents with biodegradable polymers (BP) for drug delivery, which degrade over time, and therefore hope to provide comparable long term safety to BMS while maintaining the early antirestenosis of DES. Previous studies have shown biodegradable polymer drug-eluting stents (BP-DES) is a safe and efficacious alternative to conventional durable polymer DES [4,5,6]. How-ever, uncertainty exists regarding the relative performance of BP-DES vs. BMS.

Methods

Established methods [7] were used in compliance with the PRISMA statement for reporting systematic reviews and meta-analyses in health care interventions [8].

Search Strategy

We searched Embase, PubMed, and Cochrane Central Register of Controlled Trials (CENTRAL) for studies on BP-DES until December 2013. The search strategy was formulated as the AND-combination of terms 1) Polymer 2) Stent, in Randomized controlled trials (RCTs). There was no language restriction for the search.

References of meta-analyses, review articles, and original studies identified by the electronic searches were manually checked for additional trials. For studies that did not report outcomes of interest, efforts to contact authors were performed to obtain further details. Internet-based sources of information on the results of clinical trials in cardiology www.theheart.org, www.cardiosource.com/clinicaltrials, www.clinicaltrialresults.com, and www.tctmd.com) were also searched. In addition, we searched conference abstracts of the following societies: American College of Cardiology, Transcatheter Cardiovascular Therapeutics, American Heart Association, European Society of Cardiology, Society of Cardiovascular Angiography and Intervention and Euro-PCR.

Selection Criteria

Inclusion criteria were: 1. Human studies related to PCI. 2. RCTs. 3. BMS as control. Exclusion criteria were: 1. Non-RCT; 2. Sub-study of the RCT. Two authors (Yangguang Yin and Yao Zhang) independently assessed trial bias risk and extracted data.

Data Extraction and Synthesis

Efficacy outcomes were target-lesion revascularization (TLR), target-vessel revascularization (TVR) and in-stent late loss (ISLL). Safety outcomes were death, myocardial infarction (MI) and stent thrombosis (ST). Stent thrombosis was defined as Academic Research Consortium (ARC) [9]. TLR or TVR defined as any revascularization procedure involving the target lesion or vessel owing to luminal re-narrowing in the presence of symptoms or objective signs of ischemia, respectively.

Quality Assessment

The CONSORT 2010 Statement, as a standard for the quality control assessment, was applied to evaluate the quality of the studies included. For each evaluation criterion of the CONSORT 2010 Statement, we assigned 'Adequate', 'Not Adequate', or 'Unclear' to evaluate the quality of the 7 RCTs included. The following criteria were used: Adequate indicated low bias and completely fulfilled quality standards with the least bias; Unclear indicated a lack of information or bias uncertainty; and Not Adequate was assigned if the criteria were completely unfulfilled or there was a high likelihood of bias. If a trial completely fulfilled at least six quality standards of the 10 inclusion/exclusion criteria, it was considered to be of high quality. Two reviewers (Yangguang Yin and Yao Zhang) independently evaluated and cross-checked the quality and assessed the bias of the literatures.

Statistical Methods

All statistical tests were performed using the Cochrane Collaboration's Revman5.2.6.

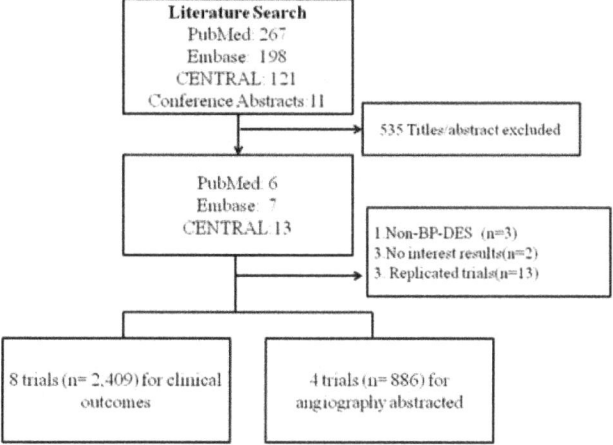

Figure 1. Flow diagram of the review process.

Table 1. Main characteristics of the included studies.

No.	Trial	FU (m)	sample DP	sample BMS	drugs DP	drugs BMS	Male (%) DP	Male (%) BMS	Age (Year+SD) DP	Age (Year+SD) BMS	DAPT (m) DP	DAPT (m) BMS	Diabets% DP	Diabets% BMS	Admission Diagnosis
1	PAINT	36	217	57	P/S	bare	64.1	66.7	59.9 10.4	58.5 9.6	12	12	31.8	26.3	CAD
2	EUROSTAR II	8	152	151	paclitaxel	bare	74.3	68.9	64.9 9.2	66.2 9.4	6	6	26.3	22.5	CAD
3	STEALTH	6	80	40	biolimus	bare	60	82.5	62.2 10.1	61.1 9.4	3	3	26.6	22.5	CAD
4	COMFOR-AMI	12	575	582	biolimus	bare	80.5	78.2	60.7 11.6	60.4 11.9	12	12	14.6	15.5	STIMI
5	EUCATAX	12	211	211	Paclitaxel	bare	83.4	79.1	63.8 10.2	64.7 12.2	6	3	23.2	16.1	CAD
6	CORACTO	24	45	46	sirolimus	bare	69.6	82.2	64.7 9.9	64.8 8.9	6	6	21.7	22.2	CTO
7	FUTURE 1	12	27	15	Everolimus	bare	85.2	86.7	64.2 8.8	65.6 9.6	6	6	3.7	0	CAD

Table 2. Vessel Size and Lesion Length of the included studies.

No.	Published	Trial	inclusion	Stent Platform DP	Stent Platform BMS	drugs DP	drugs BMS	Vessel Size DP (mm±SD)	Vessel Size BMS (mm±SD)	Lesion Length DP (mm±SD)	Lesion Length BMS (mm±SD)
1	Lemos 2012	PAINT	de novo, native, 2.5–3.5 mm; single stent ≤29 mm	SS	SS	paclitaxel	bare	3.1±0.4	3.1±0.4	NA	NA
2	Silber 2011	EUROSTAR II	de novo, native, 2.5–3.5 mm; leision ≤24 mm	CC	SS	Sirolimus	bare	2.74±0.51	2.73±0.48	21.8±4.8	22.5±5
3	Grube 2005	STEALTH	de novo, native, 2.75–4.0 mm	SS	SS	biolimus	bare	2.95±0.4	2.97±0.42	15.12±7.58	15.16±7.69
4	Räber 2012	COMFOR-AMI	STIMI	SS	SS	biolimus	bare	3.04±0.47	3.01±0.46	15.37±4.64	13.75±3.77
5	Rodriguez 2011	EUCATAX	de novo, 70% ≤stenosis	SS	SS	Paclitaxel	bare	2.75±0.5	2.85±0.5	18.19±9.73	17.77±9.57
6	Reifart 2010	CORACTO	native, CTO, 2.5–4.5 mm	SS	SS	sirolimus	bare	2.7±0.51	2.8±0.63	16.2±6.1	15.6±6.3
7	Grube 2004	FUTURE 1	de novo, 2.75–4.0 mm; leision ≤18 mm	SS	SS	Everolimus	bare	3.1±0.47	2.96±0.43	39.4±23.1	35.8±20.7

Table 3. Target Vessel, Stent Length and Stent Diameter of the included studies.

No.	Published	drugs DP	drugs BMS	RCA DP	RCA BMS	LCX DP	LCX BMS	LAD DP	LAD BMS	Stent Length DP (mm±SD)	Stent Length BMS (mm±SD)	Stent Diameter DP (mm±SD)	Stent Diameter BMS (mm±SD)
1	Lemos 2012	paclitaxel	bare	33.3	15.8	44.1	57.9	22.5	26.3	22.5±5.5	22.5±5	3.1±0.4	3.1±0.4
2	Silber 2011	Sirolimus	bare	25.5	15.8	56.6	57.9	17.9	26.3	21.8±4.8	22.5±5	3.1±0.3	3.1±0.4
3	Grube 2005	biolimus	bare	36	31.3	23.8	27	39	40.5	16.98±6.74	17.01±8.29	NA	NA
4	Räber 2012	biolimus	bare	34.1	27.5	37.8	30	28	42.5	19.03±8.76	16.23±5.53	3.2±0.4	3.2±1.1
5	Rodriguez 2011	Paclitaxel	bare	45.9	44.6	14.3	15.5	39.3	39.6	25.2±12.7	24.1±12.3	2.96±0.4	2.93±0.6
6	Reifart 2010	sirolimus	bare	17.6	25.1	18.5	23.8	62.8	48.5	21.7±5.6	20±4.8	NA	NA
7	Grube 2004	Everolimus	bare	41	27	18	13	41	60	NA	NA	NA	NA

Safety and Efficacy of Biodegradable Drug-Eluting vs. Bare Metal Stents

25

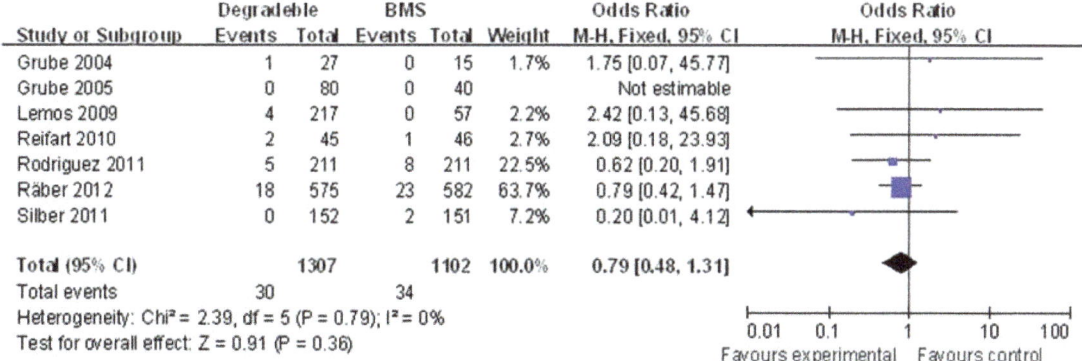

Figure 2. Individual and summary odds ratios for death in patients treated with BP-DES vs. BMS.

The chi-square test was used to examine differences in categorical variables, such as the frequencies, A P value<.05 was considered statistically significant. Summary estimate includes odds ratio (OR), Standard Mean Difference, (SMD) and its 95% confidence intervals (CI) were used as summary statistics in forest plot.

Heterogeneity among studies was determined by the Chi-square-based Q test and the I^2 statistics. A p value less than 0.05 for the Q test together with an I^2 value greater than 50% was considered a measure of severe heterogeneity. Therefore, the pooled OR estimate of each study was calculated using the fixed-effect model (the Mantel–Haenszel method); otherwise, the random-effects model (the DerSimonian and Laird method) was used. The Potential publication bias for each of the pooled study groups was assessed with a funnel plot. A two-tailed test was used to assess the funnel plot asymmetry; the significance was set at p< .05 level.

Results

Study Selection

We identified 7 RCTs that satisfied our inclusion criteria (Figure 1). [10,11,12,13,14,15,16,17] Additional follow-up data on safety and efficacy were available for PAINT trial [11]. The STEALTH trial 5 years and EUCATAX 2 years updated studies are just abstracts without strict peer review and sufficient outcomes data, and therefore excluded [18,19].

Altogether, 7 trials (n = 2,409) were finally analyzed to compare the clinical outcomes with 1,307 and 1,102 allocated to the BP-

DES and BMS, respectively. Four trials were used for angiography evaluation of ISLL. For 3-arm PAINT trial, ISLL data was abstracted to compare BP-DES (sirolimus or paclitaxel arm) to BMS, respectively.

Baseline Characteristics

The baseline characteristics are described in Table 1. Mean lesion length was 21.01±9.33 mm in the BP-DES group as compared to 20.09±8.84 mm in the BMS group. Mean vessel size was 2.94±0.45 mm in BP-DES and 2.94±0.45 mm in BMS (Table 2). Mean stent size was 3.09±0.38 mm in BP-DES and 3.08±0.63 mm in BMS. Mean stent length was 21.2±7.35 mm in the BP-DES group as compared to 20.39±6.82 mm in the BMS group (Table 3). The target vessel was 33.3% patients with RAD, 30.4% with LCX and 35.8% with LAD in the BP-DES group, as compared to 26.7% patients with RAD, 32.2% with LCX and 40.5% with LAD in the BMS group. Mean age was similar in the two groups (62.9±10.03 vs. 63.1±10.14). Men represented 73.9% of the BP-DES and 77.8% of the BMS population. There were 21.1% patients with diabetes in the BP-DES group and 17.9% in the BMS group. Mean dual anti-platelet duration was similar in the 2 groups (7.3 vs. 6.9 months).

Safety Endpoints

Death. There was no significant difference in the rate of death with BP-DES as compared with BMS: 2.29% (30/1,307) in the BP-DES group and 3.09% (34 of 1,102) in the BMS group (OR [95% CI] = 0.79 [0.48–1.31]) (Figure 2).

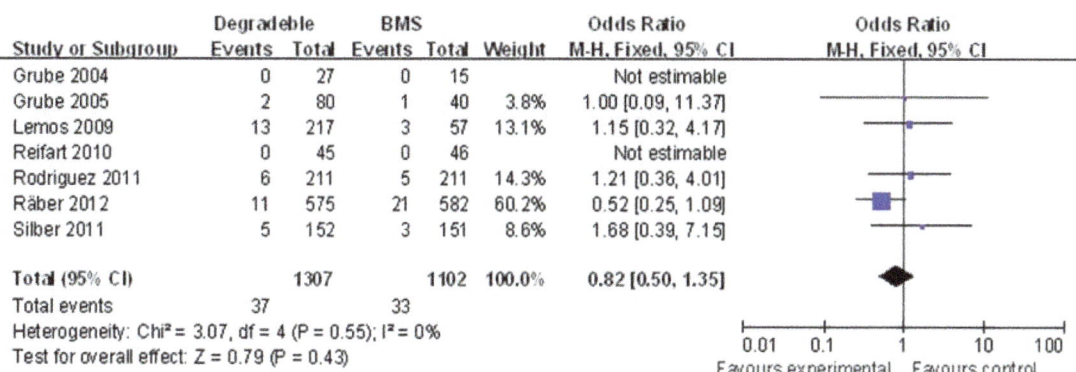

Figure 3. Individual and summary odds ratios for myocardial infarction in patients treated with BP-DES vs. BMS.

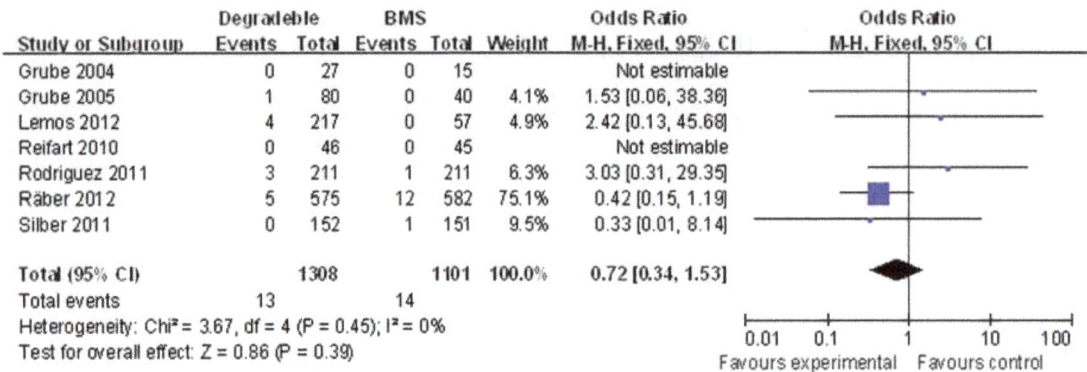

Figure 4. Individual and summary odds ratios for definite stent thrombosis (DST) in patients treated with BP-DES vs. BMS.

Myocardial infarction. There was no significant difference in the rate of MI with BP-DES as compared with BMS: 2.83% (37/1,307) in the BP-DES group and 2.99% (33/1,102) in the BMS group (OR [95% CI] = 0.82 [050–1.35]) (Figure 3).

Definite stent thrombosis. Seven studies (2,409 patients) with mean follow-up 10.5 months were included to compare the ST between BP-DES vs. BMS. There was no significant difference in the rate of total DST with BP-DES as compared with BMS: 0.99% (13/1,308) in the BP-DES group and 1.27% (14/1,101) in the BMS group (OR [95% CI] = 0.72 [0.34–1.53]) (Figure 4).

The meta-analysis did not showed a significant decreased late DST in patients treated with BP-DES (0.38%, 5/1,308) as compared to patients receiving BMS (0.18%, 2/1,101) (OR [95% CI] = 0.57 [0.23–1.40]) (Figures S1).

There was no significant difference in the rate of early DST with BP-DES as compared with BMS: 0.54% (7/1,308) in the BP-DES group and 1.59% (12/1,101) in the BMS group (OR [95% CI] = 1.19 [0.30–4.72]) (Figures S2).

Efficacy Endpoints

Target lesion revascularisation. Six studies with 2,318 patients were included. The meta-analysis showed a significant decreased TLR in patients treated with BP-DES (5.47%, 69/1,262) as compared to patients receiving BMS (11.84%, 125/1,056) (OR [95% CI] = 0.38 [0.27–0.52]) (Figure 5).

Target vessel revascularisation. Seven studies (2,409 patients) with mean follow-up 10.5 months were included. The meta-analysis showed a significant decreased TVR in patients

treated with BP-DES (6.66%, 87/1,307) as compared to patients receiving BMS (14.43%, 159/1,102) (OR [95% CI] = 0.37 [0.28–0.50]) (Figure 6).

In-stent late loss. We included 886 patients with mean follow-up 7 months. ISLL significantly decreased in BP-DES group (0.43±0.49 mm) compared to BMS group (0.85 mm±0.52). (SMD [95% CI] = −0.41 [−0.48; −0.34]), when paclitaxel arm data of PAINT trial was used as BP-DES group. (Figure 7).

The results were confirmed when sirolimus arm data of PAINT trial was used as BP-DES group (0.38±0.48 mm), comparing to BMS group (0.85 mm±0.52). (SMD [95% CI] = −0.46 [−0.53; −0.39]). (Figures S3).

Sensitivity and subgroup analyses. Sensitivity analysis was performed by removing each of the studies one at a time, which did not detected any influence of any single study on the overall results.

With regard to ISLL, the overall results in favor of BP-DES were confirmed when paclitaxel-eluting BP-DES were analyzed separately: BP-DES group (0.49±0.50 mm) compared to BMS group (0.88 mm±0.55). (SMD [95% CI] = −0.39 [−0.47; −0.32]). (Figures S4).

Subgroup analysis of outcomes between BMS and BP-BES, as well as biodegradable limus- and sirolimus eluting stents are performed, which confirmed that BP-DES is more effective in reducing ISLL, TVR and TLR, as safe as standard BMS with regard to death, ST and MI. (Figures S5–S21).

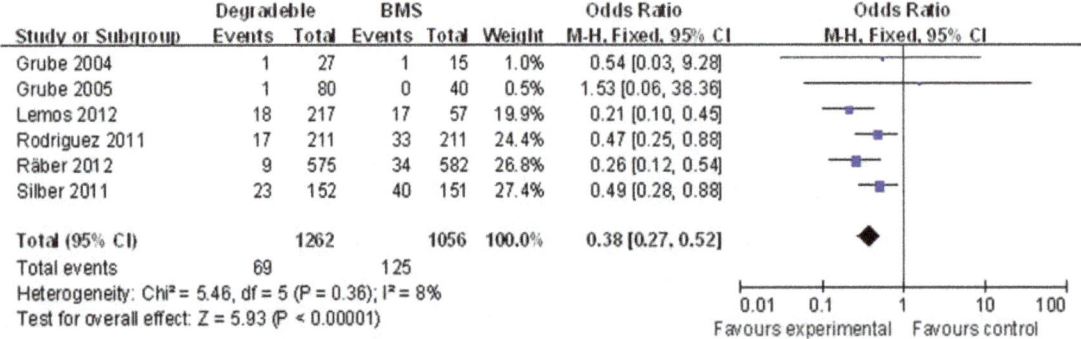

Figure 5. Individual and summary odds ratios for TLR in patients treated with BP-DES vs. BMS.

Safety and Efficacy of Biodegradable Drug-Eluting vs. Bare Metal Stents

27

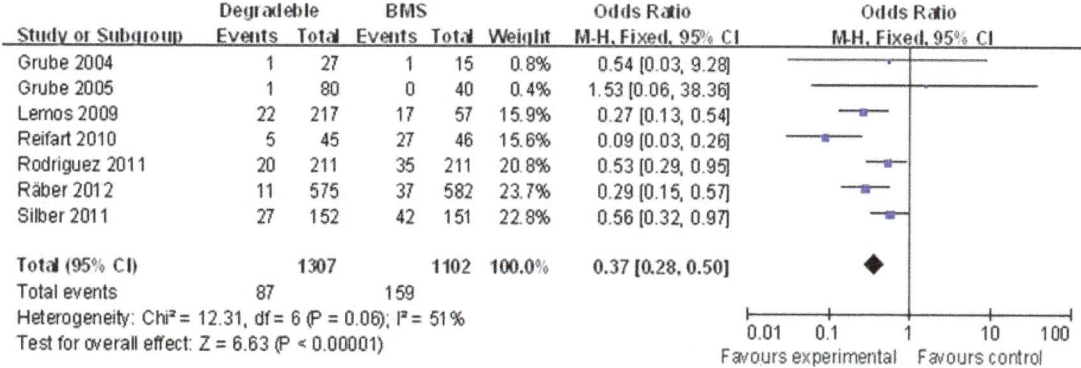

Figure 6. Individual and summary odds ratios for TVR in patients treated with BP-DES vs. BMS.

Discussion

This is the first meta-analysis that directly compared outcomes between BP-DES and BMS. The main finding is that patients allocated to BP-DES showed significantly less ISLL, TVR and TLR, with comparable MI, death, DST to those treated with BMS.

Drug-eluting stents (DES) with durable polymer coating rapidly transformed the practice of percutaneous coronary intervention (PCI), by significantly reducing rates of restenosis in comparison with bare-metal stents (BMS). [20,21] However, residual polymer in the coronary milieu induces inflammatory response at the vessel-wall and then contributes to late thrombotic stent as well as late neointimal overgrowth [22,23].

Degradable-polymer DES has been developed by providing similar controlled drug release with subsequent degradation of the polymer in 3–9 months and, therefore, appears to be a promising solution to overcome this problem [4,5]. However, at least 2 benchmarks, efficacy and safety, should be considered when appraising the results of BP-DES. First, they should demonstrate comparable, if not superior, safety results compared with BMS and DES. Second, the BP-DES should also reduce the incidence of revascularization compared with BMS, and be shown to be at least noninferior in regard to contemporary DES [6]. At present, clinical data have accumulated to support the use of biodegradable polymer stents to be a safe and efficacious alternative to conventional durable polymer DES [24,25].

Several RCTs have been investigated to compare outcomes of BP-DES vs. BMS. FUTURE I was the first prospective, single-blind, randomized trial to evaluate the safety and efficacy of everolimus-eluting stents (EES), coated with a bio-absorbable polymer, comparing with BMS [17]. In this initial clinical experience, BP-DES demonstrated a safe and efficacious method to reduce in-stent neointimal hyperplasia and restenosis. In

PAINT trial, Lemos et al tested 2 novel DES, covered with a biodegradable-polymer carrier and releasing paclitaxel or sirolimus, which were compared against a bare metal stent [10]. They found both BD-DES were effective in reducing neointimal hyperplasia and 1-year re-intervention, compared to BMS. The COMFORTABLE AMI [14] is the largest RCTs (1161 patients) to date, comparing outcomes of BP-DES vs. BMS. This study showed that the use of biolimus-eluting stents with a biodegradable polymer resulted in a lower rate of the composite of major adverse cardiac events at 1 year among patients with ST-elevation myocardial infarction undergoing primary PCI. However, all those trials comparing BP-DES vs. BMS were not powerful to reveal potential differences in low frequency events including MI, death and ST, and therefore their relative efficacy and safety remains undetermined.

The findings of the current study are novel and important for at least 2 reasons.

First, our study directly addressed the comparison of outcomes between BP-DES and BMS. We didn't show a significant difference in death, DST and MI for BP-DES, as compared to BMS. These results should be explained carefully: 1. It is our opinion that an analysis with 2,409 patients was unable to detect a significant advantage may be interpreted as a limited difference between BP-DES and BMS. 2. The low incidence of death, DST and MI has made investigating the difference of these outcomes difficult. Further large RCTs with long-term follow-up are warranted to better define the relative merits of BP-DES.

Recently, 2 large scale network studies have showed BP-DES were associated with significantly lower rates of cardiac death/MI, MI, and ST than BMS [24,25]. In our opinion, these different results should be noted and could be explained with following reasons: 1. Network analysis is a different statistic method with our meta-analysis, which allows for indirect comparisons of stents not

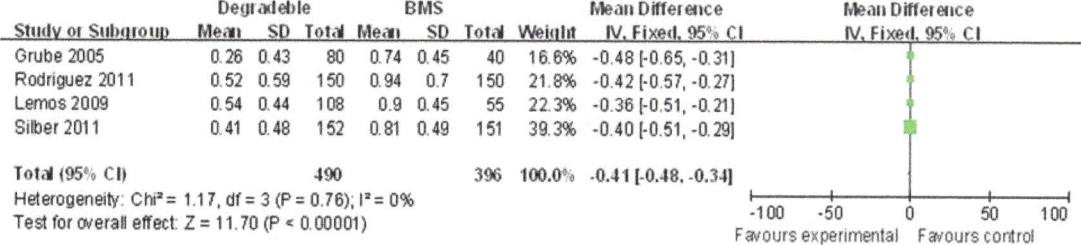

Figure 7. Standardized mean difference (SMD) for ISLL in patients treated with BP-DES vs. BMS.

in any of the individual trials (comparison of stent A vs. C by using trials comparing A vs. B and B vs. C), and may include more trials. 2. We included 7 trials of direct comparison of BP-DES vs. BMS for data abstraction. However, Palmerini et al [25] only included 1 trial (COMFORTABLE AMI) in their analysis, indicating that most of their results about BP-DES vs. BMS are based on indirect comparison. 3. Duration of antiplatelet therapy in patients treated with BD-DES and BMS differed across trials and therefore represented a confounding factor in these 2 network analysis.

Secondary, we for the first time reported an improved anti-restenotic efficacy of BP-DES vs. BMS with lower ISLL in 8 months, as well as a significant reduction of BP-DES in both TLR and TVR. This finding is supported by the results of previous network meta-analysis regarding to TVR [24,25]. Thus, similar findings with different trials further clarified the efficacy profile of BP-DES, as compare to BMS.

DES had revolutionized the practice of interventional cardiology and been implanted in the majority of PCI procedures over the past decades. However, BMS are still used especially in patients with AMI, high bleeding risk or large coronary vessel (> 3.0 mm). Thus, the findings of a reduced ISLL, TVR and TLR, as well as non-inferior safety outcomes with BP-DES as compared to BMS in our meta-analysis are clinically significant and indicating a safe and efficacious alternative to conventional BMS.

Multiple studies have shown improved safety and efficacy of second generation everolimus-eluting stent than early-generation sirolimus-eluting, paclitaxel-eluting stents, [26,27,28] and therefore, representing the standard care to which new stent designs should be compared. [29] Also, previous studies have also proved superior outcomes with EES when compared to BMS. [30,31,32] However, there is only FUTURE I trial comparing the safety and efficacy of biodegradable polymer everolimus-eluting stents (BP-EES) and BMS. This study indicated that BP-EES with biodegradable polymer could be a safe and efficacious method to reduce in-stent neointimal hyperplasia and restenosis. [17].

Biolimus is the limus analogue with the highest lipophilicity used for drug elution on currently available stent platforms. [33] Theoretically, the increased lipophilicity of the drug biolimus may provide a more rapid and homogeneous drug distribution, potentially leading to a more potent anti-inflammatory and antithrombotic local effect. In fact, previous study reported that BP-BES, as compared to PP-EES, showed similar stent coverage and apposition as assessed by OCT at 6–8 months. [34] Furthermore, meta-analysis and clinical trials proved that BP-BES are as safe and efficacious as the current standard of a thin-strut EES with a durable biocompatible polymer. [35,36,37,38] So, BP-BES may also be an alternative standard choice for comparing the stents safety and efficacy.

We compared the outcomes of BMS with BP-BES, as well as biodegradable limus- and sirolimus eluting stents. All the subgroup analysis support our conclusions that BP-DES is more effective in reducing ISLL, TVR and TLR, as safe as standard BMS with regard to death, ST and MI.

Limitations

1. The limitations of the meta-analytical approach are well known and documented. [39] 2. We didn't have data for all trials at each time period; therefore, this limited comparison of rates across time within a specific end point. 3. Inclusion criteria were not equivalent across the included trials, however, reflects the broadly inclusive nature of the included patient population. 4. Our

meta-analysis might be un-powerful to detect the difference of low incidence events such as MI, death and ST. 5. A major limitation is absence of comparisons with DES like everolimus eluting ones, which represent the standard of care for PCI.

Conclusions

BP-DES is more effective in reducing ISLL, TVR and TLR, as well as comparable with BMS in regard to death, ST and MI. Further large RCTs with long-term follow-up are warranted to better define the relative merits of BP-DES.

Supporting Information

Figure S1 Individual and summary odds ratios for late definite stent thrombosis (DST) in patients treated with BP-DES vs. BMS.

Figure S2 Individual and summary odds ratios for early definite stent thrombosis (DST) in patients treated with BP-DES vs. BMS.

Figure S3 Standardized mean difference (SMD) for ISLL in patients treated with BP-DES vs. BMS.

Figure S4 Standardized mean difference (SMD) for ISLL in patients treated with paclitaxel-eluting BP-DES vs. BMS.

Figure S5 Individual and summary odds ratios for death in patients treated with BP-BES vs. BMS.

Figure S6 Individual and summary odds ratios for myocardial infarction in patients treated with BP-BES vs. BMS.

Figure S7 Individual and summary odds ratios for TLR in patients treated with BP-BES vs. BMS.

Figure S8 Individual and summary odds ratios for TVR in patients treated with BP-BES vs. BMS.

Figure S9 Individual and summary odds ratios for early definite stent thrombosis in patients treated with BP-BES vs. BMS.

Figure S10 Individual and summary odds ratios for late definite stent thrombosis (DST) in patients treated with BP-BES vs. BMS.

Figure S11 Individual and summary odds ratios for death in patients treated with BP-limus eluting stents vs. BMS.

Figure S12 Individual and summary odds ratios for myocardial infarction in patients treated with BP-limus eluting stents vs. BMS.

Figure S13 Individual and summary odds ratios for TLR in patients treated with BP-limus eluting stents vs. BMS.

Figure S14 Individual and summary odds ratios for TVR in patients treated with BP-limus eluting stents vs. BMS.

Figure S15 Individual and summary odds ratios for early definite stent thrombosis in patients treated with BP-limus eluting stents vs. BMS.

Figure S16 Individual and summary odds ratios for late definite stent thrombosis in patients treated with BP-limus eluting stents vs. BMS.

Figure S17 Standardized mean difference (SMD) for ISLL in patients treated with BP-limus eluting stents vs. BMS.

Figure S18 Individual and summary odds ratios for death in patients treated with BP-SES vs. BMS.

Figure S19 Individual and summary odds ratios for myocardial infarction in patients treated with BP-SES vs. BMS.

Figure S20 Individual and summary odds ratios for TVR in patients treated with BP-SES vs. BMS.

Figure S21 Individual and summary odds ratios for late define stent thrombosis in patients treated with BP-SES vs. BMS.

Table S1 Protocols of dual anti-platelet therapy (DAPT).

Author Contributions

Conceived and designed the experiments: XZ. Performed the experiments: YY YZ. Analyzed the data: YY. Contributed reagents/materials/analysis tools: YZ. Wrote the paper: XZ.

References

1. Fischman DL, Leon MB, Baim DS, Schatz RA, Savage MP, et al. (1994) A randomized comparison of coronary-stent placement and balloon angioplasty in the treatment of coronary artery disease. Stent Restenosis Study Investigators. N Engl J Med 331: 496–501.
2. Bangalore S, Kumar S, Fusaro M, Amoroso N, Attubato MJ, et al. (2012) Short- and long-term outcomes with drug-eluting and bare-metal coronary stents: a mixed-treatment comparison analysis of 117 762 patient-years of follow-up from randomized trials. Circulation 125: 2873–2891.
3. Camenzind E, Steg PG, Wijns W (2007) Stent thrombosis late after implantation of first-generation drug-eluting stents: a cause for concern. Circulation 115: 1440–1455; discussion 1455.
4. Stefanini GG BR, Serruys PW, de Waha A, Meier B, Massberg S, et al. (2012) Biodegradable polymer drug-eluting stents reduce the risk of stent thrombosis at 4 years in patients undergoing percutaneous coronary intervention: a pooled analysis of individual patient data from the ISAR-TEST 3, ISAR-TEST 4, and LEADERS randomized trials. Eur Heart J 33: 1214–1222.
5. Navarese EP KJ, Castriota F, Gibson CM, De Luca G, Buffon A, et al. (2011) Safety and efficacy of biodegradable vs. durable polymer drug-eluting stents: evidence from a meta-analysis of randomised trials. EuroIntervention 7: 985–994.
6. Garg S, Bourantas C, Serruys PW (2013) New concepts in the design of drug-eluting coronary stents. Nat Rev Cardiol 10: 248–260.
7. The Cochrane Collaboration. Cochrane Handbook for Systematic Reviews of Interventions. The Cochrane Collaboration website, Available: http://www.cochrane.org/resources/handbook. Accessed 2011 March.
8. Liberati A, Altman DG, Tetzlaff J, Mulrow C, Gotzsche PC, et al. (2009) The PRISMA statement for reporting systematic reviews and meta-analyses of studies that evaluate health care interventions: explanation and elaboration. PLoS Med 6: e1000100.
9. Cutlip DE, Windecker S, Mehran R, Boam A, Cohen DJ, et al. (2007) Clinical end points in coronary stent trials: a case for standardized definitions. Circulation 115: 2344–2351.
10. Lemos PA, Moulin B, Perin MA, Oliveira LA, Arruda JA, et al. (2009) Randomized evaluation of two drug-eluting stents with identical metallic platform and biodegradable polymer but different agents (paclitaxel or sirolimus) compared against bare stents: 1-year results of the PAINT trial. Catheter Cardiovasc Interv 74: 665–673.
11. Lemos PA, Moulin B, Perin MA, Oliveira LA, Arruda JA, et al. (2012) Late clinical outcomes after implantation of drug-eluting stents coated with biodegradable polymers: 3-year follow-up of the PAINT randomised trial. EuroIntervention 8: 117–119.
12. Silber S, Gutierrez-Chico JL, Behrens S, Witzenbichler B, Wiemer M, et al. (2011) Effect of paclitaxel elution from reservoirs with bioabsorbable polymer compared to a bare metal stent for the elective percutaneous treatment of de novo coronary stenosis: the EUROSTAR-II randomised clinical trial. EuroIntervention 7: 64–73.
13. Grube E, Hauptmann KE, Buellesfeld L, Lim V, Abizaid A (2005) Six-month results of a randomized study to evaluate safety and efficacy of a Biolimus A9 eluting stent with a biodegradable polymer coating. EuroIntervention 1: 53–57.
14. Raber L, Kelbaek H, Ostojic M, Baumbach A, Heg D, et al. (2012) Effect of biolimus-eluting stents with biodegradable polymer vs bare-metal stents on cardiovascular events among patients with acute myocardial infarction: the COMFORTABLE AMI randomized trial. JAMA 308: 777–787.
15. Rodriguez AE, Vigo CF, Delacasa A, Mieres J, Fernandez-Pereira C, et al. (2011) Efficacy and safety of a double-coated paclitaxel-eluting coronary stent: the EUCATAX trial. Catheter Cardiovasc Interv 77: 335–342.
16. Reifart N, Hauptmann KE, Rabe A, Enayat D, Giokoglu K(2010) Short and long term comparison (24 months) of an alternative sirolimus-coated stent with bioabsorbable polymer and a bare metal stent of similar design in chronic coronary occlusions: the CORACTO trial. EuroIntervention 6: 356–360.
17. Grube E, Sonoda S, Ikeno F, Honda Y, Kar S, et al. (2004) Six- and twelve-month results from first human experience using everolimus-eluting stents with bioabsorbable polymer. Circulation 109: 2168–2171.
18. Ricardo Costa RM, Alexandre Abizaid, Karl E Hauptmann, Eberhard Grube (2011) STEALTH I: 5-year Follow-up from a Prospective Randomized Study of Biolimus A9-Eluting Stent with a Biodegradable Polymer Coating vs a Bare Metal Stent. JACC 58/20/Suppl B.
19. Rodriguez-Granillo AM MJ, Fernandez-Pereira C, Delacasa A, Vigo CF, Risau G, et al. (2013) Two-year reports of efficacy and safety end points from the randomised, multicentre and controlled Eucatax trial. Eurointervention website, Available: http://www.pcronline.com/eurointervention/M_issue/156. Accessed 2013.
20. Stone GW, Ellis SG, Cox DA, Hermiller J, O'Shaughnessy C, et al. (2004) A polymer-based, paclitaxel-eluting stent in patients with coronary artery disease. N Engl J Med 350: 221–231.
21. Moses JW, Leon MB, Popma JJ, Fitzgerald PJ, Holmes DR, et al. (2003) Sirolimus-eluting stents versus standard stents in patients with stenosis in a native coronary artery. N Engl J Med 349: 1315–1323.
22. Virmani R, Guagliumi G, Farb A, Musumeci G, Grieco N, et al. (2004) Localized hypersensitivity and late coronary thrombosis secondary to a sirolimus-eluting stent: should we be cautious? Circulation 109: 701–705.
23. Finn AV, Kolodgie FD, Harnek J, Guerrero LJ, Acampado E, et al. (2005) Differential response of delayed healing and persistent inflammation at sites of overlapping sirolimus- or paclitaxel-eluting stents. Circulation 112: 270–278.
24. Bangalore S, Toklu B, Amoroso N, Fusaro M, Kumar S, et al. (2013) Bare metal stents, durable polymer drug eluting stents, and biodegradable polymer drug eluting stents for coronary artery disease: mixed treatment comparison meta-analysis. BMJ 347: f6625.
25. Palmerini T, Biondi-Zoccai G, Della Riva D, Mariani A, Sabate M, et al. (2014) Clinical Outcomes with Bioabsorbable Polymer-based versus Durable Polymer-based Drug-Eluting Stents and Bare Metal Stents: Evidence from a Comprehensive Network Meta-analysis. J Am Coll Cardiol 63: 299–307.
26. Stone GW, Rizvi A, Sudhir K, Newman W, Applegate RJ, et al. (2011) Randomized comparison of everolimus- and paclitaxel-eluting stents: 2-year follow-up from the SPIRIT IV trial. J Am Coll Cardiol 58: 19–25.
27. Smits PC, Kedhi E, Royaards KJ, Joesoef KS, Wassing J, et al. (2011) 2-year follow-up of a randomized controlled trial of everolimus- and paclitaxel-eluting stents for coronary revascularization in daily practice: COMPARE. J Am Coll Cardiol 58: 11–18.
28. Palmerini T, Biondi-Zoccai G, Della Riva D, et al. (2012) Stent thrombosis with drug-eluting and bare-metal stents: evidence from a comprehensive network meta-analysis. Lancet 379: 1393–402.
29. Ormiston JA, Webster MWI (2012) Stent thrombosis: has the firestorm been extinguished? Lancet 379: 1368–69.
30. Omar A, Torguson R, Kitabata H, Pendyala LK, Loh JP, et al. (2014) Long-Term safety and efficacy of second-generation everolimus-eluting stents compared to other limus-eluting stents and bare metal stents in patients with acute coronary syndrome. Catheter Cardiovasc Interv. Wiley online library website, Available: http://onlinelibrary.wiley.com/doi/10.1002/ccd.25469/pdf Accessed 2014 Mar 12.

31. Sabaté M, Brugaletta S, Cequier A (2014) The EXAMINATION trial: 2-year results from a multicenter randomized controlled trial. JACC Cardiovasc Interv 7: 64–71.

32. Valgimigli M, Tebaldi M, Borghesi M, Vranckx P, Campo G, et al. (2014) Two-year outcomes after first- or second-generation drug-eluting or bare-metal stent implantation in all-comer patients undergoing percutaneous coronary intervention: a pre-specified analysis from the PRODIGY study. JACC Cardiovasc Interv 7: 20–8.

33. Davi G, Patrono C (2007) Platelet activation and atherothrombosis. N Engl J Med 357: 2482–2494.

34. Tada T, Kastrati A, Byrne RA, Schuster T, Cuni R, et al. (2014) Randomized comparison of biolimus-eluting stents with biodegradable polymer versus everolimus-eluting stents with permanent polymer coatings assessed by optical coherence tomography. Int J Cardiovasc Imaging 30: 495–504.

35. Zhang YJ, Zhu LL, Bourantas CV, Iqbal J, Dong SJ, et al. (2014) The impact of everolimus versus other rapamycin derivative-eluting stents on clinical outcomes in patients with coronary artery disease: A meta-analysis of 16 randomized trials.

J Cardiol. Sciencedirect website, Available: http://www.sciencedirect.com/science/article/pii/S0914508714000252. Accessed 2014 Feb 20.

36. Smits PC, Hofma S, Togni M, Vázquez N, Valdés M, et al. (2013) Abluminal biodegradable polymer biolimus-eluting stent versus durable polymer everolimus-eluting stent (COMPARE II): a randomised, controlled, non-inferiority trial. Lancet 381: 651–60.

37. Natsuaki M, Kozuma K, Morimoto T, Kadota K, Muramatsu T, et al. (2013) Biodegradable polymer biolimus-eluting stent versus durable polymer everolimus-eluting stent: a randomized, controlled, noninferiority trial. J Am Coll Cardiol 62: 181–90.

38. Separham A, Sohrabi B, Aslanabadi N, Ghaffari S (2011) The twelve-month outcome of biolimus eluting stent with biodegradable polymer compared with an everolimus eluting stent with durable polymer. J Cardiovasc Thorac Res 3: 113–6.

39. Stroup DF, Berlin JA, Morton SC, Olkin I, Williamson GD, et al. (2000) Meta-analysis of observational studies in epidemiology: a proposal for reporting. Meta-analysis Of Observational Studies in Epidemiology (MOOSE) group. JAMA 283: 2008–2012.

4

Interplay between Genetic and Clinical Variables Affecting Platelet Reactivity and Cardiac Adverse Events in Patients Undergoing Percutaneous Coronary Intervention

Jolanta M. Siller-Matula[1]*, Irene M. Lang[1], Thomas Neunteufl[1], Marek Kozinski[2], Gerald Maurer[1], Katarzyna Linkowska[3], Tomasz Grzybowski[3], Jacek Kubica[2], Bernd Jilma[4]*

1 Department of Cardiology, Medical University of Vienna, Vienna, Austria, 2 Department of Cardiology and Internal Medicine, Collegium Medicum of the Nicolaus Copernicus University, Bydgoszcz, Poland, 3 Institute of Molecular and Forensic Genetics, Collegium Medicum of the Nicolaus Copernicus University, Bydgoszcz, Poland, 4 Department of Clinical Pharmacology, Medical University of Vienna, Vienna, Austria

Abstract

Several clinical and genetic variables are associated with influencing high on treatment platelet reactivity (HTPR). The aim of the study was to propose a path model explaining a concurrent impact among variables influencing HTPR and ischemic events. In this prospective cohort study polymorphisms of CYP2C19*2, CYP2C19*17, ABCB1, PON1 alleles and platelet function assessed by Multiple Electrode Aggregometry were assessed in 416 patients undergoing percutaneous coronary intervention treated with clopidogrel and aspirin. The rates of major adverse cardiac events (MACE) were recorded during a 12-month follow up. The path model was calculated by a structural equation modelling. Paths from two clinical characteristics (diabetes mellitus and acute coronary syndrome (ACS)) and two genetic variants (CYP2C19*2 and CYP2C19*17) independently predicted HTPR (path coefficients: 0.11 0.10, 0.17, and -0.10, respectively; p<0.05 for all). By use of those four variables a novel score for prediction of HTPR was built: in a factor-weighted model the risk for HTPR was calculated with an OR of 3.8 (95%CI: 3.1–6.8, p<0.001) for a score level of ≥1 compared with a score of <1. While MACE was independently predicted by HTPR and age in the multivariate model (path coefficient: 0.14 and 0.13, respectively; p<0.05), the coexistence of HTPR and age ≥75 years emerged as the strongest predictor of MACE. Our study suggests a pathway, which might explain indirect and direct impact of variables on clinical outcome: ACS, diabetes mellitus, CYP2C19*2 and CYP2C19*17 genetic variants independently predicted HTPR. In turn, age ≥75 years and HTPR were the strongest predictors of MACE.

Editor: Christian Schulz, King's College London School of Medicine, United Kingdom

Funding: This study was partly supported by a grant from the Jubiläumsfond of the Austrian National Bank and partly by internal founding of the institution. The external funder had no role in study design, data collection and analysis, decision to publish, or preparation of the manuscript.

Competing Interests: The authors have read the journal's policy and have the following conflicts: Jolanta M. Siller-Matula has received lecture or consultant fees from AstraZeneca, Daiichi Sankyo and Eli Lilly and a research grant from Roche. Irene M. Lang has relationships with drug companies including AOPOrphan Pharmaceuticals, Actelion, Bayer, Astra-Zeneca, Servier, Cordis, Medtronic, GSK, Novartis, Pfizer and United Therapeutics. In addition, Irene Marthe Lang is an investigator in trials involving these companies, with relationships including consultancy service, research grants and membership in scientific advisory boards. Thomas Neunteufl has received lecture or consultant fees from AstraZeneca, BMS/Sanofi Aventis, Eli Lilly-Daiichi Sankyo. Marek Kozinski has received lecture fee from AstraZeneca. Gerald Maurer: none, Katarzyna Linkowska: none, Tomasz Grzybowski: none. Jacek Kubica has received a research grant from AstraZeneca. Bernd Jilma has received lecture fees from AstraZeneca.

* Email: jolanta.siller-matula@meduniwien.ac.at (JS-M); bernd.jilma@meduniwien.ac.at (BJ)

Introduction

Within the past years, platelet function studies have shown that up to 50% of clopidogrel treated patients have high on-treatment platelet reactivity (HTPR) [1]. Studies in over 20.000 of patients indicate an up to 10-fold higher risk of adverse ischemic events in patients with HTPR [2–9]. Several clinical and genetic variables are associated with HTPR. The clinical factors include obesity, renal dysfunction, diabetes, age, heart failure, inflammation and acute coronary syndromes (ACS) [10–13]. From multiple candidate genes being involved in metabolism of clopidogrel, the CYP2C19*2 (loss-of-function allele) and the CYP2C19*17 (gain-of-function mutation), have been associated with response variability to clopidogrel in some studies [12,14–19]. Whether

other polymorphisms of genes being involved in the metabolism or action of clopidogrel (e.g. the intestinal efflux transport pump P-glycoprotein pump encoded by the ABCB1 gene or the paraoxonase-1, PON1 gene) predict HTPR is a matter of debate [14,20–23].

To our knowledge, a concurrent impact among different variables influencing HTPR and ischemic events has not been reported. Therefore, the aim of the current paper was to investigate the interaction of clinical and genetic risk factors of HTPR in relation to cardiac ischemic events.

Methods

Study design

This paper reports a sub-analysis of a previously published prospective observational cohort study [24]. The study design has been reported in detail [24]. In brief, the Ethics Committee of the Medical University of Vienna approved the study protocol in accordance with the Declaration of Helsinki. Participants were included into the study between March 2007 and September 2008, and followed up for 12 months. Clinical follow up information was obtained by contacting all patients by phone and/or mail every three months, and by queries from the national death registry. Inclusion criteria were: written informed consent obtained before study entry, previous stent implantation, PCI at least 2 h after clopidogrel loading with 600 mg, age >18 years and planned treatment with clopidogrel and aspirin for 12 months. The only exclusion criterion was participation in other interventional trials. Four hundred sixteen patients with coronary artery disease (CAD) undergoing percutaneous coronary intervention (PCI) were consecutively enrolled. All patients received a clopidogrel loading dose of 600 mg followed by a daily dose of 75 mg. Blood samples from patients were obtained from the arterial sheath (6F) in the catheterization laboratory directly post PCI and at least 5 minutes after intravenous infusion of aspirin. All analyses were performed by trained laboratory technicians blinded to the results of other test and to the outcomes. The study is reported according to the STROBE (strengthening the reporting of observational studies in epidemiology) standards.

Platelet Aggregometry

Whole blood aggregation was determined using Multiple Electrode Aggregometry (MEA) on a new generation impedance aggregometer (Multiplate Analyzer, Verum Diagnostica GmbH, Munich, Germany) directly after blood sampling at the Department of Clinical Pharmacology at the Medical University of Vienna. The system detects the electrical impedance change due to the adhesion and aggregation of platelets on two independent electrode-set surfaces in the test cuvette [25]. We used hirudin as anticoagulant and adenosine diphosphate (ADP) + prostaglandin E1 (PGE1) as agonists [26]. A 1:2 dilution of whole blood anticoagulated with hirudin and 0.9% NaCl was stirred at $37°C$ for 3 min in the test cuvettes, ADP: 6.4 µM and PGE1: 9.4 nM were added and the increase in electrical impedance was recorded continuously for 6 min [27]. The mean values of the 2 independent determinations are expressed as the area under the curve of the aggregation tracing (AUC = AU*min) and reported in U (10 AU*min = 1 U). Values >48U corresponded to HTPR [24].

Genotyping

Genotyping was performed after inclusion of the last participant at the Institute of Molecular and Forensic Genetics, Collegium Medicum of the Nicolaus Copernicus University in Bydgoszcz, Poland. Genomic DNA was extracted from blood according to the standard procedures. *CYP2C19*17* (CYP2C19_-806_C>T, rs12248560) was genotyped with a commercially available validated drug metabolism genotyping assay (TaqMan Drug Metabolism Genotyping Assay C_469857_10, Life Technologies, Carlsbad, California) with the ABI Prism Sequence Detector 7000 (Life Technologies) in accordance with manufacturer's instructions. *CYP2C19*2* (CYP2C19_681_G>A; rs4244285) was genotyped with real-time allelic discrimination assay on an ABI Prism Sequence Detector 7000 (Life Technologies) according to standard procedures. Primers 5′- GATATGCAATAATTTTCCCAC-

TATCATTG-3′ and 5′-GGTGTTCTTTTACTTTCTC-CAAAATATCAC-3′ were used to amplify a sequence of the CYP2C19 gene containing the single nucleotide polymorphism 681G>A (rs4244285). The sequence of the G allele-specific probe was 5′-FAM-TTATTTCCCGGGAACC-3′ and the sequence of the A allele-specific probe was 5′-VIC-ATTATTTCCCAG-GAACC-3′. SNPs in ABCB1 (rs1045542) and PON1 (rs662) were genotyped using commercial *TaqMan SNP Genotyping Assays* (assay IDs: rs1045642: C_7586657_20; rs662: C_2548962_20) on a *ViiA 7 Real-Time PCR System* (Life Technologies) following the manufacturer's instructions. After PCR, fluorescence yield for the two different dyes was measured and presented in a two-dimensional graph to obtain the allelic discrimination plot and identify individual genotypes. Correctness of genotyping was evaluated for randomly selected samples by direct sequencing of PCR products with the use of BigDye Terminator v. 3.1 sequencing kit and 3130xl Genetic Analyzer (Life Technologies). No discrepancies were observed between real-time discrimination and sequencing strategies.

Study endpoint

The clinical endpoint was the composite of major adverse cardiac events (MACE: stent thrombosis: definite and probable, ACS and cardiac death) during a 12-month follow up. Stent thrombosis was defined according to the Academic Research Consortium criteria as the occurrence of an ACS with either angiographic or pathological confirmation of thrombosis [28]. Probable stent thrombosis was defined as any unexplained death within 30 days or target vessel myocardial infarction without angiographic confirmation of thrombosis or other identified culprit lesion [28].

Statistical analysis

Based on a 22% rate of a composite of major adverse events in the group with high on treatment platelet reactivity (HTPR) compared to 8% in the group without HTPR [29], we calculated that 416 patients in the study would provide 99.9% power to detect significant differences (one sided alpha value of <0.05). Normal distribution was tested with the Kolmogorov Smirnov test. Data are expressed as mean, standard deviation (SD), 95% confidence intervals (CI) median or interquartile range. Statistical comparisons were performed with the t test, the Mann Whitney U test and the X^2-test when applicable. Kaplan-Meier curves with the Breslow test were used for survival analyses. The Bonferroni correction was used for multiple comparisons. A multivariate Cox regression model was used to determinate independent predictors of MACE. The univariate logistic regression analysis was used to estimate variables responsible for HTPR and was a first step in the factor analysis. The effect of each variable on HTPR and MACE was tested using path analysis modelling, wherein the model fit was examined, as well as the significance of the direct and indirect effects (included variables: *CYP2C19*2, CYP2C19*17*, ABCB1 and PON1 carrier status, body mass index (BMI), diabetes mellitus, age, renal failure (creatinine clearance <60 mg/ml) and ACS at admission). Other gene environment interactions were tested in an exploratory factor analysis.

The following indicators were used to assess the goodness of fit of the models: Comparative Fit Index and Root Mean Square Error of Approximation. The maximum likelihood estimation method for structural equation modelling was used to test the conceptual model, examining the relationships among latent variables. The rationale for using the structural equation modelling instead of logistic regression in our paper is explained below. Logistic regression allows investigation of relationship

Table 1. Patient demographics.

Patient Demographics

	N = 416
Age (years)	64±12
Gender (male) n (%)	318 (76)
Risk factors/past medical history n (%)	
Body mass index (BMI; mean±SD)	28.1±5.5
Hypertension	352 (84)
Hyperlipidemia	318 (76)
Smoking	230 (55)
Family history of CAD	129 (31)
Diabetes mellitus	135 (32)
Prior PCI	197 (47)
Prior myocardial infarction	135 (31)
Peripheral arterial occlusive disease	54 (13)
Cerebrovascular disease	41(10)
Laboratory data (mean±SD)	
White blood cell count (WBC; ×10^9/L)	7.9±2.6
Platelets (x10^9/L)	224±71
C reactive protein (mg/dl)	1.3±1.2
Hemoglobin (g/dl)	13.3±1.9
Fibrinogen (mg/dl)	413±119
Creatinine (mg/dl)	1.3±0.9
Medication n (%)	
Aspirin	416 (100)
Clopidogrel	416 (100)
Proton pump Inhibitors (PPI)	317 (76)
β blockers	309 (74)
Angiotensin converting enzyme inhibitors (ACE)	219 (53)
Statins	303 (73)
Calcium channel blockers (CCB)	80 (19)
PCI data	
Elective PCI	274 (66)
PCI due to an acute coronary syndrome (ACS)	140 (34)
NSTE-ACS	67 (16)
STEMI	73 (18)
Number of stents per patient	1.7±1
Total stent length	31.8±21.7
CYP2C19*2 carrier status n (%)	126 (30)
CYP2C19*17 carrier status n (%)	165 (40)
ABCB1 carrier status n (%)	323 (77)
PON1 carrier status n (%)	210 (50)

Data are reported as Mean ± standard deviation (SD), n (number of patients) or percentages; CAD: coronary artery disease; PCI: percutaneous coronary intervention; NSTE-ACS: non ST- elevation acute coronary syndrome, STEMI: ST- elevation myocardial infarction. ABCB1: gene encoding transmembrane transporter P-glycoprotein; PON1: paroxonase 1.

between isolated independent variables and a single dependent variable. Therefore, regression analysis alone is inadequate when examining the interplay between the independent variables and several dependent variables. The structural equation modelling is more effective and more appropriate for analyzing complex models. The major difference between these two approaches is the mulicollinearity (when predictor variables are highly correlated). Whereas in a structural equation modelling, mulicollinearity is necessary, in a regression analysis mulicollinearity is problematic.

For the development of score predicting HTPR variables were selected by structural equation modeling and by forward and backward logistic regression. All statistical calculations were

Table 2. Univariate logistic regression for prediction of high on treatment platelet reactivity (HTPR).

Variable	HTPR N = 81 (20%)	no HTPR N = 321 (80%)	Regression coefficient	P value	OR	95% confidence intervals	
Age (years)	63±12	64±12	−0.014	0.225	0.986	0.964	1.009
Gender (male) n (%)	58 (72)	249 (78)	0.454	0.139	1.574	0.862	2.873
Risk factors/past medical history n (%)							
Body mass index (BMI; mean±SD)	29±5.8	28±5.2	0.036	0.141	1.036	0.988	1.086
Hypertension	66 (83)	275 (869)	−0.210	0.559	0.810	0.400	1.641
Hyperlipidemia	60 (75)	248 (78)	−0.111	0.717	0.895	0.491	1.630
Smoking	46 (58)	174 (55)	0.128	0.650	1.137	0.653	1.979
Family history of CAD	21 (26)	105 (33)	−0.313	0.276	0.731	0.416	1.285
Diabetes mellitus	36 (44)	97 (30)	0.724	0.011	2.063	1.178	3.614
Peripheral arterial occlusive disease	9 (11)	45 (14)	−0.373	0.402	0.689	0.288	1.647
Cerebrovascular disease	7 (9)	34 (11)	0.114	0.812	1.121	0.437	2.875
Glomerular filtration rate (GFR: mean±SD)	78 (31)	85 (37)	0.006	0.137	1.006	0.998	1.014
Medications (%)							
Aspirin	81 (100)	321 (100)	−0.337	0.785	0.714	0.064	7.983
Clopidogrel	81 (100)	321 (100)	−41.805	0.999	0	0	0
Statins	63 (80)	257 (84)	−0.189	0.599	0.828	0.41	1.673
β blockers	65 (83)	256 (84)	−0.052	0.892	0.95	0.45	2.003
Proton pump inhibitors	68 (87)	246 (80)	0.357	0.354	1.429	0.672	3.04
Angiotensin converting enzyme inhibitors	54 (69)	210 (69)	−0.006	0.984	0.994	0.562	1.757
Calcium channel blockers	10 (13)	68 (22)	−0.719	0.06	0.487	0.231	1.03
PCI data							
PCI due to an acute coronary syndrome (ACS)	40 (50)	92 (29)	0.378	0.006	1.459	1.116	1.907
Number of stents per patient	1.86±1.27	1.69±0.98	0.204	0.085	1.226	0.972	1.547
Total stent length	33.7±24.7	31.1±20.9	0.005	0.36	1.005	0.994	1.016
Genetic data							
CYP2C19*17	24 (30)	135 (42)	−0.616	0.038	0.540	0.302	0.966
CYP2C19*2	33 (41)	90 (28)	0.477	0.070	1.611	0.929	2.796
ABCB1 C3435T	63 (77)	250 (77)	0.057	0.859	1.059	0.561	1.997
PON1 Q192R	40 (49)	160 (50)	−0.147	0.592	0.864	0.505	1.476

ACS: acute coronary syndrome; BMI: body mass index; GFR: glomerular filtration rate; CAD: coronary artery disease; CYP: cytochrome P450; ABCB1: gene encoding transmembrane transporter P-glycoprotein; PON1: paroxonase 1.

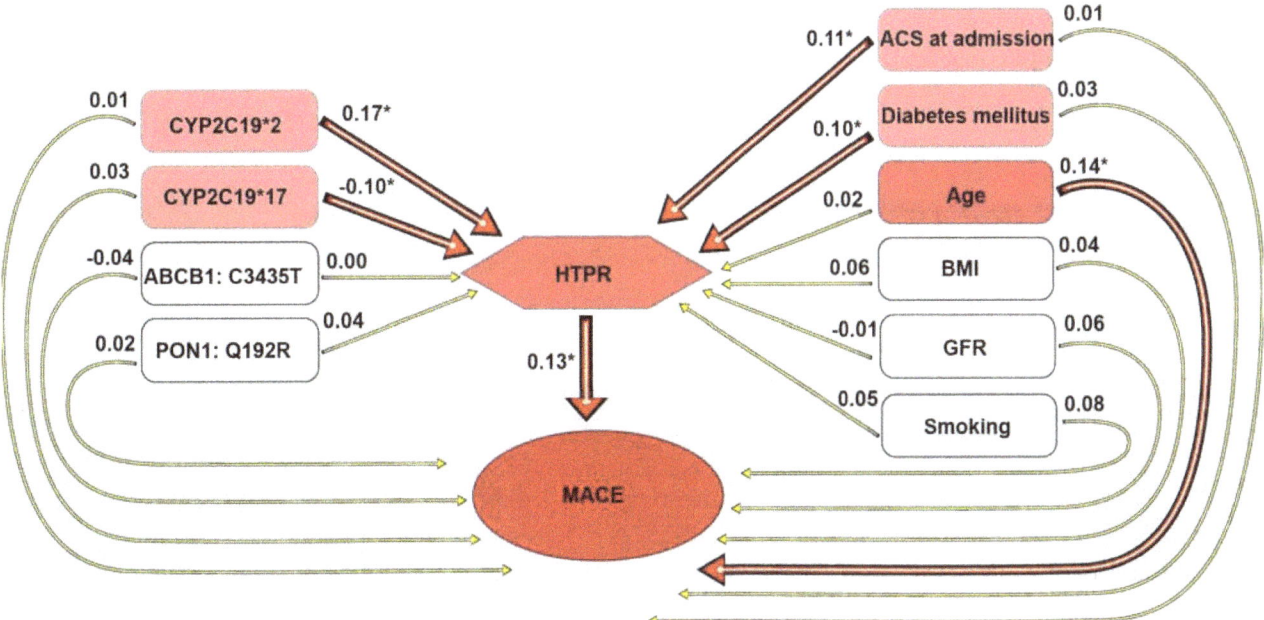

Figure 1. Path model of independent variables predicting high on treatment platelet reactivity (HTPR) and major adverse cardiac events (MACE: the composite of acute coronary syndrome, stent thrombosis and cardiac death). Paths from independent to dependent variables represent standardized estimates. *p<0.05; ACS: acute coronary syndrome; BMI: body mass index; GFR: glomerular filtration rate; CYP: cytochrome P450; ABCB1: gene encoding transmembrane transporter P-glycoprotein; PON1: paroxonase 1.

performed using commercially available statistical software (SPSS and AMOS, Version 21.0; Chicago).

Results

Patient Demographics

Patient demographics and co-medications are shown in Table 1. Two third of patients underwent non-emergent PCI and one third presented with an ACS on admission. Only five patients were lost to follow up during twelve months of follow-up.

Genotype distribution

Thirty percent of patients were *CYP2C19*2* carriers (27.6% heterozygote and 2.6% homozygote), 40% were *CYP2C19*17* carriers (33.9% heterozygote and 5.8% homozygote), 78% had an ABCB1 C3435T genotype (55.6% heterozygote and 22.0% homozygote) and 50% were carriers of PON1 Q192R allele (44.2% heterozygote and 6.3% homozygote; Table 2).

Univariate influence of baseline characteristics and genetic polymorphisms on high on treatment platelet reactivity (HTPR)

Twenty percent of patients presented with a HTPR phenotype. Diabetes mellitus (OR: 2.1; 95%CI: 1.2–3.6; p = 0.011), ACS (OR: 1.5; 95%CI: 1.2–1.9; p = 0.006) and *CYP2C19*17* genotype (OR: 0.54; 95%CI: 0.30-0-97; p = 0.038) emerged as HTPR predictors (Table 2). *CYP2C19*2* genotype predicted HTPR only at 7% significance level (OR: 1.6; 95%CI: 0.93–2.80; p = 0.07; Table 2). No other variables differed between groups.

Suggested path model explaining associations between genetic and clinical variables

Genetic and clinical variables were included into the model (Figure 1). The path model presented very good fit (Root Mean

Square Error of Approximation = 0.000, Comparative Fit Index = 1.000). The paths from genetic polymorphisms of *CYP2C19*2* and *17* (hetero or homozygote) as well as from clinical characteristics as ACS on admission and diabetes mellitus were independent predictors of HTPR (path coefficients: 0.17, -0.10, 0.11 and 0.10. respectively; p<0.05 for all; Figure 1; Table 2 and 3). In contrast, polymorphisms of ABCB1 or PON1 genes or other clinical characteristics were not depicted as independent predictors of HTPR in the model. From all included variables (genetic and clinical), only HTPR and age were independent predictors of MACE (path coefficient: 0.14 and 0.13, respectively; p<0.05; Figure 2; Table 2 and 3).

No other gene environment interactions were found.

Development of a risk score

By using of the following four factors: diabetes mellitus, ACS, *CYP2C19*2* and *CYP2C19*17* a cumulative score was formed and applied on the total patient cohort to analyze its predictive value for HTPR. To account for the unequal influence of score variables, we allocated a weighing factor of -1 to 2 to each of the variables depending on the OR (-1 = OR<0; 1 = OR>1 but <2; 2 = OR>2). In detail, **D**iabetes was weighed by factor 2, **A**CS by factor 1, **C**YP2C19*2 by factor 1 and **C**YP2C19*17 by factor -1 (DACC score). Thus, a score ranging from -1 to 4 was developed. Hereby, we found an increasing incidence of HTPR by cumulative number of score variables (Figure 2). In logistic regression analysis the risk of having HTPR was calculated with an OR of 3.8 (95%CI: 3.1–6.8, p<0.001) for a score level of ≥1 compared with a score of <1 (Figure 2).

Survival analysis

The composite of major adverse cardiac events (MACE: stent thrombosis, ACS and cardiac death) occurred in 52 patients (12.5%). Cox multivariate adjusted model confirmed that HTPR

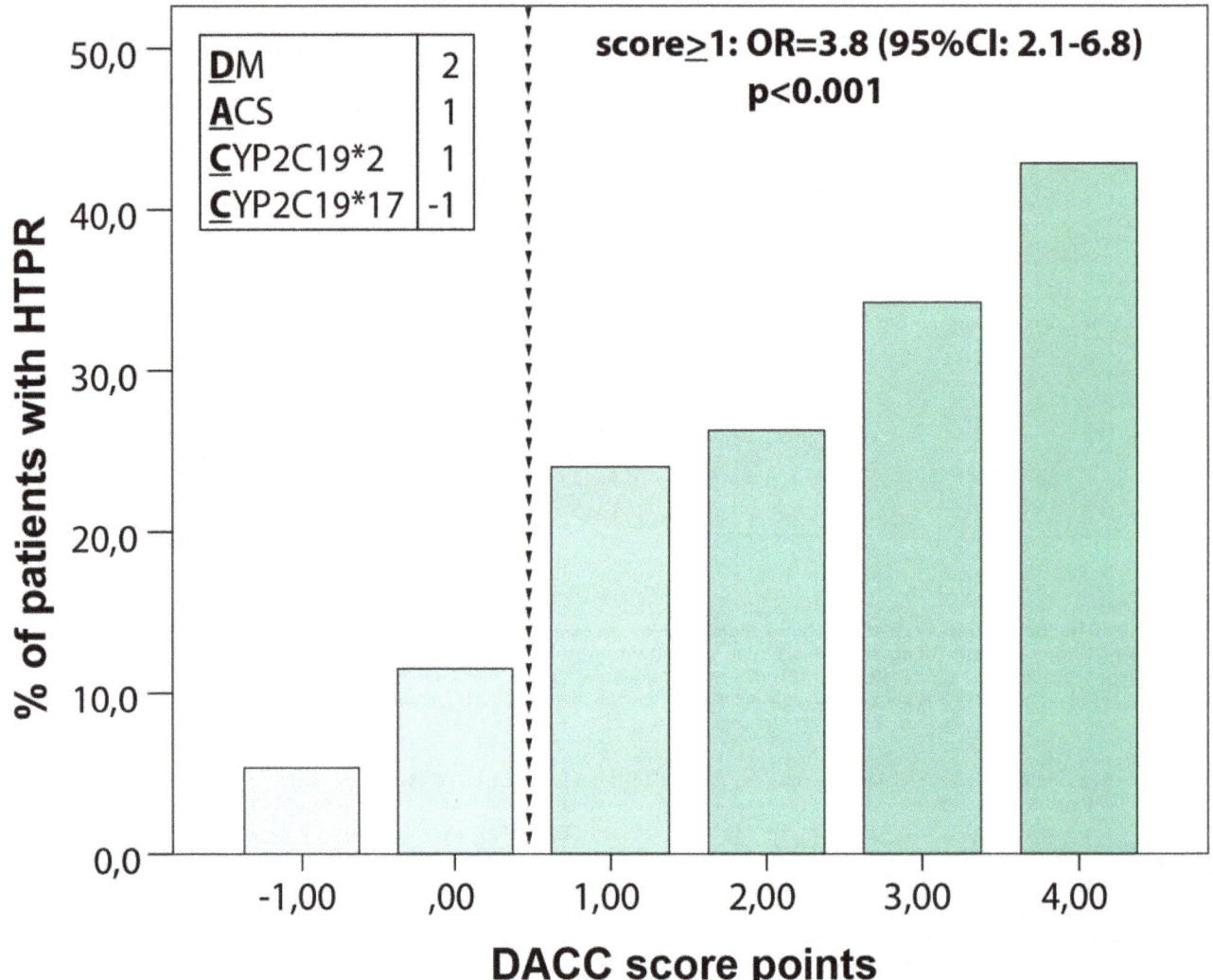

Figure 2. Incidence of increased % of patients with high on treatment platelet reactivity (HTPR) according to cumulative number of score variables. ACS: acute coronary syndrome; DM: diabetes mellitus; CYP: cytochrome P450.

and age independently predicted MACE: patients with HTPR were at 2-fold higher risk (95%CI: 1.1–3.6; p = 0.027; Table 4), whereas patients with ≥75 years of age had a 2.3-fold higher risk (95%CI: 1.3–4.4; p = 0.008; Table 4). A significant risk increase was observed after stratification of patients according to the HTPR and age: those with HTPR and age ≥75 years suffered the highest incidence of MACE: 27% during 12-month follow up (Figure 3). The lowest MACE rate occurred in patients younger than 75 years of age and without HTPR (9%; p = 0.004; Figure 3).

Adapted path model

Based on the results of the DACC score and survival analyses, we adapted the previous path model. Whereas the DACC score explained 7.0% in the variance of HTPR (p<0.001; Figure 4), HTPR and age ≥75 years explained 5.6% in the variance of MACE p = 0.004, p = 0.003; respectively; Figure 4). Although the DACC score predicted HTPR, it did not predict MACE (Figure 4).

To verify the results of the path analysis, we performed a survival analysis looking at the event rates for each DACC score and there was no statistical difference. This confirms the results of

the path analysis, which indicates that while DACC score predicts HTPR it does not predict MACE.

Discussion

The central findings of this paper investigating a concurrent impact of clinical and genetic variables on HTPR and clinical outcome are as following:

i)   Two clinical characteristics (ACS and diabetes mellitus) and two genetic variants (*CYP2C19*2* and *CYP2C19*17*) independently predicted HTPR but not MACE.

ii) By use of those four variables a score can be built, which allows estimating the probability of HTPR.

iii) While MACE was independently predicted by HTPR and age, the coexistence of HTPR and age ≥75 years emerged as the strongest predictor of MACE.

The findings of our study are interesting, since they pointed out for the first time the pathways of different variables leading to adverse outcomes. The first segment in the pathway leading to HTPR was built upon two genetic variants and two clinical

Table 3. Path modelling results.

dependent variable		path precursor	standardized estimate/path coefficient	standard error	P value
HTPR	<---	CYP2C19*2	0.165	2.814	0.001
	<---	CYP2C19*17	−0.103	2.643	0.035
	<---	ABCB1 C3435T	−0.010	3.092	0.838
	<---	PON1 Q192R	0.039	2.577	0.417
	<---	ACS at admission	0.109	1.305	0.025
	<---	Diabetes mellitus	0.096	2.755	0.048
	<---	BMI	0.062	0.244	0.207
	<---	GFR	−0.009	2.384	0.850
	<---	Smoking	0.047	2.612	0.333
	<---	Age	0.023	0.104	0.638
MACE	<---	CYP2C19*2	0.012	0.037	0.803
	<---	CYP2C19*17	0.034	0.034	0.497
	<---	ABCB1 C3435T	−0.040	0.040	0.418
	<---	PON1 Q192R	0.019	0.033	0.694
	<---	ACS at admission	0.014	0.036	0.770
	<---	Diabetes mellitus	0.033	0.017	0.508
	<---	BMI	0.041	0.003	0.409
	<---	GFR	0.061	0.031	0.224
	<---	Smoking	0.080	0.034	0.104
	<---	Age	0.141	0.001	0.004
	<---	HTPR	0.126	0.001	0.016

ACS: acute coronary syndrome; BMI: body mass index; GFR: glomerular filtration rate; CYP: cytochrome P450; ABCB1: gene encoding transmembrane transporter P-glycoprotein; PON1: paroxonase 1; HTPR: high on treatment platelet reactivity; MACE: major adverse cardiac events (MACE: the composite of acute coronary syndrome, stent thrombosis and cardiac death).

variables. The *CYP2C19*2* and *17* affect HTPR in different directions. As *CYP2C19*2* reduces clopidogrel activation, it is a positive predictor of HTPR. In contrast, *CYP2C19*17* which intensifies activation of clopidogrel, correlates negatively with HTPR. PON1 and ABCB1 polymorphism did not have an impact on HTPR. Therefore, our observation is in line with previous reports [30–33]. From several clinical variables reported to be associated with clopidogrel, only ACS and diabetes mellitus independently and positively predicted HTPR in this model. Both variables are factors known to be associated with HTPR [11,34].

The suggested pathway examined with structural equation modelling might give a satisfactory explanation why many discrepancies exist in regard to whether or not genetic factors might predict clinical outcome. The association between *CYP2C19*2* and adverse cardiovascular events postulated in some studies [12,14–18], has not been confirmed in others [24,35,36]. Our model indicates that whereas platelet function testing identifies patients with HTPR, pharmacogenomic testing provides only a weak risk marker for HTPR. Platelet function testing provides therefore more comprehensive information than genotyping, as it reflects the influence of intrinsic (co-morbidities, drug-drug interactions) and genetic factors on the response to antiplatelet drugs. Nevertheless, in patients undergoing elective PCI (RAPID GENE study) or presenting with STEMI (RAPID STEMI study) pharmacogenomic testing with a subsequent use of prasugrel has been shown to eliminate HTPR [37,38]. It is, however, still unknown whether pharmacogenomic approach will improve patient's outcome. Hopefully, undergoing trials as GIANT (NCT01134380) or TAILOR-PCI (NCT01134380) will

deliver the missing answer to the above stated question. Importantly, it is still a matter of debate to define those patient cohorts, in whom platelet function testing or pharmacogenomics testing would be of clinical importance.

The second segment in our path model leading to MACE consisted of HTPR and age. Moreover, the coexistence of HTPR and age ≥75 years was a good risk stratifier for ischemic adverse events. The association between HTPR and adverse ischemic events is well characterized [2–8]. Higher age seems to be a universal clinical marker of risk. Age as a cofactor to HTPR, was less well described. Interestingly, one would presume that more pronounced platelet inhibition would be necessary in older patients. Surprisingly, this assumption could not be confirmed in the TRITON TIMI-38 study, showing that prasugrel was not superior to clopidogrel in older patient population but caused more bleeding events [39]. The latter aspect might be due to the fact that age has been identified as a baseline risk factor associated with both bleeding and ischemic events [40].

Accordingly, the combination of HTPR and age ≥75 years predicted MACE in 27% of cases, but explained only 5.6% of the variability in the occurrence of MACE during 1 year of follow-up. Nevertheless, it is unknown how our score compares with the known models of prediction of MACE based on traditional cardiovascular risk factors, as to our knowledge, the established scores did not report the R2 value.

Our model indicates that the two genetic variants *CYP2C19*2* and *17* as well as the two clinical variables ACS and diabetes mellitus explain only 7% of the variability in platelet inhibition by clopidogrel. Similarly, previous reports showed that the

Table 4. Multiple Cox regression model for prediction major adverse cardiac events (MACE: the composite of acute coronary syndrome, stent thrombosis and cardiac death).

	Regression coefficient	P value	OR	95% confidence intervals	
HTPR	0.677	0.027	1.968	1.078	3.592
Age	0.845	0.008	2.38	1.248	4.345

HTPR: high on treatment platelet reactivity.

*CYP2C19*2* carrier status accounted only for 5–12% of the variability in the platelet response to clopidogrel [18,41]. Thus, available data suggest that other variables like unknown genetic variants or other not identified factors contribute to this phenomenon.

Based on the results of the multivariate logistic regression and the structural equation modelling we developed a DACC score for prediction of HTPR. Interestingly, only four variables: two genetic variants and two clinical variables were necessary, to build the score. What was even more interesting, one point in the score was already satisfactory for prediction of HTPR. Three to four points in the DACC score predicted HTPR with a probability of 35–40%. This can be directly interpolated to the clinical practice: even without genetic testing it is probable by a factor 5 that a diabetic patient presenting with an ACS (3 score points) will have a HTPR. If this is the case, and if the patient is older than 75 years

of age, the probability to develop MACE increases by factor 3 as compared to a younger patient without HTPR. Based on this example, the score might be useful in the clinical practice. Noteworthy, another score for prediction of HTPR has been already proposed. The weighted PREDICT score includes ACS, diabetes mellitus, left ventricular function, renal failure, age and *CYP2C19*2* genotype, ranging a maximum of 165 points [42]. The disadvantage of the PREDICT score might be the limited availability of left ventricular function tests and a somehow challenging 2-step calculation algorithm with a requirement of a nomogram for estimation of HTPR probability. Nevertheless, both scores might offer a complementary information. Prospective studies would be required to test the usefulness of the scores in order to improve the management of antiplatelet agents and the net clinical outcome in the routine use.

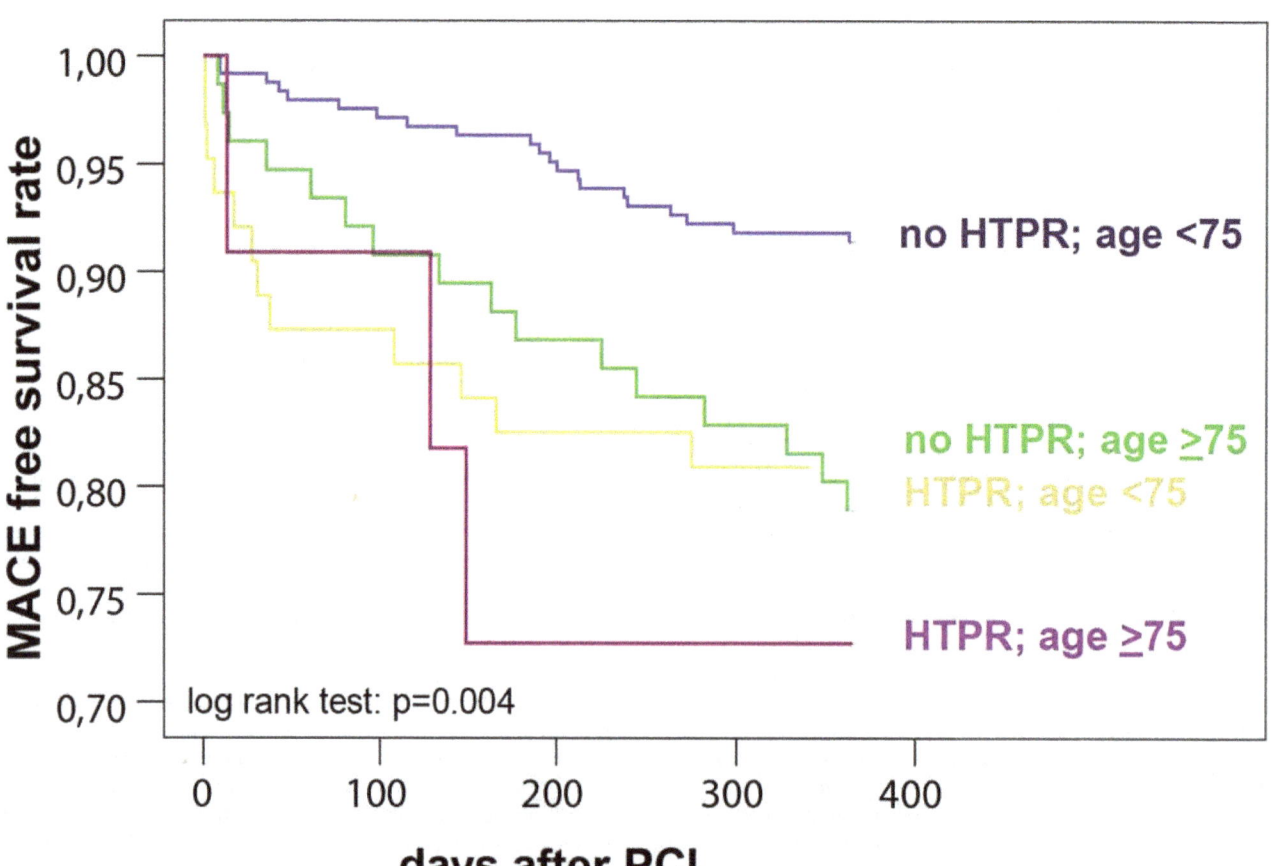

Figure 3. Survival analysis according to the high on treatment platelet reactivity (HTPR) and age. MACE: major adverse cardiac events: the composite of acute coronary syndrome, stent thrombosis and cardiac death; PCI: percutaneous coronary intervention.

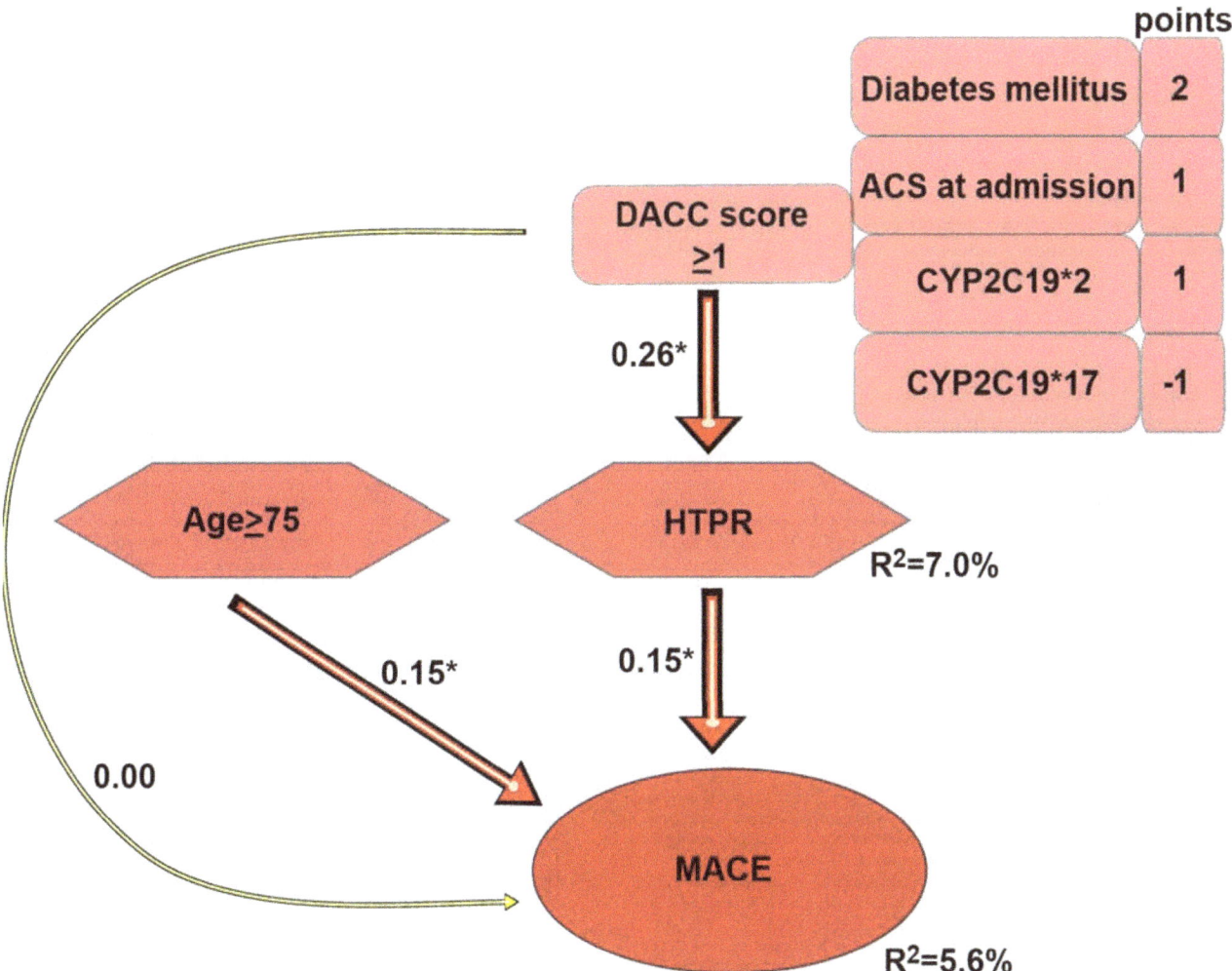

Figure 4. Adapted path model including the DACC score as an independent variable predicting high on treatment platelet reactivity (HTPR); Age and HTPR as independent predictors of major adverse cardiac events (MACE: the composite of acute coronary syndrome, stent thrombosis and cardiac death). Paths from independent to dependent variables represent standardized estimates. *p<0.05; ACS: acute coronary syndrome; CYP: cytochrome P450.

Until now, only geno- and phenotyping but not scoring systems were used to personalize the antiplatelet therapy. Several studies have demonstrated that HTPR can be reduced with higher loading or maintenance doses of clopidogrel, or by switching to prasugrel or ticagrelor. Administration of a 150 mg maintenance dose of clopidogrel or up to four repeated loading doses of clopidogrel resulted in more intense inhibition of platelet aggregation in a major subset of patients but not in all [9,43,44]. Novel P2Y$_{12}$ receptor inhibitors such as prasugrel or ticagrelor also achieved a stronger platelet inhibition in patients with HTPR under clopidogrel [9,45,46]. With regard to genotype-based personalized treatment, increased loading doses of clopidogrel up to 900 mg or maintenance doses up to 300 mg have been show to overcome clopidogrel non-responsiveness in heterozygous carriers of *CYP2C19*2* allele but not in homozygous carriers [47,48]. Although more potent platelet inhibitors prasugrel and ticagrelor became available in the ACS setting, our findings might still be important. Firstly, because clopidogrel is still the only authorized agent in patients undergoing elective PCI. Secondly, clopidogrel is widely used in ACS patients in some countries due to an economic impact since clopidogrel generics have entered into the market. Furthermore, recent studies in patients suffering from an ACS suggest that HTPR also occurs in patients treated with prasugrel or ticagrelor, especially in the early phase of treatment [49].

Limitations

We are aware of the fact that the antiplatelet drug response is a multifactorial phenomenon, which cannot be solely explained by identified risk factors, because baseline differences in platelet aggregation are even observed in patients naive to antiplatelet treatment. As a further limitation, additional procedural factors during coronary intervention that might play an important role (e.g. type of lesion or procedure al time) or further genetic variants (e.g. ITGB3 encoding the integrin Beta3 of the GpIIb/IIIa receptor, P2Y$_{12}$ receptor or insulin receptor substrate IRS-1) were not considered in our study. Moreover, due to the limited sample size, the study would not have enough power to include into the model and score the differentiation between homo- and hetero-zygotes of the *CYP2C19*2* or *17** polymorphisms or to test the predictors of bleeding events. Most importantly, the absence of a validation cohort makes the generalizability of the DACC score difficult to predict.

Conclusion

Our study suggests a pathway, which might explain the association between the genetic and clinical variables influencing the phenotype of response to clopidogrel. Furthermore, the proposed model also shows indirect and direct impact of several variables on clinical outcome: ACS, diabetes mellitus, CYP2C19*2 and CYP2C19*17 genetic variants independently

predicted HTPR. In turn, age ≥75 years and HTPR were the strongest predictors of MACE. Further studies are needed to investigate the usefulness of our finding.

Author Contributions

Conceived and designed the experiments: JSM BJ IL TN GM. Performed the experiments: JSM KL. Analyzed the data: JSM. Contributed reagents/materials/analysis tools: KL TG JSM MK. Wrote the paper: JSM BJ TN IL JK MK TG KL GM.

References

1. Siller-Matula JM, Trenk D, Schror K, Gawaz M, Kristensen SD, et al. (2013) Response Variability to P2Y12 Receptor Inhibitors: Expectations and Reality. JACC Cardiovasc Interv 6: 1111–1128.
2. Geisler T, Zurn C, Simonenko R, Rapin M, Kraibooj H, et al. (2010) Early but not late stent thrombosis is influenced by residual platelet aggregation in patients undergoing coronary interventions. Eur Heart J 31: 59–66.
3. Gurbel PA, Erlinge D, Ohman EM, Neely B, Neely M, et al. (2012) Platelet function during extended prasugrel and clopidogrel therapy for patients with ACS treated without revascularization: the TRILOGY ACS platelet function substudy. Jama 308: 1785–1794.
4. Buonamici P, Marcucci R, Migliorini A, Gensini GF, Santini A, et al. (2007) Impact of platelet reactivity after clopidogrel administration on drug-eluting stent thrombosis. J Am Coll Cardiol 49: 2312–2317.
5. Gori AM, Marcucci R, Migliorini A, Valenti R, Moschi G, et al. (2008) Incidence and clinical impact of dual nonresponsiveness to aspirin and clopidogrel in patients with drug-eluting stents. J Am Coll Cardiol 52: 734–739.
6. Gurbel PA, Bliden KP, Hayes KM, Yoho JA, Herzog WR, et al. (2005) The relation of dosing to clopidogrel responsiveness and the incidence of high post-treatment platelet aggregation in patients undergoing coronary stenting. J Am Coll Cardiol 45: 1392–1396.
7. Cuisset T, Frere C, Quilici J, Barbou F, Morange PE, et al. (2006) High post-treatment platelet reactivity identified low-responders to dual antiplatelet therapy at increased risk of recurrent cardiovascular events after stenting for acute coronary syndrome. J Thromb Haemost 4: 542–549.
8. Siller-Matula JM, Christ G, Lang IM, Delle-Karth G, Huber K, et al. (2010) Multiple Electrode Aggregometry predicts stent thrombosis better than the VASP assay. J Thromb Haemost 8: 351–359.
9. Siller-Matula JM, Francesconi M, Dechant C, Jilma B, Maurer G, et al. (2013) Personalized antiplatelet treatment after percutaneous coronary intervention: the MADONNA study. Int J Cardiol 167: 2018–2023.
10. Angiolillo DJ (2009) Antiplatelet therapy in diabetes: efficacy and limitations of current treatment strategies and future directions. Diabetes Care 32: 531–540.
11. Geisler T, Grass D, Bigalke B, Stellos K, Drosch T, et al. (2008) The Residual Platelet Aggregation after Deployment of Intracoronary Stent (PREDICT) score. J Thromb Haemost 6: 54–61.
12. Cayla G, Hulot JS, O'Connor SA, Pathak A, Scott SA, et al. (2011) Clinical, angiographic, and genetic factors associated with early coronary stent thrombosis. Jama 306: 1765–1774.
13. Neubauer H, Kaiser AF, Endres HG, Kruger JC, Engelhardt A, et al. (2011) Tailored antiplatelet therapy can overcome clopidogrel and aspirin resistance—the BOchum CLopidogrel and Aspirin Plan (BOCLA-Plan) to improve antiplatelet therapy. BMC Med 9: 3.
14. Hulot JS, Collet JP, Cayla G, Silvain J, Allanic F, et al. (2011) CYP2C19 but not PON1 genetic variants influence clopidogrel pharmacokinetics, pharmacodynamics, and clinical efficacy in post-myocardial infarction patients. Circ Cardiovasc Interv 4: 422–428.
15. Giusti B, Gori AM, Marcucci R, Saracini C, Sestini I, et al. (2009) Relation of cytochrome P450 2C19 loss-of-function polymorphism to occurrence of drug-eluting coronary stent thrombosis. Am J Cardiol 103: 806–811.
16. Collet JP, Hulot JS, Pena A, Villard E, Esteve JB, et al. (2009) Cytochrome P450 2C19 polymorphism in young patients treated with clopidogrel after myocardial infarction: a cohort study. Lancet 373: 309–317.
17. Mega JL, Close SL, Wiviott SD, Shen L, Hockett RD, et al. (2009) Cytochrome p-450 polymorphisms and response to clopidogrel. N Engl J Med 360: 354–362.
18. Shuldiner AR, O'Connell JR, Bliden KP, Gandhi A, Ryan K, et al. (2009) Association of cytochrome P450 2C19 genotype with the antiplatelet effect and clinical efficacy of clopidogrel therapy. Jama 302: 849–857.
19. Kubica A, Kozinski M, Grzesk G, Fabiszak T, Navarese EP, et al. (2011) Genetic determinants of platelet response to clopidogrel. J Thromb Thrombolysis 32: 459–466.
20. Bouman HJ, Schomig E, van Werkum JW, Velder J, Hackeng CM, et al. (2011) Paraoxonase-1 is a major determinant of clopidogrel efficacy. Nat Med 17: 110–116.
21. Sibbing D, Koch W, Massberg S, Byrne RA, Mehilli J, et al. (2011) No association of paraoxonase-1 Q192R genotypes with platelet response to clopidogrel and risk of stent thrombosis after coronary stenting. Eur Heart J 32: 1605–1613.
22. Trenk D, Hochholzer W, Fromm MF, Zolk O, Valina CM, et al. (2011) Paraoxonase-1 Q192R polymorphism and antiplatelet effects of clopidogrel in patients undergoing elective coronary stent placement. Circ Cardiovasc Genet 4: 429–436.
23. Simon T, Steg PG, Becquemont L, Verstuyft C, Kotti S, et al. (2011) Effect of paraoxonase-1 polymorphism on clinical outcomes in patients treated with clopidogrel after an acute myocardial infarction. Clin Pharmacol Ther 90: 561–567.
24. Siller-Matula JM, Delle-Karth G, Lang IM, Neunteufl T, Kozinski M, et al. (2012) Phenotyping vs. genotyping for prediction of clopidogrel efficacy and safety: the PEGASUS-PCI study. J Thromb Haemost 10: 529–542.
25. Kozinski M, Bielis L, Wisniewska-Szmyt J, Boinska J, Stolarek W, et al. (2011) Diurnal variation in platelet inhibition by clopidogrel. Platelets 22: 579–587.
26. Kasprzak M, Kozinski M, Bielis L, Boinska J, Plazuk W, et al. (2009) Pantoprazole may enhance antiplatelet effect of enteric-coated aspirin in patients with acute coronary syndrome. Cardiol J 16: 535–544.
27. Siller-Matula JM, Miller I, Gemeiner M, Plasenzotti R, Bayer G, et al. (2012) Continuous thrombin infusion leads to a bleeding phenotype in sheep. Thromb Res 130: 226–236.
28. Cutlip DE, Windecker S, Mehran R, Boam A, Cohen DJ, et al. (2007) Clinical end points in coronary stent trials: a case for standardized definitions. Circulation 115: 2344–2351.
29. Parodi G, Marcucci R, Valenti R, Gori AM, Migliorini A, et al. (2011) High residual platelet reactivity after clopidogrel loading and long-term cardiovascular events among patients with acute coronary syndromes undergoing PCI. JAMA 306: 1215–1223.
30. Campo G, Parrinello G, Ferraresi P, Lunghi B, Tebaldi M, et al. (2011) Prospective evaluation of on-clopidogrel platelet reactivity over time in patients treated with percutaneous coronary intervention relationship with gene polymorphisms and clinical outcome. J Am Coll Cardiol 57: 2474–2483.
31. Sibbing D, Koch W, Gebhard D, Schuster T, Braun S, et al. (2010) Cytochrome 2C19*17 allelic variant, platelet aggregation, bleeding events, and stent thrombosis in clopidogrel-treated patients with coronary stent placement. Circulation 121: 512–518.
32. Jeong YH, Tantry US, Kim IS, Koh JS, Kwon TJ, et al. (2011) Effect of CYP2C19*2 and *3 loss-of-function alleles on platelet reactivity and adverse clinical events in East Asian acute myocardial infarction survivors treated with clopidogrel and aspirin. Circ Cardiovasc Interv 4: 585–594.
33. Campo G, Ferraresi P, Marchesini J, Bernardi F, Valgimigli M (2011) Relationship between paraoxonase Q192R gene polymorphism and on-clopidogrel platelet reactivity over time in patients treated with percutaneous coronary intervention. J Thromb Haemost 9: 2106–2108.
34. Siller-Matula JM, Delle-Karth G, Christ G, Neunteufl T, Maurer G, et al. (2013) Dual non-responsiveness to antiplatelet treatment is a stronger predictor of cardiac adverse events than isolated non-responsiveness to clopidogrel or aspirin. Int J Cardiol 167: 430–435.
35. Wallentin L, James S, Storey RF, Armstrong M, Barratt BJ, et al. (2010) Effect of CYP2C19 and ABCB1 single nucleotide polymorphisms on outcomes of treatment with ticagrelor versus clopidogrel for acute coronary syndromes: a genetic substudy of the PLATO trial. Lancet 376: 1320–1328.
36. Bhatt DL, Pare G, Eikelboom JW, Simonsen KL, Emison ES, et al. (2012) The relationship between CYP2C19 polymorphisms and ischaemic and bleeding outcomes in stable outpatients: the CHARISMA genetics study. Eur Heart J.
37. Roberts JD, Wells GA, Le May MR, Labinaz M, Glover C, et al. (2012) Point-of-care genetic testing for personalisation of antiplatelet treatment (RAPID GENE): a prospective, randomised, proof-of-concept trial. Lancet.
38. So DYF, Wells G, McPherson R, Labinaz M, Glover C, et al. (2013) A Pharmacogenomic approach to antiplatelet therapy in STEMI patients: reassessment of anti-platelet therapy using an individualized strategy in patents with ST-elevation myocardial infarction (The RAPID STEMI study). J Am Coll Cardiol 61: doi:10.1016/S0735-1097(1013)60006-60006.
39. Wiviott SD, Braunwald E, McCabe CH, Montalescot G, Ruzyllo W, et al. (2007) Prasugrel versus clopidogrel in patients with acute coronary syndromes. N Engl J Med 357: 2001–2015.

40. Siller-Matula JM (2012) Hemorrhagic complications associated with aspirin: an underestimated hazard in clinical practice? Jama 307: 2318–2320.

41. Hochholzer W, Trenk D, Fromm MF, Valina CM, Stratz C, et al. (2010) Impact of cytochrome P450 2C19 loss-of-function polymorphism and of major demographic characteristics on residual platelet function after loading and maintenance treatment with clopidogrel in patients undergoing elective coronary stent placement. J Am Coll Cardiol 55: 2427–2434.

42. Geisler T, Schaeffeler E, Dippon J, Winter S, Buse V, et al. (2008) CYP2C19 and nongenetic factors predict poor responsiveness to clopidogrel loading dose after coronary stent implantation. Pharmacogenomics 9: 1251–1259.

43. Angiolillo DJ, Bernardo E, Sabate M, Jimenez-Quevedo P, Costa MA, et al. (2007) Impact of platelet reactivity on cardiovascular outcomes in patients with type 2 diabetes mellitus and coronary artery disease. J Am Coll Cardiol 50: 1541–1547.

44. von Beckerath N, Kastrati A, Wieczorek A, Pogatsa-Murray G, Sibbing D, et al. (2007) A double-blind, randomized study on platelet aggregation in patients treated with a daily dose of 150 or 75 mg of clopidogrel for 30 days. Eur Heart J 28: 1814–1819.

45. Kozinski M, Obonska K, Stankowska K, Navarese EP, Fabiszak T, et al. (2014) Prasugrel overcomes high on-clopidogrel platelet reactivity in the acute phase of acute coronary syndrome and maintains its antiplatelet potency at 30-day follow-up. Cardiol J doi: 10.5603/CJ.a2014.0026.: in press.

46. Storey RF, Bliden KP, Ecob R, Karunakaran A, Butler K, et al. (2011) Earlier recovery of platelet function after discontinuation of treatment with ticagrelor compared with clopidogrel in patients with high antiplatelet responses. J Thromb Haemost 9: 1730–1737.

47. Mega JL, Hochholzer W, Frelinger AL, 3rd, Kluk MJ, Angiolillo DJ, et al. (2011) Dosing clopidogrel based on CYP2C19 genotype and the effect on platelet reactivity in patients with stable cardiovascular disease. Jama 306: 2221–2228.

48. Collet JP, Hulot JS, Anzaha G, Pena A, Chastre T, et al. (2011) High doses of clopidogrel to overcome genetic resistance: the randomized crossover CLOVIS-2 (Clopidogrel and Response Variability Investigation Study 2). JACC Cardiovasc Interv 4: 392–402.

49. Alexopoulos D, Xanthopoulou I, Gkizas V, Kassimis G, Theodoropoulos KC, et al. (2012) Randomized Assessment of Ticagrelor Versus Prasugrel Antiplatelet Effects in Patients with ST-Segment-Elevation Myocardial Infarction. Circ Cardiovasc Interv 5: 797–804.

5

The Impact of Endothelial Progenitor Cells on Restenosis after Percutaneous Angioplasty of Hemodialysis Vascular Access

Chih-Cheng Wu[1,5,8], **Po-Hsun Huang**[2,6,7,8,9]*, **Chao-Lun Lai**[1,5], **Hsin-Bang Leu**[1,4,9], **Jaw-Wen Chen**[2,3,9,10], **Shing-Jong Lin**[2,3,6,7,8,9]

1 Cardiovascular center, National Taiwan University Hospital, Hsinchu Branch, Hsinchu, Taiwan, 2 Division of Cardiology, Taipei Veterans General Hospital, Taipei, Taiwan, 3 Department of Medical Research and Education, Taipei Veterans General Hospital, Taipei, Taiwan, 4 Healthcare and Management Center, Taipei Veterans General Hospital, Taipei, Taiwan, 5 School of Medicine, National Taiwan University, Taipei, Taiwan, 6 Department of Medicine, National Yang-Ming University, Taipei, Taiwan, 7 Institute of Clinical Medicine, National Yang-Ming University, Taipei, Taiwan, 8 School of Medicine, National Yang-Ming University, Taipei, Taiwan, 9 Cardiovascular Research Center, National Yang-Ming University, Taipei, Taiwan, 10 Institute and Department of Pharmacology, National Yang-Ming University, Taipei, Taiwan

Abstract

Objective: We prospectively investigate the relation between baseline circulating endothelial progenitor cells and the subsequent development of restenosis after angioplasty of hemodialysis vascular access.

Background: Effect of angioplasty for hemodialysis vascular access is greatly attenuated by early and frequent restenosis. Circulating endothelial progenitor cells (EPCs) play a key role in vascular repair but are deficient in hemodialysis patients.

Method: After excluding 14 patients due to arterial stenosis, central vein stenosis, and failed angioplasty, 130 patients undergoing angioplasty for dysfunctional vascular access were prospectively enrolled. Flow cytometry with quantification of EPC markers (defined as $CD34^+$, $CD34^+KDR^+$, $CD34^+KDR^+CD133^+$) in peripheral blood immediately before angioplasty procedures was used to assess circulating EPC numbers. Patients were followed clinically for up to one year after angioplasty.

Results: During the one-year follow-up, 95 patients (73%) received interventions for recurrent access dysfunction. Patients in the lower tertile of $CD34^+KDR^+$ cell count had the highest restenosis rates (46%) at three month (early restenosis), compared with patients in the medium and upper tertiles of $CD34^+KDR^+$ cell count (27% and 12% respectively, p = 0.002). Patients in the lower tertile of $CD34^+KDR^+$ cell count received more re-interventions during one year. Patients with early restenosis had impaired EPC adhesive function and increased senescence and apoptosis. In multivariate analysis, the $CD34^+KDR^+$ and $CD34^+KDR^+CD133^+$ cell counts were independent predictors of target-lesion early restenosis.

Conclusion: Our results suggest that the deficiency of circulating EPCs is associated with early and frequent restenosis after angioplasty of hemodialysis vascular access.

Editor: Alberico Catapano, University of Milan, Italy

Funding: This study was supported by grants from the National Taiwan University Hospital, Hsinchu Branch (HCH100-4, HCH101-13), and the UST-UCSD International Centre of Excellence in Advanced Bio-engineering NSC-100-2911-I-009-101-A2. The funders had no role in study design, data collection and analysis, decision to publish, or preparation of the manuscript.

Competing Interests: The authors have declared that no competing interests exist.

* Email: huangbs@vghtpe.gov.tw

Introduction

A functioning vascular access greatly influences the survival and quality of life of patients undergoing hemodialysis. Vascular accesses are subject to failure and the underlying pathology is usually a stenosis due to venous intimal hyperplasia. [1] Endovascular interventions are useful in restoring the function of vascular access. [2] Nonetheless, their benefits are attenuated by a high restenosis rate, far more aggressive than that of arterial lesions in non-uremic patients. Physiological and anatomical differences between arteries and veins, continuous hemodynamic stress, repeated puncture, uremia and endothelial dysfunction have all

been proposed as possible causes. [1] However, in all patients, it is not precisely known how much the listed factors contribute to the high restenosis rates.

Maintenance of the integrity and function of the endothelium has been shown to play a pivotal role in the prevention of restenosis after angioplasty. [3] Accumulating evidence suggests that circulating endothelial progenitor cells (EPCs) incorporate into sites of endothelial denudation. [4] The circulating EPCs reflect not only repair capacity but also the health of the endothelium. [5] Clinical studies have shown that circulating EPC numbers are decreased and associated with vascular events in hemodialysis patients. [6,7] However, limited data are available about the role of EPCs for venous intimal hyperplasia in hemodialysis patients.

Accordingly, we conducted this prospective study to evaluate the impact of circulating EPC number and function on the outcome of vascular access.

Methods

Ethical statements

The study was based on the Declaration of Helsinki (edition 6, revised 2000). Written informed consent was obtained from all study participants, and the study was approved by the Institutional Review Board of our hospital (Hsinchu General Hospital Institutional Review Board, No. HCGH99G005 and National Taiwan University Hospital Hsinchu Branch Institutional Review Board, No. HCGH100G003).

Study participants

From January 2010 to July 2011, a series of patients with dysfunctional hemodialysis vascular access scheduled for percutaneous intervention were prospectively enrolled. Patients were referred based on one or more of the following criteria: clinical signs suggesting fistula dysfunction, reduction of flow rate and increased venous pressure during dialysis. Participants had to have received regular dialysis treatment for at least 6 months without clinical evidence of acute or chronic inflammation, recent myocardial infarction, unstable angina, or circulatory congestion. According to the same criteria, 26 patients who had normal functioning vascular access for at least two years were invited as the uremic control group. Another 30 non-uremic patients who received cardiac catheterization examination with patent coronary arteries were invited as the non-uremic control group.

Study protocol

Patients eligible for this study were scheduled for diagnostic fistulography and angioplasty on a mid-week non-dialysis day. Baseline characteristics and blood samples were collected on the morning of fistulography. After diagnostic fistulography or angioplasty, patients with insignificant stenosis (less than 50% diameter stenosis), thrombosed fistulas, arterial side stenosis, central vein lesions, or those who failed to obtain anatomic success after angioplasty were excluded. Diagnostic fistulography and angiograms of the angioplasty procedures were independently reviewed by another expert angiographer who was unaware of the patients' clinical and analytic data. The degree of stenosis was evaluated by two orthogonal planes and the greatest degree of stenosis was used for subsequent anatomical measurements. Anatomic measurements were made with use of a calibrated reference maker or computer-assisted edge detection software within the angiographic imaging system. The reference vessel was defined as an adjacent segment of normal vein located upstream from the target lesion. The degree of stenosis was reported as the maximum diameter reduction compared to the reference vessel diameter.

Laboratory methods

Blood samples were drawn after a 12 hour overnight fast and cessation of medications before diagnostic procedures. Plasma biochemical parameters were analyzed by standard laboratory methods. Assessment of the circulating EPCs by flow cytometry was performed by researchers blinded to clinical data. [8–10] A volume of 1000-μL peripheral blood was incubated for 30 minutes in the dark with Allophycocyanin (APC)-conjugated monoclonal antibody against human KDR (R&D, Minneapolis, MN, USA),

Phycoerythrin (PE)-conjugated monoclonal antibody against human CD133 (Miltenyi Biotec, Germany), and Fluorescein isothiocyanate (FITC)-conjugated monoclonal antibodies against human CD34 (Becton Dickinson Pharmingen, USA). After incubation, cells were lysed, washed with phosphate-buffered saline (PBS), and fixed in 2% paraformaldehyde before analysis. Each analysis included 150,000 events. The number of cells was normalized and expressed as a percentage (%) of cells and cells per 1×10^5 mononuclear cells (MNC). To assess the reproducibility of EPC measurements, circulating EPCs were measured from 2 separate blood samples in 10 subjects, and there was a strong correlation between the two measurements (r = 0.90, P<0.001).

Human EPC culture and functional studies

Peripheral blood samples for EPC culture were obtained from twenty of the study participants, ten from the early restenosis group (restenosis developed within three months after angioplasty) and ten from the late restenosis group (restenosis within 4–12 months after angioplasty), matched by age and types of vascular access. These samples were collected retrospectively while vascular accesses were functioning well after angioplasty. Total MNCs were isolated by density gradient centrifugation with Histopaque-1077 (Sigma, St. Louis, MO, USA). [11] Briefly, MNCs (5×10^6) were plated in 2 ml endothelial growth medium (EGM-2 MV Cambrex, East Rutherford, NJ, USA) on fibronectin-coated 6-well plates. After 4 days of culturing, the medium was changed and non-adherent cells were removed; attached EPCs appeared elongated with a spindle shape. EPCs were collected and used for the functional assays in this study.

Fibronectin adhesion test were assessed as previous described. [12] Cellular aging was determined with a Senescence Cell Staining kit (Sigma). TUNEL assay (Terminal deoxynucleotidyl transferase mediated deoxyuridine triphosphate nick-end labeling) was performed using the In Situ Cell Death Detection kit (Roche Diagnostics, Basel, Switzerland) according to the instructions of the manufacturers (**Methods S1**).

Follow-up and definitions

After the angioplasty procedure, all the participants of this study were prospectively followed for one year under the same protocol at respective hemodialysis centers. Medications of the participants were continued or adjusted according to their original indications but not for the maintenance of their vascular accesses. Follow-up surveillance included physical examination and dynamic venous pressure monitoring at each hemodialysis session, and transonic examination of access blood flow rate immediately after the intervention followed by monthly examinations. The referring nephrologists were blinded to the EPC levels of their patients. When abnormal clinical or hemodynamic parameters fulfilling the original referral criteria were detected, patients were referred for repeat fistulography and angioplasty as appropriate.

Anatomic success was defined as less than 30% residual stenosis. Clinical success was defined as an improvement from baseline in clinical or hemodynamic parameters indicative of access dysfunction. Success of the procedure was defined as the combination of anatomic and clinical success. Target-lesion restenosis was defined as more than 50% diameter reduction of the original target lesion. Primary patency of vascular access was defined as time until the next intervention on the access of any kind; secondary patency of vascular access was defined as time from the intervention until surgical revision or abandonment of the access.

Statistical analysis

All data are presented as means ± standard deviations or percentages. Categorical data were compared using the Chi-square test with Yates' correction and Fisher's exact test as appropriate. Continuous variables were tested for a normal distribution by the Kolmogorov-Smirnov test. For normally distributed data, means between categories were compared by one-way analysis-of-variance. For non-normally distributed data, the Kruskal-Wallis test was used for comparison between categories. We made the assumption of three times relative risk of restenosis according to a previous study about the role of CD34$^+$ cell counts on cardiovascular events in hemodialysis patients. [7] There were 39 restenosis events in the 130 patients enrolled in our study. With the assumption of a hazard ratio for restenosis = 3.0, alpha level = 0.05, and power = 80%, each group needs 16 restenosis events by the log rank test. Thus, we stratified our patients into tertiles to compare the relative risk or restenosis between tertiles of CD34$^+$KDR$^+$ cell counts. The primary patency of the whole access in each group was estimated by the Kaplan-Meier method and differences were assessed using the log-rank test. Proportions of patients with early restenosis, late restenosis, and no restenosis were compared by Chi-square test. Cox regression analysis was used for estimating the relative hazard of vascular access events by tertile of CD34$^+$KDR$^+$ cell count with subjects in the lower tertile of CD34$^+$KDR$^+$ cell count as the reference group. All variables with P<0.2 in the univariate analysis (including use of calcium channel blocker, side of access, location of access, nature of access, diameter of access and post-dilatation stenosis) and traditional cardiovascular risk factors (including age, hypertension, diabetes mellitus, dyslipidemia, and smoking) were entered into a multivariate analysis to determine independent predictors. A P value of less than 0.05 was considered to be statistically significant. Statistical analysis was performed with the use of SPSS software, version 20.0 for Windows.

Results

Baseline characteristics of study participants

One hundred and forty-four patients with dysfunctional vascular access were enrolled prior to the diagnostic procedures. After diagnostic fistulography and angioplasty, fourteen patients were excluded: five due to central vein lesions; two due to arterial lesions, five due to thrombosed lesions, and two due to a failed angioplasty procedure. Therefore, the study group consisted of 130 patients. All patients underwent one-year clinical follow-up after the angioplasty procedure apart from six patients who died before the end of one-year.

As shown in **Figure 1**, the circulating EPCs were gated with monocytes and defined as CD34$^+$, CD34$^+$KDR$^+$, and CD34$^+$KDR$^+$CD133$^+$, respectively. Compared to the non-uremic control group, patient with dysfunctional vascular access had significantly lower CD34$^+$ cells (50±60 vs. 83±54 cells/10^5 MNCs, p = 0.014), CD34$^+$KDR$^+$ cells (9±9 vs. 20±15 cells/10^5 MNCs, p<0.001), and CD34$^+$KDR$^+$CD133$^+$ cells (6±6 vs. 15±15, p<0.001). Compared to the uremic control group, patients with dysfunction vascular access had a trend of lower CD34$^+$ cell counts (50±60 vs. 61±31 cells/10^5 MNCs, p = 0.66), CD34$^+$KDR$^+$ cell counts (9±9 vs. 10±5 cells/10^5 MNCs, p = 0.88), and CD34$^+$KDR$^+$CD133$^+$ cell counts (6±6 vs. 10±5, p = 0.08) but the difference didn't reach statistical significance (**Figure 2**).

Endothelial progenitor cell counts and baseline variables

Participants with abnormal vascular access function were stratified into tertiles according to their baseline CD34$^+$KDR$^+$ cell count (lower, <4.0; medium, 4.0 to 9.0; upper, >9.0 cells/10^6 MNCs). The baseline characteristics of study participants and vascular accesses were shown in **Table 1**. In terms of baseline characteristics, only albumin level and white cell count were associated with tertile of baseline CD34$^+$KDR$^+$ cell count. In addition to CD34$^+$KDR$^+$ cells, we also estimated surface marker CD133$^+$ cells, which were expressed as a subfraction of immature EPCs. Increased age and white cell count were associated with a higher CD34$^+$KDR$^+$CD133$^+$ cell count.

Incidence of vascular and clinical events (Table 2)

At the end of one year follow-up, 95 patients underwent a re-intervention; 94 of whom had a restenosis at the same location. All the patients with target lesion restenosis received re-interventions and were included in the re-intervention group as well. Nine patients lost their vascular access and six patients died during the follow-up period: three patients due to cardiovascular causes (myocardial infarction or sudden cardiac death) and the others due to non-cardiovascular causes.

Because the majority of patients had target-lesion restenosis at the end of one-year follow-up, the vascular access events were further stratified according the presence and timing of target-lesion restenosis: early restenosis (within 3 months), late restenosis (between 4–12 months) and no restenosis (within 12 months). The same time frame was applied in the stratification of vascular access re-intervention. Patients in the lower tertile of CD34$^+$KDR$^+$ cell count had the highest rate of early restenosis and re-intervention. In contrast, patients in the highest tertile of CD34$^+$KDR$^+$ cell count possessed the highest proportions of late or no restenosis compared to the other two tertiles, although they did not achieve statistical significance. The discrepancy in cumulative primary patency rates between EPC groups was largest at three months and then declined as the follow-up period extended (**Table 2 and Figure 3**).

As shown in Figure 3, patients in the lower tertile of EPC received an average of 3.4±2.8 interventions in one year, which was higher than those in the medium tertile (2.6±2.5, P = 0.15) and the upper tertile (1.5±1.5, P = 0.004). As presented in **Table 3**, patients with target-lesion early restenosis had significantly lower CD34$^+$KDR$^+$ and CD34$^+$KDR$^+$CD133$^+$ cell counts, but not CD34$^+$ cell counts, than those with late restenosis.

Characterization of human EPC and function

The peripheral blood mononuclear cells (MNCs) that were initially seeded on fibronectin-coated wells were round in shape. After the medium was changed on day 4, attached EPCs had an elongated and spindle shape. The EPCs were characterized as adherent cells positive for acetylated low-density lipoprotein (AcLDL) uptake and lectin binding by direct fluorescent staining and immunohistochemical staining. Most of the EPCs expressed endothelial and hematopoietic stem cell markers, CD34, VE-cadherin, CD133, Kinase insert domain receptor (KDR), and CD31 (**Figure 4A**), which are considered critical markers of EPCs.

There were no significant differences in clinical or access characteristics between the two groups of patients, except for lower CD34$^+$KDR$^+$ and CD34$^+$KDR$^+$CD133$^+$ cell counts in the early restenosis group. (**Table S1**) Patients with early restenosis had attenuated EPC adhesive function compared to those with late restenosis (9.7±2.3 vs. 17.7±3.3 cells/HPF, P<0.001; **Figure 4B**). Patients with early restenosis also had higher

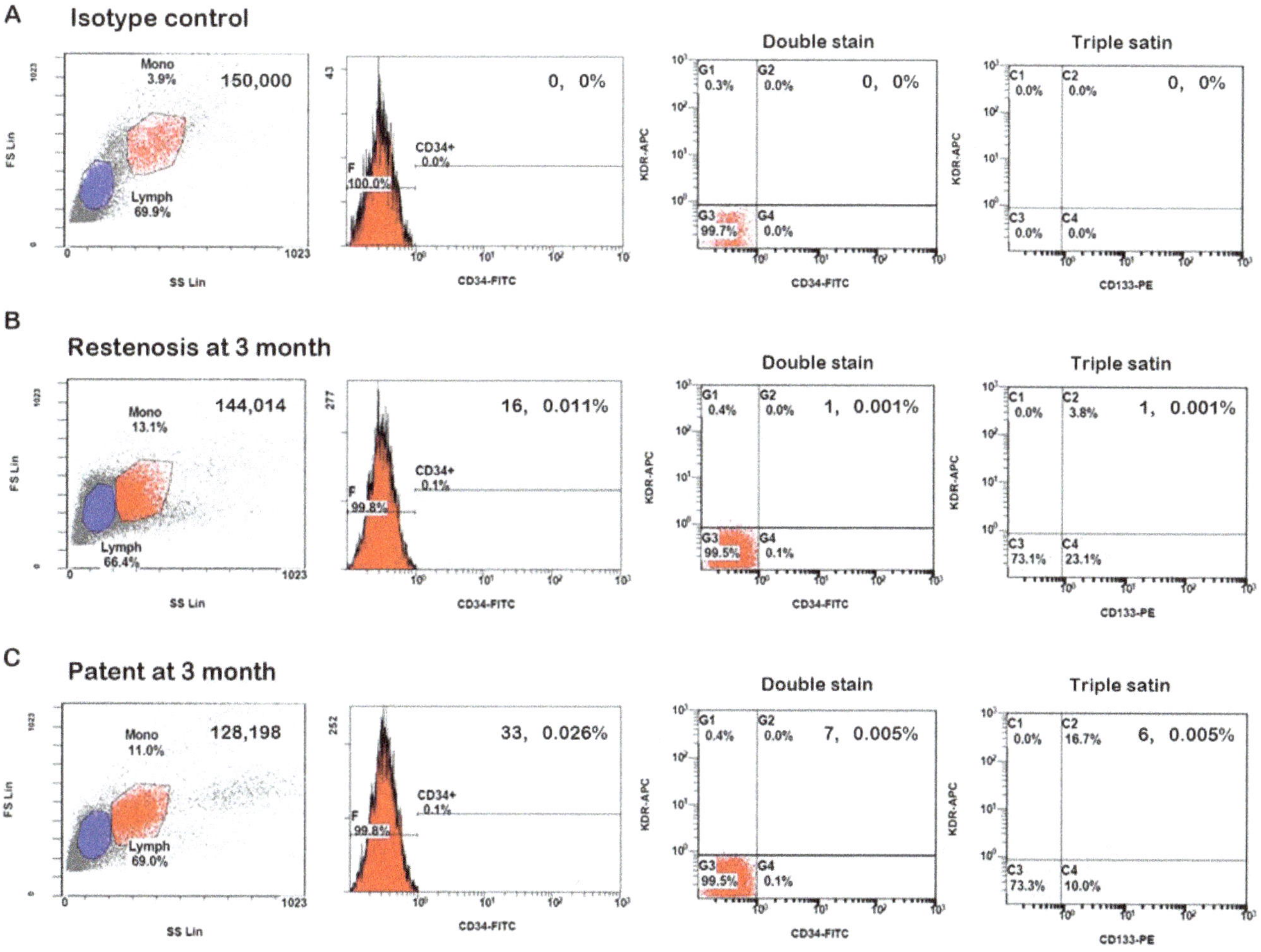

A **Isotype control**

B **Restenosis at 3 month**

C **Patent at 3 month**

Figure 1. Representative flow cytometry analysis. Panels show mononuclear cells (MNCs) that were gated by forward/sideward scatter (FSC/SSC) in isotype controls (A), patients with restenosis (B), and patients without (C) restenosis at 3 months. The numbers of circulating endogenous progenitor cells (EPCs) were defined as CD34$^+$, CD34$^+$KDR$^+$, and CD34$^+$KDR$^+$CD133$^+$, respectively.

percentage of senescence-associated β-galactosidase-positive EPCs (65.5±18.0% vs. 37.6±10.7, P<0.001, **Figure 4C**) and TUNEL-positive EPCs (29.7±8.2% vs. 12.7±5.5, P<0.001; **Figure 4D**) that that with late restenosis.

Univariate analysis for factors associated with target-lesion early restenosis

In univariate Cox regression analysis, the incidence of target-lesion early restenosis was not associated with demographic factors, cardiovascular risk factors, medications, or biochemical profiles; but significantly associated with access factors, including upper-arm access (hazard ratio [HR], 2.31, 95% confidence interval [CI], 1.09–4.92, p = 0.030), right-sided access (HR, 2.94; CI, 1.03–4.34, p = 0.043), graft access (HR, 2.22; CI, 1.03–4.34, p = 0.020), post-dilatation stenosis (HR, 1.01; 95% CI, 1.00–1.01, p = 0.032), and baseline level of circulating EPCs, including CD34$^+$KDR$^+$ cell count (HR, 0.91; CI, 0.85–0.98, p = 0.013) or tertiles (high vs. low, HR, 0.20; 95% CI, 0.08–0.53, p = 0.001) and CD34$^+$KDR$^+$CD133$^+$ cell count (HR, 0.89; CI, 0.80–0.98, p = 0.024) or tertiles (high vs. low, HR, 0.25; CI, 0.11–0.59, p = 0.002) (**Table S2**).

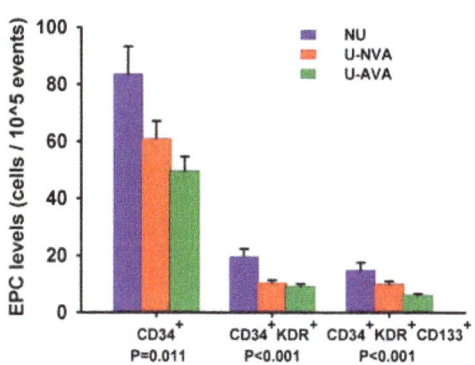

Figure 2. Circulating EPC counts between different groups. Comparisons of EPCs counts between the non-uremic controls (NU), uremic controls (normal vascular access function without interventions in previous two years, U-NVA), and uremic patients with abnormal vascular access function referred for interventions (U-AVA). (Values presented as mean ± standard error).

Table 1. Baseline characteristics of patients and vascular accesses.

| Characteristic | Total (N = 130) | Tertiles of CD34$^+$KDR$^+$ Cell Count | | | P value |
		Lower (N = 43)	Medium (N = 44)	Upper (N = 43)	
Age (yr)	66±13	71±12	65±12	63±14	0.06
Gender (men/women)	47/83	14/29	20/24	13/30	0.31
Risk factors					
Hypertension (%)	76(58%)	24(56%)	26(59%)	26(60%)	0.90
Diabetes (%)	48(37%)	15(35%)	17(39%)	16(37%)	0.94
Dyslipidemia (%)	23(18%)	11(26%)	4(9%)	8(19%)	0.13
Current smoker (%)	15(11%)	5(11%)	6(14%)	4(9%)	0.71
Cardiovascular disease (%)	26(20%)	12(28%)	8(18%)	6(14%)	0.25
Biochemical data					
Cholesterol (mg/dl)	166±40	170±38	164±48	163±33	0.71
Triglycerides (mg/dl)	161±108	177±106	147±99	159±117	0.51
Albumin (g/dl)	3.9±0.5	3.8±0.5	3.8±0.4	4.1±0.4	0.004
Hemoglobin (g/dl)	10.8±1.4	10.7±1.7	10.8±1.3	10.9±1.2	0.88
WBC (10^3/μL)	6.7±2.0	7.2±2.7	5.8±1.4	7.1±1.5	0.01
Calcium (mg/dl)	9.4±1.2	9.1±1.7	9.6±0.9	9.6±0.9	0.16
Phosphate (mg/dl)	4.4±1.3	4.3±1.3	4.4±1.5	4.6±1.1	0.53
Kt/V	1.46±0.30	1.28±0.30	1.62±0.30	1.63±0.27	0.07
Medications					
Anti-platelet	50(43%)	15(38%)	17(47%)	18(46%)	0.64
Nitrates	22(19%)	9(23%)	7(19%)	6(15%)	0.72
β-blocker	23(50%)	7(18%)	7(19.4%)	9(23%)	0.82
Calcium blocker	34(30%)	11(28%)	12(33%)	11(28%)	0.83
ACEI/ARB	23(20%)	6(15%)	8(22.2%)	9(23%)	0.62
Lipid-lowering agents	18(16%)	5(13%)	5(14%)	8(21%)	0.58
Erythropoietin (U/kg/week)	80±36	78±40	79±37	82±34	0.94
Access/lesion					
Shunt age (month)	48±44	42±31	58±57	45±40	0.30
Prosthetic graft	70(54%)	20(47%)	22(50%)	28(65%)	0.18
Upper arm access	19(15%)	7(16%)	8(18%)	4(9%)	0.50
Right arm access	32(25%)	13(30%)	10(23%)	9(21%)	0.60
Diameter (mm)	7.2±1.3	7.1±1.2	7.3±1.4	7.2±1.2	0.76
Pre-stenosis (%)	73±15	71±15	75±15	72±14	0.47
Post-stenosis (%)	22±17	24±17	23±16	21±19	0.78
CD34$^+$KDR$^+$ cells/10^{5}MNCs	9.2±9.4	2.3±1.2	6.3±1.3	19.1±10.4	<0.001

ACEI, angiotensin converting enzyme inhibitor; ARB, angiotensin receptor blocker; Kt/V, urea clearance; MNC, mononuclear cell; WBC, white blood cell.
P for ANOVA or Kruskal-Wallis test in continuous variables and p for Chi-square test in categorical variables.

Multivariate analysis for factors associated with target-lesion early restenosis

A multivariate Cox regression analysis with adjustment for covariates confirmed a significant association of CD34$^+$KDR$^+$ cell tertile (high vs. low, HR, 0.24, CI, 0.08–0.76, p = 0.016) and CD34$^+$KDR$^+$CD133$^+$ cell tertile (high vs. low, HR, 0.23, CI, 0.08–0.64, p = 0.005) with the development of target-lesion early restenosis. In addition, use of calcium channel blockers, side of access and nature of access were identified as independent predictors of early restenosis as well (**Table 4**).

Discussion

Main findings

Our study showed the impact of circulating EPCs on restenosis of hemodialysis vascular access. Deficiency of CD34$^+$KDR$^+$ cells was significantly associated with an increased risk of early restenosis. Patients in the lower CD34$^+$KDR$^+$ cell tertile were four times as likely to experience restenosis compared to those in the upper tertile. In addition, patients with early restenosis were more likely to have impaired EPC adhesive function, and increased cellular apoptosis and senescence. In the clinical setting, uremic patients usually have a cluster of cardiovascular risk factors, which significantly influence the number and function of

Table 2. Vascular access and clinical events during follow-up period.

Event	Total (N = 130)	Tertiles of CD34$^+$KDR$^+$ Cell Count			P value
		Low (N = 43)	Medium (N = 44)	High (N = 43)	
Vascular access event					
Target-lesion restenosis					
Early restenosis	37(28%)	20(46%)	12(27%)	5(12%)	0.002
Late restenosis	57(44%)	14(33%)	19(43%)	24(56%)	0.09
No restenosis	36(28%)	9(21%)	13(30%)	14(33%)	0.46
Access re-intervention					
Early re-intervention	39(30%)	20(46%)	13(30%)	6(14%)	0.004
Late re-intervention	56(43%)	14(33%)	18(41%)	24(56%)	0.09
No re-intervention	35(27%)	9(21%)	13(29%)	13(30%)	0.56
Access primary patency rate					
At 3 months	70%	53%	70%	86%	0.004
At 6 months	41%	30%	39%	56%	0.009
At 12 months	27%	21%	29%	30%	0.50
Access secondary patency rate					
At 12 months	93%	94%	86%	98%	0.09
Clinical event					
Death (any cause)	6(5%)	1(2%)	3(7%)	2(5%)	0.61
Death (cardiac cause)	3(2%)	1(2%)	2(5%)	0(0%)	0.37
Hospitalization (any cause)	21(16%)	8(19%)	10(23%)	3(7%)	0.12
Hospitalization (cardiac cause)	11(9%)	5(12%)	5(11%)	1(2%)	0.21

Timing of restenosis or re-intervention: early, within 3 months; late, within 4–12 months; P for Chi-square test.

EPCs. [6] Our study has demonstrated for the first time that there is an association between circulating EPCs and the aggressive venous intimal hyperplasia of hemodialysis vascular access, independent of traditional risk factors.

Possible mechanisms from animal studies

Angioplasty is associated with mechanical vascular injury, followed by an intensive local inflammatory response, platelet activation, thrombus formation, and intimal hyperplasia. [13] Endothelial disruption is considered to be the primary event in the initiation of restenosis after balloon angioplasty. [14] Besides acting as a mechanical barrier protecting smooth cell migration, a functional endothelium modulates local hemostasis and thrombolysis, and regulates smooth muscle cell proliferation. [14] The importance of endothelial integrity has been demonstrated in animal studies, suggesting that a functionally intact endothelium is

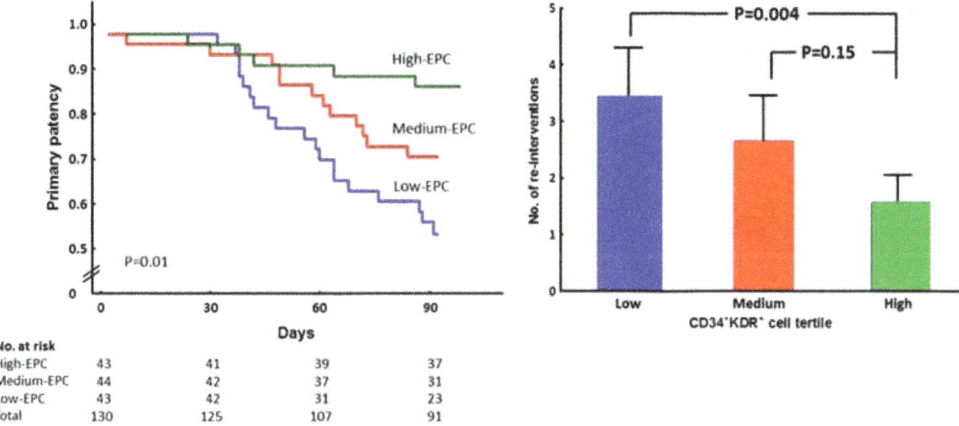

No. at risk

High-EPC	43	41	39	37
Medium-EPC	44	42	37	31
Low-EPC	43	42	31	23
Total	130	125	107	91

Figure 3. Kaplan-Meier analyses at three months and frequency of re-intervention at one year stratified by EPC tertiles. Left: The figure demonstrates the proportion of patients without target-lesion early restenosis according to their baseline circulating CD34$^+$KDR$^+$ cell count. Patients are divided into tertiles (low, medium, high) according to their baseline circulating CD34$^+$KDR$^+$ cell count. Right: Frequency of re-interventions at one year after angioplasty stratified by baseline circulating CD34$^+$KDR$^+$ cell count. (Values presented as mean ± standard error).

Table 3. Comparisons of EPC levels according to the presence and timing of target-lesion restenosis at one year.

EPC	All patients (N = 130)			Restenosis patients (N = 94)		
	Patent (N = 36)	Restenosis (N = 94)	P value	Late (N = 57)	Early (N = 37)	P value
EPC (%)						
CD34$^+$	0.062±0.082	0.044±0.047	0.12	0.043±0.038	0.046±0.057	0.77
CD34$^+$KDR$^+$	0.012±0.017	0.009±0.010	0.33	0.012±0.012	0.005±0.005	<0.001
CD34$^+$KDR$^+$CD133$^+$	0.009±0.017	0.007±0.007	0.27	0.008±0.008	0.004±0.003	<0.001
EPC (cells/10^{5}MNCs)						
CD34$^+$	63±83	45±47	0.13	44±39	46±57	0.89
CD34$^+$KDR$^+$	9±7	9±10	0.90	12±12	5±5	<0.001
CD34$^+$KDR$^+$CD133$^+$	6±5	6±6	0.85	8±7	4±3	<0.001

EPC, endothelial progenitor cell; MNCs: mononuclear cells.
Timing of restenosis: early restenosis, within 3 months; late, restenosis within 4–12 months.

requisite for the inhibition of intimal hyperplasia. [14,15] Accordingly, it is believed that faster re-endothelialization may inhibit the formation of intimal hyperplasia. [16] The traditional paradigm of re-endothelialization is based on the proliferation and migration of pre-existing mature adjacent endothelial cells. Increasing evidence suggests that the injured endothelium is regenerated by circulating EPCs and that the levels of EPCs reflect vascular repair capacity. These cells are derived from the bone marrow and can be mobilized into the peripheral circulation in response to many stimuli, including tissue ischemia and vascular damage, through the release of growth factors and cytokines. [4,15,16] In animal studies, Werner et al demonstrated that bone marrow-derived progenitor cells home in to areas of endothelial denudation. [17] Furthermore, intravenous injection of these EPCs can accelerate re-endothelialization and decrease neo-intimal hyperplasia. [18] These animal studies provided mechan-

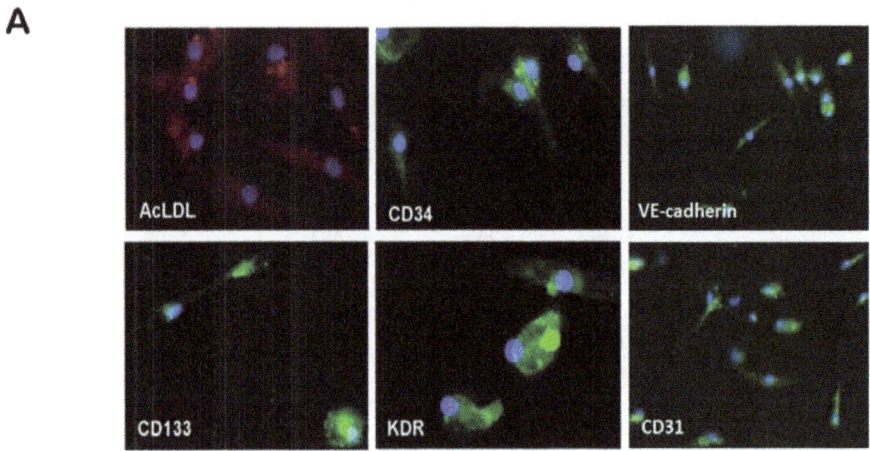

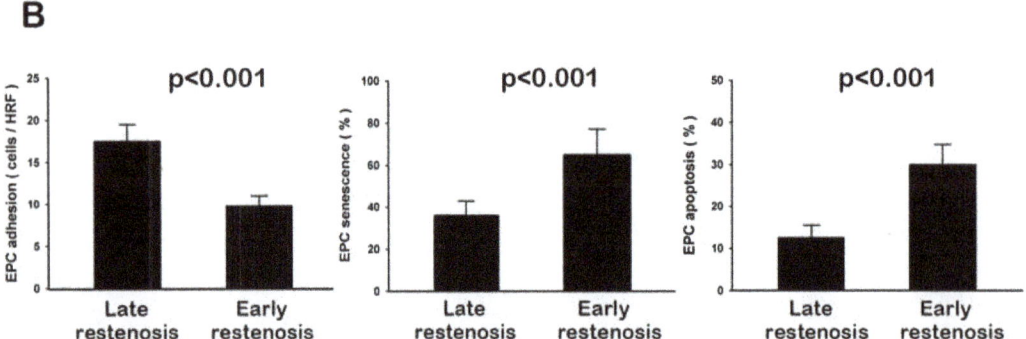

Figure 4. Morphology and functional study. Morphological characterization of human endothelial progenitor cells (EPCs) from peripheral blood (A) and comparisons of the EPC adhesive function (B), senescence assay (C), and apoptosis assay (D) in participants stratified by early (within 3 months) or late (within 4–12 months) restenosis. Values presented as mean ± standard deviation.

Table 4. Multivariate Cox regression analysis for factors predicting target-lesion early restenosis.

Factors	Unit of increase	Hazard Ratio	95% CI	P value
CD34⁺KDR⁺ cells entered as a continuous variable				
Use of CCB	Yes vs. no	0.31	0.11–0.87	0.025
Side of access	Left vs. right	0.23	0.07–0.79	0.020
Nature of access	Native vs. graft	0.40	0.18–0.92	0.030
CD34⁺KDR⁺ cells	1 cell/10⁵ MNCs	0.89	0.81–0.97	0.011
CD34⁺KDR⁺ cells entered as a categorical variable				
Use of CCB	Yes vs. no	0.33	0.12–0.88	0.027
Side of access	Left vs. right	0.26	0.08–0.88	0.031
Nature of access	Native vs. graft	0.38	0.16–0.86	0.020
CD34⁺KDR⁺ cells	High vs. low	0.24	0.08–0.76	0.016
CD34⁺KDR⁺CD133⁺cells entered as a continuous variable				
Use of CCB	Yes vs. no	0.37	0.14–0.99	0.049
Side of access	Left vs. right	0.21	0.06–0.74	0.015
Nature of access	Native vs. graft	0.37	0.16–0.84	0.018
CD34⁺KDR⁺CD133⁺cells	1 cell/10⁵ MNCs	0.82	0.72–0.94	0.003
CD34⁺KDR⁺CD133⁺cells entered as a categorical variable				
Use of CCB	Yes vs. no	0.35	0.13–0.94	0.037
Side of access	Left vs. right	0.22	0.06–0.76	0.017
Nature of access	Native vs. graft	0.37	0.16–0.84	0.017
Post-stenosis (%)	1%	1.02	1.00–1.05	0.047
CD34⁺KDR⁺CD133⁺cells	High vs. low	0.23	0.08–0.64	0.005

CCB, calcium channel blocker; CI, confidence interval; MNC, mononuclear cell.
Age, hypertension, diabetes, smoking, dyslipidemia, use of calcium channel blocker, side of access, nature of access, diameter of access, post-angioplasty stenosis were entered as covariates.

ical basis for the association between the circulating EPCs and intimal hyperplasia.

Evidence from clinical studies

In retrospective studies, George et al demonstrated a reduced number and adhesive function of EPCs in patients with proliferative type in-stent restenosis; Matsuo et al also showed reduced EPC numbers and senescence function in patients with in-stent restenosis. [19,20] In addition, some studies have demonstrated mobilization of EPCs after angioplasty, providing indirect evidence that EPCs may participate in the response to vascular injury. [17] Despite this, conflicting results exist in regards to the relationship between EPC mobilization and subsequent restenosis. [21] Using baseline EPC levels, our study demonstrated that a reduced number of baseline EPCs is an aggravating factor for venous intimal hyperplasia in uremic patients.

Besides being a marker of vascular repair capacity, circulating EPCs are also a surrogate marker for endothelial dysfunction and vascular health. [5] Accordingly, it is possible that deficiency of circulating EPCs may be just a marker of cumulative cardiovascular risk, rather than a direct mediator of intimal hyperplasia. This distinction is important because modulation of EPCs will be beneficial only if it is a 'disease maker'. Our data favors that EPC deficiency may not only be a marker of intimal hyperplasia for the following reasons. First, most of the cardiovascular risk factors were not correlated with the number of EPCs in our hemodialysis patients. Second, our data is consistent with previous studies demonstrating that cardiovascular risk factors do not predict

venous intimal hyperplasia of hemodialysis vascular accesses [22–24].

Early vs. late restenosis

Compared to the 30% restenosis rate after coronary angioplasty [4], the 72% target-lesion restenosis rate in our study confirms the aggressive nature of venous intimal hyperplasia. Although the group with high EPC levels had a better patency rate initially, this difference vanished rapidly within one year. This late catch-up phenomenon suggests that rapid re-endothelialization only delays but does not stop the development of intimal hyperplasia. This is further supported by our observation that no difference in EPC counts between patients with late or no restenosis. Our explanation is biologically plausible as the inflammatory activation and intimal hyperplasia develop earlier than re-endothelialization. According to the animal models of restenosis, the inflammation and cellular proliferation phase occur rapidly after balloon injury, usually within days to weeks. [25] In contrast, the regeneration of the endothelium usually takes weeks to months to complete. [14] In consequence, EPCs seem to play a more significant role in the early stage after angioplasty. After the critical point of re-endothelialization, uremia or hemodialysis-related factors may dominate the development of restenosis, such as endothelial dysfunction, systemic inflammation, repeated punctures of vascular access and less well-defined elastic lamina of veins.

Comparisons of EPCs of uremic patients between different studies

It is difficult to compare studies because different surface markers or units have been used to measure EPCs. EPC counts in our study were expressed as a fraction of the number of events, rather than events per microliter. We believe this unit is more appropriate for hemodialysis patients because of the substantial variation in fluid status. Although low circulating $CD34^+$ cells have been found to be associated with all-cause and cardiovascular mortality in uremic patients [7], we didn't find a similar association in our study. Furthermore, $CD34^+$ cells were not associated with the presence or timing of restenosis in our study as well. This marker is common to a variety of progenitor cells, including smooth muscle progenitor cells, not only endothelial progenitor cells. [26] In a recent animal study using $CD34^+$ antibodies to accelerate endothelialization of synthetic grafts, intimal hyperplasia was also stimulated. [27] The dichotomy implies that $CD34^+$ antibodies may attract cells with potential transforming into smooth muscle cell or myofibroblasts as well. EPCs represent only a minor cell population in whole blood, and the choice of markers is very important. Because CD34 and KDR are also expressed on circulating mature endothelial cells, surface marker CD133 was used to ensure the identity of EPCs. Despite the rarity of these cells in the circulation, a significant correlation was still observed between counts of these cells and restenosis. There is still confusion about the cell markers used for EPC. The putative EPCs identified by surface marker CD34, KDR, and CD133 in this study are not certainly EPC but also various amounts of hematopoietic stem cells and circulating endothelial cells. These cells could only be discriminated by extensive gene expression analysis or use of a variety of functional assays. [28,29] Nonetheless, these meticulous methods are not often applied and no simple universal definition exists at the present time. [30,31] Therefore, putative EPCs in the study were still identified by the panel of CD34, KDR, and CD133 markers, which have been widely used in publications and consistently used as a surrogate marker for cells displaying regenerative properties in human study.

Limitations

Our study has several limitations that should be considered when interpreting our results. Only pre-procedure EPC levels were measured and the effect of EPC activation, migration, and homing was not evaluated. Second, we were not able to demonstrate increased EPC homing and migration to the injured endothelium, as has been demonstrated in animal studies. Third, there is still no universal definition of EPCs. KDR is not exclusively a marker of EPC but also expressed on hematopoietic stem cells and circulating mature endothelial cells. [29] Various methods to more specifically identify EPCs are emerging but they were not applicable when the study was conducted. [30,31] Forth, the number of EPCs per 150,000 events analyzed in peripheral blood is relatively low in hemodialysis patients and analysis of more blood amount may be helpful to improve the yield rate. Finally and most importantly, despite our observation of association between EPCs and early restenosis, this is not a sufficient evidence for their causal relationship. Further study to

evaluate the effect of EPC manipulation and explore the underlying pathway was needed to prove the mechanical link.

Clinical implications and conclusion

Although the contribution of EPC deficiency to restenosis remains to be proven, EPC-capturing stents are undergoing clinical evaluation as a coronary intervention. [32] The most relevant clinical implication of our study is that deficiency of certain circulating EPCs is possibly pathogenic for the rapid venous intimal hyperplasia observed in hemodialysis patients. Based on this putative mechanism, methods of modifying EPC number or function, including physical exercise, pharmacological modulation (statin, GSF), infusion of autologous EPCs, capturing EPC to the denuded endothelium, may have the potential to delay the development of restenosis. [13] Studies aimed at modulating the number or function of more specific EPCs is warranted not only to clarify the causal role of EPCs but also as a potential strategy to decrease the frequency. In addition, $CD34^+KDR^+$ cells may serve as a biomarker for patients vulnerable to restenosis. It will be helpful in therapeutic planning, such as aggressive monitoring, EPC-modulating intervention, or early surgical revision. Finally, EPCs seems to play a significant role only in the development of early restenosis. In consequence, therapeutic approach to modulating EPC may focus on this critical period of re-endothelialization.

In conclusion, this study demonstrated for the first time that deficiency of circulating EPCs predicts early restenosis of hemodialysis vascular access. Our observation supports a significant role of circulating EPCs on intimal hyperplasia in human, as that was demonstrated in previous animal models. Further studies to clarify their pathogenic role in human by therapeutic approach are warranted.

Acknowledgments

We would like to thank the following hemodialysis centers for the referral and follow-up of patients: Hemodialysis center of Nanmen Hospital and Zen-Tz hospital; Hung-Zen Hemodialysis clinic, and Ansn Hemodialysis Clinic.

Author Contributions

Conceived and designed the experiments: CCW PHH. Performed the experiments: CCW PHH. Analyzed the data: CCW CLL. Contributed reagents/materials/analysis tools: HBL JWC SJL. Wrote the paper: CCW.

References

1. Roy-Chaudhury P, Sukhatme VP, Cheung AK (2006) Hemodialysis vascular access dysfunction: a cellular and molecular viewpoint. J Am Soc Nephrol 17: 1112–1127.
2. Bittl JA (2010) Catheter interventions for hemodialysis fistulas and grafts. J Am Coll Cardiol Intv 3: 1–11.
3. Inoue T, Croce K, Morooka T, Sakuma M, Node K, et al. (2011) Vascular Inflammation and Repair Implications for Re-Endothelialization, Restenosis, and Stent Thrombosis. J Am Coll Cardiol Intv 4: 1057–1066.
4. Werner N, Priller J, Laufs U, Endres M, Böhm M, et al. (2002) Bone Marrow–Derived Progenitor Cells Modulate Vascular Reendothelialization and Neointimal Formation. Arterioscler Thromb Vasc Biol 22: 1567–1572.

5. Hill JM, Zalos G, Halcox JPJ, Schenke WH, Waclawiw MA, et al. (2003) Circulating Endothelial Progenitor Cells, Vascular Function, and Cardiovascular Risk. N Engl J Med 348: 593–600.

6. de Groot K, Bahlmann FH, Sowa J, Koenig J, Menne J, et al. (2004) Uremia causes endothelial progenitor cell deficiency. Kidney Int 66: 641–646.

7. Maruyama S, Taguchi A, Iwashima S, Ozaki T, Yasuda K, et al. (2008) Low circulating CD34+ cell count is associated with poor prognosis in chronic hemodialysis patients. Kidney Int 74: 1603–1609.

8. Vasa M, Fichtlscherer S, Aicher A, Adler K, Urbich C, et al. (2001) Number and Migratory Activity of Circulating Endothelial Progenitor Cells Inversely Correlate With Risk Factors for Coronary Artery Disease. Circ Res 89: e1–e7.

9. Chiang CH, Huang PH, Chung FP, Chen ZY, Leu HB, et al. (2012) Decreased circulating endothelial progenitor cell levels and function in patients with nonalcoholic fatty liver disease. PLoS One 7: e31799.

10. Chiang CH, Huang PH, Chiu CC, Hsu CY, Leu HB, et al. (2014) Reduction of circulating endothelial progenitor cell level is associated with contrast-induced nephropathy in patients undergoing percutaneous coronary and peripheral interventions. PLoS One 9: e89942.

11. Huang PH, Chen YH, Tsai HY, Chen JS, Wu TC, et al. (2010) Intake of red wine increases the number and functional capacity of circulating endothelial progenitor cells by enhancing nitric oxide bioavailability. Arterioscler Thromb Vasc Biol 30: 869–877.

12. Fadini GP, Baesso I, Albiero M, Sartore S, Agostini C, et al. (2008) Technical notes on endothelial progenitor cells: ways to escape from the knowledge plateau. Atherosclerosis 197: 496–503.

13. Padfield GJ, Newby DE, Mills NL (2010) Understanding the role of endothelial progenitor cells in percutaneous coronary intervention. J Am Coll Cardiol 55: 1553–1565.

14. Kipshidze N, Dangas G, Tsapenko M, Moses J, Leon MB, et al. (2004) Role of the endothelium in modulating neointimal formation: vasculoprotective approaches to attenuate restenosis after percutaneous coronary interventions. J Am Coll Cardiol 44: 733–739.

15. Marboeuf P, Corseaux D, Mouquet F, Van Belle E, Jude B, et al. (2008) Inflammation triggers colony forming endothelial cell mobilization after angioplasty in chronic lower limb ischemia. J Thromb Haemost 6: 195–197.

16. Asahara T, Murohara T, Sullivan A, Silver M, van der Zee R, et al. (1997) Isolation of putative progenitor endothelial cells for angiogenesis. Science 275: 964–967.

17. Banerjee S, Brilakis E, Zhang S, Roesle M, Lindsey J, et al. (2006) Endothelial progenitor cell mobilization after percutaneous coronary intervention. Atherosclerosis 189: 70–75.

18. Mills NL, Tura O, Padfield GJ, Millar C, Lang NN, et al. (2009) Dissociation of phenotypic and functional endothelial progenitor cells in patients undergoing percutaneous coronary intervention. Heart 95: 2003–2008.

19. George J, Herz I, Goldstein E, Abashidze S, Deutch V, et al. (2003) Number and adhesive properties of circulating endothelial progenitor cells in patients with in-stent restenosis. Arterioscler Thromb Vasc Biol 23: e57–60.

20. Matsuo Y, Imanishi T, Hayashi Y, Tomobuchi Y, Kubo T, et al. (2006) The Effect of Senescence of Endothelial Progenitor Cells on In-stent Restenosis in Patients Undergoing Coronary Stenting. Intern Med 45: 581–587.

21. Pelliccia F, Cianfrocca C, Rosano G, Mercuro G, Speciale G, et al. (2010) Role of endothelial progenitor cells in restenosis and progression of coronary atherosclerosis after percutaneous coronary intervention: a prospective study. J Am Coll Cardiol Intv 3: 78–86.

22. Wu CC, Wen SC, Yang CW, Pu SY, Tsai KC, et al. (2009) Plasma ADMA predicts restenosis of arteriovenous fistula. J Am Soc Nephrol 20: 213–222.

23. Rajan DK, Bunston S, Misra S, Pinto R, Lok CE (2004) Dysfunctional autogenous hemodialysis fistulas: outcomes after angioplasty–are there clinical predictors of patency? Radiology 232: 508–515.

24. Wu C-C, Wen S-C, Yang C-W, Pu S-Y, Tsai K-C, et al. (2010) Baseline plasma glycemic profiles but not inflammatory biomarkers predict symptomatic restenosis after angioplasty of arteriovenous fistulas in patients with hemodialysis. Atherosclerosis 209: 598–600.

25. Otsuka F, Finn AV, Yazdani SK, Nakano M, Kolodgie FD, et al. (2012) The importance of the endothelium in atherothrombosis and coronary stenting. Nat Rev Cardiol 9: 439–453.

26. Stam F, van Guldener C, Becker A, Dekker JM, Heine RJ, et al. (2006) Endothelial Dysfunction Contributes to Renal Function–Associated Cardiovascular Mortality in a Population with Mild Renal Insufficiency: The Hoorn Study. J Am Soc Nephrol 17: 537–545.

27. Rotmans JI, Heyligers JM, Verhagen HJ, Velema E, Nagtegaal MM, et al. (2005) In vivo cell seeding with anti-CD34 antibodies successfully accelerates endothelialization but stimulates intimal hyperplasia in porcine arteriovenous expanded polytetrafluoroethylene grafts. Circulation 112: 12–18.

28. Kraan J, Sleijfer S, Foekens JA, Gratama JW (2012) Clinical value of circulating endothelial cell detection in oncology. Drug Discov Today 17: 710–717.

29. Yoder MC (2012) Human endothelial progenitor cells. Cold Spring Harb Perspect Med 2: a006692.

30. Lanuti P, Santilli F, Marchisio M, Pierdomenico L, Vitacolonna E, et al. (2012) A novel flow cytometric approach to distinguish circulating endothelial cells from endothelial microparticles: relevance for the evaluation of endothelial dysfunction. J Immunol Methods 380: 16–22.

31. Kraan J, Strijbos MH, Sieuwerts AM, Foekens JA, den Bakker MA, et al. (2012) A new approach for rapid and reliable enumeration of circulating endothelial cells in patients. J Thromb Haemost 10: 931–939.

32. Nakazawa G, Granada JF, Alviar CL, Tellez A, Kaluza GL, et al. (2010) Anti-CD34 Antibodies Immobilized on the Surface of Sirolimus-Eluting Stents Enhance Stent Endothelialization. J Am Coll Cardiol Intv 3: 68–75.

6

Effects of Intra-Aortic Balloon Counterpulsation Pump on Mortality of Acute Myocardial Infarction

Liwen Ye[1¶]**, Minming Zheng**[2,3¶]**, Qingwei Chen**[1]*****, Guiqion Li**[1]**, Wei Deng**[1]**, Dazhi Ke**[1]

1 Department of Geriatrics Cardiology, the Second Affiliated Hospital of Chongqing Medical University, Chongqing, China, 2 Chongqing Ophthalmology Research Center for the Senile, the Second Affiliated Hospital of Chongqing Medical University, Chongqing, China, 3 Department of Ophthalmology, the Second Affiliated Hospital of Chongqing Medical University, Chongqing, China

Abstract

Background: Several randomized controlled trials (RCTs) have evaluated the effect of intra-aortic balloon counterpulsation pump(IABP) on the mortality of acute myocardial infarction (AMI).

Objectives: To analyze the relevant RCT data on the effect of IABP on mortality and the occurrence of bleeding in AMI.

Data Sources: Published RCTs on the treatment of AMI by IABP were retrieved in searches of Medline, EMBASE, Cochrane and other related databases. The last search was conducted on July 20, 2014.

Study Eligibility Criteria: Randomized clinical trials comparing IABP to controls as treatment for AMI.

Participants: Patients with AMI.

Synthesis Methods: The primary endpoint was mortality, and the secondary endpoint was bleeding events. To account for to heterogeneity, a random-effects model was used to analyze the study data.

Results: Ten trials with a total population of 973 patients that were included in the analysis showed no significant difference in 2-month mortality between the IABP and the control groups. The 6-month mortality in the IABP group was not significantly lower than in the control group in the four RCTs that enrolled 59 AMI patients with CS. But in the four that enrolled AMI 66 patients without CS, the data showed opposite conclusion.

Conclusions: IABP cannot reduce within 2 months and 6–12 months mortality of AMI patients with CS as well as within 2 months mortality of AMI patients without CS, but can reduce 6–12 months mortality of AMI patients without CS. In addition, IABP can increase the risk of bleeding.

Editor: Katriina Aalto-Setala, University of Tampere, Finland

Funding: The authors have no support or funding to report.

Competing Interests: The authors have declared that no competing interests exist.

* Email: chenqwcq@126.com

¶ LY and MZ are co-first authors on this work.

Introduction

Intra-aortic balloon counterpulsation pump(IABP) can increase blood flow in the coronary artery and the brain while reducing afterload and cardiac oxygen consumption [1]. Kantrowitz [2] first reported the clinical application of IABP. Because IABP can quickly improve the effect of patients' clinical symptom, so this technology causes people's attention. Although numerous percutaneous circulation support equipments are applied, the effect of IABP in adjuvant therapy of AMI patients is still controversial. Some previous studies show that IABP benefits for high-risk patients with AMI, but most of these studies are non-randomized and retrospective, with serious selection bias and poor credibility. However, in some other studies, the effectiveness of IABP in adjuvant therapy for severe patients with AMI has not been ensured [14,18].

The American College of Cardiology and American Heart Association (ACC/AHA) guidelines recommend IABP for patients with unstable angina and non-ST-elevation myocardial infarction UA/NSTEMI with severe ischemia [3]. However, the curative effect of IABP as a treatment of AMI is still unresolved, and it is not clear whether time and cardiogenic shock (CS) influence its effectiveness. To evaluate the curative effect systematically, we performed a meta-analysis of randomized controlled trials (RCTs) on the treatment of AMI by IABP.

Methods

1. Data sources and search strategy

theThe Medline, EMBASE, Cochrane databases, and related websites were searched without restriction by publication date or publication status; however, only articles published in English were selected. The search keywords included intra-aortic balloon counterpulsation, intra-aortic balloon pump, percutaneous coronary intervention, acute coronary syndrome, acute myocardial infarction, IABP, IABC, PCI, and ACS. The last search was conducted on July 20, 2014.

2. Selection criteria

To ensure the quality of the meta-analysis, the following selection and exclusion criteria were applied to assess the RCTs that were retrieved during the searches. Only published RCTs that enrolled AMI patients treated with drugs or PCI (percutaneous coronary intervention) were eligible. Only studies of IABP as an intervention for circulatory support were included, and only if the methods, study dates, sample size, and results were clearly and completely described. Trials that were non- or incompletely randomized, that included patients with coronary syndromes other than AMI, or patients treated with coronary artery bypass grafting, that compared IABP with other percutaneous circulation support equipment, or with unclear data reporting were excluded.

3. Data extraction and management

In the selected articles, all-cause mortality was the primary endpoint used to assess the curative effect of IABP on AMI. Bleeding was a secondary endpoint used to assess IABP safety. The patients in the selected RCTs were divided into subgroups whether with or without CS to account for treatment effects depending on the patients' condition. Mortality was evaluated in two subgroups depending on follow-up duration: mortality within 2 months (i.e., in-hospital, at 1 month, and at 2 months), and mortality within 6–12 months.

4. Methodology/quality assessment

The RCT quality was assessed independently by two reviewers. The 12 RCTs that were selected were assessed using the Cochrane Collaboration bias risk tool, which considers the following six criteria: proper random sequence generation, concealment of subjects' group allocation, blinding during outcomes assessment, complete recording and reporting of outcomes data, and lack of experimental bias.

5. Statistical analysis

The data were analyzed using Review Manager 5.1. Endpoints were treated as dichotomous outcomes, and odds ratios (ORs) with 95% confidence intervals (CIs) were taken as a statistical indicator of the curative effect and safety of IABP in AMI. When the event of interest did not occur, the treatment effect of that study was treated as not estimable [9].

The Breslow–Day χ^2 test ($p<0.1$) and the I^2 statistic were used to test heterogeneity of the 13 included studies. An I^2 of less than 25%, indicated low, $25\%<I^2<50\%$ moderate, $p>0.1$; and $I^2>50$, a high degree of heterogeneity [4]. When $I^2<50\%$, a fixed-effects Mantel-Haenzel model was used to analyze the data, and when $I^2>50\%$, the DerSimonian and Laird random-effects model was found better than the former model. Publication bias was evaluated using funnel plots [5].

Results

1. Study sample selection characteristics

A total of 641 potentially eligible publications were retrieved during the searches, and 524 articles not associated with treatment of AMI with IABP were excluded by browsing the title or abstract (Figure 1). After further screening, an additional 104 articles were excluded, including 86 non-RCTs, 13 animal experiments, four case reports, and two articles involving other assist devices. The remaining 13 articles satisfied the selection criteria. The 13 studies enrolled 2237 AMI patients; 1112 were treated with IABP (the treatment group) and 1125 patients were not treated with IABP (the control group). The characteristics of the 13 articles are shown in Table 1. In four of the studies, participants in the IABP were AMI patients with CS; however, in the other eight studies, the patients did not have CS.

Acorrding to the PRISMA Statement [6], A flow diagram (Figure 1) and a 27-item checklist (Checklist S1) for transparent reporting of a systematic review were used to included in the papper.

2. Risk of bias within studies

The 13 selected RCTs provided complete dates of conduct and were free of selective reporting of results or risk of bias. However, three of the RCTs [8,17,18] did not clearly describe the methods of randomization or concealment of group allocation (Table 2).

3. Mortality within 2 months

Ten trials with a total of 973 AMI patients reported 2-month mortality. The I^2 statistic showed that study heterogeneity was significant ($p = 0.03$, $I^2 = 53\%$), and thus the random-effects model of DerSimonian and Laird was selected to analyze the data. There was no significant difference in 2-month mortality between the IABP group and the control group (three RCTs enrolled AMI patients with CS (OR = 0.67, 95% CI: 0.28–1.64; $p = 0.39$). Seven RCTs enrolled AMI without CS (OR = 1.60, 95% CI: 0.52–4.90; $p = 0.41$.). (Figure 2).

4. Mortality within 6–12 months

Seven trials, with a total sample size of 1500, reported 6–12-month mortality. The study results did not show significant heterogeneity (P = 0.21, $I^2 = 27\%$), and thus the fixed-effects Mantel–Haenzel model was used for data analysis. The 6-month mortality in the IABP group was not significantly lower than in the control group in the four RCTs that enrolled AMI patients with CS (OR = 0.90, 95% CI: 0.67–1.21; $p = 0.49$). But in the four that enrolled AMI patients without CS, the data showed opposite conclusion(OR = 0.53, 95% CI: 0.30–0.93; $p = 0.03$). (Figure 3). The funnel diagram was proximally symmetrical, which indicated no publication bias (Figure 4).

5. Bleeding events

A total of eight RCTs with a total sample size of 1485 reported bleeding events. The study results did not show significant heterogeneity ($p = 0.85$, $I^2 = 0\%$) and indicated that the risk of bleeding occurring in IABP patients in IABP was higher than in the control group (OR = 1.66, 95% CI: 1.25–2.20; $p<0.01$) (Figure 5).

Discussion

This meta-analysis of 12 RCTs investigating treatment of AMI by IABP indicated that (1)IABP can not reduce within 2 months and 6–12 months mortality of AMI patients with cardiac shock (CS), as well as within 2 months mortality of AMI patients without CS, (2)but can reduce 6–12 months mortality of AMI patients without CS. (3)However, IABP increased the risk of bleeding.

Existing research shows that IABP increases blood supply to the coronary artery and the brain, reduces afterload, and eventually decreases cardiac oxygen consumption [1,2]. It can thus be considered as an adjuvant method for treatment of AMI. The difference in results for short- (1–2 months) and long-term (6–12

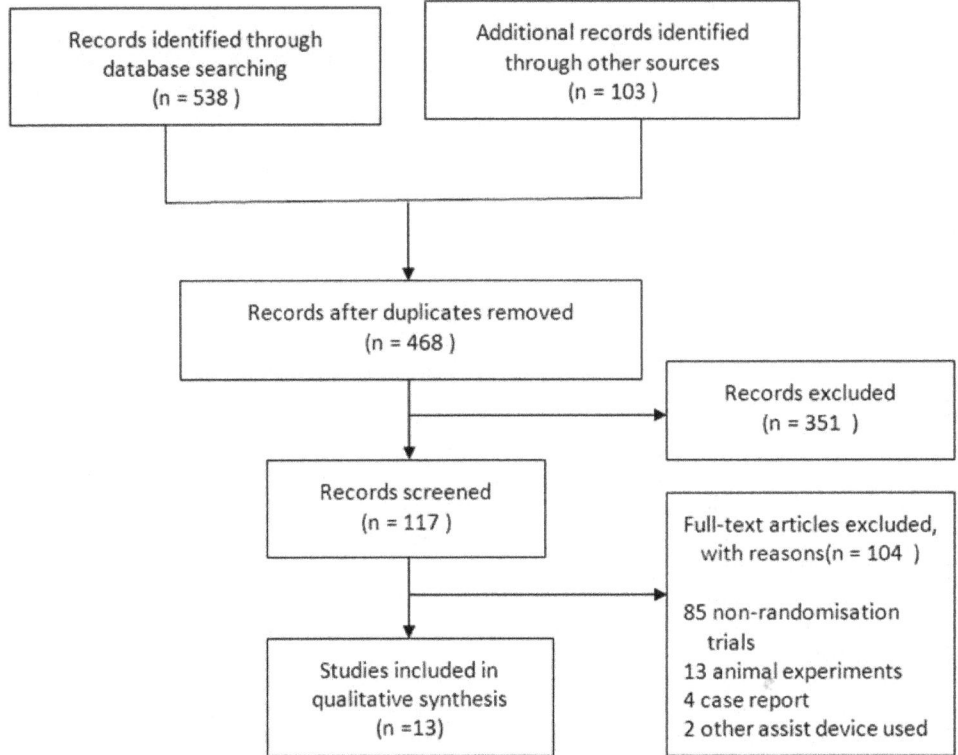

Figure 1. Meta-Analyses statement for trial selection.

months) follow-up indicates that treatment of AMI with IABP may be associated with some slow, compensatory mechanism of myocardial repair, but the specific mechanism is still not clear. A study by Chang [20], showed that in 2 months, the granulation scar tissue in the infarct area changed into connective tissue. In 2–3 months, the infarct area changed into a complete, acellular fibrous scar. These changes in scar tissue are consistent with the effect of IABP on mortality in this meta-analysis and suggest that IABP treatment may be affected by some unknown factors associated with scar formation. More experiments should be conducted to determine the mechanism. Although IABP can reduce AMI patient mortality in the first 6–12 months, it also increases the risk of bleeding. This mechanism is also not clear, thus further studies are needed.

Since 1980s, IABP is widely used in clinic. AMI is commonly seen in internal medicine, and about 7%~10% of AMI patients with CS has high mortality rate, through timely and effective treatment is performed. Coronary artery recanalization is the key to treat AMI, but in theory IABP can be used to better ensure sufficient blood supply and improve cardiac function of patients so as to save more myocardium and eventually further reduce the adverse consequence of AMI for patients. But, in the process of actual clinical research, the role of IABP is still controversial.

SHOCK registered study [21] and NRMI registered study [22] confirm that application of IABP obviously benefits patients. SHOCK research retrospectively analyzes 856 patients AMI combined with cardiac shock and shows that mortality rate in the hospital of IABP group is better than that of non IABP group (50% vs72%, P<0.0001). NRMI study evaluates American 23180 patients with AMI combined with cardiac shock registered, with total mortality of 70%; 31% of the patients are undergone IABP; among patients with venous thrombolysis, the application of IABP

is significantly correlated to case fatality rate (67% vs49%, P<0.05); thrombolysis combined with IABP treatment can reduce the risk of death by 18% (OR0.82; 95%CI 0.72–0.93), but this study also puts forward that application of IABP is not obviously effective in emergency angioplasty(45% vs 47%).

Zeymer [23] retrospectively analyzed 653 cases of patients with acute STEMI and non acute STEMI combined with cardiac shock in 176 European medical centers from May, 2005 to April, 2008, showing only 25% of the patients with IABP in PCI surgery, and there was no significant difference in survival rate between IABP group and non IABP group(OR 1.47; 95% CI 0.97–2.21, P = 0.07). Zeymer [24] carried out a retrospective analysis on 55008 cases of ACS patients (1913 cases combined with shock)with PCI treatment from January, 2006 to December, 2011, among of whom, 487 cases were undergone IABP treatment. The mortality in the hospital for patients with IABP and without IABP was 43.5% and 37.4%, respectively (P = 0.0004), showing the application of IABP is obviously associated with higher fatality rate(OR 1.45,95%CI 1.15–1.84).

Valk [25] retrospectively analyzed 437 AMI patients with IABP from 1999 to 2004 (1990–2004 as the first stage, 1995–1999 as the second stage and 2000–2004 as the third stage), whose results showed that the amount of shock patients in three stages was not different; with the increase of ABP treatment, 30 d case fatality rate was reduced to 26% from 41%; about half of the patients still alive after ten years' follow-up.

In this meta-analysis, major adverse cardiac events (MACEs) were not analyzed because the details of relevant events have not been reported in most published studies. A retrospective study [26] including 1490 AMI patients showed that the occurrence of MACEs in AMI patients with CS was significantly reduced by treatment with IABP (14.5% in the IABP group vs. 35.1% in the

Table 1. Characteristics of the included articles.

Author(Year)	Patients(n)	Gender(male(%))		Mean age(y)		Inclusion criteria	Adjunctive therapy		IABP after AMI(h)	IABP duration(h)	Follow-up time duration(d)
		IABP	Control	IABP	Control		IABP	Control			
Flaherty 1985 [7]	20	9(90.0)	9(90.0)	52.0	52.0	AMI without CS	IABP+TT	TT	5.0±2.6	34±25	60
Gu 2011 [8]	106	29(56.9)	36(65.5)	67.4	66.6	AMI without CS	IABP+PCI	PCI	5.3±1.9	52±17	30;180
Kono 1996 [9]	45	20(87.0)	16(72.7)	54.0	60.0	AMI without CS	IABP+PTCA	PTCA	2.5±0.5	48	21
Li 2007 [10]	39	12(60.0)	12(63.1)	67.4	64.9	AMI with CS	IABP+PCI	PCI	NR	72	360
Ohman 1994 [11]	182	73(75.6)	64(74)	56.0	55.0	AMI without CS	IABP+TT	TT	<24	12	9
Ohman 2005 [12]	57	23(77.0)	20(74.0)	68.0	67.0	AMI with CS	IABP+PCI	PCI	0.5(0.3–0.9), AR	34(24–68)	30;180
Patel 2011 [13]	337	132(82.0)	144(81.8)	56.1	57.7	AMI without CS	IABP+PCI	PCI	3.4(2.4–4.5)	22.1 (16.8–26.1)	180
Perera 2010 [14]	301	122(81.0)	117(78.0)	71.0	71.0	AMI without CS	IABP+PCI	PCI	<24 h, AR	4–24	30;180
Prondzinsky 2010 [15]	40	14(73.6)	17(80.9)	62.1	66.1	AMI with CS	IABP+PCI	PCI	13.91±3.06	96	4
Stone 1997 [16]	437	158(74.9)	170(75.2)	64.7	63.7	AMI without CS	IABP+PTCA	PTCA	12	47.9±28.0	30
Thiele 2013 [17]	595	299(66.9)	296(70.6)	UC	UC	AMI with CS	IABP+PCI	PCI	UC	UC	12
Vijayalakshmi 2007 [18]	33	14(82.3)	14(87.5)	39.8	44.7	AMI without CS	IABP+PCI	PCI	7.1±5.5	48	30
Waksman 1993 [19]	45	14(58.3)	15(71.4)	66.8	67.8	AMI with CS	IABP+TT	TT	3	228	30;180

AR:after randomization; CS:cardiogenic shock; IABP:intra-aortic balloon counterpulsation pump; NR, not reported; PTCA:percutaneous transluminal coronary angioplasty; TT: thrombolytic therapy; U, Unclear.

Table 2. Methodological quality assessment of the included articles.

Author	Random sequence generation (selection bias)	Allocation concealment(selection bias)	Blinding? (performance bias and detection bias)	Incomplete outcome data addressed?	Free of selective reporting? (reporting bias)	Free of other bias?
Flaherty 1985 [7]	Y	Y	Y	N	Y	Y
Gu 2011 [8]	U	U	Y	Y	Y	Y
Kono 1996 [9]	Y	Y	N	Y	Y	Y
Li 2007 [10]	Y	Y	Y	Y	Y	Y
Ohman 1994 [11]	Y	Y	Y	Y	Y	Y
Ohman 2005 [12]	Y	Y	Y	Y	Y	N
Patel 2011 [13]	Y	Y	Y	Y	Y	Y
Perera 2010 [14]	Y	Y	Y	Y	Y	Y
Prondzinsky 2010 [15]	Y	Y	N	Y	Y	Y
Stone 1997 [16]	Y	Y	Y	Y	N	Y
Thiele 2013 [17]	Y	Y	N	Y	Y	Y
Vijayalakshmi 2007 [18]	U	U	N	Y	Y	Y
Waksman 1993 [19]	U	U	N	Y	Y	Y

N:No; U:Unclear; Y:Yes.

control group, $p = 0.009$), and that IABP was also beneficial in AMI patients with decreased left ventricular function. Barron et al. [27] carry out a NRMI-2 study involved 23,180 AMI patients with CS, of whom, 7268 patients were performed with IABP treatment. The result shows that the mortality rate of patients with IABP treatment is significantly lower than that of patients with

thrombolytic therapy (67% vs49%). Unfortunately, most of the published studies were not RCTs. Besides, some studies with large sample sizes have yielded conflicting results [16,28].

Although similar meta-analyses have been published, their conclusions differ from those provided here. In a meta-analysis based on six RCTs (two of which included patients with

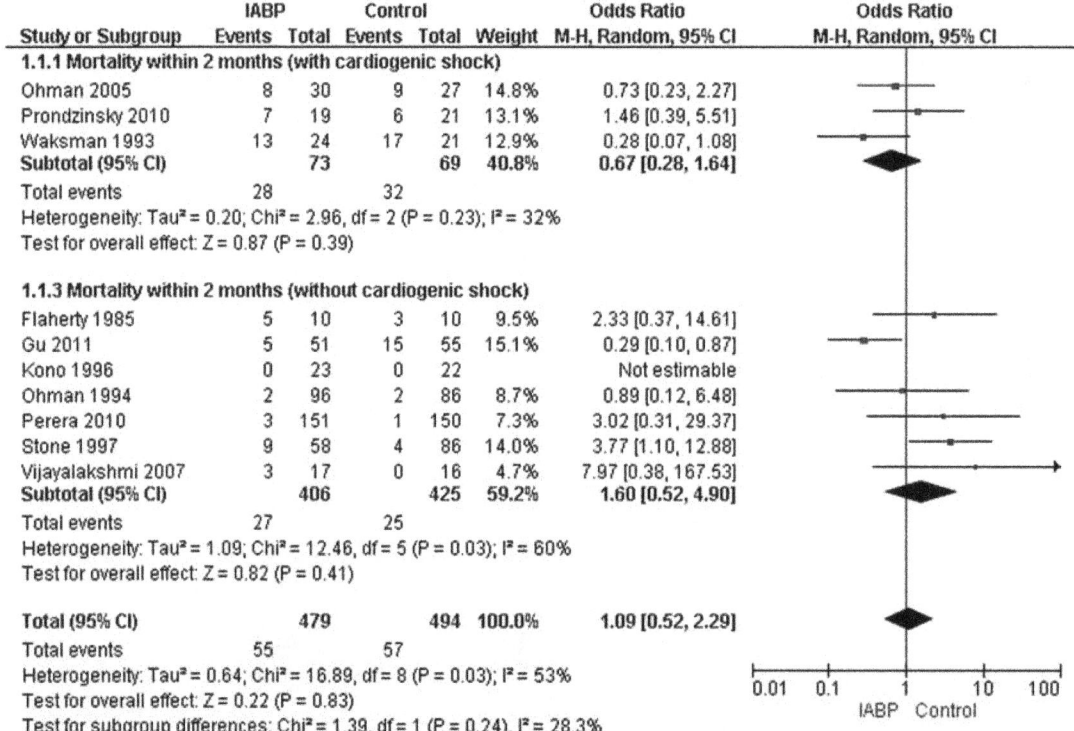

Figure 2. Forest plot of studies evaluating curative effect of IABP in mortality within 2 months.

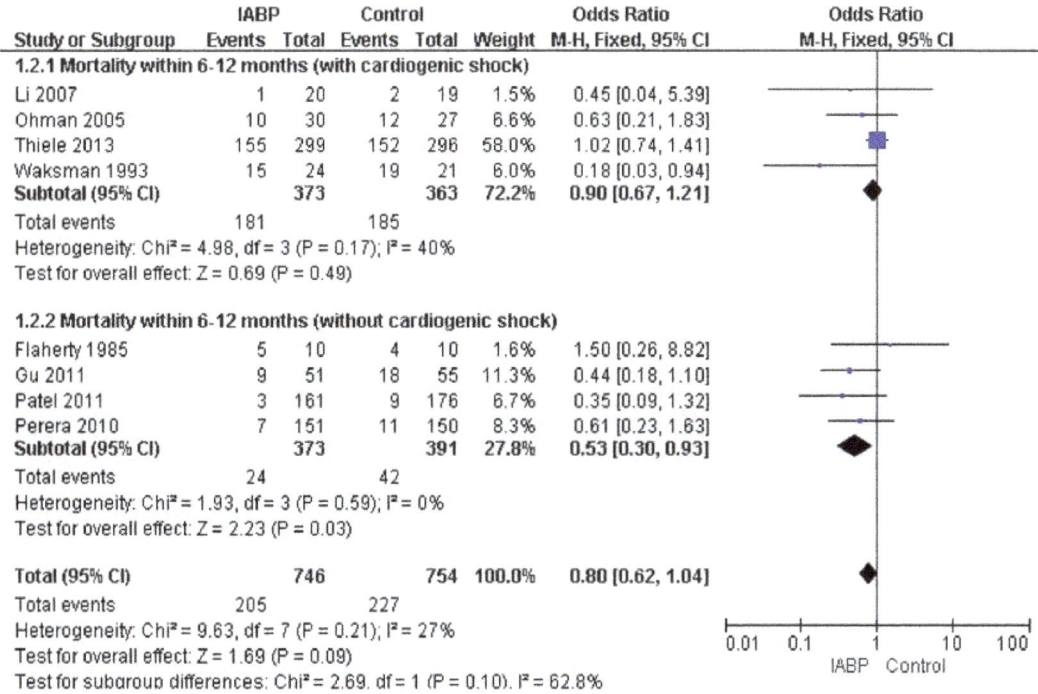

Figure 3. Forest plot of studies evaluating curative effect of IABP in mortality within 6–12 months.

percutaneous left ventricular assist devices in the control group), no convincing benefit was observed with IABP therapy in AMI patients with CS [29]. Another meta-analysis concluded that IABP did not reduce mortality in AMI patients without CS, but the data were not divided into subgroups based on follow-up duration [30]. Briefly, those analyses concluded that IABP might not benefit AMI patients. However, in this analysis, we came to the opposite conclusion when the data were stratified by different durations of follow-up. Without analyzing different follow-up time, a meta-analysis showed that IABP can not improve LVEF or reduce the occurrence of angina or infarction on AMI patients without CS

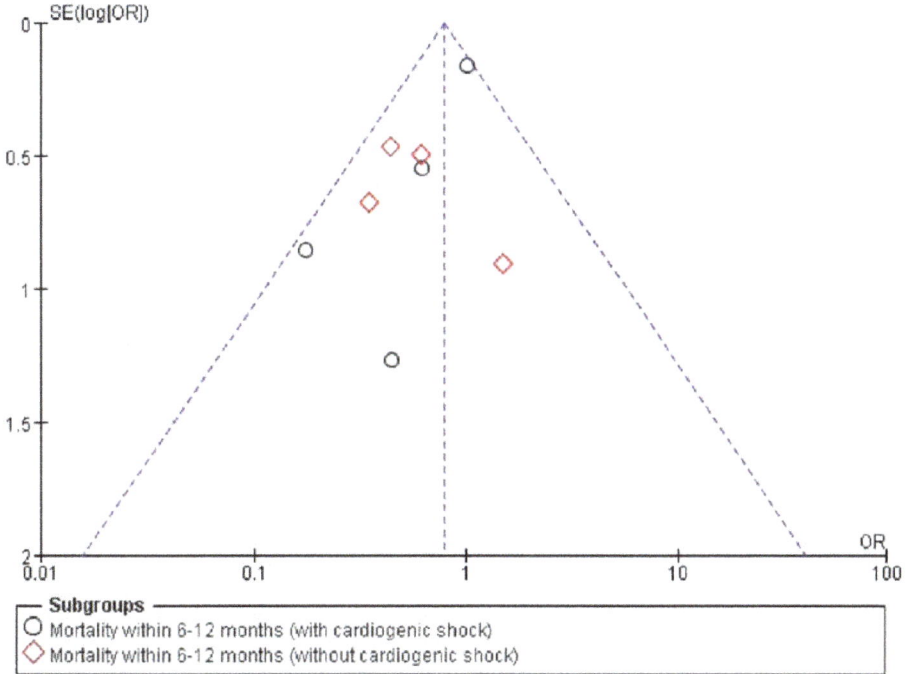

Figure 4. Funnel plot of mortality within 6–12 months.

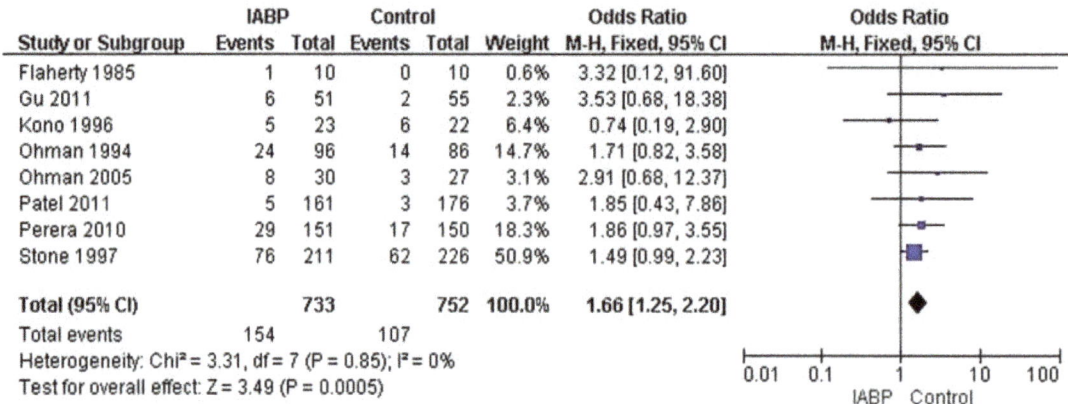

Study or Subgroup	IABP Events	Total	Control Events	Total	Weight	Odds Ratio M-H, Fixed, 95% CI
Flaherty 1985	1	10	0	10	0.6%	3.32 [0.12, 91.60]
Gu 2011	6	51	2	55	2.3%	3.53 [0.68, 18.38]
Kono 1996	5	23	6	22	6.4%	0.74 [0.19, 2.90]
Ohman 1994	24	96	14	86	14.7%	1.71 [0.82, 3.58]
Ohman 2005	8	30	3	27	3.1%	2.91 [0.68, 12.37]
Patel 2011	5	161	3	176	3.7%	1.85 [0.43, 7.86]
Perera 2010	29	151	17	150	18.3%	1.86 [0.97, 3.55]
Stone 1997	76	211	62	226	50.9%	1.49 [0.99, 2.23]
Total (95% CI)		**733**		**752**	**100.0%**	**1.66 [1.25, 2.20]**
Total events	154		107			

Heterogeneity: Chi² = 3.31, df = 7 (P = 0.85); I² = 0%
Test for overall effect: Z = 3.49 (P = 0.0005)

Figure 5. Forest plot of studies evaluating curative effect of IABP in bleeding events.

[31]. However, IABP reduced the mortality of AMI patients with CS, but it increased the incidence of stroke and bleeding.

The present study differs from similar, previously published meta-analyses in that (1) it includes the most recent RCTs; (2) follow-up time was divided into two periods so that the impact of follow-up time can be assessed; and (3) the AMI patients were divided into subgroups with and without CS, thus making it easier to analyze the mechanism of treatment of AMI with IABP.

The present analysis also has certain limitations. (1) The basic therapies for the patients included in the selected studies were different. (2) Both the start-time and duration of IABP differed in the selected studies. (3) The sample sizes of some of the RCTs were relatively small. (4) The quality of some studies was relatively low. (5) The follow-up time in most studies was not sufficiently long. (6) MACEs were not analyzed statistically. To solve these problems, more high-quality clinical studies with longer follow-up time and more detailed records are needed. To confirm the curative effect and safety of IABP in AMI patients, more rigorous studies with larger sample sizes, longer follow-up time and more detailed records should be conducted.

Conclusions

IABP can not reduce within 2 months and 6–12 months mortality of AMI patients with CS, as well as within 2 months mortality of AMI patients without CS, but can reduce 6–12 months mortality of AMI patients without CS. In addition, IABP can increase the risk of bleeding.

Acknowledgments

I would like to express my great gratitude to my colleagues for all their assistance in carrying out this study. I would like to thank Li Wang and Qingzhi Wu for their helpful suggestions.

Author Contributions

Conceived and designed the experiments: LY MZ QC. Performed the experiments: LY MZ. Analyzed the data: LY GL WD. Contributed reagents/materials/analysis tools: LY DK QC. Wrote the paper: LY MZ.

References

1. Kern MJ, Aguirre F, Bach R, Donohe T, Siegel R, et al. (1993) Augmentation of coronary blood flow by intra-aortic balloon pumping in patients after coronary angioplasty. Circulation 87:500–511.
2. Kantrowitz A, Tjønneland S, Freed PS, Phillips SJ, Butner AN, et al. (1968) Initial clinical experience with intraaortic balloon pumping in cardiogenic shock. JAMA 203:113–118.
3. Anderson JL, Adams CD, Antman EM, Bridges CR, Califf RM, et al. (2011) ACC/AHA Practice Guideline.2011 ACCF/AHA focused update incorporated into the ACC/AHA 2007 Guidelines for the management of patients with unstable angina/Non–ST-Elevation myocardial infarction. a report of the American College of Cardiology Foundation/American Heart Association Task Force on Practice Guidelines. Circulation 123:e426–e579.
4. Higgins JP, Thompson SG, Deeks JJ, Altman DG (2003) Measuring inconsistency in meta-analyses. BMJ 327:557–560.
5. Sterne JA, Egger M, Smith GD (2001) Systematic reviews in health care: investigating and dealing with publication and other biases in meta-analysis. BMJ 323:101–105.
6. Moher D, Liberati A, Tetzlaff J, Altman DG, The PRISMA Group (2009) Preferred reporting items for systematic reviews and Meta-Analyses: The PRISMA Statement. PLoS Med 6(7): e1000097. doi:10.1371/journal.pmed.1000097.
7. Flaherty JT, Becker LC, Weiss JL, Brinker JA, Bulkley BH, et al. (1985) Results of a randomized prospective trial of intraaortic balloon counterpulsation and intravenous nitroglycerin in patients with acute myocardial infarction. J Am Coll Cardiol 6:434–446.
8. Gu J, Hu W, Xiao H, Feng X, Song Z, et al. (2011) Prophylactic intra-aortic balloon pump reduces C-reactive protein levels and early mortality in high-risk

patients undergoing percutaneous coronary intervention. Acta Cardiol 66:499–504.
9. Kono T, Morita H, Nishina T, Fujita M, Onaka H, et al. (1996) Aortic counterpulsation may improve late patency of the occluded coronary artery in patients with early failure of thrombolytic therapy. J Am Coll Cardiol 28:876–881.
10. Li J, Xue H, Wang B, Zhang HY, Yin L, et al. (2007) Effect of prolonged intra-aortic balloon pumping in patients with cardiogenic shock following acute myocardial infarction. Medical Science Monitor 23:CR270–274.
11. Ohman EM, George BS, White CJ, Kern MJ, Gurbel PA, et al. (1994) Use of aortic counterpulsation to improve sustained coronary artery patency during acute myocardial infarction. Results of a randomized trial. The Randomized IABP Study Group. Circulation 90:792–799.
12. Ohman EM, Nanas J, Stomel RJ, Leesa MA, Nielsen DWT, et al. (2005) Thrombolysis and counterpulsation to improve survival in myocardial infarction complicated by hypotension and suspected cardiogenic shock or heart failure: results of the TACTICS Trial. Journal of Thrombosis and Thrombolysis 19:33–39.
13. Patel MR, Smalling RW, Thiele H, Barnhart HX, Zhou Y, et al. (2011) Intra-aortic balloon counterpulsation and infarct size in patients with acute anterior myocardial infarction without shock:The CRISP AMI randomized trial. JAMA 306:1329–1337.
14. Perera D, Stables R, Thomas M, Booth J, Pitt M, et al. (2010) Elective intra-aortic balloon counterpulsation during high-risk percutaneous coronary intervention a randomized controlled trial. JAMA 304:867–874.
15. Prondzinsky R, Lemm H, Swyter M, Wegener N, Unverzagt S, et al. (2010) Intra-aortic balloon counterpulsation in patients with acute myocardial

infarction complicated by cardiogenic shock: the prospective, randomized IABP SHOCK Trial for attenuation of multiorgan dysfunction syndrome. Person-Centered and Experiential Psychotherapies 38:152–160.

16. Stone GW, Marsalese D, Brodie BR, Griffin JJ, Donohue B, et al. (1997) A prospective, randomized evaluation of prophylactic intraaortic balloon counterpulsation in high risk patients with acute myocardial infarction treated with primary angioplasty fn1. J Am Coll Cardiol 29:1459–1467.

17. Thiele H, Zeymer U, Neuman F, Ferenc M, Olbrich H, et al. (2013) Intra-aortic balloon counterpulsation in acute myocardial infarction complicated by cardiogenic shock (IABP-SHOCK II): final 12 month results of a randomised, open-label trial. Lancet 382:1638–1645.

18. Vijayalakshmi K, Kunadian B, Whittaker VJ, Wright RA, Hall JA, et al. (2007) Intra-aortic counterpulsation does not improve coronary flow early after PCI in a high-risk group of patients: observations from a randomized trial to explore its mode of action. J Invasive Cardiol 19:339–346.

19. Waksman R, Weiss AT, Gotsman MS, Hasin Y (1993) Intra-aortic balloon counterpulsation improves survival in cardiogenic shock complicating acute myocardial infarction. Eur Heart J. 14:71–74.

20. Chang J; Nair V; Luk A, Butany J (2013) Pathology of myocardial infarction. Diagnostic Histopathology 19:7–12.

21. Sanborn TA, Sleeper LA, Bates ER, Jacobs AK, Boland J, et al. (2000) Impact of thrombolysis, intra-aortic balloon pump counterpulsation, and their combination in cardiogenic shock complicating acute myocardial infarction: a report from the SHOCK Trial Registry. Should we emergently revascularize Occluded Coronaries for cardiogenic shock? J Am Coll Cardiol 36(3suppl A):1123–1129.

22. Barron HV, Every NR, Parsons LS, Angeja B, Goldberg RJ, et al. (2001) The use of intra-aortic balloon counterpulsation in patients with cardiogenic shock complicating acute myocardial infarction: data from the National Registry of Myocardial Infarction 2. Am Heart J 141:933–939.

23. Zeymer U, Bauer T, Hamm C, Zahn R, Weidinger F, et al. (2011) Use and impact of intra-aortic balloon pump on mortality in patients with acute myocardial infarction complicated by cardiogenic shock: results of the Euro Heart Survey on PCI. Euro Intervention 7:437–441.

24. Zeymer U, Hochadel M, Hauptmann KE, Wiegand K, Schuhmacher B, et al. (2013) Intra-aortic balloon pump in patients with acute myocardial infarction complicated by cardiogenic shock: results of the ALKK-PCI registry. Clin Res Cardiol 102:223–227.

25. Valk SDA, Cheng JM, den Uil CA, Lagrand WK, van der Ent M, et al. (2011) Encouraging survival rates in patients with acute myocardial infarction treated with an intra-aortic balloon pump. Neth Heart J 19:112–118.

26. Brodie BR, Stuckey TD, Hansen C, Muncy D (1999) Intra-aortic balloon counterpulsation before primary percutaneous transluminal coronary angioplasty reduces catheterization laboratory events in high-risk patients with acute myocardial infarction. Am J Cardiol 84:18–23.

27. Barron HV, Every NR, Parsons LS, Angeja B, Goldberg RJ, et al. (2001) The use of intra-aortic balloon counterpulsation in patients with cardiogenic shock complicating acute myocardial infarction: Data from the National Registry of Myocardial Infarction 2. Am Heart J 141:933–939.

28. Van't Hof AW, Liem AI, Boer MJ, Hoorntje JC, Suryapranata H, et al. (1999) A randomized comparison of intra-aortic balloon pumping after primary coronary angioplasty in high risk patients with acute myocardial infarction. Eur Heart J 20:659–665.

29. Unverzagt S, Machemer MT, Solms A, Thiele H, Burkhoff D, et al. (2011) Intra-aortic balloon pump counterpulsation (IABP) for myocardial infarction complicated by cardiogenic shock. Cochrane Database Of Systematic Reviews (Online) 7. Available: http://onlinelibrary.wiley.com/doi/10.1002/14651858. CD007398.pub2/abstract. Assessed 19 July 2010.

30. Cassese S, Waha A, Ndrepepa G, Ranftl S, King L, et al. (2012) Intra-aortic balloon counterpulsation in patients with acute myocardial infarction without cardiogenic shock. A meta-analysis of randomized trials. Am Heart J 164:58–65.

31. Bahekar A, Singh M, Singh S, Bhuriya R, Ahmad K, et al. (2012) Cardiovascular outcomes using intra-aortic balloon pump in high-risk acute myocardial infarction with or without cardiogenic shock: A Meta-Analysis. J Cardiovasc Pharmacol Ther 17:144–156.

7

Chronic Total Occlusions in Sweden – A Report from the Swedish Coronary Angiography and Angioplasty Registry (SCAAR)

Truls Råmunddal[1][*][9], **Loes Hoebers**[2][9], **Jose P. S. Henriques**[2], **Christian Dworeck**[1], **Oskar Angerås**[1], **Jacob Odenstedt**[1], **Dan Ioanes**[1], **Göran Olivecrona**[3], **Jan Harnek**[3], **Ulf Jensen**[4], **Mikael Aasa**[4], **Risto Jussila**[4], **Stefan James**[5], **Bo Lagerqvist**[5], **Göran Matejka**[1], **Per Albertsson**[1], **Elmir Omerovic**[1]

1 Department of Cardiology, Sahlgrenska University Hospital, Gothenburg, Sweden, 2 Department of Cardiology, Academic Medical Center, Amsterdam, The Netherlands, 3 Department of Coronary Heart Disease, Skåne University Hospital, Scania, Sweden, 4 Department of Cardiology, Stockholm South General Hospital, Stockholm, Sweden, 5 Department of Medical Sciences, Uppsala University, Uppsala, Sweden

Abstract

Introduction: Evidence for the current guidelines for the treatment of patients with chronic total occlusions (CTO) in coronary arteries is limited. In this study we identified all CTO patients registered in the Swedish Coronary Angiography and Angioplasty Registry (SCAAR) and studied the prevalence, patient characteristics and treatment decisions for CTO in Sweden.

Methods and Results: Between January 2005 and January 2012, 276,931 procedures (coronary angiography or percutaneous coronary intervention) were performed in 215,836 patients registered in SCAAR. We identified all patients who had 100% luminal diameter stenosis known or assumed to be ≥3 months old. After exclusion of patients with previous coronary artery bypass graft (CABG) surgery or coronary occlusions due to acute coronary syndrome, we identified 16,818 CTO patients. A CTO was present in 10.9% of all coronary angiographies and in 16.0% of patients with coronary artery disease. The majority of CTO patients were treated conservatively and PCI of CTO accounted for only 5.8% of all PCI procedures. CTO patients with diabetes and multivessel disease were more likely to be referred to CABG.

Conclusion: CTO is a common finding in Swedish patients undergoing coronary angiography but the number of CTO procedures in Sweden is low. Patients with CTO are a high-risk subgroup of patients with coronary artery disease. SCAAR has the largest register of CTO patients and therefore may be valuable for studies of clinical importance of CTO and optimal treatment for CTO patients.

Editor: Ingo Ahrens, University Hospital Medical Centre, Germany

Funding: The SCAAR registry is sponsored by the Swedish Health Authorities only and is independent of commercial funding. No current funding sources for this study. The funders had no role in study design, data collection and analysis, decision to publish, or preparation of the manuscript.

Competing Interests: Dr Stefan James has during the last 3 years received institutional research grants from Medtronic, Terumo Inc,Vascular Solutions and served as an advisory board member for Medtronic. Dr Jose P.S. Henriques has received unrestricted research grant from Abbott Vascular. Dr Elmir Omerovic serves as an advisory board member for Astra Zeneca and has received lecturing fees from Medtronic and Astra Zeneca. All other co-authors have no disclosures or potential conflicts of interest.

* Email: truls@wlab.gu.se

9 These authors contributed equally to this work.

Introduction

Chronic total occlusions (CTO) are difficult to treat with percutaneous coronary intervention (PCI) [1]. Revascularization of CTO demands expert skills, longer procedural time and is associated with higher procedural risks such as coronary perforation, contrast nephropathy, radiation exposure, and loss of collateral circulation [1,2]. According to the European and American guidelines, PCI of CTO has class-IIa recommendation (weight of evidence in favour of the treatments usefulness/efficacy) [3,4] but this recommendation is based on small retrospective studies and on expert consensus.

The true prevalence of a CTO in the general population is unknown and few studies have addressed this question. In observational studies, a CTO was found in approximately one third of the patients referred for coronary angiography [5–7]. However, these studies were based on low number of patients and participating hospitals, and may therefore be prone to selection bias. To date, no epidemiological study has investigated the prevalence and clinical characteristics of CTO patients at the nationwide level.

The Swedish Coronary Angiography and Angioplasty Registry (SCAAR) is a prospective national registry that collects data about all patient undergoing coronary angiography and PCI in Sweden [8]. Therefore, we identified all CTO patients registered in SCAAR and studied prevalence, patient characteristics and treatment decision for CTO in Sweden.

Methods

Swedish Coronary Angiography and Angioplasty Registry (SCAAR)

The SCAAR registry was established in 1999 after the unification of Swedish Coronary Angiography registry (Acta Coronaria) and the Swedish Coronary Angioplasty registry (SCAP). SCAAR, which is a part of the national SWEDEHEART registry, holds data on all consecutive patients from all centres that perform coronary angiography and PCI in Sweden. The registry is independent of commercial funding and is sponsored by the Swedish Health Authorities only. The technology has been developed and administered by the Uppsala Clinical Research Center. Since 2001, SCAAR has been Internet-based, with recording of data online through an Internet interface in the catheterization laboratory; data are transferred in an encrypted format to a central server at the Uppsala Clinical Research Center.

In total, there are 30 hospitals with cardiac catheterization facilities in Sweden of which 9 are university hospitals. In SCAAR, a coronary angiography procedure is described by approximately 50 variables while a PCI procedure allows for is described by approximately 200 variables. The information about clinical characteristics and procedural details is entered into the registry immediately after the procedure by the PCI physician after the review of clinical information.

Ethics statement

The study was approved by the regional ethical review board of Gothenburg University, Gothenburg,Sweden. The regional ethical review board waived the need for written informed consent from the participants according to Swedish legislation and because data were de-identified and anonymized before analysis.

Definitions

We defined CTO as 100% luminal diameter stenosis and the absence of antegrade flow known or assumed to be ≥3 months duration [6,9,10]. Coronary artery disease was defined as a luminal narrowing ≥50% on angiography. Procedural success after PCI treatment of the coronary lesion is defined as residual stenosis <50%, decreased grade of stenosis after intervention by at least 20%, normal blood flow and no serious complications.

Study cohort

We used two different methods to identify CTO patients in SCAAR between January 2005 and January 2012.

The first method is based on the information about %-luminal stenosis at the level of coronary segments that was introduced in 2005. From this date onwards, the information derived from a diagnostic coronary angiogram can also be used to determine if a coronary segment was totally occluded. In order to differentiate between acute and chronic occlusions, we excluded patients who underwent a procedure for acute coronary syndrome in whom the occlusion was located in the same coronary artery as the culprit vessel. Furthermore, we excluded patients who underwent a procedure in the same vessel within the previous 3 months. The CTO patients identified by this method constitute the *coronary segment subcohort*.

The second method is based on the separate variable by which PCI operators classify a treated occlusion either as a chronic occlusion ≥3 months duration or as an acute/subacute occlusion ≤3 months duration.

The patients with previous coronary artery bypass graft (CABG) surgery were excluded from analysis as the patency of the graft could not be determined. The study was scrutinised and approved by the ethics board according to the Swedish law and regulations.

Total CTO cohort

The total CTO cohort contains all CTO patients identified by either of the two methods (**Figure 1**). Patients and procedures in which the same CTO lesion was registered through both methods or at multiple occasions were identified and duplicate observations were excluded from the analysis. For each patient, the procedure where the CTO was observed first was selected.

Coronary segment subcohort

We also present data from the subcohort of patients who were identified according to whether they had a 100% luminal stenosis and considered to be a CTO based on the above mentioned inclusion criteria. We compared patient characteristics and treatment decisions between patients with significant coronary artery disease in whom a CTO was observed or not. Prevalence of a CTO was calculated only from the coronary segment subcohort and in relation to three different denominators: the number of unique procedures, the number of unique patients and the number of unique patients with significant coronary artery disease.

Validation of CTO

Validation of the CTO definition was performed in a subgroup of 955 patients from one university hospital (Sahlgrenska University Hospital) and from three county hospitals (Norra Älvsborgs Hospital, Borås Hospital, Skövde Hospital). This subgroup represents 5.7% of all identified CTO patients in SCAAR in the study period. The patients were randomly selected by means of random number generator using Stata software (Version 12.1, StataCorp, College Station, Texas, USA). The validation procedure was conducted by a panel consisting of five experienced interventional cardiologists. The panellists examined individual coronary angiograms according to a monitoring plan defined in advance. Each angiogram was evaluated in regard to whether the patient had previous CABG, whether the treated occlusion was ≥3 months old and whether 100% segmental stenosis on angiogram was an occlusion ≥3 months old. The results from the validation procedure were then compared to the data entered in SCAAR.

Statistical analysis

Differences in baseline characteristics between the groups were tested by the χ^2 test for categorical variables while Mann–Whitney U test and Kruskal-Wallis test were used for comparison of continuous non-normally distributed variables. We used Shapiro-Wilks test to test for normal distribution. Tests for trends were made using linear contrasts of means in a one-way analysis of variance model for numerical data and the Armitage-Cohrane trend test for categorical data. We used logistic regression with test for linear trend to evaluate whether annual incidence of CTO and success rate for PCI of CTO changed during the study period. Statistical significance was defined as a P-value<0.05. All analyses were performed using Stata software (Version 13.1, StataCorp, College Station, Texas, USA).

Results

Prevalence of CTO in Sweden

As of January 2012, 497,572 procedures (coronary angiographies and PCIs) performed in 348,863 patients were registered in SCAAR. The numbers of PCIs and coronary angiographies

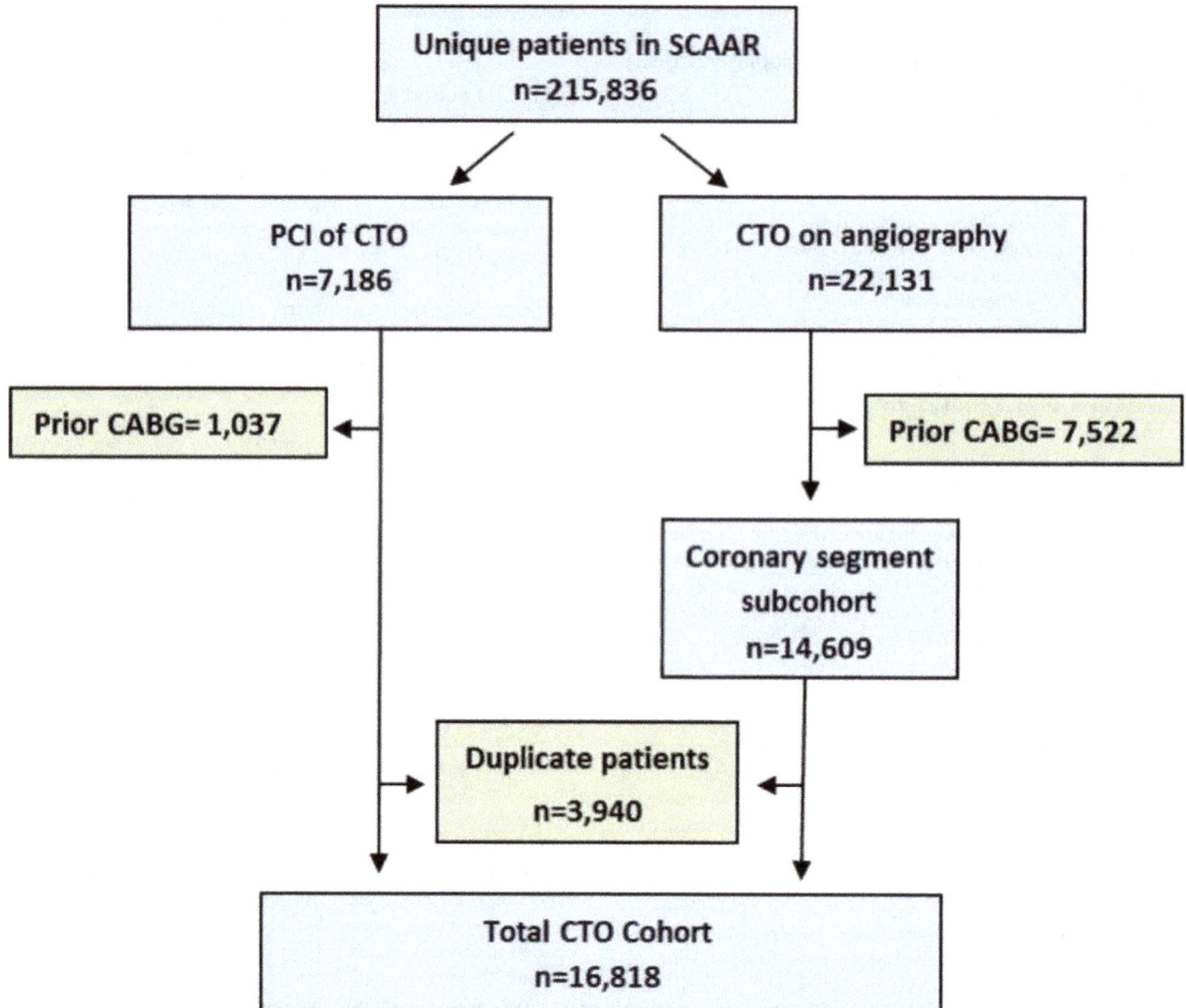

Figure 1. Flow chart for identification and selection of CTO patients in SCAAR. Based on the selection methods we have defined two CTO groups. The first group - *the total CTO cohort*- contains all CTO patients recognized by one or both methods during the period. The second group is the subcohort that contains the patients in whom a CTO was identified through the %-luminal stenosis on the coronary segments – *the coronary segment subcohort*.

increased since 1999 (**Figure 2**). The annual rate of PCIs for CTO remained low (~1200 in 2011).

Between January 2005 and January 2012, Swedish interventionalists completed 276,931 procedures in 215,836 patients. The total number of CTO patients without previous CABG during the same period was 16,818 and these patients constitute the total CTO cohort (**Figure 1**).

Information about age of the treated CTO was missing in 0.8% (n = 1077) of all procedures. Of the 134,087 reported PCIs, 7,816 (5.8%) involved the treatment of a CTO. These procedures were performed in 29 different hospitals on 7,186 unique patients of whom 6,149 without prior CABG. Almost half (43%) of all CTO procedures were performed at university hospitals. Data on procedural success was missing in 12 procedures (0.2%). The overall success rate was 53.1%. The annual success rate did not change significantly during the study period with 54.4% in 2005 and 56.6% in 2012 (OR 1.02, 95% CI 0.99–1.06; P = 0.15 test for linear trend).

Complete information about luminal %-stenosis was available in 160,159 (57.8%) angiographies of which 144,744 were from in patients without previous CABG. A CTO was observed in 10.6% of angiographies from 126,745 patients. Of these patients, 14,609 had at least one CTO resulting in a prevalence of 11.5%. Coronary artery disease was diagnosed in 91,154 patients of which 16.0% had a CTO. In patients who underwent multiple procedures, the CTO was diagnosed on the first diagnostic angiogram in 90% of the cases. The annual number of diagnosed CTO in patients undergoing coronary angiography decreased gradually by 25% from 11.5% in 2005 to 8.6% in 2012 (OR 0.97; 95% CI 0.96–0.98; P<0.001 test for linear trend). In patients with significant coronary artery disease, CTO decreased by 12% from 17.2 in 2005 to 15.1 in 2012 (OR 0.95; 95% CI 0.94–0.96; P< 0.001 test for linear trend).

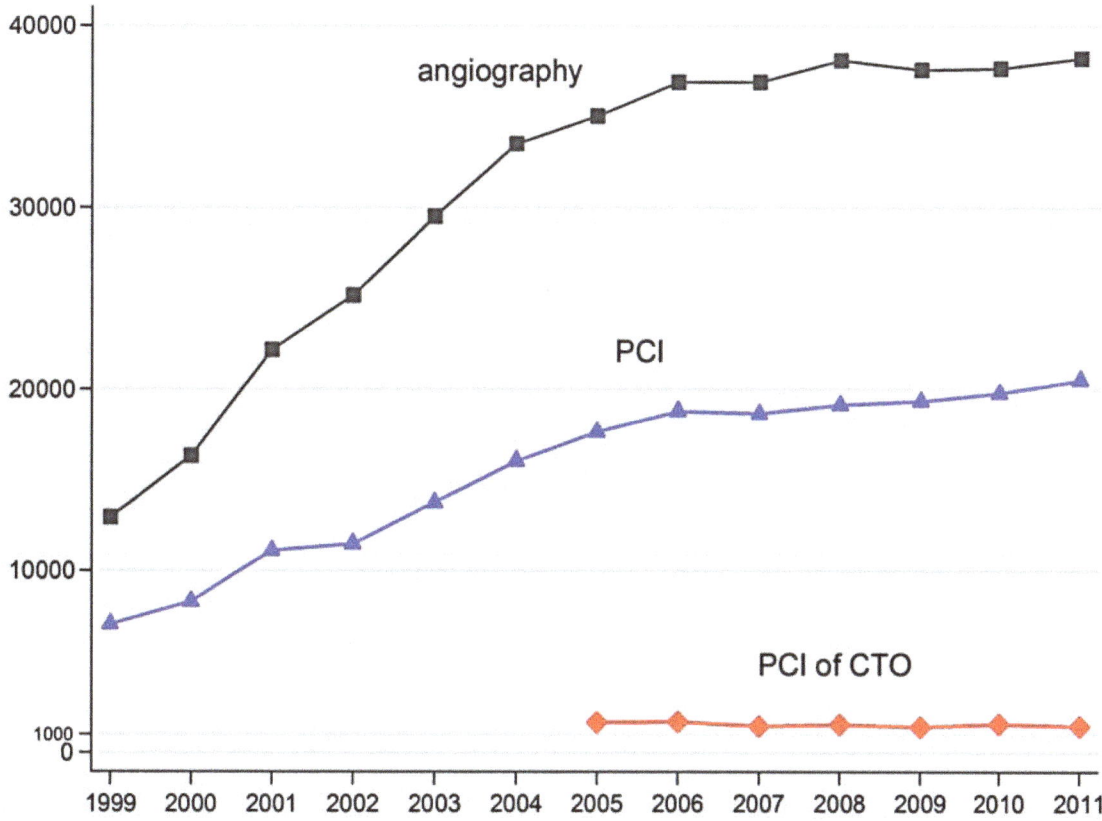

Figure 2. Annual number of coronary angiographies, PCI's, and PCI's performed in CTO patients in Sweden reported in SCAAR since 1999.

Patient characteristics

The clinical characteristics of all CTO patients - the total CTO cohort - registered in SCAAR since 2005 are summarized in **Table 1**. The majority of CTO patients were male. The high occurrence of previous MI (37%) and the presence of traditional cardiovascular risk factors make CTO patients a high-risk population.

Table 2 shows the baseline demographic and angiographic characteristics of patients with coronary artery disease stratified for the presence of a CTO on angiography (coronary segment subcohort). CTO patients were more often males and were more likely to have risk factors including previous MI. In addition, the extent of coronary artery disease was more severe in CTO patients with more multivessel and left main disease. Although CTO was diagnosed in the majority of cases during a coronary angiography for stable angina, a substantial proportion was diagnosed in patients with acute coronary syndrome. Furthermore, patients with a CTO more often presented in cardiogenic shock at presentation for STEMI compared to patients without a CTO. The CTO was more frequently located in the right coronary artery (RCA) followed by the left anterior descending artery (LAD) and left circumflex artery (LCx) (**Figure 3**). In approximately 14%, CTOs were observed in more than one vessel of which only 0.1% included the left main.

Treatment of CTO patients

Table 3 shows the differences in baseline demographic and angiographic characteristics of CTO patients identified through the coronary segment stenosis, according to the received treatment at baseline. After diagnosis, the majority of the CTO patients (56%) received medical treatment only. The CTO patients who received invasive treatment were evenly distributed between PCI (22.3%) and referral for CABG (21.7%). CTO patients, who received medical treatment only, had more often previous MI, presented more often with STEMI, had a lower creatinine clearance and had less severe angina symptoms in comparison to the patients who were treated invasively for a CTO. Patients who were referred for CABG were more often male with a higher prevalence of cardiovascular risk factors including diabetes, had less often previous MI or PCI, presented more often with stable angina and suffered more frequently from extensive coronary artery disease than CTO patients treated with PCI. CTO patients treated for stable angina received medical treatment in 41.6%, PCI in 20.6% and CABG in 37.8%. CTO patients who were treated for acute coronary syndrome received medical treatment in 28.6%, PCI in 71.2%, and were referred to CABG in 0.2%. Procedure-related complications were reported in 5.4% CTO patients treated with PCI. The following complications were reported: death (0%), major bleeding (1.3%), stroke (0.3%), pericardial tamponade (0.4%) renal insufficiency (0.7%), emergency PCI (0.1%), emergency CABG (0%), procedure-related MI (1.1%), anaphylactic reaction (0.1%), other (1.4%)

Validation of CTO

The validation analysis revealed 36 (3.8%) erroneously classified patients. Of these, 18 patients did not have a 100% occluded coronary artery on the coronary angiogram. Another 5 patients

Table 1. Baseline characteristics of the total CTO cohort in SCAAR at the time of diagnosis based on data collected during the period 2005–2012.

	All CTO patients (n = 16,818)	Missing %
Male (%)	77.5	0.0
Age (median, IQR)	68 (60–76)	0.2
Diabetes (%)	23.9	1.0
Hypertension (%)	61.9	2.5
Hyperlipidemia (%)	62.7	2.9
Smoking status (%)		6.2
Current smoker	19.9	
Previous smoker	40.2	
Previous MI (%)	37.2	3.8
Previous PCI (%)	18.4	0.1
Cardiogenic shock (%)*	10.2	1.2
Creatinine Clearance (ml/min)	81 (61–104)	28.2
CCS class (%)**		7.0
I	9.0	
II	52.2	
III	37.4	
IV	1.4	
Indication (%)		0.0
Stable CAD	45.5	
Unstable CAD/NSTEMI	27.5	
STEMI	14.3	
Other	12.7	
Extent of CAD (%)		1.1
1 vessel	20.4	
2 vessel	35.1	
3 vessel	36.1	
Left main disease***	8.4	

CAD: coronary artery disease, CCS: Canadian cardiovascular society, CTO: chronic total occlusion, IQR: inter quartile range, MI: myocardial infarction, (N)STEMI: (non-)ST-elevation myocardial infarction, PCI: percutaneous coronary intervention.
* Cardiogenic shock only displayed for the indication STEMI.
**CCS class only displayed for the indication stable CAD.
*** Left main (LM) disease includes: LM+1 vessel, LM+2 vessel and LM+3 vessel.

had prior CABG and 13 patients had acute or subacute coronary occlusions.

Discussion

In this study, we identified and studied 16,818 CTO patients in SCAAR. We found CTO in every tenth patient undergoing coronary angiography, and that the prevalence of CTO in Sweden decreased by one quarter in these patients between January 2005 and January 2012.

The true prevalence of a CTO in the general population is unknown and not well studied. In a few older studies based on small populations, CTO prevalence was 35% [7] and 52% [5] in patients with significant coronary artery disease. In a recent study from Canada based on 1697 patients, CTO prevalence was 14.7% in all patients undergoing angiography [6]. However, our study shows that the prevalence of CTO was 11.5% in Sweden. The reason for the difference in CTO prevalence between Sweden and other countries may be due to selection bias. While all previous studies were based on selected and relatively small populations,

SCAAR holds information from all hospitals that perform coronary angiography and PCI in Sweden which reduces selection bias. Another explanation may be that prevalence of CTO differs between the countries due to variance in severity of coronary artery disease, treatment algorithms for acute coronary syndromes and organization of health care system [11].

Our study shows that CTO patients are a high-risk population with more traditional cardiovascular risk factors, multivessel disease, history of MI and PCI, which is in accordance with previous reports [1,6,9]. Furthermore, a substantial number (14%) of patients had multiple CTO's in separate vessels.

Majority of CTO patients had stable angina but approximately 40% had acute coronary syndrome at the time when CTO was diagnosed. Overall, 56% of the CTO patients were treated with medical treatment initially. The remaining patients were evenly distributed between percutaneous and surgical revascularization similar to the Canadian study [9]. The success rate for CTO procedures in all Swedish hospitals was 53% which is lower than 70% and 80% reported by others [2,6,12]. However, the success

Table 2. Baseline characteristics of patients from coronary segment subcohort with coronary artery disease, stratified for the presence of a CTO observed on angiography.

	CTO observed (n = 14,609)	Missing %	CTO not observed (n = 76,545)	Missing %	P-value
Male gender (%)	77.7	0	70.6	0.0	<0.01
Age (median, IQR)	68 (61–76)	0.2	68 (60–75)	0.2	<0.01
Diabetes (%)	24.0	1.0	18.6	0.8	<0.01
Hypertension (%)	62.0	2.4	52.5	2.0	<0.01
Hyperlipidemia (%)	61.9	2.8	44.4	2.5	<0.01
Smoking status (%)		5.8		5.5	<0.01
Current smoker	20.0		21.6		
Previous smoker	40.0		35.0		
Previous MI (%)	37.0	3.8	16.5	2.3	<0.01
Previous PCI (%)	17.5	0.1	10.7	0.05	<0.01
Cardiogenic shock(%)*	10.1	1.0	3.5	1.3	<0.01
Creatinine Clearance	80	28.2	81	34.2	<0.01
(ml/min)	(60–103)		(62–103)		
CCS class (%)**		6.9		5.5	0.19
I	9.3		9.6		
II	53.4		54.7		
III	36.0		34.5		
IV	1.3		1.2		
Indication (%)		0		0	<0.01
Stable CAD	44.5		17.1		
Unstable CAD/NSTEMI	26.3		49.6		
STEMI	15.1		26.0		
Other	14.0		7.3		
Extent of CAD (%)		1.5		1.2	<0.01
1 vessel	17.4		48.7		
2 vessel	35.1		25.9		
3 vessel	38.3		17.2		
Left main disease***	9.2		8.2		

CAD: coronary artery disease, CCS: Canadian cardiovascular society, CTO: chronic total occlusion, IQR: inter quartile range, MI: myocardial infarction, (N)STEMI: (non-)ST-elevation myocardial infarction, PCI: percutaneous coronary intervention.
* Cardiogenic shock only displayed for the indication STEMI.
**CCS class only displayed for the indication stable CAD.
*** Left main (LM) disease includes: LM+1 vessel, LM+2 vessel and LM+3 vessel.

rate in this study is based on all CTO procedures performed in our country rather than in a single hospital or smaller registries in other studies. The average success of 53% in SCAAR is unlikely to be representative for low- versus high-volume CTO centers [2,10]. Among the 30 hospitals reporting to SCAAR there are only a few high-volume centres with a dedicated CTO program and less than half of the CTO procedures in Sweden were performed at university hospitals. Some evidence suggest that procedural success is closely related to operator experience [13]. However, the recommendation that CTO procedures should be concentrated to dedicated high-volume hospitals needs stronger evidence.

Although CTO patients are common in clinical work, the evidence for the current guidelines and clinical practice is limited. The need for randomized clinical trials in this patient population is pressing; however, only a few such trials are initiated and on-going [12,14]. Until evidence from randomized trials becomes available we will need to identify and utilize the information available from

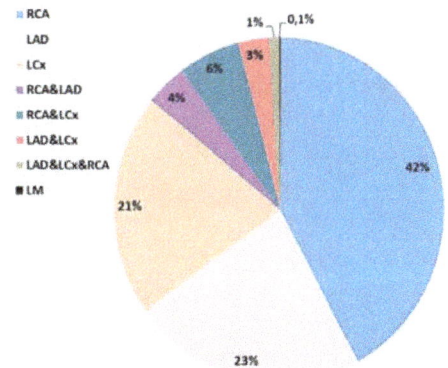

Figure 3. Coronary location of CTO observed at angiography.
RCA = right coronary artery, LAD = left descending coronary artery, LCx = left circumflex coronary artery, LM = left main.

Table 3. Baseline characteristics of CTO patients from coronary segment subcohort according to the treatment strategy.

	No PCI of CTO (n=8,182)		PCI of CTO (n=3,251)		Referral for CABG (n=3,172)		
	(%)	Missing (%)	(%)	Missing (%)	(%)	Missing (%)	P-value
Male gender	76.2	0	76.5	0	82.9	0	<0.01
Age (median, IQR)	69 (61–77)	0.2	66 (59–74)	0.2	68 (61–74)	0.2	<0.01
Diabetes	24.0	1.1	21.0	1.2	26.9	0.4	<0.01
Hypertension	61.6	3.0	59.8	2.3	65.2	1.5	<0.01
Hyperlipidemia	58.6	3.4	60.2	2.7	71.2	1.3	<0.01
Smoking status		7.0		5.0		3.6	<0.01
Current smoker	21.4		20.7		15.5		
Previous smoker	39.4		39.5		42.1		
Previous MI	41.3	4.1	33.4	3.5	29.4	3.2	<0.01
Previous PCI	19.9	0.1	20.3	0.2	8.3	0.03	<0.01
Cardiogenic Shock**	10.0	1.0	10.4	0.9	0	0	0.84
Creatinine Clearance (ml/min)	77 (57–101)	31.6	85 (65–109)	26.1	82 (64–102)	21.8	<0.01
CCS class*		7.1		4.6		7.8	<0.01
I	13.2		8.6		5.3		
II	55.2		56.3		49.8		
III	30.3		34.3		43.3		
IV	1.4		0.8		1.6		
Indication		0		0		0	<0.01
Stable CAD	33.1		41.3		77.4		
Unstable CAD/NSTEMI CAD/NSTEMI	31.1		39.8		0.4		
STEMI	21.7		13.5		0		
Other	14.2		5.5		22.2		
Extent of CAD (%)		1.2		1.3		1.3	<0.01
1 vessel	14.9		36.5		4.2		
2 vessel	40.9		39.6		15.8		
3 vessel	37.9		21.1		56.8		
Left main disease***	6.3		2.8		23.2		

CAD: coronary artery disease, CCS: Canadian cardiovascular society, CTO: chronic total occlusion, IQR: inter quartile range, MI: myocardial infarction, (N)STEMI: (non-)ST-elevation myocardial infarction, PCI: percutaneous coronary intervention.
* Cardiogenic shock only displayed for the indication STEMI.
**CCS class only displayed for the indication stable CAD.
*** Left main (LM) disease includes: LM+1 vessel, LM+2 vessel and LM+3 vessel.
Data about initial treatment strategy were missing in four CTO patients.

contemporary databases and quality registries. The SCAAR registry with its distinctive structure covering the whole Swedish nation provides unique possibility to study several important features of CTO's including epidemiology, patients characteristic as well as health outcomes. It contains information about both past and current treatment strategies of these complex patients not only from specialized centers, but also from all hospitals that preforms PCI. Given these circumstances, the SCAAR registry can be an important instrument to address many key questions in CTO.

The prevalence of CTO in Sweden decreased by one quarter during the study period. We hypothesize that this primarily reflects the increasing rate of timely revascularisation with PCI of patients with acute coronary syndrome – STEMI and non-STEMI. Because the prevalence decreased by 25% while the number of procedures remained unchanged, the proportion of CTO procedures increased by the same percentage. Besides the decreased prevalence, the relatively low annual rate of CTO procedures in Sweden may be related to improved treatment of symptoms, better quality of life, fear of complications, technical complexity, and low evidence-level.

There are some important limitations that need to be addressed. First, this is an observational study and as such it provides only associative evidence, not causative. Second, we cannot rule out the possibility of selection bias, as only hospitalized patients are included in the registry. Substantial proportion of missing data in the coronary segment subcohort may have resulted in biased estimate on CTO prevalence. Third, patients with missing data tend to have higher risk and their exclusion from the analysis might have produced biased results. Fourth, we cannot exclude the possibility that some occlusions had duration of less than three months, however the validation of CTO diagnosis and procedures in SCAAR have shown that only 3.8% were erroneously classified.

Conclusions

SCAAR is the largest database of CTO patients to date. CTO is a frequent finding in Swedish population and is diagnosed in every 10th patient undergoing coronary angiography. The prevalence of CTO has decreased by one quarter. Patients with a CTO represent a high risk subgroup of CAD patients. SCAAR may be a valuable source of data in the process of evidence-building in the CTO field.

Acknowledgments

We would like to acknowledge Rosie Perkins for excellent support and scientific editing.

Author Contributions

Conceived and designed the experiments: TR EO LH JPSH CD DI JO OA UJ MA RJ SJ BL GO JH PA GM. Analyzed the data: TR EO LH JPSH CD DI JO OA UJ MA RJ SJ BL GO JH PA GM. Wrote the paper: TR EO LH JPSH CD DI JO OA UJ MA RJ SJ BL GO JH PA GM.

References

1. Grantham JA, Marso SP, Spertus J, House J, Holmes DR Jr, et al. (2009) Chronic total occlusion angioplasty in the United States. JACC Cardiovascular Interventions 2: 479–486.
2. Galassi AR, Tomasello SD, Reifart N, Werner GS, Sianos G, et al. (2011) In-hospital outcomes of percutaneous coronary intervention in patients with chronic total occlusion: insights from the ERCTO (European Registry of Chronic Total Occlusion) registry. EuroIntervention 7: 472–479.
3. Task Force on Myocardial Revascularization of the European Society of C, the European Association for Cardio-Thoracic S, European Association for Percutaneous Cardiovascular I, Kolh P, Wijns W, et al. (2010) Guidelines on myocardial revascularization. Eur J Cardiothorac Surg 38 Suppl: S1–S52.
4. Members WC, Levine GN, Bates ER, Blankenship JC, Bailey SR, et al. (2011) 2011 ACCF/AHA/SCAI Guideline for Percutaneous Coronary Intervention: A Report of the American College of Cardiology Foundation/American Heart Association Task Force on Practice Guidelines and the Society for Cardiovascular Angiography and Interventions. Circulation 124: e574–e651.
5. Christofferson RD, Lehmann KG, Martin GV, Every N, Caldwell JH, et al. (2005) Effect of chronic total coronary occlusion on treatment strategy. AmJCardiol 95: 1088–1091.
6. Fefer P, Knudtson ML, Cheema AN, Galbraith PD, Osherov AB, et al. (2012) Current perspectives on coronary chronic total occlusions: the Canadian Multicenter Chronic Total Occlusions Registry. JAmCollCardiol 59: 991–997.
7. Kahn JK (1993) Angiographic suitability for catheter revascularization of total coronary occlusions in patients from a community hospital setting. AmHeart J 126: 561–564.
8. Angeras O, Albertsson P, Karason K, Ramunddal T, Matejka G, et al. (2013) Evidence for obesity paradox in patients with acute coronary syndromes: a report from the Swedish Coronary Angiography and Angioplasty Registry. Eur Heart J 34: 345–353.
9. Prasad A, Rihal CS, Lennon RJ, Wiste HJ, Singh M, et al. (2007) Trends in outcomes after percutaneous coronary intervention for chronic total occlusions: a 25-year experience from the Mayo Clinic. J Am Coll Cardiol 49: 1611–1618.
10. Mehran R, Claessen BE, Godino C, Dangas GD, Obunai K, et al. (2011) Long-term outcome of percutaneous coronary intervention for chronic total occlusions. JACC Cardiovasc Interv 4: 952–961.
11. Fox KA, Goodman SG, Klein W, Brieger D, Steg PG, et al. (2002) Management of acute coronary syndromes. Variations in practice and outcome; findings from the Global Registry of Acute Coronary Events (GRACE). Eur Heart J 23: 1177–1189.
12. Joyal D, Afilalo J, Rinfret S (2010) Effectiveness of recanalization of chronic total occlusions: a systematic review and meta-analysis. Am Heart J 160: 179–187.
13. Thompson CA, Jayne JE, Robb JF, Friedman BJ, Kaplan AV, et al. (2009) Retrograde techniques and the impact of operator volume on percutaneous intervention for coronary chronic total occlusions an early US experience. JACC Cardiovasc Interv 2: 834–842.
14. van der Schaaf RJ, Claessen BE, Hoebers LP, Verouden NJ, Koolen JJ, et al. (2010) Rationale and design of EXPLORE: a randomized, prospective, multicenter trial investigating the impact of recanalization of a chronic total occlusion on left ventricular function in patients after primary percutaneous coronary intervention for acute ST-elevation myocardial infarction. Trials 11: 89.

8

Transradial versus Transfemoral Approach in Patients Undergoing Percutaneous Coronary Intervention for Acute Coronary Syndrome. A Meta-Analysis and Trial Sequential Analysis of Randomized Controlled Trials

Raffaele Piccolo[1], Gennaro Galasso[1]*, Ernesto Capuano[1], Stefania De Luca[1], Giovanni Esposito[1], Bruno Trimarco[1], Federico Piscione[2]

1 Department of Advanced Biomedical Sciences, Federico II University, Naples, Italy, 2 Department of Medicine and Surgery, University of Salerno, Salerno, Italy

Abstract

Background: Transfemoral approach (TFA) remains the most common vascular access for percutaneous coronary intervention (PCI) in many countries. However, in the last years several randomized trials compared transradial approach (TRA) with TFA in patients with acute coronary syndrome (ACS), but only few studies were powered to estimate rare events. The aim of the current study was to clarify whether TRA is superior to TFA approach in patients with ACS undergoing percutaneous coronary intervention. A meta-analysis, meta-regression and trial sequential analysis of safety and efficacy of TRA in ACS setting was performed.

Methods and Results: Medline, the Cochrane Library, Scopus, scientific session abstracts and relevant websites were searched. Data concerning the study design, patient characteristics, risk of bias, and outcomes were extracted. The primary endpoint was death. Secondary endpoints were: major bleeding and vascular complications. Outcomes were assessed within 30 days. Eleven randomized trials involving 9,202 patients were included. Compared with TFA, TRA significantly reduced the risk of death (odds ratio [OR] 0.70; 95% confidence interval [CI], 0.53–0.94; $p = 0.016$), but this finding was not confirmed in trial sequential analysis, indicating that sufficient evidence had not been yet reached. Furthermore, TRA compared with TFA reduced the risk of major bleeding (OR 0.60; 95% CI, 0.41–0.88; $p = 0.008$) and vascular complications (OR 0.35; 95% CI, 0.28–0.46; $p < 0.001$); these findings were supported by trial sequential analyses.

Conclusions: In patients with ACS undergoing PCI, a lower risk of death was observed with TRA. Nevertheless, the association between mortality and TRA in ACS setting should be interpreted with caution because it is based on insufficient evidence. However, because of the clinical relevance associated with major bleeding and vascular complications reduction, TRA should be recommended as first-choice vascular access in patients with ACS undergoing cardiac catheterization.

Editor: Bernardo Cortese, Cliniche Humanitas Gavazzeni, Italy

Funding: The authors have no support or funding to report.

Competing Interests: The authors have declared that no competing interests exist.

* E-mail: gengalas@unina.it

Introduction

Percutaneous coronary intervention (PCI) represents a cornerstone for the treatment of patients with acute coronary syndrome (ACS). Currently, transfemoral approach (TFA) is the most common access for PCI in many countries [1]. During the last two decades, transradial approach (TRA) emerged as a valid alternative to TFA, because of earlier ambulation, shorter hospital stay and possibly reduced bleeding risk [2]. Despite these advantages, TRA for catheterization was performed infrequently (<3%) in the United States between 2005 and 2009 [3]. The reasons of this uncommon use remain uncertain, but could include familiarity with TFA and concerns for the longer learning curve of TRA, along with increased radiation exposure [4]. In the last years, several randomized clinical trials compared these two approaches in patients with ACS, but only few studies were adequately powered to allow a reliable estimation of rare events. Furthermore, recent meta-analyses assessing the role of TRA in ACS setting excluded patients with non-ST-segment elevation myocardial infarction, which represents the most frequent ACS presentation [5,6]. Therefore, the aim of the current study was to perform a meta-analysis and trial sequential analysis of randomized trials evaluating the clinical outcomes following TRA versus TFA across the whole spectrum of ACS.

Methods

Data sources and searches

We searched Medline, the Cochrane Library, Scopus, scientific session abstracts (published in Circulation, Journal of the

American College of Cardiology, European Heart Journal and The American Journal of Cardiology), and relevant websites (www.acc.org, www.americanheart.org, www.europcronline.com, www.escardio.org, www.clinicaltrialresults.org, www.tctmd.com and www.theheart.org). The reference list of relevant studies was additionally scanned. No language, publication date, or publication status restrictions were imposed. The last search was run on 15th June, 2013. The following search terms were matched: "femoral", "radial", "transradial", "transfemoral", "percutaneous coronary intervention", "randomized", "acute coronary syndrome", "myocardial infarction", "unstable angina", "non-ST-segment elevation", "ST-segment elevation".

Study selection

To be included, the citation had to meet the following criteria: 1) random treatment allocation; 2) inclusion of patients with ACS; and 3) the use of TRA in the experimental arm. Exclusion criteria were: 1) ongoing studies; 2) irretrievable data and 3) trials not reporting death occurrence during follow-up. Complete electronic search strategy for Medline (PubMed) and The Cochrane Library was reported in the Supporting Information.

Data Extraction and Quality Assessment

Two investigators (R.P. and G.G.) independently assessed reports for eligibility at title and/or at abstract level, with divergences resolved with a third reviewer (F.P.); studies that met inclusion criteria were selected for further analysis. The risk of bias was evaluated by the same two reviewer authors, in accordance with The Cochrane Collaboration methods and considering the following methodological items: random sequence generation, allocation concealment, blinding of participants and personnel, blinding of outcome assessment, incomplete outcome data, selective reporting, other bias and sample size calculation. We did not use a quality score, since this practice has been previously discouraged [7].

The primary endpoint of this meta-analysis was death within 30 days. Secondary endpoints were: major bleeding and vascular complications. Per protocol definitions of clinical endpoints were reported in the Table S1 in File S1.

Data Synthesis and Analysis

Statistical analysis was performed with STATA 11 statistical software (STATA Corp, College Station, Texas, USA). The κ statistic was used to assess agreement between reviewers for study selection. Odds ratio (OR) and 95% confidence intervals (95% CI) were used as summary statistics. The pooled OR was calculated by using the fixed effects Mantel-Hænzel model, while, in case of significant heterogeneity across studies, the random effects DerSimonian and Laird model was reported instead. In case of statistical significance, the number needed to treat (NNT) and the number of avoided events per 1,000 treated patients were provided. The Breslow-Day chi-squared test was calculated to test the statistical evidence of heterogeneity across the studies (p< 0.1). In addition, we used the I^2 statistic, which describes the percentage variation across studies that is due to heterogeneity rather than chance. As a guide, I^2 values <25% indicated low, 25–50% indicated moderate, and >50% indicated high heterogeneity [8]. The influence of single studies on the summary estimates was examined graphically by checking how the elimination of each study affected the resulting summary estimate of OR. We assessed the possibility of small-study effects by visual inspection of funnel plot asymmetry. Because graphical evaluation can be subjective, we performed both Harbord [9] and Peters tests [10], as formal statistical tests for publication bias. A weighted random-effect meta-regression analysis was used to evaluate relationship between the risk of study endpoints and the following study-level covariates: age, sex, year of publication, enrolling centres (single- vs. multi-centre), sample size (<150 patients vs. ≥150 patients), proportion of primary PCI, glycoprotein IIb/IIIa inhibitors use and crossover rates to TFA. Furthermore, the relationship between the magnitude of risk reduction with TRA and the baseline risk for bleeding/vascular complications was also investigated with the *metareg* command, as previously described [11].

Trial sequential analysis was performed according to the monitoring boundaries approach [12,13], by using TSA version 0.9 beta (www.ctu.dk/tsa). This is a methodology that combines an a priori information size calculation for a meta-analysis with the adaptation of monitoring boundaries to evaluate the accumulating evidence [14]. The information size calculation is similar to the sample size calculation in a single trial, allowing a quantification of the reliability of cumulative data in meta-analyses. Trial sequential analysis was obtained with alfa set to 5%, power to 80% and including the control event proportion observed in the meta-analysis. For death, major bleeding and vascular complication we chose a 20%, 35% and 50% relative risk reduction, respectively.

The study was realized in compliance with the Preferred Reporting Items for Systematic reviews and Meta-Analyses (PRISMA) statement [15].

Results

As reported in Figure 1, we screened the title and/or the abstract of 321 potentially eligible publications. Of these, 240 citations were excluded because they were not relevant to this study or were duplicated publications. Eighty-one studies were thus assessed for eligibility and 70 records were discarded because the inclusion criteria were not met. Finally, eleven trials [16–26] were included in this meta-analysis, enrolling a total of 9,202 patients (4,583 or 49.3% randomly assigned to TRA and 4,619 or 50.7% randomly assigned to TFA). The interobserver agreement for study selection was very good, with κ = 0.95. The main characteristics of the included studies are summarized in Table 1. The risk of bias among studies is reported in Table 2. Anticoagulation was obtained with heparin in the vast majority of patients.

Clinical outcomes

A total of 200 patients died (2.15%). As reported in Figure 2A, TRA was associated with a significant reduction in death as compared to TFA (1.81% vs. 2.53%, respectively, OR 0.70; 95% CI, 0.53–0.94; p = 0.016). No heterogeneity was found among trials (I^2 = 0%; 95% CI, 0–65%; p_{het} = 0.94). Visual inspection of funnel plot did not reveal a skewed distribution for death, suggesting the absence of small-study effects (Figure 3). Moreover, both Harbord (p = 0.93) and Peters tests (p = 0.18) were not significant. The NNT to prevent one death with TRA was 136.3 and 7.3 (95% CI, 1.6–11.7) deaths were prevented in each 1,000 patients treated; these data were based on an OR = 0.70 applied to the control group event rate.

Trial sequential analysis showed a lack of sufficient evidence of a benefit of TRA for the reduction of death. Only the 33% (8,949 out of 26,836) of the required sample size was accrued to detect a 20% relative risk reduction for death (Figure 2B).

Major bleeding was reported in a total of 116 patients (1.25%). As shown in Figure 4A, TRA significantly reduced major bleeding complications as compared with TFA (0.94% vs. 1.58%, respectively, OR 0.60; 95% CI, 0.41–0.88; p = 0.008). No heterogeneity was found across trials (I^2 = 0%; 95% CI, 0–65%; p_{het} = 0.83). The NNT to prevent one major bleeding with TRA

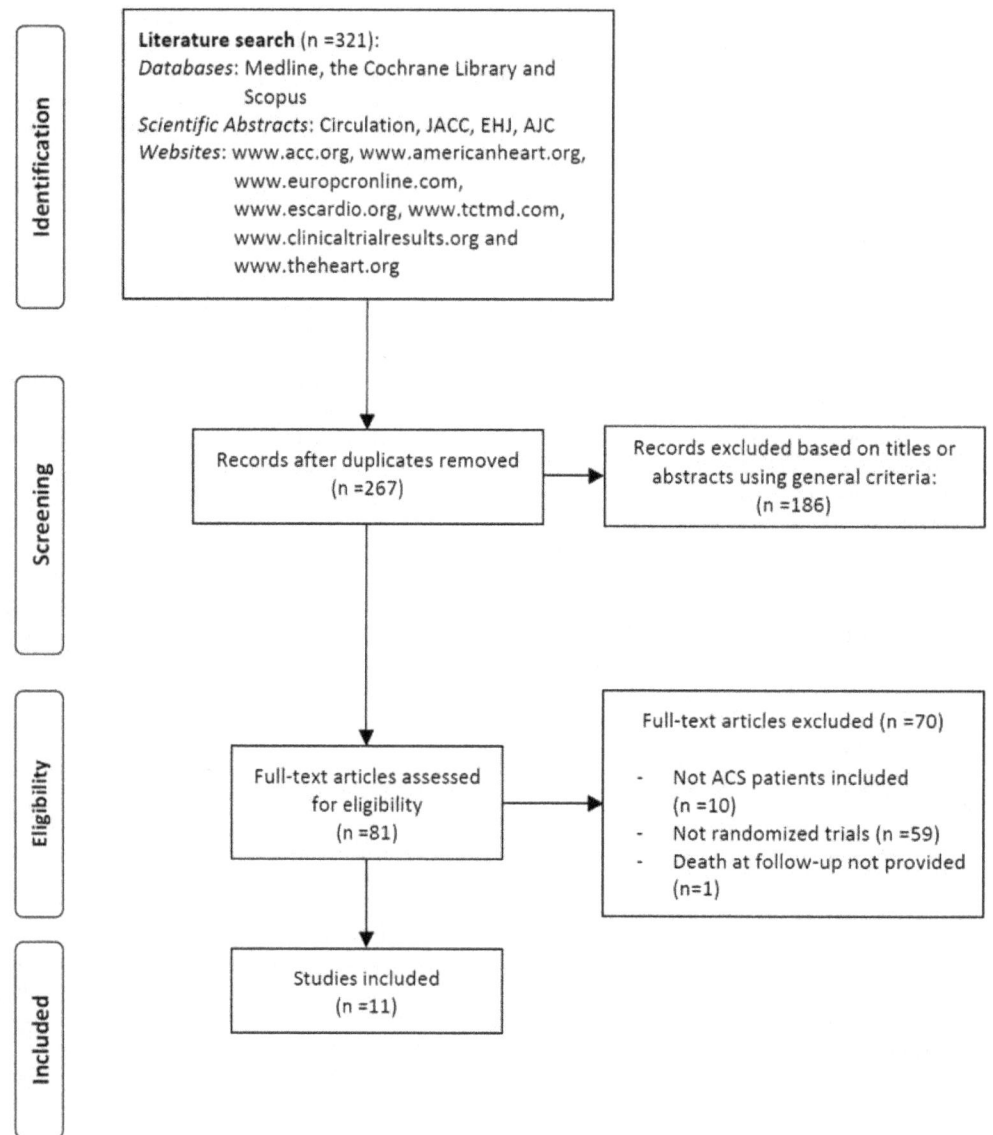

Figure 1. Flow diagram of trial selection. ACS, acute coronary syndrome.

was 160.8 and 6.2 (95% CI, 1.9–9.2) major bleedings were prevented in each 1,000 patients treated; these data were based on an OR = 0.60 applied to the control group event rate.

In trial sequential analysis, despite the required information size was not met (13,368 patients), the cumulative Z-curve crossed the trial sequential monitoring boundary, indicating that sufficient evidence exists for a 35% reduction in the relative risk of major bleeding with TRA (Figure 4B).

Data about vascular complications were available for 9,053 patients (98%). A total of 318 patients (3.51%) had vascular complications. As reported in Figure 5A, TRA was associated with a significant reduction in vascular complications (1.88% vs. 5.12% OR 0.35; 95% CI, 0.28–0.46; p<0.001). No heterogeneity was found across trials ($I^2 = 0\%$; 95% CI, 0–62%; $p_{het} = 0.74$). The NNT to prevent one vascular complication with TRA was 30.8 and 32.4 (95% CI, 27.1–36.6) vascular complications were prevented in each 1,000 patients treated; these data were based on an OR = 0.35 applied to the control group event rate.

Trial sequential analysis confirmed that TRA is superior to TFA in reducing vascular complications (Figure 5B).

Influence analysis and meta-regression

Influence analysis demonstrated that no single study significantly altered the summary ORs for the endpoints, because one at a time study omission did not result in a movement of the point estimate outside the 95% CI (Figures S1–S3 in File S1).

None of the study-level covariates significantly influenced the risk of study endpoints at meta-regression analysis (Table S2 in File S1). Furthermore, we did not find a significant relationship between TRA-related risk reduction in major bleeding and major bleeding events in the TFA population (p = 0.64), as well as TRA-related risk reduction in vascular complications and the vascular complication events in the TFA population (p = 0.81) (Figure 6).

Table 1. Main Characteristics of included trials.

Trial	Year of publication	Period of enrollment	Multi-centre	Patients number TFA	Patients number TRA	Mean age (years) TFA	Mean age (years) TRA	Male (%) TFA	Male (%) TRA	ACS type	Rescue PCI (%) TFA	Rescue PCI (%) TRA	Follow-up	Gp IIb/IIIa inhibitors (%) TFA	Gp IIb/IIIa inhibitors (%) TRA	Type of Gp IIb/IIIa inhibitors	Hemostasis TFA	Hemostasis TRA	Crossover (%) TFA	Crossover (%) TRA
FARMI (16)	2007	2004-05	No	57	57	60	58	86	82.5	STEMI	49.1	35.1	In-hospital	100	100	Abciximab	manual compression	manual compression	1.8	12.3
Gan et al. (17)	2009	2004-07	Yes	105	90	52.3	53.6	80	81.1	STEMI	0	0	In-hospital	34.3	31.1	N.A.	manual compression	manual compression	0	1.1
Hou et al. (18)	2010	2005-08	No	100	100	66.2	64.9	69	72	STEMI	0*	0*	30-day	20	28	Tirofiban	manual compression	TR-Band	0	4
Mann et al. (19)	1998	1997	No	77	65	62	63	78	65	STEMI NSTEMI UA	N.A.	N.A.	In-hospital	10	15	Abciximab	manual compression + compression FemoStop	radial artery compression device	0	13.8
RADIAL-AMI (20)	2005	N.A.	Yes	25	25	58	52	0	76	STEMI	68	64	30-day	92	95	Abciximab Tirofiban Eptifibatide	manual compression (92%). VCD (8%).	manual compression	0	4
RADIAMI (21)	2009	2005-06	No	50	50	59.1	59.9	48.5	51.5	STEMI	0	0	In-hospital	42	44	Abciximab	manual compression	TR-Band	2	8
RADIAMI II (22)	2011	2006-08	No	59	49	57.6	62.1	63	65	STEMI	0*	0*	In-hospital	54	51	Abciximab	StarClose device	TR-Band	1.7	4.1
RIFLE-STEACS (23)	2012	2009-11	Yes	501	500	65	65	71.9	74.8	STEMI	7	8.2	30-day	69.9	67.4	N.A.	N.A.	N.A.	2.8	9.6
RIVAL (24)	2011	2006-10	Yes	3,514	3,507	62	62	72.9	74.1	STEMI NSTEMI UA	11.1	10.6	30-day	24	25.3	N.A.	manual compression (74.4%). VCD (25.6%)	N.A.	0.9	7
TEMPURA (25)	2003	1999-2001	No	72	77	67	66	81.9	80.5	STEMI	0*	0*	In-hospital	0†	0†	-	manual compression	manual compression	0	1.5
Wang et al. (26)	2012	2008-10	No	59	60	60.2	59.8	83.1	86.7	STEMI‡	N.A.	N.A.	In-hospital	50.8	55	Tirofiban	manual compression	manual compression	1.7	6.7

* Only patients treated with primary PCI were enrolled.
†Glycoprotein IIb/IIIa inhibitors were not given in any of the patients because not approved for clinical use in Japan.
‡STEMI patients receiving routine early PCI within 12 hours after thrombolysis were enrolled.
PCI, Percutaneous coronary intervention; ACS, Acute coronary syndrome; STEMI, ST-segment elevation myocardial infarction; NSTEMI, Non-ST-segment elevation myocardial infarction; UA, Unstable angina; TFA, Transfemoral approach; TRA, Transradial approach; VCD, vascular closure devices; N.A., Not available data.

Table 2. Risk of bias assessment.

Trial Name	Random sequence generation	Allocation concealment	Blinding of participants and personnel	Blinding of outcome assessment	Incomplete outcome data	Selective reporting	Other bias	Sample size calculation
FARMI (16)	Unclear risk	Unclear risk	High risk	High risk	Low risk	Low risk	Low risk	No
Gan et al. (17)	Unclear risk	Unclear risk	High risk	High risk	Low risk	Low risk	Low risk	No
Hou et al. (18)	Unclear risk	Unclear risk	High risk	High risk	Low risk	Low risk	Low risk	No
Mann et al. (19)	Unclear risk	Unclear risk	High risk	High risk	Low risk	Low risk	High risk	No
RADIAL-AMI (20)	Low risk	Low risk	High risk	High risk	Low risk	Low risk	Low risk	Yes
RADIAMI (21)	High risk	High risk	High risk	High risk	Low risk	Low risk	Low risk	No
RADIAMI II (22)	High risk	High risk	High risk	High risk	Low risk	Low risk	Low risk	No
RIFLE-STEACS (23)	Low risk	Low risk	High risk	Low risk	Low risk	Low risk	Low risk	Yes
RIVAL (24)	Low risk	High risk	High risk	Low risk	Low risk	Low risk	Low risk	Yes
TEMPURA (25)	Unclear risk	Unclear risk	High risk	High risk	Low risk	Low risk	Low risk	Yes
Wang et al. (26)	Low risk	Low risk	High risk	High risk	Low risk	Low risk	Low risk	Yes

Discussion

The main findings of this study are that: TRA compared with TFA reduced the risk of major bleeding and vascular complications in patients with ACS; despite the meta-analysis showed a reduced risk of death with TRA, there is no definite evidence supporting this association as demonstrated by trial sequential analysis; the meta-regression analysis suggested that the benefit with TRA, in terms of bleeding and vascular complications, was irrespective of the patient risk profile.

The incidence of recurrent ischemic events in patients with ACS has been drastically reduced by the combination of multiple antithrombotic agents, along with the early use of coronary angiography with a view to revascularization [27]. Nevertheless, the benefit derived from these therapies led to an increase in the rates of bleeding complications. In the recent years, several studies demonstrated that bleeding occurrence in patients undergoing PCI is associated with a worse prognosis in terms of death, myocardial infarction, and stroke [28]. At this regard, TRA has the potential to decrease bleeding events, primarily by reducing vascular complications [29]. The main results of this study including 11 randomized trials with a total of 9,202 patients were in accordance with previous meta-analyses that dealt exclusively with patients with ST-elevation myocardial infarction [5,6,30]. However, these meta-analyses were limited by the inclusion of the ST-elevation myocardial infarction subgroup of the RIVAL trial [24], in which randomization was not stratified by clinical presentation.

Despite we found a 30% reduction in the odds of death in favour of TRA, with about 7 deaths prevented per 1,000 patients treated, this finding was not confirmed in trial sequential analysis, which disclosed an insufficient evidence for this association. Indeed, current available data do not conclusively support a 20% relative risk reduction in mortality with TRA, since only one third of the required study population was accrued in this study. Thus, trial sequential analysis should be implemented when a meta-analysis is performed, since many apparently conclusive meta-analyses may become inconclusive when the statistical analyses take into account the risk of random error due to repetitive testing.

In contrast with previous meta-analyses [5,6], we reported for the first time a significant reduction in the risk of major bleeding in TRA group, attributable to the higher statistical power of this study. Trial sequential analysis showed a sufficient evidence for this association, despite the required information size was not reached (9,202 out of 13,368 patients). At this regard, a possible advantage of this methodological tool is that it may prevent the initiation of unnecessary trials when firm evidence has been gained [13].

The decreased risk of major bleeding, along with the dramatic reduction in vascular complications, might provide an explanation to the possible risk reduction in death. In this respect, a large pooled analysis of three randomized trials including ACS patients found that approximately 1 in 10 patients who developed major bleeding died during the first 30 days after hospitalization compared with 1 in 40 of those who did not develop major bleeding [31]. Consistently, an analysis of the ACUITY (Acute Catheterization and Urgent Intervention Triage strategy) trial showed that both major bleeding and myocardial infarction have a similar association with mortality, carrying a similar risk of death in the first year following presentation with an ACS [32]. In addition, Doyle et al. found that patients experiencing major femoral bleeding after PCI had a higher mortality at long-term follow-up, due to an excess of death during the first 30 days [33].

A.

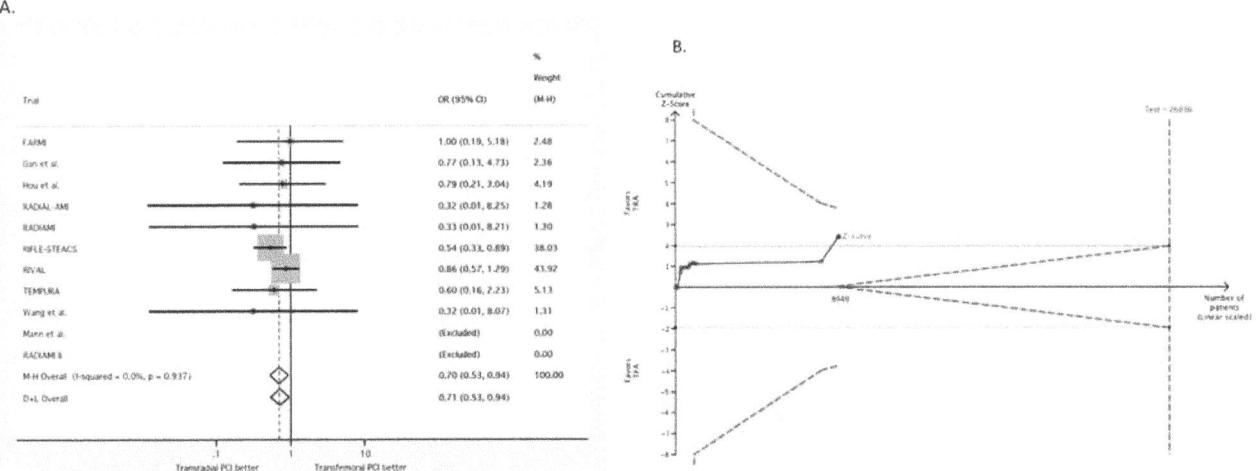

B.

Figure 2. Effect of transradial vs. transfemoral approach on death. 2A. Odds ratio of death with transradial vs. transfemoral approach. The squares and the horizontal lines indicate the OR and the 95% CIs for each trial included; the size of each square is proportional to the statistical weight of a trial in the meta-analysis; diamond indicates the effect estimate derived from meta-analysis, with the centre indicating the point estimate and the left and the right ends the 95% CI. M-H, Mantel-Hænzel model; D+L, DerSimonian and Laird model. **2B.** Trial sequential analysis for death. Heterogeneity adjusted information size of 26,836 participants calculated on basis of death of 2.53% in the transfemoral group, relative risk reduction 20%, $\alpha = 5\%$, $\beta = 20\%$, $I^2 = 0\%$. Solid green cumulative Z-curve did not cross red dashed trial sequential monitoring boundaries for benefit or harm. Horizontal dotted green lines illustrate traditional level of statistical significance (p = 0.05).

However, the relationship between major bleeding after PCI and death is likely to be multifactorial. Major bleeding could directly increase the risk of death by causing hemodynamic compromise and could lead clinicians to discontinue antithrombotic agents. Bleeding also may reduce oxygen delivery to the myocardium and anaemia-induced erythropoietin release may promote a systemic prothrombotic state. Furthermore, despite increased haemoglobin levels, transfusion does not increase tissue oxygenation and its use is associated with a poor outcome in PCI patients [34]. Several non-randomized studies supported the association between bleeding reduction with TRA and mortality. In the PRESTO ACS (Comparison of Early Invasive and Conservative Treatment in Patients with Non-ST-Elevation Acute Coronary Syndromes) vascular substudy [35], TRA compared with TFA was associated with a decrease in bleeding complications and death or reinfarction at 1-year. Accordingly, a recent analysis of the HORIZONS-AMI (Harmonizing Outcomes with RevascularIZatiON and Stents) trial demonstrated a significant reduction in major bleeding and in the composite of death or reinfarction at 30-day with TRA compared with TFA [36].

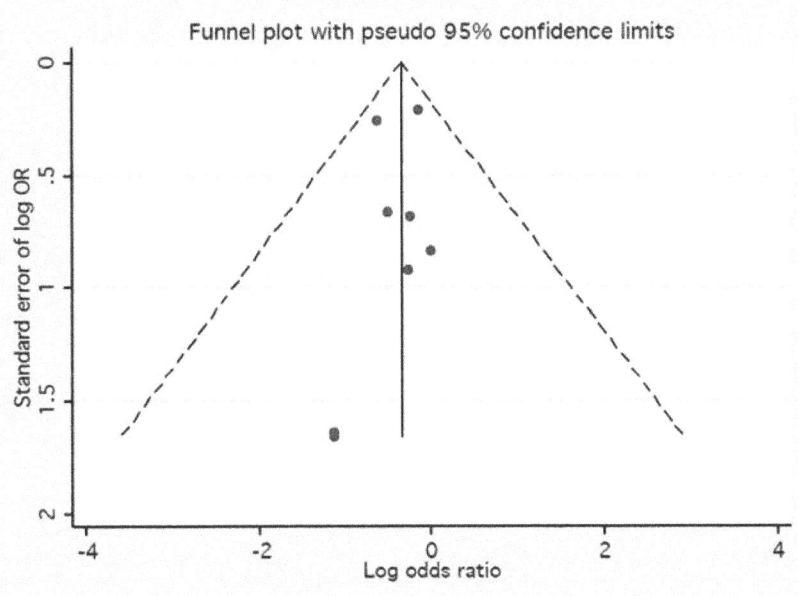

Figure 3. Funnel plot for the primary endpoint.

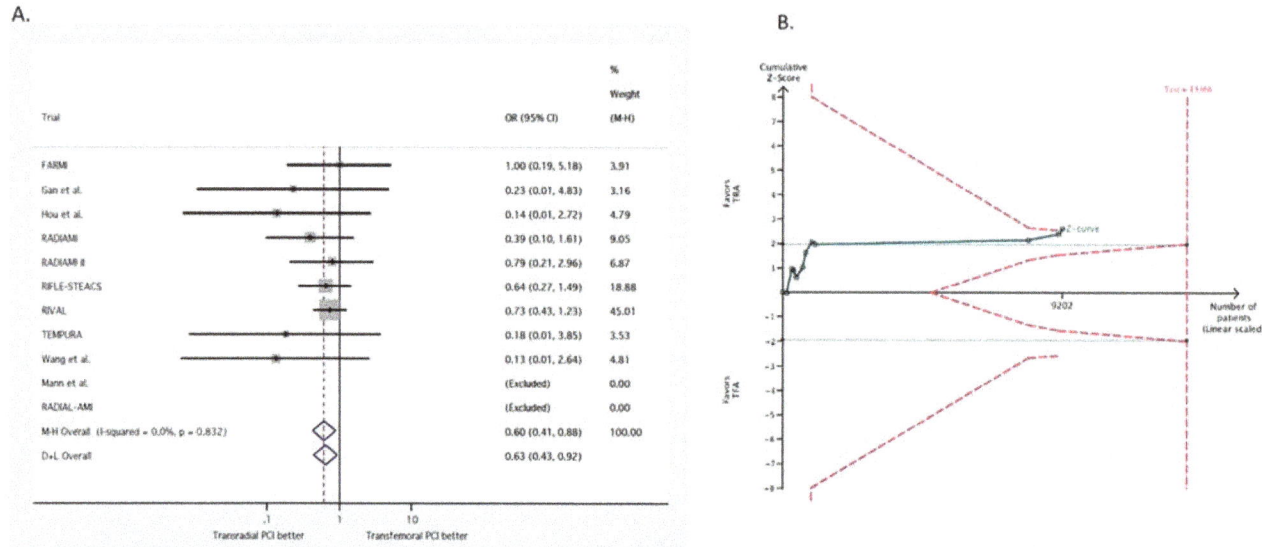

Figure 4. Effect of transradial vs. transfemoral approach on major bleeding. 4A. Odds ratio of major bleeding with transradial vs. transfemoral approach. **4B.** Trial sequential analysis for major bleeding. Heterogeneity adjusted information size of 13,368 participants calculated on basis of major bleeding of 1.58% in the transfemoral group, relative risk reduction 35%, $\alpha = 5\%$, $\beta = 20\%$, $I^2 = 0\%$. Solid green cumulative Z-curve crossed both red dashed trial sequential monitoring and information size boundaries, thereby confirming that transradial approach is superior to transfemoral approach in reducing vascular complications. Horizontal dotted green lines illustrate traditional level of statistical significance (p = 0.05).

Meta-regression analysis showed consistent results in single- versus multi-centre trials. This was an important finding since single-centre trials are usually associated with a larger treatment effects than multi-centre trials [37]. In addition, we found that TRA may decrease the risk of major bleeding and vascular complications independently from the patient risk profile, in a "one-size fits-all" manner (Figure 6). Although these findings should be considered hypothesis generating, they may be due to

the fact that vascular access-related complications are almost eliminated with TRA, as also supported by trial sequential analysis. Accordingly, access site bleeding is the most common source of bleeding complications in patients undergoing PCI and it is associated with a 2-fold increase in 1-year mortality [38]. However, the reduction in the risk of major bleeding did not lead to a parallel risk reduction of death, probably because access-site bleeding is associated with a lower risk of death than non-access-

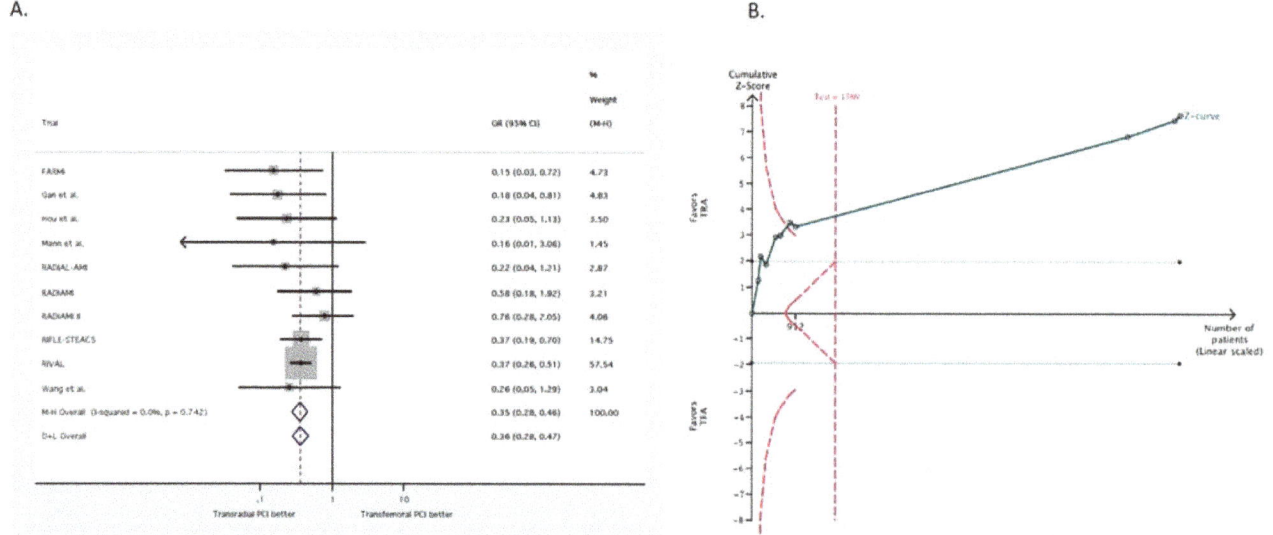

Figure 5. Effect of transradial vs. transfemoral approach on vascular complications. 5A. Odds ratio of vascular complications with transradial vs. transfemoral approach. **5B.** Trial sequential analysis for vascular complications. Heterogeneity adjusted information size of 1,769 participants calculated on basis of major bleeding of 5.12% in the transfemoral group, relative risk reduction 50%, $\alpha = 5\%$, $\beta = 20\%$, $I^2 = 0\%$. Solid green cumulative Z-curve crossed the red dashed monitoring boundaries, demonstrating sufficient evidence reached for 35% reduction in the risk of major bleeding with transradial approach. Horizontal dotted green lines illustrate traditional level of statistical significance (p = 0.05).

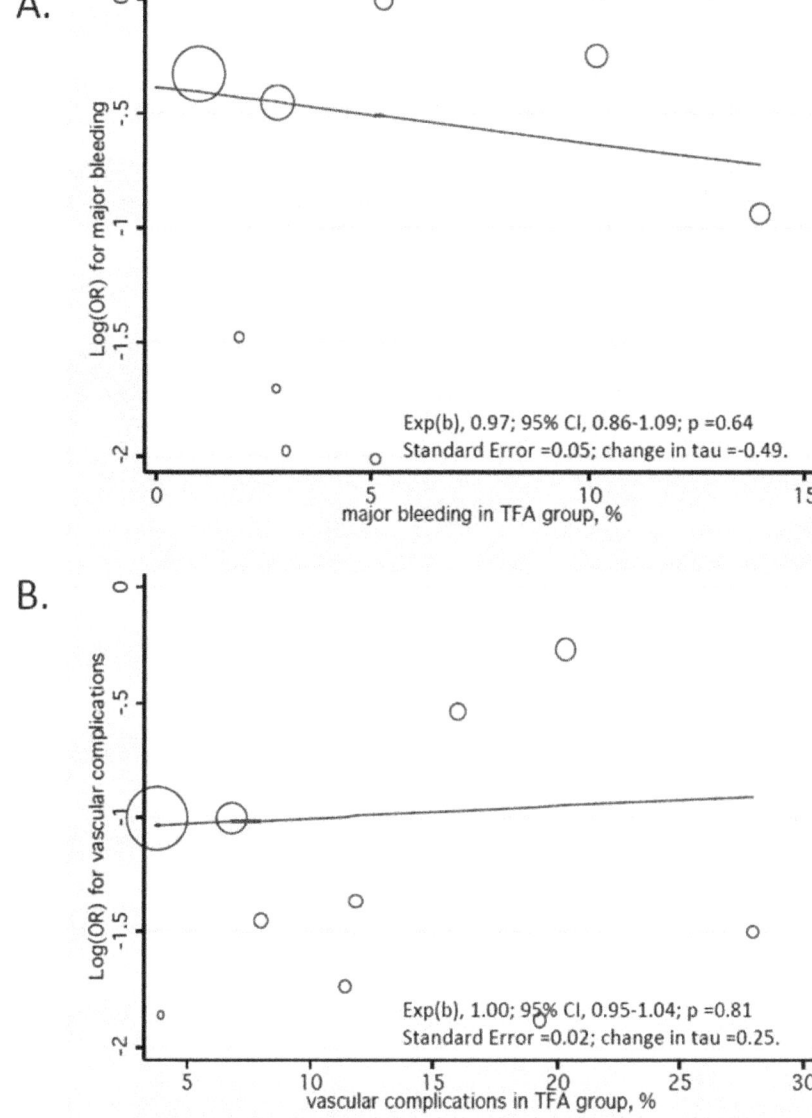

A.

Exp(b), 0.97; 95% CI, 0.86-1.09; p =0.64
Standard Error =0.05; change in tau =-0.49.

B.

Exp(b), 1.00; 95% CI, 0.95-1.04; p =0.81
Standard Error =0.02; change in tau =0.25.

Figure 6. Meta-regression analysis for major bleeding (A) and vascular complications (B). The size of circles is proportional to the weight of each study in the fitted random-effects meta-regression. TFA, transfemoral.

site bleeding. In fact, among more than 3 millions of patients included in the Cath PCI Registry [39], in-hospital mortality was 2.73% vs. 1.87% for access-site vs. no bleeding, and 8.25% vs. 1.87% for non-access-site vs. no bleeding. However, none of the included trials used contemporary transfemoral closure systems that are known to consistently reduce vascular complications by more than 50% [40]. At this regard, the ARISE (AngioSeal versus the Radial approach In acute coronary SyndromE) trial will help to define the role of a vascular closure device as a bleeding avoidance strategy in patients with ACS [41]. A final remark about vascular complications is related to sheath size used for both TRA and TFA. In fact, in the Leipzig registry [42], radial artery occlusion was documented with vascular ultrasound in 30.5% and 13.7% of patients treated with 6-F and 5-F sheaths, respectively. Similar results may be achieved through 5-F TFA [43].

Study limitations

First, this is a meta-analysis at the study level and we could not properly assess the role of confounding factors. Second, all included trials were performed by experienced operators skilled in TRA, thus limiting the external validity of the results of this meta-analysis for centres mainly performing transfemoral procedures. This reinforces the need for dedicated training programs for TRA, especially in teaching hospitals [44]. On the other hand, patients undergoing PCI from the TFA by default radial operators may be at higher risk of vascular access-site complication [45]. Third, this meta-analysis provides clinical follow-up within 30 days and it is still underpowered to evaluate the risk of death as demonstrated by trial sequential analysis. Thus, larger trials and longer follow-up data are needed to establish whether the observed benefit in mortality persists over time. Fourth, because of the frequent use of glycoprotein IIb/IIIa inhibitors in the included studies, it remains largely unknown whether the use of bivalirudin, that has been associated with lower bleeding events [46], may offset the greater risk of bleeding and vascular complications associated with TFA. Fifth, despite crossover rates to TFA did not influence study endpoints, the effect of crossover to TFA in patients undergoing primary PCI remains uncertain. At this regard, despite the risk of mortality with TRA is reduced even with longer door-to-balloon times [47], caution should be exercised in centres transitioning from a routine TFA to TRA in primary PCI setting. Six, patients with cardiogenic shock or hemodynamic instability were excluded from the most of trials. Therefore, the potential benefits of TRA in this setting are not well established. Finally, clinical data in patients with non-ST-elevation ACS derive from the RIVAL trial [24], in which the benefit of TRA was not manifest in this subgroup. Thus, further research with dedicated, adequately powered trials is needed to establish whether the benefit of TRA over TFA can be extended to patients with non-ST-elevation ACS.

Conclusions

This study demonstrated that the use of TRA in patients with ACS undergoing invasive management was associated with a significant reduction in the risk of major bleeding and vascular complications, as compared with TFA. The robustness of these findings was confirmed by trial sequential analysis. The clinical benefit, in terms of major bleeding or vascular complications, might translate in a lower risk of death with TRA. Nevertheless, the association between mortality and TRA in ACS setting should be interpreted cautiously because it is based on insufficient evidence, as demonstrated by trial sequential analysis.

However, because of the clinical relevance associated with major bleeding and vascular complications reduction, TRA should be recommended as first-choice vascular access in patients with ACS undergoing cardiac catheterization.

Author Contributions

Conceived and designed the experiments: RP GG BT FP. Analyzed the data: RP GG SDL EC GE. Wrote the paper: RP GG FP.

References

1. Rao SV, Ou FS, Wang TY, Roe MT, Brindis R, et al. (2008) Trends in the prevalence and outcomes of radial and femoral approaches to percutaneous coronary intervention: a report from the National Cardiovascular Data Registry. JACC Cardiovasc Interv 1: 379–386.
2. Rao SV, Cohen MG, Kandzari DE, Bertrand OF, Gilchrist IC (2010) The transradial approach to percutaneous coronary intervention: historical perspective, current concepts, and future directions. J Am Coll Cardiol 55: 2187–2195.
3. Subherwal S, Peterson ED, Dai D, Thomas L, Messenger JC, et al. (2012) Temporal trends in and factors associated with bleeding complications among patients undergoing percutaneous coronary intervention: a report from the National Cardiovascular Data CathPCI Registry. J Am Coll Cardiol 59: 1861–1869.
4. Brasselet C, Blanpain T, Tassan-Mangina S, Deschildre A, Duval S, et al. (2008) Comparison of operator radiation exposure with optimized radiation protection devices during coronary angiograms and ad hoc percutaneous coronary interventions by radial and femoral routes. Eur Heart J 29: 63–70.
5. Jang JS, Jin HY, Seo JS, Yang TH, Kim DK, et al. (2012) The transradial versus the transfemoral approach for primary percutaneous coronary intervention in patients with acute myocardial infarction: a systematic review and meta-analysis. EuroIntervention 8: 501–510.
6. Joyal D, Bertrand OF, Rinfret S, Shimony A, Eisenberg MJ (2012) Meta-analysis of ten trials on the effectiveness of the radial versus the femoral approach in primary percutaneous coronary intervention. Am J Cardiol 109: 813–818.
7. Juni P, Witschi A, Bloch R, Egger M (1999) The hazards of scoring the quality of clinical trials for meta-analysis. JAMA 282: 1054–1060.
8. Higgins JP, Thompson SG, Deeks JJ, Altman DG (2003) Measuring inconsistency in meta-analyses. BMJ 327: 557–560.
9. Harbord RM, Egger M, Sterne JA (2006) A modified test for small-study effects in meta-analyses of controlled trials with binary endpoints. Stat Med 25: 3443–3457.
10. Peters JL, Sutton AJ, Jones DR, Abrams KR, Rushton L (2006) Comparison of two methods to detect publication bias in meta-analysis. JAMA 295: 676–680.
11. Piccolo R, Cassese S, Galasso G, De Rosa R, D'Anna C, et al. (2011) Long-term safety and efficacy of drug-eluting stents in patients with acute myocardial infarction: a meta-analysis of randomized trials. Atherosclerosis 217: 149–157.
12. Brok J, Thorlund K, Wetterslev J, Gluud C (2009) Apparently conclusive meta-analyses may be inconclusive—Trial sequential analysis adjustment of random error risk due to repetitive testing of accumulating data in apparently conclusive neonatal meta-analyses. Int J Epidemiol 38: 287–298.
13. Wetterslev J, Thorlund K, Brok J, Gluud C (2008) Trial sequential analysis may establish when firm evidence is reached in cumulative meta-analysis. J Clin Epidemiol 61: 64–75.
14. Thorlund K, Devereaux PJ, Wetterslev J, Guyatt G, Ioannidis JP, et al. (2009) Can trial sequential monitoring boundaries reduce spurious inferences from meta-analyses? Int J Epidemiol 38: 276–286.
15. Moher D, Liberati A, Tetzlaff J, Altman DG (2009) Preferred reporting items for systematic reviews and meta-analyses: the PRISMA statement. Ann Intern Med 151: 264–269, W264.
16. Brasselet C, Tassan S, Nazeyrollas P, Hamon M, Metz D (2007) Randomised comparison of femoral versus radial approach for percutaneous coronary intervention using abciximab in acute myocardial infarction: results of the FARMI trial. Heart 93: 1556–1561.
17. Gan L, Lib Q, Liuc R, Zhaoc Y, Qiuc J, et al. (2009) Effectiveness and feasibility of transradial approaches for primary percutaneous coronary intervention in patients with acute myocardial infarction. Journal of Nanjing Medical University 23: 270–274.
18. Hou L, Wei YD, Li WM, Xu YW (2010) Comparative study on transradial versus transfemoral approach for primary percutaneous coronary intervention in Chinese patients with acute myocardial infarction. Saudi Med J 31: 158–162.
19. Mann T, Cubeddu G, Bowen J, Schneider JE, Arrowood M, et al. (1998) Stenting in acute coronary syndromes: a comparison of radial versus femoral access sites. J Am Coll Cardiol 32: 572–576.
20. Cantor WJ, Puley G, Natarajan MK, Dzavik V, Madan M, et al. (2005) Radial versus femoral access for emergent percutaneous coronary intervention with adjunct glycoprotein IIb/IIIa inhibition in acute myocardial infarction—the RADIAL-AMI pilot randomized trial. Am Heart J 150: 543–549.
21. Chodor P, Krupa H, Kurek T, Sokal A, Swierad M, et al. (2009) RADIal versus femoral approach for percutaneous coronary interventions in patients with Acute Myocardial Infarction (RADIAMI): A prospective, randomized, single-center clinical trial. Kardiol Pol 67:
22. Chodor P, Kurek T, Kowalczuk A, Swierad M, Was T, et al. (2011) Radial vs femoral approach with StarClose clip placement for primary percutaneous coronary intervention in patients with ST-elevation myocardial infarction. RADIAMI II: a prospective, randomised, single centre trial. Kardiol Pol 69: 763–771.
23. Romagnoli E, Biondi-Zoccai G, Sciahbasi A, Politi L, Rigattieri S, et al. (2012) Radial versus femoral randomized investigation in ST-segment elevation acute coronary syndrome: the RIFLE-STEACS (Radial Versus Femoral Randomized Investigation in ST-Elevation Acute Coronary Syndrome) study. J Am Coll Cardiol 60: 2481–2489.
24. Jolly SS, Yusuf S, Cairns J, Niemela K, Xavier D, et al. (2011) Radial versus femoral access for coronary angiography and intervention in patients with acute coronary syndromes (RIVAL): a randomised, parallel group, multicentre trial. Lancet 377: 1409–1420.
25. Saito S, Tanaka S, Hiroe Y, Miyashita Y, Takahashi S, et al. (2003) Comparative study on transradial approach vs. transfemoral approach in primary stent implantation for patients with acute myocardial infarction: results of the test for myocardial infarction by prospective unicenter randomization for access sites (TEMPURA) trial. Catheter Cardiovasc Interv 59: 26–33.
26. Wang YB, Fu XH, Wang XC, Gu XS, Zhao YJ, et al. (2012) Randomized Comparison of Radial Versus Femoral Approach for Patients With STEMI Undergoing Early PCI Following Intravenous Thrombolysis. J Invasive Cardiol 24: 412–416.
27. Fox KA, Steg PG, Eagle KA, Goodman SG, Anderson FA Jr., et al. (2007) Decline in rates of death and heart failure in acute coronary syndromes, 1999-2006. JAMA 297: 1892–1900.

28. Doyle BJ, Rihal CS, Gastineau DA, Holmes DR Jr. (2009) Bleeding, blood transfusion, and increased mortality after percutaneous coronary intervention: implications for contemporary practice. J Am Coll Cardiol 53: 2019–2027.

29. Nathan S, Rao SV (2012) Radial versus femoral access for percutaneous coronary intervention: implications for vascular complications and bleeding. Curr Cardiol Rep 14: 502–509.

30. Vorobcsuk A, Konyi A, Aradi D, Horvath IG, Ungi I, et al. (2009) Transradial versus transfemoral percutaneous coronary intervention in acute myocardial infarction Systematic overview and meta-analysis. Am Heart J 158: 814–821.

31. Eikelboom JW, Mehta SR, Anand SS, Xie C, Fox KA, et al. (2006) Adverse impact of bleeding on prognosis in patients with acute coronary syndromes. Circulation 114: 774–782.

32. Mehran R, Pocock SJ, Stone GW, Clayton TC, Dangas GD, et al. (2009) Associations of major bleeding and myocardial infarction with the incidence and timing of mortality in patients presenting with non-ST-elevation acute coronary syndromes: a risk model from the ACUITY trial. Eur Heart J 30: 1457–1466.

33. Doyle BJ, Ting HH, Bell MR, Lennon RJ, Mathew V, et al. (2008) Major femoral bleeding complications after percutaneous coronary intervention: incidence, predictors, and impact on long-term survival among 17,901 patients treated at the Mayo Clinic from 1994 to 2005. JACC Cardiovasc Interv 1: 202–209.

34. Chatterjee S, Wetterslev J, Sharma A, Lichstein E, Mukherjee D (2012) Association of Blood Transfusion With Increased Mortality in Myocardial Infarction: A Meta-analysis and Diversity-Adjusted Study Sequential Analysis. Arch Intern Med: 1–8.

35. Sciahbasi A, Pristipino C, Ambrosio G, Sperduti I, Scabbia EV, et al. (2009) Arterial access-site-related outcomes of patients undergoing invasive coronary procedures for acute coronary syndromes (from the ComPaRison of Early Invasive and Conservative Treatment in Patients With Non-ST-ElevatiOn Acute Coronary Syndromes [PRESTO-ACS] Vascular Substudy). Am J Cardiol 103: 796–800.

36. Genereux P, Mehran R, Palmerini T, Caixeta A, Kirtane AJ, et al. (2011) Radial access in patients with ST-segment elevation myocardial infarction undergoing primary angioplasty in acute myocardial infarction: the HORIZONS-AMI trial. EuroIntervention 7: 905–916.

37. Dechartres A, Boutron I, Trinquart L, Charles P, Ravaud P (2011) Single-center trials show larger treatment effects than multicenter trials: evidence from a meta-epidemiologic study. Ann Intern Med 155: 39–51.

38. Verheugt FW, Steinhubl SR, Hamon M, Darius H, Steg PG, et al. (2011) Incidence, prognostic impact, and influence of antithrombotic therapy on access and nonaccess site bleeding in percutaneous coronary intervention. JACC Cardiovasc Interv 4: 191–197.

39. Chhatriwalla AK, Amin AP, Kennedy KF, House JA, Cohen DJ, et al. (2013) Association between bleeding events and in-hospital mortality after percutaneous coronary intervention. JAMA 309: 1022–1029.

40. Gregory D, Midodzi W, Pearce N (2013) Complications with Angio-Seal vascular closure devices compared with manual compression after diagnostic cardiac catheterization and percutaneous coronary intervention. J Interv Cardiol 26: 630–638.

41. de Andrade PB, LA EM, Tebet MA, Rinaldi FS, Esteves VC, et al. (2013) Design and rationale of the AngioSeal versus the Radial approach In acute coronary SyndromE (ARISE) trial: a randomized comparison of a vascular closure device versus the radial approach to prevent vascular access site complications in non-ST-segment elevation acute coronary syndrome patients. Trials 14: 435.

42. Uhlemann M, Mobius-Winkler S, Mende M, Eitel I, Fuernau G, et al. (2012) The Leipzig prospective vascular ultrasound registry in radial artery catheterization: impact of sheath size on vascular complications. JACC Cardiovasc Interv 5: 36–43.

43. Buchler JR, Ribeiro EE, Falcao JL, Martinez EE, Buchler RD, et al. (2008) A randomized trial of 5 versus 7 French guiding catheters for transfemoral percutaneous coronary stent implantation. J Interv Cardiol 21: 50–55.

44. Leonardi RA, Townsend JC, Bonnema DD, Patel CA, Gibbons MT, et al. (2012) Comparison of percutaneous coronary intervention safety before and during the establishment of a transradial program at a teaching hospital. Am J Cardiol 109: 1154–1159.

45. Rafie IM, Uddin MM, Ossei-Gerning N, Anderson RA, Kinnaird TD (2014) Patients undergoing PCI from the femoral route by default radial operators are at high risk of vascular access-site complications. EuroIntervention 9: 1189–1194.

46. De Luca G, Cassetti E, Verdoia M, Marino P (2009) Bivalirudin as compared to unfractionated heparin among patients undergoing coronary angioplasty: A meta-analyis of randomised trials. Thromb Haemost 102: 428–436.

47. Baklanov DV, Kaltenbach LA, Marso SP, Subherwal SS, Feldman DN, et al. (2013) The prevalence and outcomes of transradial percutaneous coronary intervention for ST-segment elevation myocardial infarction: analysis from the National Cardiovascular Data Registry (2007 to 2011). J Am Coll Cardiol 61: 420–426.

9

Admission Lipoprotein-Associated Phospholipase A$_2$ Activity Is Not Associated with Long-Term Clinical Outcomes after ST-Segment Elevation Myocardial Infarction

Pier Woudstra[1], Peter Damman[1], Wichert J. Kuijt[1], Wouter J. Kikkert[1], Maik J. Grundeken[1], Peter M. van Brussel[1], An K. Stroobants[2], Jan P. van Straalen[2], Johan C. Fischer[2], Karel T. Koch[1], José P. S. Henriques[1], Jan J. Piek[1], Jan G. P. Tijssen[1], Robbert J. de Winter[1]*

1 Heart Center, Academic Medical Center – University of Amsterdam, Amsterdam, The Netherlands, 2 Department of Clinical Chemistry, Academic Medical Center – University of Amsterdam, Amsterdam, The Netherlands

Abstract

Background: Lipoprotein-associated phospholipase A$_2$ (Lp-PLA$_2$) activity is a biomarker predicting cardiovascular diseases in a real-world. However, the prognostic value in patients undergoing primary percutaneous coronary intervention (pPCI) for ST-segment elevation myocardial infarction (STEMI) on long-term clinical outcomes is unknown.

Methods: Lp-PLA$_2$ activity was measured in samples obtained prior to pPCI from consecutive STEMI patients in a high-volume intervention center from 2005 until 2007. Five years all-cause mortality was estimated with the Kaplan-Meier method and compared among tertiles of Lp-PLA2 activity during complete follow-up and with a landmark at 30 days. In a subpopulation clinical endpoints were assessed at three years. The prognostic value of Lp-PLA$_2$, in addition to the Thrombolysis In Myocardial Infarction or multimarker risk score, was assessed in multivariable Cox regression.

Results: The cohort (n = 987) was divided into tertiles (low <144, intermediate 144–179, and high >179 nmol/min/mL). Among the tertiles differences in baseline characteristics associated with long-term mortality were observed. However, no significant differences in five years mortality in association with Lp-PLA$_2$ activity levels were found; intermediate versus low Lp-PLA$_2$ (HR 0.97; CI 95% 0.68–1.40; p = 0.88) or high versus low Lp-PLA$_2$ (HR 0.75; CI 95% 0.51–1.11; p = 0.15). Both in a landmark analysis and after adjustments for the established risk scores and selection of cases with biomarkers obtained, non-significant differences among the tertiles were observed. In the subpopulation no significant differences in clinical endpoints were observed among the tertiles.

Conclusion: Lp-PLA$_2$ activity levels at admission prior to pPCI in STEMI patients are not associated with the incidence of short and/or long-term clinical endpoints. Lp-PLA$_2$ as an independent and clinically useful biomarker in the risk stratification of STEMI patients still remains to be proven.

Editor: Giuseppe Danilo Norata, University of Milan, Italy

Funding: The Lp-PLA2 sample kits were provided by Anton Jansen, diaDexus Inc. The work was funded by the Heart Center, Academic Medical Center – University of Amsterdam. The Lp-PLA2 sample kits were provided by Anton Jansen, diaDexus Inc. The funders had no role in study design, data collection and analysis, decision to publish, or preparation of the manuscript.

Competing Interests: The Lp-PLA2 sample kits were provided by Anton Jansen, diaDexus Inc.

* E-mail: r.j.dewinter@amc.uva.nl

Introduction

Lipoprotein-associated phospholipase A$_2$ (Lp-PLA$_2$) is an enzyme secreted by monocyte-derived macrophages, T-lymphocytes, and mast cells, and bound mainly to LDL cholesterol, in particular small, dense LDL particles [1]. It is strongly expressed in the necrotic core and surrounding macrophages around vulnerable and ruptured atherosclerotic plaques [2]. Lp-PLA$_2$ plays a major role in the pathophysiology of atherosclerosis, from initiation up to the development of cardiovascular complications [3]. In a meta-analysis of studies including patients with or without vascular disease, higher Lp-PLA$_2$ mass or activity levels were linked to an increased mortality [4]. However, the clinical application of Lp-PLA$_2$ mass or activity measurements remains subject of debate [5].

Within the spectrum of acute coronary syndrome (ACS), the prognosis of ST-segment elevation myocardial infarction (STEMI) patients (excluding shock cases) who are revascularized promptly with primary percutaneous coronary intervention (pPCI) is widely perceived as being good [6]. Over the years, the prognosis of STEMI patients has improved, although a significant proportion of these patients die before any medical contact [7]. However, patients at high risk for recurrent events remain challenging subgroups. The identification of these high risk subgroups could be helpful in further improvement of the prognosis of STEMI patients. A simple multimarker risk score based on estimated glomerular filtration rate (eGFR), glucose and N-terminal pro-brain natriuretic peptide (NTproBNP) could identify a subgroup of patients at high risk for mortality [8,9]. These biomarkers respectively reflect renal function, glucose metabolism and left ventricular dysfunction. Among other known predictors of outcome in STEMI are several inflammatory markers such as interleukin-6 and −10 [10], and the controversial CRP [11,12]. The Lp-PLA$_2$ activity assay was made available to be the first to analyse the prognostic value of admission Lp-PLA$_2$ on long-term clinical endpoints in patients presenting with STEMI treated with pPCI. Because of the existing data on the prognostic value of inflammatory markers and the knowledge of Lp-PLA$_2$, we hypothesized that Lp-PLA$_2$ activity can potentially contribute to the prognostic value of our multiple biomarker approach.

Hence, in the current analyses we investigate the independent prognostic value of Lp-PLA$_2$ activity on long-term mortality in patients undergoing primary percutaneous coronary intervention (pPCI) for STEMI.

Methods

Source Population and Procedure Characteristics

Data from consecutive STEMI patients who underwent pPCI in a large tertiary hospital were included between January 1, 2005, and January 5, 2007. The pPCI and adjunctive pharmacological treatment was performed according to American College of Cardiology, American Heart Association, and European Society of Cardiology guidelines. In general, patients were eligible for pPCI if they had ischemic chest pain, onset of symptoms less than 12 hours, and at least 1 mm of ST-segment elevation in 2 contiguous leads on the 12-lead electrocardiogram. Patients received aspirin (500 mg), clopidogrel (300 to 600 mg), and unfractionated heparin (5,000 IU). Glycoprotein IIb/IIIa inhibitors were used at the discretion of the operator. If a coronary stent was implanted, clopidogrel was prescribed for a minimum of 1 month to patients after a bare-metal stent placement and for a minimum of 6 months after a drug-eluting stent placement.

In the catheterization laboratory database all data regarding procedural and angiographic characteristics were collected prospectively. The data were entered by interventional cardiologists and trained nurses as part of routine care. The database was consulted for information on baseline patient demographics and angiographic characteristics.

Ethics Statement

The study was performed under the tenets of the Helsinki declaration, local laws and regulations. The biomarker measurements were performed in de-identified plasma aliquots obtained from the Academic Medical Centre (AMC) Cathlab Biobank, remaining from routine clinical blood sampling. The clinical follow-up was obtained from patient file review. No formal patient informed consent was obtained for the biomarker measurements according to local laws and regulations at the time of the blood drawings. The Cathlab Biobank was approved by the Biobank Instutional Review Board of the AMC – University of Amsterdam. The Dutch Medical Research Involving Human Subjects Act (WMO) did not apply to the clinical follow-up in this study according to the AMC – University of Amsterdam Medical Ethical

Review Committee (METC). As a result no formal informed consent was mandatory for the follow-up [13].

Biomarkers

Blood samples were routinely drawn as part of patient care immediately after insertion of the arterial sheath, before the introduction of the catheter, for assessment of cardiac troponin T (cTnT), C-reactive protein (CRP), glucose, NT-proBNP, and plasma creatinine. Blood samples were centrifuged without undue delay and analyzed. Both cTnT and NT-proBNP were measured using a Hitachi modular E-170 analyzer (Roche Diagnostics GmbH, Mannheim, Germany). CRP was measured with an immunoturbidimetric assay on a Hitachi modular P-800 (Roche Diagnostics GmbH, Mannheim, Germany). Glucose and plasma creatinin were measured with an enzymatic assay on a Hitachi modular P-800 analyzer (Roche Diagnostics GmbH, Mannheim, Germany). Lipid levels were not measured routinely. The eGFR was calculated according to the Cockcroft and Gault formula. Remaining plasma aliquots were coded and stored at −70°C after centrifugation.

Routine Follow-up

Information on five years vital status obtained from the institutional database, which was synchronized with the Dutch national population registry as part of routine quality control of patient care. The follow-up for all patients was censored at five years of follow-up. Clinical follow-up was available in a subpopulation, including myocardial infarction, cardiac death, stroke and revascularization, up to three years. In short, subjects were included into the subpopulation if a valid activated partial thromboplastin time was available post-procedure, as described earlier [14].

Study Population and Subpopulation

The complete cohort consists of all consecutive STEMI patients (n = 1340) who underwent pPCI between January 1, 2005, and January 5, 2007. Only the first pPCI was included in the case of a patient with multiple pPCIs within the study period. STEMI patients with cardiogenic shock (n = 85) and patients undergoing rescue PCI after failed thrombolysis (n = 10) were excluded.

In a total of 1012 patients with available plasma aliquots and complete biomarker measurements prior to pPCI Lp-PLA$_2$ activity was measured. In the subpopulation a complete 3-year clinical follow-up was available (n = 567).

Lp-PLA$_2$ Activity Measurements

The Lp-PLA$_2$ activity levels were measured in de-identified plasma aliquots which were remaining from the routinely taken blood samples at baseline procedure. The samples were stored at −80°C and were thaw in a fridge at 4°C overnight and centrifuged at 2000 g at 18°C for 10 minutes prior to analysis. Lp-PLA$_2$ activity levels were measured using the DiaDexus assay (diaDexus Inc., California, USA) on an Architect C8000 (Abbott Laboratories. Illinois, U.S.A.). The detection range of this assay was at least 0.2–450 nmol/min/mL and the inter assay coefficient of variation was 3.6–5.5%. Samples with high serum indices (hemolyses >0.30 and/or icteria >273 and/or lipemia >4.4) were excluded from further analysis (n = 25).

Endpoints

The main outcome measure for our current analysis was all-cause mortality before the end of follow-up at five years. The secondary outcome measures were the clinical endpoints at three

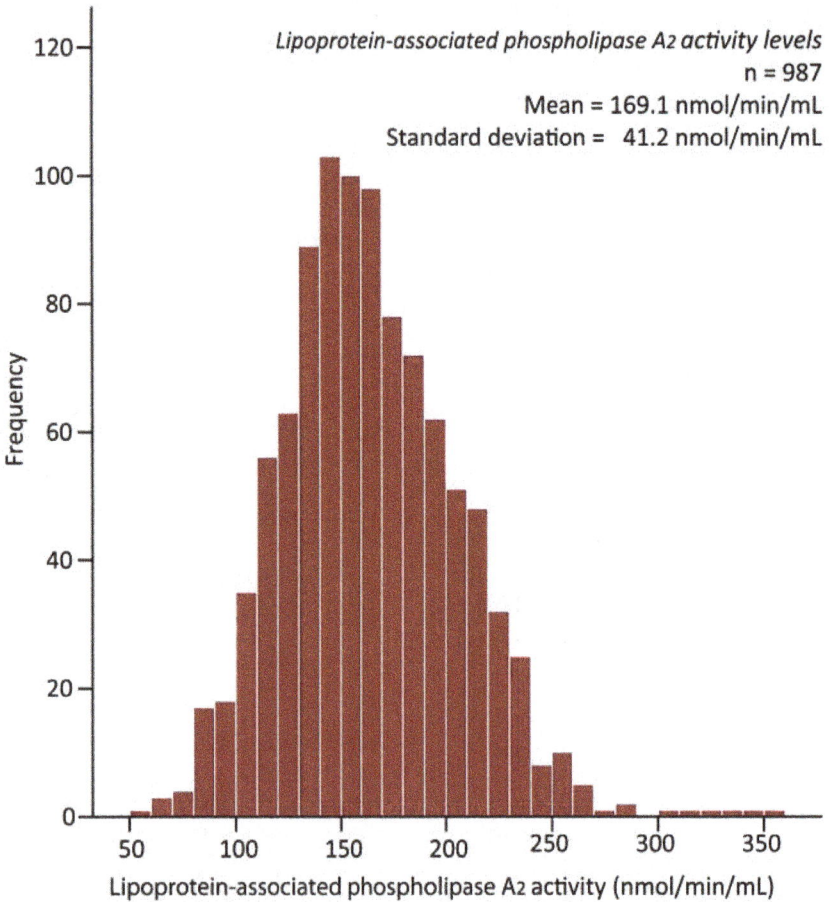

Figure 1. Histogram of Lp-PLA₂ activity levels in the complete cohort. Histogram showing distribution of measured lipoprotein-associated phospholipase A₂ activity levels. **nmol/min/mL**, nanomol per minute per milliliter.

years of follow-up, including 1) a device oriented composite endpoint of target vessel failure including cardiac death, myocardial infarction, and target vessel revascularization 2) a composite patient oriented endpoint of cardiac death and myocardial infarction. Furthermore, individual endpoints including all-cause mortality, cardiac death, myocardial infarction, stroke, and target vessel revascularization were assessed.

Statistical Analysis

The study population was divided into three equal groups based on the tertiles of Lp-PLA₂ activity levels. Tertiles were chosen because of its easy interpretation and sufficient group sizes of more than 300 patients, besides comparability with earlier published studies. Normally distributed continuous variables were reported as mean±SD and compared with the one-way ANOVA. Skewed distributed continuous variables were reported as median and interquartile range and compared with the Kruskal-Wallis test. Categorical variables were reported as number and percentage, and compared with the chi-square test.

Clinical endpoints rates were assessed by the Kaplan-Meier method and censored at date of event or last follow-up date. Clinical endpoints were compared across the Lp-PLA₂ categories using the log-rank test. The prognostic value of the Lp-PLA₂ was assessed by investigating the relationship between mortality and

the Lp-PLA₂ activity in Cox proportional-hazards analyses using the lowest tertile as the reference. The proportional hazard assumption was verified by visual estimation in a log of survival time graph. An univariate analysis of Lp-PLA₂ tertiles, and a multivariable analysis including variables associated with mortality was performed. Variables associated with mortality were depicted according the Thrombolysis In Myocardial Infarction (TIMI) risk score including age, body mass index, history of diabetes mellitus, history of hypertension, systolic blood pressure, heart frequency, anterior infarction, and symptom to open vessel time [15]. In addition, a multivariable analysis with the multimarker risk score, including eGFR, glucose and NTproBNP, was performed. Furthermore, the interactions between Lp-PLA₂ activity levels and significant different baseline variables in mortality were assessed in a Cox-regression model. For the study population and subpopulation versus the excluded patients inverse probability weighting (IPW) was utilized [16]. The propensity score for the IPW was calculated by logistic regression including the significant different variables between the selected populations and the non-selected population (P<0.05). IPW score was entered into the Cox-regression model as an independent variable to assess the possible impact of the selection out of the complete cohort on the prognostic value of Lp-PLA₂ activity on clinical outcomes.

Table 1. Baseline Characteristics.

Tertiles LpPLA$_2$ activity (nmol/min/mL)	Low (<144)	Intermediate (144–179)	High (>179)	P value
	n = 324	n = 331	n = 332	
Demographics				
Age (years)	62±13	63±13	61±13	0.07
Sex (male)	195(60.2%)	243(73.4%)	179(84.0%)	<0.001
Body mass index (kg/m^2)	27.0±4.9	26.6±4.2	26.4±3.4	0.19
Clinical history				
Prior myocardial infarction	65(20.1%)	42(12.7%)	23(6.9%)	<0.001
Prior PCI	52(16.0%)	26(7.9%)	16(4.8%)	<0.001
Prior CABG	11(3.4%)	7(2.1%)	5(1.5%)	0.26
Risk factors				
Current cigarette smoking	112(34.6%)	146(44.1%)	160(48.2%)	0.001
Hypertension	116(35.8%)	98(29.6%)	88(26.5%)	0.03
Dyslipidemia	94(29.0%)	68(20.5%)	63(19.0%)	<0.01
Diabetes mellitus	66(20.4%)	38(11.5%)	24(7.2%)	<0.001
Medication				
Aspirin	290(89.5%)	272(82.2%)	268(80.7%)	<0.01
Statin	84(25.9%)	52(15.7%)	35(10.5%)	<0.001
TIMI risk score factors				
Time to treatment* (minutes)	186(133–275)	176(128–266)	188(134–270)	0.81
Anterior infarction	110(34.0%)	137(41.4%)	155(46.7%)	<0.01
Systolic blood pressure (mmHg)	133±28	133±27	133±28	0.96
Heart rate (beats/min)	78±18	76±17	77±18	0.16
Biomarkers				
Troponin T (µg/l)	0.04(0.04–0.18)	0.04(0.04–0.21)	0.07(0.04–0.29)	0.03
Glucose (mmol/l)	9.0±3.4	8.8±3.0	8.4±3.0	0.03
NT-proBNP (ng/l)	144(57–499)	160(57–556)	144(53–778)	0.93
eGFR (ml/min)	103±42	103±38	109±41	0.03
CRP (mg/l)	3.1(1.5–8.3)	3.1(1.4–6.8)	3.3(1.3–8.1)	0.26
Multimarker risk score**	12±3	12±3	12±4	0.59
Angiographic risk factors	n = 268	n = 285	n = 288	
Thrombus pre-procedure	168(62.7%)	187(65.6%)	172(59.7%)	0.35
TIMI flow pre-procedure	0.80±1.17	0.75±1.15	0.85±1.17	0.61
TIMI flow post-procedure	2.87±0.48	2.87±0.48	2.86±0.48	0.99

Values are number(%), mean (SD) or median (interquartile range).
CABG, coronary artery bypass grafting; **CRP**, C-reactive protein; **eGFR**, estimated glomerular filtration rate; **Lp-PLA$_2$**, Lipoprotein-associated phospholipase A$_2$; **NT-proBNP**, N-terminal pro-brain natriuretic peptide; **PCI**, percutaneous coronary intervention; **TIMI**, Thrombolysis In Myocardial Infarction.
* Time of onset of symptoms to open vessel.
** According to Damman et. al. JACC 2011.

Results

Study Population

In the current analysis 987 patients with valid Lp-PLA$_2$ activity measurements were included. The mean (±SD) Lp-PLA$_2$ activity was 163.9 nmol/min/mL (±41.3) in this cohort with a near to normal distribution (Figure 1). The patient cohort was divided into tertiles with Lp-PLA$_2$ activity cut-offs of <144, 144–179, and >179 nmol/min/mL. In patients with and without statins on admission Lp-PLA$_2$ activity was respectively 146.5 (±37.2) nmol/min/mL and 167.5 (±41.2) nmol/min/mL. The mean age was 62 (±13) and 72.6% of the patients were male.

In general it should be noticed that there is a significant difference in the prevalence of several baseline characteristics among the Lp-PLA$_2$ activity tertiles, which were all associated with clinical outcomes in a STEMI population (Table 1). Importantly, Lp-PLA$_2$ activity was both positive and inverse associated with the baseline variables associated with adverse outcomes.

The baseline characteristics for the selected study population showed a significant higher incidence of dyslipidemia and aspirin use, and a significant lower incidence of prior coronary artery bypass grafting (CABG) compared with the patients not selected from the complete cohort (Table 2).

Table 2. Baseline characteristics complete cohort, study population and subpopulation.

	Complete cohort	Non-study population (Lp-PLA$_2$ activity unavailable)	Study vs. non-study population	Study population (Lp-PLA$_2$ activity available)		
				Subpopulation (Clinical follow-up)	Non-subpopulation (Mortality only)	Sub vs. non-sub population
	$n=1340$	$n=354$	P value	$n=567$	$n=420$	P value
Demographics						
Age (years)	62±13	62±13	0.62	62±13	62±13	0.46
Sex (male)	968(72.2%)	252(71.2%)	0.63	400(70.5%)	317(75.5%)	0.09
Body mass index (kg/m^2)	26.6±4.2	26.5±4.2	0.72	26.6±4.3	26.7±4.0	0.81
Clinical history						
Prior myocardial infarction	181(13.5%)	51(14.4%)	0.59	69(12.2%)	61(14.5%)	0.28
Prior PCI	121(9.0%)	27(7.6%)	0.33	45(7.9%)	49(11.7%)	0.048
Prior CABG	39(2.9%)	16(4.5%)	0.04	11(1.9%)	12(2.9%)	0.35
Risk factors						
Current cigarette smoking	563(42.0%)	145(41.0%)	0.66	248(43.7%)	170(40.5%)	0.31
Hypertension	409(30.5%)	108(30.5%)	1.00	181(31.9%)	121(28.8%)	0.29
Dyslipidemia	286(21.3%)	62(17.5%)	0.04	130(22.9%)	95(22.6%)	0.91
Diabetes mellitus	165(12.3%)	38(10.7%)	0.35	75(13.2%)	53(12.6%)	0.78
Medication						
Aspirin	1107(82.6%)	278(78.5%)	0.02	485(85.5%)	345(82.1%)	0.15
Statin	228(17.0%)	57(16.1%)	0.62	80(14.1%)	91(21.7%)	<0.01
TIMI risk score factors						
Time to treatment* (minutes)	186(132–267)	191(130–262)	0.99	182(130–269)	188(135–271)	0.52
Anterior infarction	530(39.6%)	129(36.4%)	0.18	251(44.3%)	151(36.0%)	<0.01
Systolic blood pressure (mmHg)	132±29	130±31	0.17	133±27	133±29	0.93
Heart rate (beats/min)	77±18	78±19	0.70	78±18	76±17	0.07
Biomarkers						
Troponin T (μg/l)				0.05(0.04–0.21)	0.04(0.04–0.24)	0.68
Glucose (mmol/l)				8.9±3.1	8.6±3.2	0.15
NT-proBNP (ng/l)				149(55–621)	151(58–606)	0.90
eGFR (ml/min)				104±40	105±40	0.71
CRP (mg/l)				2.9(1.4–7.0)	3.7(1.5–8.8)	0.02
Multimarker risk score**				12±3	12±3	0.63

Table 2. Cont.

	Complete cohort	Non-study population (Lp-PLA$_2$ activity unavailable)	Study vs. non-study population	Study population (Lp-PLA$_2$ activity available)		Sub vs. non-sub population
				Subpopulation (Clinical follow-up)	Non-subpopulation (Mortality only)	
			P value			*P* value
	n = 1340	n = 354		n = 567	n = 420	
	n = 1111	n = 270		n = 516	n = 325	
Angiographic risk factors						
Thrombus pre-procedure	682(61.4%)	154(44.4%)	0.21	197(60.6%)	330(64.0%)	0.18
TIMI flow pre-procedure	0.8±1.16	0.79±1.17	0.96	0.82±1.19	0.78±1.14	0.63
TIMI flow post-procedure	2.87±0.48	2.87±0.49	0.73	2.88±0.45	2.86±0.50	0.63

Values are number(%), mean (SD) or median (interquartile range).
CABG, coronary artery bypass grafting; **CRP**, C-reactive protein; **eGFR**, estimated glomerular filtration rate; **Lp-PLA$_2$**, Lipoprotein-associated phospholipase A$_2$; **NT-proBNP**, N-terminal pro-brain natriuretic peptide; **PCI**, percutaneous coronary intervention; **TIMI**, Thrombolysis In Myocardial Infarction.
* Time of onset of symptomps to open vessel.
** According to Damman et. al. JACC 2011.

Subpopulation

In the subpopulation, 567 patients with a valid Lp-PLA$_2$ activity measurement and a complete clinical follow-up were included. The mean ($\pm$SD) Lp-PLA$_2$ activity was 162.7$\pm$39.2 nmol/min/mL versus 165.5$\pm$43.9 nmol/min/mL in the non-subpopulation (p = 0.29).

Compared with those not selected for the subpopulation, the baseline characteristics in the subpopulation were significantly different for a history of PCI, anterior infarct, for the use of statin and CRP-levels (Table 2).

Study Population: Association between Lp-PLA$_2$ Activity and Mortality

During the complete follow-up 162 deaths occurred. In the univariate analysis no differences were observed when comparing the intermediate with the lowest category (HR 0.97; CI 95% 0.68–1.40; p = 0.88) or the highest with the lowest category (HR 0.75; CI 95% 0.51–1.11; p = 0.15) (Table 3–4, Figure 2). The proportional hazard assumptions were formally violated in the log of survival time graphs, however this was expected because of very parallel and similar curves among the tertiles. Therefore these formal violations do not alter the conclusions of the analyses. Furthermore, in the interaction analyses only heart frequency did have a modest statistical significant interaction with Lp-PLA$_2$ categories in mortality (HR1.012, CI95% 1.001–1.023, P = 0.026).

The following variables were included in the regression analysis to calculate the IPW score to correct for the selection of the study population out of the complete cohort; Prior CABG, history of dyslipidemia, and aspirin use. When the IPW score was introduced into the Cox-regression model no substantial changes in hazard ratios of Lp-PLA$_2$ activity were observed (intermediate versus low [HR 0.96; CI 95% 0.67–1.38; p = 0.82] and high versus low [HR 0.74; CI 95% 0.51–1.10; p = 0.33]) with an non-significant association for the IPW score for the selection from the complete cohort (HR 2.28; CI 95% 0.44–11.8; p = 0.33).

When a landmark analysis was performed, comparable mortality rates were observed at 30 days (intermediate versus low [HR 1.32; CI 95% 0.67–2.57; p = 0.42] and high versus low [HR 0.84; CI 95% 0.40–1.76; p = 0.64]) (Figure 3). Furthermore, at follow-up from 30 days until the end of follow-up non-significant differences between the groups were observed (intermediate versus low [HR 0.85; CI 95% 0.55–1.32; p = 0.48] and high versus low [HR 0.72; CI 95% 0.46–1.14; p = 0.16]) (Figure 3).

When established risk factors comprised in the TIMI risk score were added in a multivariate analysis, no differences were observed between the intermediate versus the low category (HR 1.07; CI 95% 0.69–1.67; p = 0.76) or the high versus the low category (HR 0.74; CI 95% 0.45–1.24; p = 0.25) (Table 3). Lastly, when adjusted for the multimarker risk score which was a significant predictor for mortality (HR 1.42; CI 95% 1.27–1.39; p<0.001), no differences were observed in the intermediate versus the low category (HR 0.94: CI 95% 0.65–1.35; p = 0.72) or the high versus the low category (HR 0.88; CI 95% 0.60–1.29; p = 0.51) (Table 3).

Subpopulation: Association between Lp-PLA$_2$ Activity and Clinical Endpoints

In the subpopulation no significant differences were found among the tertiles in the occurrence of the composite endpoint of cardiac death and MI (low 17.4%, intermediate 20.3%, high 14.4%, p = 0.27). The composite endpoint of target vessel failure was not significantly different among the groups (low 20.2%, intermediate 22.8%, high 17.8%, p = 0.41). In addition, the

Table 3. Unadjusted and adjusted hazard ratios for all-cause mortality at 5-years follow-up for the complete study population with available Lp-PLA$_2$ activity.

	All cause mortality		
	HR	(95% CI)	P value
Unadjusted			
Low Lp-PLA$_2$ activity (<144)		Reference	
Medium Lp-PLA$_2$ activity (144–179)	0.97	(0.68–1.40)	0.88
High Lp-PLA$_2$ activity (>179)	0.75	(0.51–1.11)	0.15
Adjusted for IPW selected population*			
Low Lp-PLA$_2$ activity (<144)		Reference	
Medium Lp-PLA$_2$ activity (144–179)	0.96	(0.67–1.38)	0.82
High Lp-PLA$_2$ activity (>179)	0.74	(0.51–1.10)	0.13
IPW selected population	2.28	(0.44–11.8)	0.33
Adjusted for TIMI risk factors**			
Low Lp-PLA$_2$ activity (<144)		Reference	
Medium Lp-PLA$_2$ activity (144–179)	1.07	(0.69–1.66)	0.75
High Lp-PLA$_2$ activity (>179)	0.75	(0.46–1.21)	0.23
Age	1.07	(1.06–1.09)	<0.001
Body mass index	1.00	(0.95–1.04)	0.84
History of diabetes mellitus	1.10	(0.68–1.77)	0.70
History of hypertension	1.17	(0.78–1.75)	0.45
Systolic blood pressure at admission	0.99	(0.99–1.00)	0.04
Heart frequency at admission	1.03	(1.02–1.04)	<0.001
Anterior myocardial infarction	0.94	(0.64–1.38)	0.76
Symptom to open vessel time	1.00	(1.00–1.00)	0.04
Adjusted for mutimarker score			
Low Lp-PLA$_2$ activity (<144)		Reference	
Medium Lp-PLA$_2$ activity (144–179)	0.94	(0.65–1.35)	0.72
High Lp-PLA$_2$ activity (>179)	0.88	(0.60–1.29)	0.51
Multimarker score	1.42	(1.34–1.50)	<0.001

Values are hazard ratio's (95% confidence interval).
IPW, inverse probability weighting; **Lp-PLA$_2$**, Lipoprotein-associated phospholipase A$_2$; **TIMI**, Thrombolysis In Myocardial Infarction.
*IPW for selection cases with biomarkers available from complete cohort.
**established by Damman et. al. JACC 2011.

individual endpoints were not significantly different among the tertiles (Table 4).

The following variables were included in the regression analyses to calculate the IPW to correct for the selection of the subpopulation out of the study population; Prior PCI, statin use, anterior infarction, and CRP level. The IPW score for selection from the complete cohort was entered into the Cox-regression models without any significant changes in hazard ratios for all events among the tertiles, and no significant association of the IPW score with the endpoints.

Discussion

The current analyses provide no evidence for an association of Lp-PLA$_2$ activity, measured at admission before pPCI for STEMI, with long-term all-cause mortality. In a subgroup, no associations between Lp-PLA$_2$ activity and clinical endpoints at 3 years, including cardiac death, MI, stroke, or revascularization, were observed. The results were consistent when corrected for known predictors of mortality in STEMI patients.

Cardiovascular Disease and Lp-PLA$_2$

Prospective epidemiological studies have investigated the association between circulating Lp-PLA$_2$ and the subsequent risk of vascular disease outcomes. A large meta-analysis did combine the individual records of 32 available prospective studies [4]. In short, Lp-PLA$_2$ activity and mass were associated with each other and with the risk of coronary heart disease, similar in magnitude to that with non-HDL cholesterol or systolic blood pressure in this population. These observations were true for the complete group of healthy individuals, and for patients with a history of stable vascular disease. However, in the subgroup of patients with acute ischemic events there was no association between baseline value of Lp-PLA$_2$ and vascular disease outcomes. The results of this meta-analysis are in accordance with the results of the current study, although the patient groups differ significantly.

Acute Ischemic Disease and Lp-PLA$_2$

Several studies have been published with regard to Lp-PLA$_2$ mass and activity levels in ACS (Table 5). One of the first studies to be published was the Olmsted County registry which prospectively

Table 4. Cumulative event rates for 3 and 5 years follow-up.

Tertiles Lp-PLA₂ activity (nmol/min/mL)	Low (<144)		Intermediate (144–179)		High (>179)		P value*
5-years follow-up	n = 324		n = 331		n = 332		
All-cause mortality	58	18.1%	58	17.6%	46	13.9%	0.29
0–30 days	15	4.9%	20	6.1%	13	4.3%	0.42
30 - end of follow up	43	14.1%	38	12.3%	33	10.4%	0.37
3-years follow-up	n = 182		n = 203		n = 182		
Composites							
Cardiac Death and MI	31	17.4%	41	20.3%	26	14.4%	0.27
Cardiac Death, MI and TVR	36	20.2%	46	22.8%	32	17.8%	0.41
Individual endpoints							
All-cause mortality	23	12.7%	30	14.8%	19	10.5%	0.42
Non-cardiac death	10	5.8%	7	3.8%	7	4.1%	0.60
Cardiac death	13	7.3%	23	11.4%	12	6.7%	0.18
Myocardial infarction	23	13.5%	23	12.1%	15	8.6%	0.35
Stroke	8	4.6%	5	2.7%	5	2.9%	0.52
Target vessel revascularization	7	4.1%	7	3.8%	7	4.0%	0.99

Values are n (%).
MI, Myocardial infarction; **Lp-PLA₂,** Lipoprotein-associated phospholipase A₂; **TIMI,** Thrombolysis In Myocardial Infarction; **TVR,** Target vessel revascularization.
*According to log-rank by Kaplan-Meier estimates.

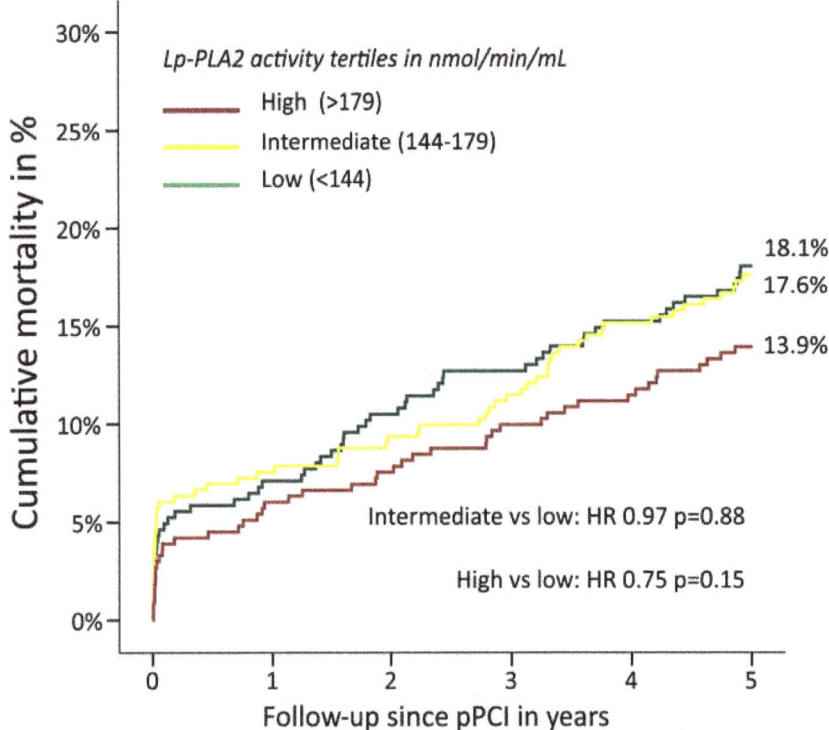

Figure 2. Kaplan-Meier estimates for mortality according to Lp-PLA₂ activity categories. Kaplan-Meier estimates showing overall mortality from pPCI until the end of follow-up. Non-significantly different hazard ratios shown according to Cox regression estimates. **HR**, Hazard ratio; **Lp-PLA₂**, Lipoprotein-associated phospholipase A₂ activity; **nmol/min/mL**, nanomol per minute per milliliter; **pPCI**, Primary percutaneous coronary intervention.

identified and followed patients (n = 271) who experienced a MI between 2003 en 2005 [17]. Lp-PLA$_2$ mass was measured in frozen samples early after MI. After adjustment for age and sex, the hazard ratios for death in the middle an upper Lp-PLA$_2$ tertiles were 2.20 (95% CI; 0.88–5.54) and 4.93 (95% CI; 2.10–11.60), compared with the lowest tertile (P_{trend} <0.001). In this

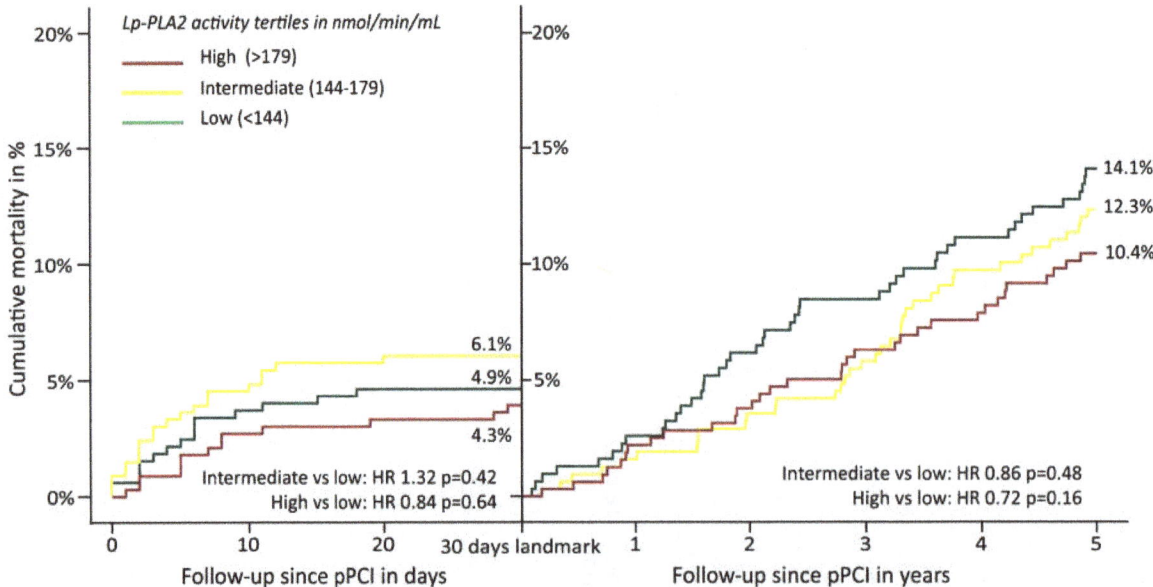

Figure 3. Landmark Kaplan-Meier estimates for mortality according to Lp-PLA₂ activity categories. Kaplan-Meier estimates showing overall mortality with a landmark at thirty days follow-up. Non-significantly different hazard ratios shown for both follow-up periods according to Cox regression estimates. **HR**, Hazard ratio; **Lp-PLA₂**, Lipoprotein-associated phospholipase A₂ activity; **nmol/min/mL**, nanomol per minute per milliliter; **pPCI**, Primary percutaneous coronary intervention.

Table 5. Previous studies in acute coronary syndrome.

Authors	Year of publication	Journal	Number of patients	Population	Sampling moment	Follow-up	Hazard ratio/event rate mortality	
							Lp-PLA$_2$ Mass	Lp-PLA$_2$ activity
Gerber et al.	2006	Arterioscler Thromb Vasc Biol	271	MI	Baseline	1 year	Lowest vs. Middle and High tertiles 1.92 (0.77–4.82), 3.48 (1.49–8.14) Ptrend = 0.003	na
O'Donoghue et al.	2006	Circulation	3648	ACS	Enrollment post-PCI	Mean 24 months	na	Quintiles, adjusted 0.65 (0.33–1.28, high vs low p = 0.21)
Oldgren et al.	2007	Eur Heart J.	2266	ACS	Post-randomization	1 year	Tertiles, high vs low 1.4 (0.77–2.5, p = 0.3)	na
Ryu et al.	2012	Circulation	2587	ACS	mean 63 hours	16 weeks	Doubling of level 1.07 (0.72–1.58, p = 0.17)	Doubling of level 0.91 (0.52–1.59, p = 0.73)
Stankovic et al.	2012	Clin. Lab	100	ACS	Admission	30 days	Low vs. High (463 ng/mL) 0% vs. 18.6% (p < 0.001)	na

study, Lp-PLA$_2$ mass levels measured shortly after MI were strongly and independently associated with one year mortality and provided incremental value in risk discrimination over traditional predictors. To best of our knowledge this is the only study to report a positive association between Lp-PLA$_2$ levels in the direct timeframe of acute ischemic disease and mortality.

Three large studies reported non-significant associations between baseline Lp-PLA$_2$ levels in ACS and outcomes. The first was the PROVE IT-TIMI 22 (PRavastatin Or atorVastatin Evaluation and Infarction Therapy – Thrombolysis) trial, in which Lp-PLA$_2$ activity levels were measured at baseline (n = 3648) and 30 days (n = 3265) in patients randomized to atorvastatin 80 mg/d or pravastatin 40 mg/d after ACS [18]. The baseline Lp-PLA$_2$ levels measured after the initial ACS event did not predict for the risk of recurrent cardiovascular events (death, myocardial infarction, unstable angina, revascularization, or stroke) at a follow-up from 18 to 36 months (mean 24 months). Though, Lp-PLA$_2$ activity levels at 30 days were lowered with high-dose statin therapy and Lp-PLA$_2$ activity levels were associated with an increased risk of cardiovascular events.

Second, in non-ST-segment elevation ACS patients in FRISC II (Fast Revascularisation during InStability in Coronary artery disease, n = 1326) and GUSTO IV (Global Utilization of STrategies to Open occluded arteries, n = 904) trials Lp-PLA$_2$ mass levels were measured at randomization [19]. In the pooled dataset, and in both studies separately, no significant association was found between Lp-PLA$_2$ levels and 1 year mortality (HR 1.4 CI 95%: 0.77–2.5, p = 0.3 for the natural logarithm of Lp-PLA$_2$).

The results of the MIRACL (Myocardial Ischemia Reduction with Acute Cholesterol Lowering) trial on the assessed biomarkers were reported [20]. In this trial Lp-PLA$_2$ mass and activity were measured at baseline (24 hours to 96 hours after hospital admission) and after 16 weeks of treatment with atorvastatin 80 mg/day or placebo in patients with ACS (n = 2587). Baseline levels of Lp-PLA$_2$ were not associated with the primary efficacy endpoint of death, myocardial infarction or unstable angina at 16 weeks.

Lastly, a study in STEMI patients measured Lp-PLA$_2$ mass in 100 patients at admission [21]. Low and high Lp-PLA$_2$ mass levels (low: <463 ng/mL, n = 67; and high: ≥463 ng/mL, n = 33) were associated with 30-day outcomes. PCI was performed within 6 hours after onset of symptoms. Both mortality and MACE rates were significantly lower in the low Lp-PLA$_2$ group versus the high Lp-PLA$_2$ group. Moreover, multiple logistic regression analysis identified the plasma Lp-PLA$_2$ level as an independent predictor of MACE (OR 1.011; 95%CI 1.001–1.013; p = 0.037). Although this analysis shows an significant prognostic value of a high Lp-PLA$_2$ at baseline, several limitations need to be mentioned; Lp-PLA$_2$ mass is only measured in a small group of patients in a very low volume center with a possible long delay to PCI, up-to 6 hour, with a very short follow-up. Although contradicting, the observations in our analyses are strengthened by the long-term follow-up in a high volume contemporary practice with a very short time from onset to measurement in a very large population. An alternative explanation could be the absence of an elevation of Lp-PLA$_2$ in the early acute phase, in which our measurements were performed. In the above study a longer time to treatment could have induced a possible selection bias, with patients with a long time-to-PCI having both a worse prognosis and a higher Lp-PLA$_2$.

The current study adds to our knowledge being the first to report on the prognostic value of admission Lp-PLA$_2$ on long-term clinical endpoints in patients presenting with STEMI treated with pPCI. In addition, this analysis reflects the prognostic value of Lp-PLA$_2$ activity in contemporary practice. Furthermore, the prospectively collected samples were obtained before pPCI in consecutive patients without other study related interventions, as was apparent in several of the earlier studies [18–20]. The results of the current study are generally in line with previous results in above mentioned study populations. One of the possible explanations for the lack of predictive value could be found in the absence of an elevation of Lp-PLA$_2$ in the early acute phase. This argument is supported by the lack of association in our analyses between the onset of symptoms to open vessel time and Lp-PLA$_2$ levels. In contrast, it could also be postulated that the Lp-PLA$_2$ activity raise in the acute phase dilutes the prognostic effect. As a result, prognostic value of activity levels could than only be observed at follow-up, such as for example in PROVE IT-TIMI 22 [18].

Biological Role of Lp-PLA$_2$

Studies on the biological role of Lp-PLA$_2$ are contradictory, showing both anti-atherogenic and pro-atherogenic functions, and not completely clarified yet. The anti-atherogenic role of Lp-PLA$_2$ was indicated by evidence showing that it plays a role in the enzymatic catabolism of biologically active oxidized phospholipids (oxPLs) in LDL and degradation of platelet activating factor [3]. However, more recent evidence suggests an anti-inflammatory role for oxPLs and as a result Lp-PLA$_2$ might promote inflammation by the hydrolysis of oxPLs [1,22]. In a patient setting Lp-PLA$_2$ deficiency has been described in the Japanese population, being associated with increased risk of developing atherosclerosis and its clinical manifestations including myocardial infarction and stroke [23,24]. These results support the concept of a protective effect of Lp-PLA$_2$.

Clinical Implications

The current analysis implicates that Lp-PLA$_2$ has no role in prognostication in the acute phase of an ACS. Notably, several baseline characteristics associated with long-term outcomes are significantly different among the tertiles. However, these differences did not influence the prognosis of the groups, probably because there was a mix of variables with positive associations and with negative associations with regard to clinical outcomes [17,18]. In contrast, it has a prognostic role in stable vascular disease or stabilized ACS, and might therefore be a potential therapeutic or preventive target. First promising results have been published on inhibitors of forms of phospholipase A$_2$ [25,26]. Currently large multicenter trials are undertaken with these new drug compounds to prove clinical benefits of phospholipase A$_2$ inhibitors in large scale populations [27–29]. Notably, the phase III STABILITY (STabilisation of Atherosclerotic plaque By Initiation of darapLadIb TherapY) randomized controlled trial on the efficacy of a Lp-PLA$_2$ inhibitor has recently been terminated on the basis of no likelihood of efficacy at the time of a prespecified interim analysis.

Limitations

Several limitations of the current study deserve to be mentioned. First, the Lp-PLA$_2$ levels have been assessed in frozen serum samples retrospectively and routine lipids levels are not available. However, all baseline data and samples were collected systematically and prospectively. Second, there is a potential selection bias

because of the exclusion of patients with missing or incomplete biomarkers. However, although some significant differences among baseline variables were observed, the IPW corrected analyses did not change the outcomes. The near normal distribution of Lp-PLA$_2$ activity is another argument to expect this cohort to be a representative sample. Third, the proportional hazard assumption is violated, limiting the interpretation of the Cox-models and hazard ratios. However, the violation is mainly caused by overlapping and parallel survival curves at each time point, as a result small changes by change cause violations of the assumption without any consequences for the clinical interpretation of the results or conclusions of the analyses. Fourth, only Lp-PLA$_2$ activity levels, and no Lp-PLA$_2$ mass, have been evaluated. Nonetheless, a previous study showed a good correlation between Lp-PLA$_2$ mass and Lp-PLA$_2$ activity with similar assays [20]. Fifth, information on vital status in the study population was obtained from the Dutch national population registry, wherein information on the cause of death is not available. Finally, only from a subpopulation follow-up including additional clinical endpoints was available. However, overall baseline characteristics were comparable, in the subpopulation no differences in clinical endpoints were found among the tertiles, and there was a similar distribution of mortality in the subpopulation compared with mortality at five years follow-up in the complete cohort. Furthermore, the analyses corrected for the IPW score for selection from the total cohort show similar results.

Conclusion

The levels of Lp-PLA$_2$ activity in STEMI patients before pPCI are associated, both positive and inversely, with differences in baseline patient characteristics which have been associated with cardiovascular mortality. However, the Lp-PLA$_2$ activity levels obtained in the acute phase of STEMI are not associated with short- or long-term clinical endpoints, including mortality, myocardial infarction, stroke or target vessel revascularization. Lp-PLA$_2$ as an independent and clinically useful biomarker in the risk stratification of STEMI patients still remains to be proven.

Acknowledgments

We would like to thank all interventional cardiologists and catheterization laboratory nurses for data collection.

Author Contributions

Conceived and designed the experiments: PW PD. Performed the experiments: PW PD W. J. Kuijt AKS JPS JCF. Analyzed the data: PW PD W. J. Kuijt W. J. Kikkert MJG PMB KTK JPSH AKS JPS JCF JJP JGPT RJW. Contributed reagents/materials/analysis tools: AJS JPS JCF. Wrote the paper: PW PD JGPT RJW. Contributed to the collection and interpretation of data; revising manuscript draft adding important intellectual content and approved the final manuscript version for submission: KTK JPSH AKS JPS JCF JJP JGPT RJW.

References

1. Tselepis AD, Dentan C, Karabina SA, Chapman MJ, Ninio E (1995) PAF-degrading acetylhydrolase is preferentially associated with dense LDL and VHDL-1 in human plasma. Catalytic characteristics and relation to the monocyte-derived enzyme. Arterioscler Thromb Vasc Biol 15: 1764–1773.

2. Kolodgie FD, Burke AP, Skorija KS, Ladich E, Kutys R et al. (2006) Lipoprotein-associated phospholipase A2 protein expression in the natural progression of human coronary atherosclerosis. Arterioscler Thromb Vasc Biol 26: 2523–2529.

3. Mallat Z, Lambeau G, Tedgui A (2010) Lipoprotein-associated and secreted phospholipases A in cardiovascular disease: roles as biological effectors and biomarkers. Circulation 122: 2183–2200.

4. Thompson A, Gao P, Orfei L, Watson S, Di Angelantonio E et al. (2010) Lipoprotein-associated phospholipase A(2) and risk of coronary disease, stroke, and mortality: collaborative analysis of 32 prospective studies. Lancet 375: 1536–1544.

5. Stein EA (2012) Lipoprotein-associated phospholipase A(2) measurements: mass, activity, but little productivity. Clin Chem 58: 814–817.

6. Biasucci LM, Della Bona R (2011) Prognostic biomarkers in ST-segment elevation myocardial infarction: a step toward personalized medicine or a tool in search of an application? J Am Coll Cardiol 57: 37–39.

7. de Vreede-Swagemakers JJ, Gorgels AP, Dubois-Arbouw WI, van Ree JW, Daemen MJ et al. (1997) Out-of-hospital cardiac arrest in the 1990's: a population-based study in the Maastricht area on incidence, characteristics and survival. J Am Coll Cardiol 30: 1500–1505.

8. Damman P, Beijk MA, Kuijt WJ, Verouden NJ, van Geloven N et al. (2011) Multiple biomarkers at admission significantly improve the prediction of mortality in patients undergoing primary percutaneous coronary intervention for acute ST-segment elevation myocardial infarction. J Am Coll Cardiol 57: 29–36.

9. Kampinga MA, Damman P, van der Horst IC, Woudstra P, Kuijt WJ et al. (2012) Survival of patients after ST-elevation myocardial infarction: external validation of a predictive biomarker model. Clin Chem 58: 1063–1064.

10. Ammirati E, Cannistraci CV, Cristell NA, Vecchio V, Palini AG et al. (2012) Identification and predictive value of interleukin-6+ interleukin-10+ and interleukin-6- interleukin-10+ cytokine patterns in ST-elevation acute myocardial infarction. Circ Res 111: 1336–1348.

11. Smit JJ, Ottervanger JP, Slingerland RJ, Kolkman JJ, Suryapranata H et al. (2008) Comparison of usefulness of C-reactive protein versus white blood cell count to predict outcome after primary percutaneous coronary intervention for ST elevation myocardial infarction. Am J Cardiol 101: 446–451.

12. Bogaty P, Boyer L, Simard S, Dauwe F, Dupuis R et al. (2008) Clinical utility of C-reactive protein measured at admission, hospital discharge, and 1 month later to predict outcome in patients with acute coronary disease. The RISCA (recurrence and inflammation in the acute coronary syndromes) study. J Am Coll Cardiol 51: 2339–2346.

13. Kikkert WJ, Zwinderman AH, Vis MM, Baan J, Jr., Koch KT et al. (2013) Timing of Mortality After Severe Bleeding and Recurrent Myocardial Infarction in Patients With ST-Segment-Elevation Myocardial Infarction. Circ Cardiovasc Interv 6: 391–398.

14. Kikkert WJ, van Nes SH, Lieve KV, Dangas GD, van Straalen J et al. (2013) Prognostic value of post-procedural aPTT in patients with ST-elevation myocardial infarction treated with primary PCI. Thromb Haemost 109: 961–970.

15. Morrow DA, Antman EM, Charlesworth A, Cairns R, Murphy SA et al. (2000) TIMI risk score for ST-elevation myocardial infarction: A convenient, bedside, clinical score for risk assessment at presentation: An intravenous nPA for treatment of infarcting myocardium early II trial substudy. Circulation 102: 2031–2037.

16. Hirano K, Imbens GW, Ridder G (2003) Efficient Estimation of Average Treatment Effects Using the Estimated Propensity Score. Econometrica 71: 1161–1189.

17. Gerber Y, McConnell JP, Jaffe AS, Weston SA, Killian JM et al. (2006) Lipoprotein-associated phospholipase A2 and prognosis after myocardial infarction in the community. Arterioscler Thromb Vasc Biol 26: 2517–2522.

18. O'Donoghue M, Morrow DA, Sabatine MS, Murphy SA, McCabe CH et al. (2006) Lipoprotein-associated phospholipase A2 and its association with cardiovascular outcomes in patients with acute coronary syndromes in the PROVE IT-TIMI 22 (PRavastatin Or atorVastatin Evaluation and Infection Therapy-Thrombolysis In Myocardial Infarction) trial. Circulation 113: 1745–1752.

19. Oldgren J, James SK, Siegbahn A, Wallentin L (2007) Lipoprotein-associated phospholipase A2 does not predict mortality or new ischaemic events in acute coronary syndrome patients. Eur Heart J 28: 699–704.

20. Ryu SK, Mallat Z, Benessiano J, Tedgui A, Olsson AG et al. (2012) Phospholipase A2 Enzymes, High-Dose Atorvastatin, and Prediction of Ischemic Events Following Acute Coronary Syndromes. Circulation.

21. Stankovic S, Asanin M, Trifunovic D, Majkic-Singh N, Miljkovic A et al. (2012) Utility of lipoprotein-associated phospholipase A2 for prediction of 30-day major adverse coronary event in patients with the first anterior ST-segment elevation myocardial infarction treated by primary percutaneous coronary intervention. Clin Lab 58: 1135–1144.

22. Bochkov VN, Kadl A, Huber J, Gruber F, Binder BR et al. (2002) Protective role of phospholipid oxidation products in endotoxin-induced tissue damage. Nature 419: 77–81.

23. Yamada Y, Ichihara S, Fujimura T, Yokota M (1998) Identification of the G994–> T missense in exon 9 of the plasma platelet-activating factor acetylhydrolase gene as an independent risk factor for coronary artery disease in Japanese men. Metabolism 47: 177–181.

24. Yamada Y, Yoshida H, Ichihara S, Imaizumi T, Satoh K et al. (2000) Correlations between plasma platelet-activating factor acetylhydrolase (PAF-AH) activity and PAF-AH genotype, age, and atherosclerosis in a Japanese population. Atherosclerosis 150: 209–216.

25. Rosenson RS, Hislop C, McConnell D, Elliott M, Stasiv Y et al. (2009) Effects of 1-H-indole-3-glyoxamide (A-002) on concentration of secretory phospholipase A2 (PLASMA study): a phase II double-blind, randomised, placebo-controlled trial. Lancet 373: 649–658.

26. Serruys PW, Garcia-Garcia HM, Buszman P, Erne P, Verheye S et al. (2008) Effects of the direct lipoprotein-associated phospholipase A(2) inhibitor darapladib on human coronary atherosclerotic plaque. Circulation 118: 1172–1182.

27. Nicholls SJ, Cavender MA, Kastelein JJ, Schwartz G, Waters DD et al. (2011) Inhibition of Secretory Phospholipase A(2) in Patients with Acute Coronary Syndromes: Rationale and Design of the Vascular Inflammation Suppression to Treat Acute Coronary Syndrome for 16 Weeks (VISTA-16) Trial. Cardiovasc Drugs Ther.

28. O'Donoghue ML, Braunwald E, White HD, Serruys P, Steg PG et al. (2011) Study design and rationale for the Stabilization of pLaques usIng Darapladib-Thrombolysis in Myocardial Infarction (SOLID-TIMI 52) trial in patients after an acute coronary syndrome. Am Heart J 162: 613–619.

29. White H, Held C, Stewart R, Watson D, Harrington R et al. (2010) Study design and rationale for the clinical outcomes of the STABILITY Trial (STabilization of Atherosclerotic plaque By Initiation of darapLadib TherapY) comparing darapladib versus placebo in patients with coronary heart disease. Am Heart J 160: 655–661.

10

Efficacy of Short-Term High-Dose Statin Pretreatment in Prevention of Contrast-Induced Acute Kidney Injury: Updated Study-Level Meta-Analysis of 13 Randomized Controlled Trials

Joo Myung Lee[1⑨], **Jonghanne Park**[1⑨], **Ki-Hyun Jeon**[1], **Ji-hyun Jung**[1], **Sang Eun Lee**[1], **Jung-Kyu Han**[1], **Hack-Lyoung Kim**[2], **Han-Mo Yang**[1], **Kyung Woo Park**[1], **Hyun-Jae Kang**[1], **Bon-Kwon Koo**[1], **Sang-Ho Jo**[3], **Hyo-Soo Kim**[1,4*]

1 Department of Internal Medicine and Cardiovascular Center, Seoul National University Hospital, Seoul, Korea, 2 Cardiovascular Center, Seoul National University, Boramae Medical Center, Seoul, Korea, 3 Division of Cardiology, Department of Internal Medicine, Hallym University Sacred Heart Hospital, Anyang-si, Gyeonggi-do, Korea, 4 Department of Molecular Medicine and Biopharmaceutical Sciences, Graduate School of Convergence Science and Technology, Seoul National University, Seoul, Korea

Abstract

Background: There have been conflicting results across the trials that evaluated prophylactic efficacy of short-term high-dose statin pre-treatment for prevention of contrast-induced acute kidney injury (CIAKI) in patients undergoing coronary angiography (CAG). The aim of the study was to perform an up-to-date meta-analysis regarding the efficacy of high-dose statin pre-treatment in preventing CIAKI.

Methods and Results: Randomized-controlled trials comparing high-dose statin versus low-dose statin or placebo pre-treatment for prevention of CIAKI in patients undergoing CAG were included. The primary endpoint was the incidence of CIAKI within 2–5days after CAG. The relative risk (RR) with 95% CI was the effect measure. This analysis included 13 RCTs with 5,825 total patients; about half of them (n = 2,889) were pre-treated with high-dose statin (at least 40 mg of atorvastatin) before CAG, and the remainders (n = 2,936) pretreated with low-dose statin or placebo. In random-effects model, high-dose statin pre-treatment significantly reduced the incidence of CIAKI (RR 0.45, 95% CI 0.35–0.57, p<0.001, $I^2 = 8.2\%$, NNT 16), compared with low-dose statin or placebo. The benefit of high-dose statin was consistent in both comparisons with low-dose statin (RR 0.47, 95% CI 0.34–0.65, p<0.001, $I^2 = 28.4\%$, NNT 19) or placebo (RR 0.34, 95% CI 0.21–0.58, p<0.001, $I^2 = 0.0\%$, NNT 16). In addition, high-dose statin showed significant reduction of CIAKI across various subgroups of chronic kidney disease, acute coronary syndrome, and old age (≥60years), regardless of osmolality of contrast or administration of N-acetylcystein.

Conclusions: High-dose statin pre-treatment significantly reduced overall incidence of CIAKI in patients undergoing CAG, and emerges as an effective prophylactic measure to prevent CIAKI.

Editor: Giuseppe Remuzzi, Mario Negri Institute for Pharmacological Research and Azienda Ospedaliera Ospedali Riuniti di Bergamo, Italy

Funding: This study was supported by grants from the Bio & Medical Technology Development Program of the National Research Foundation (NRF) funded by the Korean government (2010-0020258) and from the IRICT, Seoul National University Hospital (A062260), sponsored by the Ministry of Health and Welfare, Republic of Korea. The funders had no role in study design, data collection and analysis, decision to publish, or preparation of the manuscript.

Competing Interests: The authors have declared that no competing interests exist.

* Email: hyosoo@snu.ac.kr

⑨ These authors contributed equally to this work.

Introduction

Contrast-induced acute kidney injury (CIAKI) is a well-recognized complication of coronary angiography (CAG) with iodinated contrast medium and is the third leading cause of hospital-acquired acute renal failure. CIAKI has been known to be associated with prolonged hospitalization, increased costs, and increased short and long-term morbidity and mortality. [1] The incidence of CIAKI varies widely depending on the patient's underlying co-morbidities, definition criteria, and preventive strategies. But, certain subgroup of coronary heart disease patients, especially with acute coronary syndrome or chronic kidney disease, showed higher risk for the CIAKI. [2,3] Investigators have examined several strategies to prevent CIAKI, such as fenolopam, mannitol, theophylline, iloprost, furosemide, dopamine, hemofiltration, ascorbic acid, and N-acetylcystein (NAC). [4] However, none of the agents were proved to be effective in preventing CIAKI. [4,5] Currently, recommendations of the

European Society of Cardiology/European Association for Cardio-Thoracic Surgery (ESC/EACTS) or the ACCF/AHA/SCAI guideline are limited to the prophylactic intravenous hydration, use of iso- or low-osmolar contrast agents, and reduced dosages of contrast agents to prevent occurrence of CIAKI. [6,7] Since a few observational studies suggested that 3-hydroxyl-3-methylglutaryl coenzyme A reductase inhibitors (statins) may reduce CIAKI incidence, several RCTs have evaluated the potential benefit of statin in prevention of CIAKI. [8,9]Statin's postulated mechanism of kidney protection was through its pleotropic effects, i.e. antioxidant, anti-inflammatory, and anti-thrombotic actions. However, these previous RCTs and meta-analysis of high-dose statin pre-treatment showed disappointing results. [10–12] Recently, three RCTs with relatively large sample size (NAPLES II, PRATO-ACS, TRACK-D trial) have reported promising results favoring prophylactic efficacy of high-dose statin in prevention of CIAKI. [13–15] Considering insufficient evidences regarding efficacy of high-dose statin pre-treatment and prognostic importance of CIAKI, we therefore performed a systematic review and comprehensive meta-analysis of all published randomized control trials, in order to evaluate the efficacy of high-dose statin pre-treatment to reduce the incidence of CIAKI in various clinical situations including overall population, chronic kidney disease, or acute coronary syndrome.

Methods

Data Sources and Searches

Relevant published or unpublished studies were independently searched in PubMed, Cochrane Central Register of Controlled Trials, EMBASE, the United States National Institutes of Health registry of clinical trials (www.clinicaltrials.gov), and relevant websites (www.crtonline.org, www.clinicaltrialresults.com, www.tctmd.com, www.cardiosource.com, and www.pcronline.com) were also searched. Detailed search strategy was presented in the Method S1. The electronic search strategy was complemented by manual review of reference lists of included articles. References of recent reviews, editorials, and meta-analyses were also examined. No restrictions were imposed on language, study period, or sample size.

Study Selection

We included RCTs assessing preventive strategies for CIAKI that met following criteria. First, we selected studies which enrolled adult patients undergoing CAG with or without percutaneous coronary intervention (PCI). Second, the intervention was high-dose statin (defined as a daily dose of at least 40 mg of Atorvastatin or equivalent dose of available statins including Simvastatin, Pitavastatin, Fluvastatin, Lovastatin, Pravastatin, or Rosuvastatin), compared with low-dose statin (defined as a daily dose of less than 40 mg of Atorvastatin or equivalent dose of available statins), placebo or none of medication pre-treatment. In cases where a concomitant prophylactic measures were used (for example, NAC, sodium bicarbonate, or other preventive medications), both arms must have shared the same concomitant prophylactic measures, with only a difference in statin protocol. Finally, the incidences of post-procedural CIAKI were reported in both arms, regardless of its definition or the timing of data collection. We excluded RCTs conducted on pediatric patients (including neonates and preterm infants) and randomized crossover trials that assigned patients to both high-dose and low-dose or placebo arms.

Data Extraction and Quality Assessment

Data extraction and quality assessment was performed as previously described. [16] Summarized data as reported in the published manuscripts were used in the analysis. A standardized form was used to extract characteristics of trials, study design (including randomization sequence generation, allocation concealment, crossover between assigned groups, number of post-randomization withdrawals or follow-up loss), number of study patients, age, eligibility criteria of each trials, definition of CIAKI in each trials, baseline serum creatinine and estimated glomerular filtration rates (eGFR), mean change of serum creatinine after procedure, total cumulative dose of statin before procedure, protocols for statin treatment, hydration protocols, type or mean dosage of radio-contrast agents, the proportion of diabetes mellitus, hypertension, chronic kidney disease, timing of data collection, length of follow-up, adverse events data associated with statin treatment reported on an intention-to-treat basis. We primarily focused our analysis on the effect of prophylactic treatment with high-dose statin on the incidence of CIAKI, not on the surrogate markers of inflammation or oxidative stress. The quality of eligible RCTs was assessed using the Cochrane Collaboration's tool for assessing the risk of bias for RCTs (Table S1 in File S1). Because most previous meta-analyses have reported the methodological quality of each trial using the Jadad score, we also provided this score, as well as the Cochran Collaboration's tool, for each RCT. [17] Two investigators (JML and JP) independently performed screening of titles and abstracts, identified duplicates, reviewed full articles, and determined their eligibility. Disagreements were resolved by discussions. The last search was performed in February 2014.

Outcomes and Definitions

The primary outcome was the incidence of post-procedural CIAKI within 2–5 days after index procedure. Secondary outcomes included the incidence of post-procedural CIAKI, stratified according to the various subgroups for example, type of contrast agents (iso-osmolar or low-osmolar) used, mean age of the study patients, presence of underlying chronic kidney disease, patients with acute coronary syndrome, NAC usage, or placebo control. All of the patients and outcomes were analyzed according to the originally assigned group.

Data Synthesis and Analysis

Data synthesis and analsysis was performed as described in detail previously [16], The primary outcome was analyzed by both a random effects model and a fixed effects model. Relative risks (RR) with 95% confidence interval (CI) were presented as summary statistics. The pooled RR was calculated with the DerSimonian and Laird method for random effects model, as well as the Mantel–Haenszel method for fixed effects model. [18] To evaluate the effect of progressive chronological change in study design, such as study population, protocol of statin pre-treatment, hydration protocols or concomitant prophylactic medications including NAC or sodium bicarbonate, we evaluated the impact of publication date on the overall effect of pooled RRs for incidence of CIAKI by a cumulative meta-analysis. Stratified subgroup analyses were performed to assess treatment effects according to the control group (low-dose statin, placebo, or no medication), type of contrast agent, mean age of the patients, underlying chronic kidney disease, acute coronary syndrome, and usage of NAC along with tests for interaction derived from random effects meta-regression. Statistical heterogeneity was assessed by Cochran's Q via a χ^2 test and was quantified with the I^2 test. [19] Publication bias was assessed by funnel plot asymmetry, along with Egger's and Begg's test. The κ statistic was used to assess agreement between investigators for study selection. Results were considered statistically significant at 2-sided p<0.05. Statistical analysis was performed with the use of STATA/SE 12.0 (Stata Corp LP, College Station, Texas, USA). The present study was performed in compliance with the Preferred Reporting Items for Systematic Reviews and Meta-Analyses (PRISMA) guidelines and the review protocol has not been registered (Checklist S1). [20]

Results

Search Results

We identified 465 citations from searches as previously described. Among these, 24 studies were retrieved for detailed evaluation, of which 13 RCTs met inclusion criteria (Figure 1). [11–15,21–28] These 13 RCTs included a total of 5,825 adult patients, 2,889 (49.6%) of which were allocated to the high-dose statin group and 2,936 (50.4%) of which were allocated to the control group (low-dose statin or placebo group). The characteristics of 11 excluded studies after full article review are summarized in the Method S2. The inter-observer agreement for study selection was high (κ = 0.92).

Trial Characteristics

The main characteristics of the individual studies are summarized in Table 1 and 2. All trials reported the incidence of CIAKI within 2-5days from index procedure using contrast agents. Four trials exclusively enrolled the patients with chronic kidney disease, which was defined as eGFR of less than 60 ml/min/1.73 m² in

PROMISS, Toso et al, and NAPLES II trial, and eGFR of between 30–90 ml/min/1.73 m² in TRACK-D trial. [11–14] Only one trial (TRACK-D) exclusively enrolled type 2 diabetes mellitus patients, whereas the others enrolled the patients regardless of diabetes mellitus. [14] Among the 13 trials, 4 trials compared high-dose statin versus low-dose statin pre-treatment. [21,22,25,27] Majority of trials used Atorvastin, whereas 2 trials [11,21] used Simvastatin, and 2 trials [14,15] used Rosuvastatin. Total cumulative dose of statin in high-dose statin group ranged from 40 mg to 560 mg of Atorvastatin equivalent dose from 1 to 7 days before CAG. The detailed medication protocols in each included trials are summarized in Table 1. The definition of CIAKI slightly differed across trials. Ten trials [11,14,15,21, 22,24–28] used an increase in serum creatinine of ≥0.5mg/dL or ≥25% from baseline within 48–72 hours after radiocontrast exposure, whereas 2 trials [12,23] regarded an absolute increase in serum creatinine of ≥0.5 mg/dL within 5 days as their primary definition of CIAKI. One trial (NAPLES II) used an increase in serum cystatin C ≥10% from baseline, which was used in this analysis, although they reported the incidence of CIAKI on the base of the change in serum creatinine as secondary outcomes. [13] All trials evaluated patients with coronary artery disease undergoing CAG with or without percutaneous coronary intervention. Among the trials, 5 studies [15,21,26–28] exclusively enrolled the patients with acute coronary syndrome including unstable angina and non ST-segment elevation myocardial infarction, and 2 of these 5 studies [21,28] further included the patients with ST-segment elevation myocardial infarction. Four trials [12,13,15,24] used NAC (600 mg or 1200 mg twice daily) as additional preventive measure of CIAKI in both arms, and 1 trial

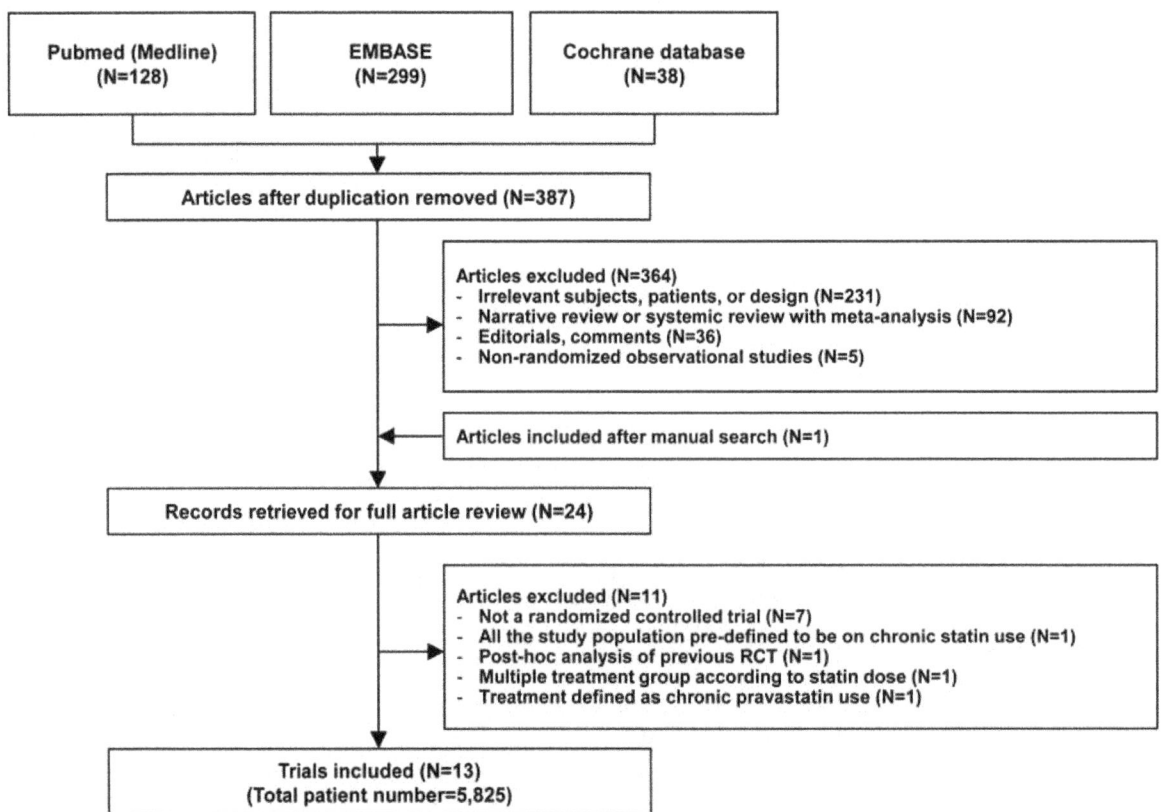

Figure 1. Flow diagram of trial selection. Abbreviations: RCT, randomized controlled trial.

Table 1. Characteristics of the study, trial characteristics and protocols.

Trial (Year)	Patients number		Inclusion criteria	Definition of CIN	Medication Protocols		Contrast agent	Contrast volumes (mean), ml		Hydration protocols
	Statin (N=2889)	Control (N=2936)			Statin	Control		Statin	Control	
PROMISS (2008)	118	118	CKD patients undergoing CAG or PCI, CrCl≤60 mL/min or SCr≥ 1.1 mg/dL	Increase of SCr≥ 0.5 mg/dL or ≥25% at 48 hours	Simvastatin 40 mg bid, 1 day pre-procedure and 1 day post-procedure	Placebo	Visipaque (iodixanol)	173.3	190.9	NS 1 mg/kg/h for 12 h before and 12 h after procedure
Toso et al. (2009)	152	152	CKD patients undergoing CAG or PCI, CrCl<60 mL/min	Increase of SCr≥ 0.5 mg/dl within 5 days.	Atorvastatin 80 mg/day 2 days pre-procedure and 2 days post-procedure, NAC 1200 mg bid from 1 day before to 1 day post-procedure	Placebo + NAC 1200 mg bid from 1day before to 1 day post-procedure	Visipaque (iodixanol)	151.0	164.0	NS 1 ml/kg/h for 12 h before and after the procedure
Xinwei et al. (2009)	113	115	ACS (UA/NSTEMI) including STEMI patients undergoing PCI	Increase of SCr≥ 0.5 mg/dL or ≥25% at 48 hours	Simvastatin 80 mg/ day from admission to the day before, 20 mg/day after procedure	Simvastatin, 20 mg/day from admission to the end	Visipaque (iodixanol) for CKD, Omnipaque (iohexol) for non-CKD	227.0	240.0	NS 1 ml/kg/h for 6 to 12 h before and 12 h after procedure
Zhou Xia et al. (2009)	50	50	Patients undergoing CAG or PCI	Increase of SCr≥ 0.5 mg/dL or ≥ 25% at 72 hours	Atorvastatin 80 mg/ day before for 1day,10 mg/day for 6days after procedure	Atorvastatin 10 mg/day for 7 days	Iopamidol 370 mg/ml	118.7	112.9	NS 1000 mL infusion, for 12 h before and 12 h after intervention
Acikel et al. (2010)	80	80	Patients undergoing elective CAG or PCI (excluding ACS), LDL≥ 70 mg/dl, eGFR≥60 ml/min/ 1.73 m²	Increase of SCr≥ 0.5 mg/dL at 48 hours	Atorvastatin 40 mg/ day 3 days pre-procedure and 2 days post-procedure	None	Omnipaque(iohexol)	105.0	103.0	NS 1 ml/kg/h starting 4 h before and continuing until 24 h after procedure
Ozhan et al. (2010)	60	70	Patients undergoing CAG or PCI, eGFR≥70 ml/min/1.73 m² or SCr≤1.5 mg/dL	Increase of SCr≥ 0.5 mg/dL or ≥25% at 48 hours	Atorvastatin 80 mg 1 day pre-procedure and 2 days post-procedure, NAC 600 mg bid pre-procedure	No statin pre-procedure, NAC 600 mg bid pre-procedure	Iopamidol	97.0	93.0	NS 1000 ml infusion during 6 h after procedure
Hua et al. (2010)	76	97	Patients undergoing CAG or PCI	Increase of SCr≥ 0.5 mg/dL or ≥25% at 72 hours	Atorvastatin 80 mg/day pre-procedure	Atorvastatin 20 mg/day pre-procedure	Iopromide	173.0	177.0	NR
ARMYDA-CIN (2011)	120	121	ACS (UA/NSTEMI) Patients undergoing CAG or PCI (excluding high-risk NSTEMI requiring emergency PCI), SCr≤3 mg/dl	Increase of SCr≥ 0.5 mg/dL or ≥25% at 48 hours	Atorvastatin 80 mg (12 h before) → 40 mg (2 h before), 40 mg for 2days after procedure	Placebo before procedure → Atorvastatin 40 mg for 2days after procedure	Xenetix (iobitridol)	209.0	213.0	For patients CrCl < 60 ml/min, NS 1 ml/ kg/h for 12 h before and 24 h after intervention

Table 1. Cont.

Trial (Year)	Patients number		Inclusion criteria	Definition of CIN	Medication Protocols		Contrast agent	Contrast volumes (mean), ml		Hydration protocols
	Statin (N = 2889)	Control (N = 2936)			Statin	Control		Statin	Control	
Wei Li et al. (2012)	78	83	STEMI patients undergoing emergency PCI within 12 hours of symptom onset	Increase of SCr≥ 0.5 mg/dL or ≥25% at 72 hours	Atorvastatin 80 mg loading pre-procedure, long-term 40 mg/day after procedure	Placebo 801mg loading pre-procedure, long-term 40 mg/day after procedure	Ultravist 370 (iopromide)	100.0	103.6	NS 1 ml/kg/h before the procedure and for 12 h after the procedure
NAPLES II (2012)	202	208	CKD patients undergoing CAG or PCI, eGFR<60 ml/min/1.73 m²	Increase of Serum Cystatin C concentration ≥10% at 24 hours	Atorvastatin 80 mg before procedure, NAC 1200 mg bid the day before and the day of procedure	No statin pre-procedure, NAC 1200 mg bid the day before and the day of procedure	Visipaque (iodixanol)	177.0	184.0	Sodium bicarbonate solution (154 mEq/L), initial bolus of 3 mL/kg/h for 1 h before procedure, 1 mL/kg/h during and for 6 h after the procedure
CAO et al. (2012)	90	90	Patients undergoing CAG or PCI	Increase of SCr≥ 0.5 mg/dL or ≥25% at 72 hours	Atorvastatin 40 mg/day from 3days before procedure, 20 mg/day after procedure	Atorvastatin 20 mg/day from 3days before procedure, 20 mg/day after procedure	NR	162.3	158.9	NR
PRATO-ACS (2014)	252	252	ACS (UA/NSTEMI) patients undergoing CAG or PCI (excluding STEMI and high-risk NSTEMI requiring emergency PCI), SCr≤ 3 mg/dl	Increase of SCr≥ 0.5 mg/dL or ≥25% at 72 hours	Rosuvastatin 40 mg loading → 20 mg/day before procedure, Rosuvastatin 20 mg/day continued after procedure, NAC 1200 mg bid the day before and the day of procedure	No statin pre-procedure, Atorvastatin 40 mg/day after procedure, NAC 1200 mg bid the day before and the day of procedure	Visipaque (iodixanol)	149.7	138.2	NS 1 ml/kg/h for 12 h both before and after the procedure. Hydration rate was reduced to 0.5 ml/kg/h in both arms for patients with LVEF <40%
TRACK-D (2014)	1498	1500	Stage 2 or 3 CKD and type II DM patients undergoing CAG or PCI, eGFR ≥30 ml/min/1.73 m² and < 90 ml/min/1.73 m² (excluded stage 0,1,4,5 CKD patients)	Increase of SCr≥ 0.5 mg/dL or ≥25% at 72 hours	Rosuvastatin 10 mg/day from 2 days before to 3 days after procedure → continued after procedure	No statin pre-procedure, Rosuvastatin 10 mg. day 3 days after procedure	Visipaque (iodixanol)	120.0	110.0	NS 1 ml/kg/h started 12 h before and continued for 24 h after procedure

Abbreviations: ACS, acute coronary syndrome; CAG, coronary angiography; CIN, contrast induced nephropathy; CKD, chronic kidney disease; CrCl, creatinine clearance; DM, diabetes mellitus; eGFR, estimated glomerular filtration rate; LDL, low-density lipoprotein; LVEF, left ventricular ejection fraction; NAC, N-acetylcystein; NR, not reported; NS, normal saline (isotonic saline, 0.9%); NSTEMI, non ST-segment elevation myocardial infarction; PCI, percutaneous coronary intervention; SCr, serum creatinine; STEMI, ST-segment elevation myocardial infarction; UA, unstable angina.

Table 2. Characteristics of the study, baseline characteristics.

Trial (Year)	Mean age, year		Mean baseline SCr (mg/dL)		Mean baseline eGFR (ml/min)		Male proportion	Diabetes Mellitus proportion	Hypertension proportion	Additional measures
	Statin	Control	Statin	Control	Statin	Control				
PROMISS (2008)	65	66	1.29	1.25	53.46	55.40	72.5%	25.9%	63.2%	None
Toso et al. (2009)	75	76	1.20	1.18	46.00	46.00	64.5%	21.1%	60.5%	NAC
Xinwei et al. (2009)	65	66	0.82	0.83	86.50	93.60	36.0%	20.6%	63.6%	None
Zhou Xia et al. (2009)	60	61	1.04	1.08	76.88	70.54	59.0%	20.0%	75.0%	None
Acikel et al. (2010)	59	61	0.84	0.85	97.70	97.00	63.8%	24.4%	58.1%	None
Ozhan et al. (2010)	54	55	0.88	0.88	92.00	89.00	59.2%	16.2%	22.3%	NAC
Hua et al. (2010)	65	65	1.34	1.40	68.20	66.70	67.1%	26.6%	74.6%	None
ARMYDA-CIN (2011)	65	66	1.04	1.04	79.80	77.00	77.6%	28.2%	75.1%	None
Wei Li et al. (2012)	66	65	0.93	0.93	NR	NR	75.8%	28.0%	80.7%	None
NAPLES II (2012)	70	70	1.32	1.29	42.00	43.00	54.4%	41.2%	86.3%	NAC, bicarbonate
CAO et al. (2012)	63	63	0.85	0.83	109.60	106.80	57.2%	21.7%	37.2%	None
PRATO-ACS (2014)	66	66	0.95	0.96	69.90	69.30	65.7%	21.2%	55.8%	NAC
TRACK-D (2014)	62	61	1.08	1.07	74.16	74.43	65.2%	100.0%	71.9%	None

Abbreviations: ACS, acute coronary syndrome; CAG, coronary angiography; CIN, contrast induced nephropathy; CKD, chronic kidney disease; CrCl, creatinine clearance; DM, diabetes mellitus; eGFR, estimated glomerular filtration rate; LDL, low-density lipoprotein; LVEF, left ventricular ejection fraction; NAC, N-acetylcystein; NR, not reported; NS, normal saline (isotonic saline, 0.9%); NSTEMI, non ST-segment elevation myocardial infarction; PCI, percutaneous coronary intervention; SCr, serum creatinine; STEMI, ST-segment elevation myocardial infarction; UA, unstable angina.

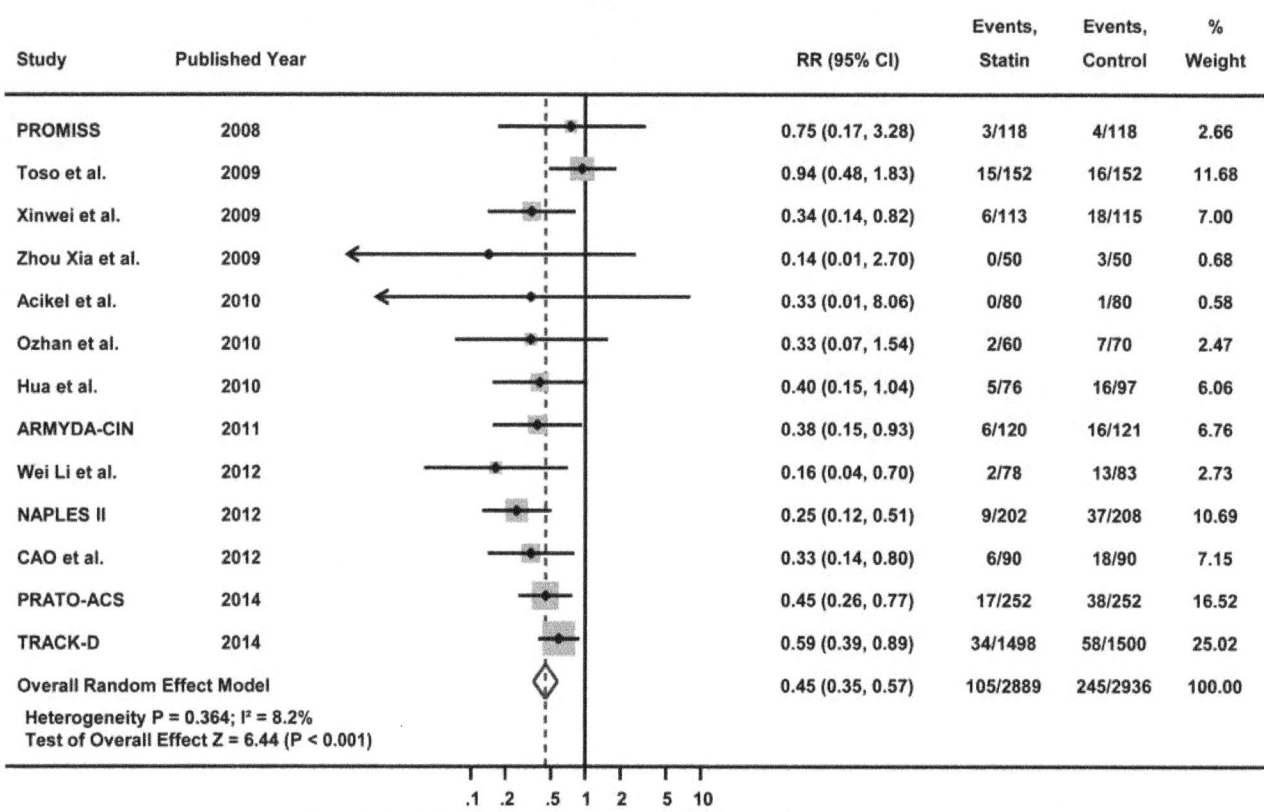

Figure 2. The effect of high-dose statin on the incidence of contrast-induced acute kidney injury by random effects model. Forest plot with relative risks for the incidence of contrast-induced acute kidney injury associated with high-dose statin pre-treatment, compared with control group (low-dose statin or placebo) for individual trials and the pooled population. Abbreviations: CI, confidence intervals; RR, relative risks.

[13] used sodium bicarbonate solution as primary hydration protocol.

Risk of Bias within Trials

Figure S1 in File S1 shows the risk of bias graph illustrating the proportion of studies with each of the judgments ('Yes', 'No', 'Unclear') for each entry in the Cochrane Collaboration's tool. A full description of the summary of risk of bias judgments of each study is available in Figure S2 and Table S1 in File S1. All of the included trials were RCTs and no substantial risk of bias was observed in random sequence generation. The included trials showed relatively high methodological quality. Among the 13 RCTs, 5 trials [11,12,15,26,28] had double-blinded design, whereas others were open-label or non-blinded trials. However, all trials used objective findings (serum creatinine or cystatin C) to define the primary endpoint (the incidence of CIAKI), the authors, therefore, judged that the outcomes were not likely to be influenced by lack of blinding.

Effect of Statin on the Incidence of Contrast-Induced Acute Kidney Injury

As shown in Figure 1, this meta-analysis included 13 RCTs [11–15,21–28], all of which provided the incidence of CIAKI. Figure 2 illustrates the RRs of individual study and pooled RR in regards to the incidence of CIAKI, the primary outcome. The overall incidence of CIAKI in the intention-to-treat population was 3.6% (105/2889) in high-dose statin group and 8.3% (245/2936) in control group, respectively. In pooled analysis using

random effects model, patients receiving high-dose statin pre-treatment had 55% less risk of CIAKI compared with the control group (RR 0.45, 95% CI 0.35–0.57, p<0.001) (Figure 2). A fixed effects model yielded a similar result (RR 0.44, 95% CI 0.35–0.55, p<0.001) (Figure S3 in File S1). The number needed to treat (NNT) of high-dose statin was 16 in random effects model which means that treatment of 16 patients with high-dose statin will reduce 1 event of CIAKI. There was no significant heterogeneity in either the random effects or the fixed effects model ($I^2 = 8.2\%$, heterogeneity p = 0.364 for both random and fixed effects model). Since 4 trials compared high-dose versus low-dose statin group and 9 trials compared high-dose versus placebo or no treatment, we performed stratified analysis according to the type of treatment (Figure 3). High-dose statin significantly reduced the risk of CIAKI by 53% (RR 0.47, 95% CI 0.34–0.65, p<0.001, $I^2 = 28.4\%$, heterogeneity p = 0.192) or 66% (RR 0.34, 95% CI 0.21–0.58, p<0.001, $I^2 = 0.0\%$, heterogeneity p = 0.931), when compared with placebo or low-dose statin group, respectively.

Visual estimation of the funnel plot indicated no apparent publication or small study effect bias with the support of the Egger's test (p = 0.128) and Begg's test (p = 0.625) (Figure S4 in File S1). No individual study unduly influenced the pooled estimate of high-dose statin for the incidence of CIAKI (Figure S5 in File S1). Cumulative meta-analysis, which sorts trials chronologically, showed no apparent progressive shift of pooled estimate of high-dose statin from a negative to a positive effect, despite of differences in practice patterns or patient populations from 2008 to 2014 (Figure S6 in File S1). Along with the

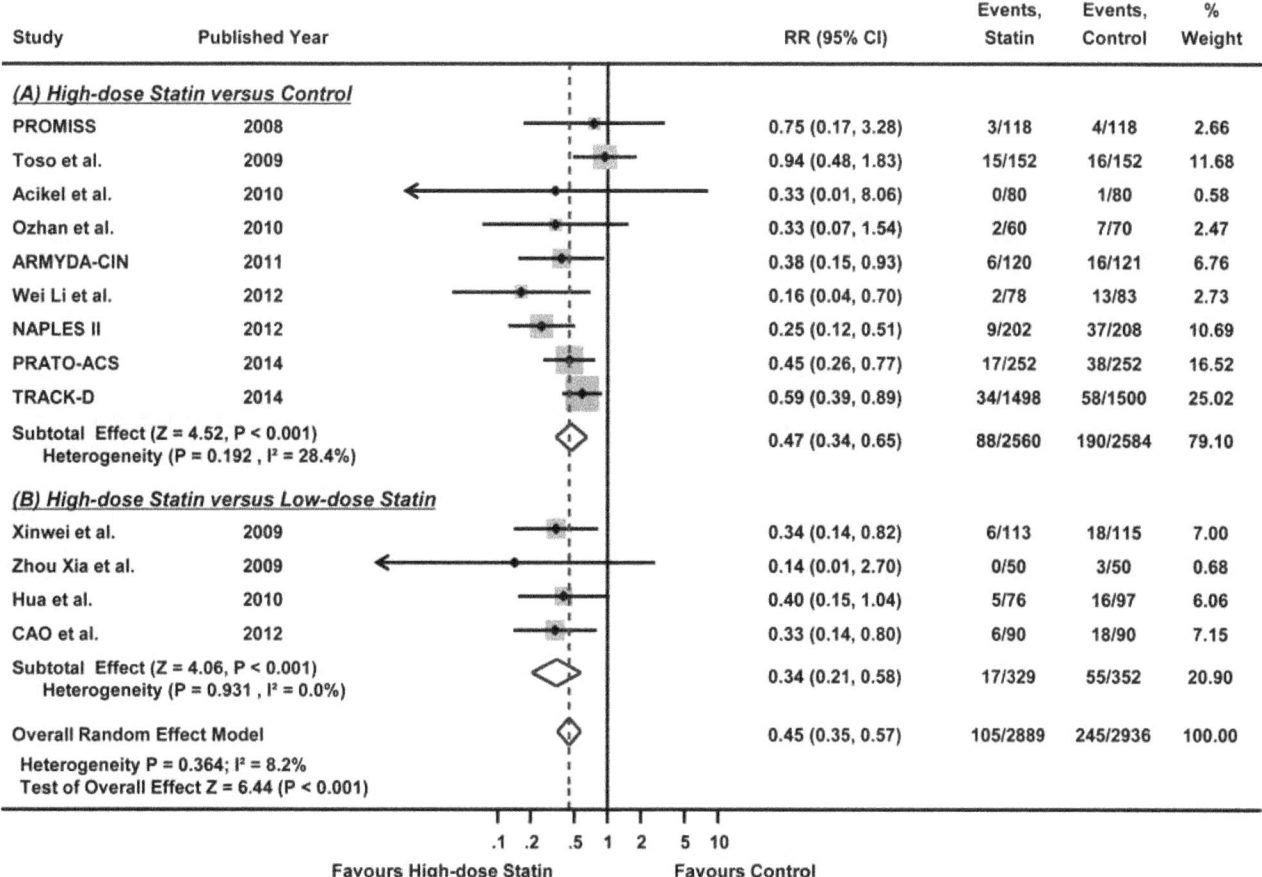

Figure 3. The effect of high-dose statin on the incidence of contrast-induced acute kidney injury, stratified according to the high-dose versus low-dose statin or high-dose versus placebo. Forest plot with relative risks for the incidence of contrast-induced acute kidney injury associated with (A) high-dose statin versus low-dose statin or (B) high-dose statin versus placebo for individual trials and the pooled population. Abbreviations: CI, confidence intervals; RR, relative risks.

significantly reduced incidence of CIAKI in high-dose statin group, mean change of post-procedural serum creatinine was also significantly lower in the high-dose statin group, compared with control group (SMD −0.37, 95% CI −0.59 to −0.15, p = 0.001) (Figure S7 in File S1).

Subgroup Analysis

The results of subgroup analysis are presented in Figure 4. The beneficial effect of high-dose statin pre-treatment was consistent across all the subgroups, except the subgroup of age less than 60 years old. The high-dose statin showed significantly less development of CIAKI in the patients with old age (≥60 years old), underlying chronic kidney disease, or acute coronary syndrome. When the high-risk subgroup was defined with the patients with chronic kidney disease or acute coronary syndrome, the high-dose statin showed also significant beneficial effect in reducing CIAKI in both high-risk and low-risk subgroup. In addition, the protective effect of high-dose statin was also significant regardless of the osmolality of the contrast agents (iso- or low-osmolar) or concomitant treatment of NAC. Lastly, high-dose statin significantly reduced the incidence of CIAKI compared with placebo or low-dose statin. The NNT of high-dose statin ranged from 12 to 26 (Figure 4). Detailed results of pooled analysis in each subgroup are summarized in the Figure S8-S12 in File S1.

Discussion

The results of this meta-analysis indicate that high-dose statin pre-treatment in patients undergoing CAG with or without PCI significantly reduced the incidence of CIAKI, compared with control (placebo or low-dose statin). The beneficial effect of high-dose statin was obvious in various subgroups of patients including underlying chronic kidney disease, acute coronary syndrome, or old age (≥60 years). The effect of high-dose statin was also clear regardless of type of contrast agent or concomitant treatment of NAC.

This study is the most up-to-date comprehensive meta-analysis with improved statistical power to address the effect of statin for CIAKI prevention in CAG. [10,29–33] The inconclusive results of previous meta-analyses regarding the efficacy of statin pre-treatment, might mainly originate from the limited sample size of included trials. [29–31] Some of these studies included both randomized and non-randomized clinical trials, which might have led to potential bias. [10,32] In the most recent meta-analysis by Li et al. [33], the authors showed significant benefit of statin pre-treatment in reducing the incidence of CIAKI. However, they argued that statin pre-treatment had no protective effect in the patients with underlying chronic kidney disease (RR 0.79, 95% CI 0.47–1.32, p = 0.37), however, the included studies in this subgroup analysis were only 3 studies with total sample size of

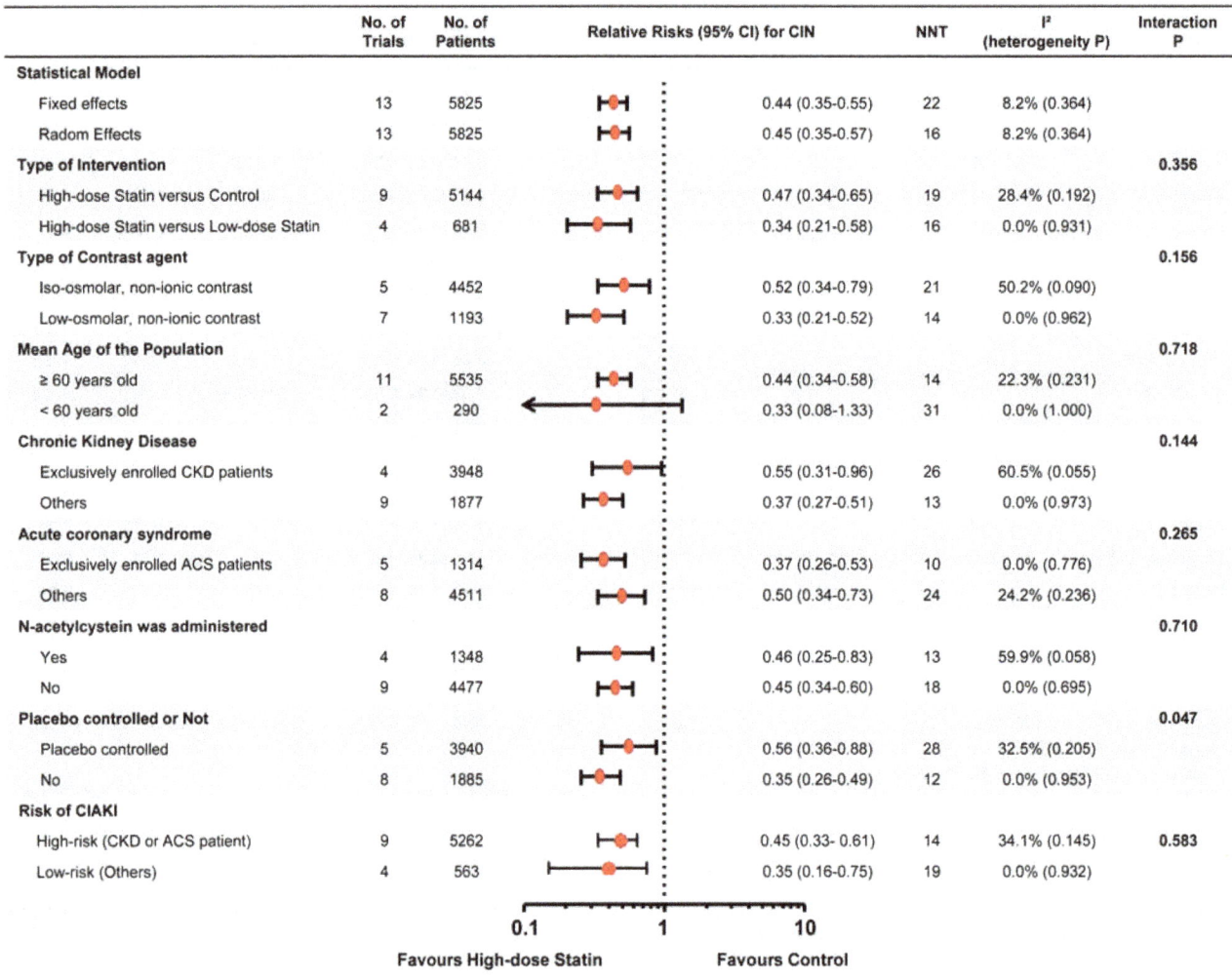

	No. of Trials	No. of Patients	Relative Risks (95% CI) for CIN		NNT	I² (heterogeneity P)	Interaction P
Statistical Model							
Fixed effects	13	5825		0.44 (0.35-0.55)	22	8.2% (0.364)	
Radom Effects	13	5825		0.45 (0.35-0.57)	16	8.2% (0.364)	
Type of Intervention							0.356
High-dose Statin versus Control	9	5144		0.47 (0.34-0.65)	19	28.4% (0.192)	
High-dose Statin versus Low-dose Statin	4	681		0.34 (0.21-0.58)	16	0.0% (0.931)	
Type of Contrast agent							0.156
Iso-osmolar, non-ionic contrast	5	4452		0.52 (0.34-0.79)	21	50.2% (0.090)	
Low-osmolar, non-ionic contrast	7	1193		0.33 (0.21-0.52)	14	0.0% (0.962)	
Mean Age of the Population							0.718
≥ 60 years old	11	5535		0.44 (0.34-0.58)	14	22.3% (0.231)	
< 60 years old	2	290		0.33 (0.08-1.33)	31	0.0% (1.000)	
Chronic Kidney Disease							0.144
Exclusively enrolled CKD patients	4	3948		0.55 (0.31-0.96)	26	60.5% (0.055)	
Others	9	1877		0.37 (0.27-0.51)	13	0.0% (0.973)	
Acute coronary syndrome							0.265
Exclusively enrolled ACS patients	5	1314		0.37 (0.26-0.53)	10	0.0% (0.776)	
Others	8	4511		0.50 (0.34-0.73)	24	24.2% (0.236)	
N-acetylcystein was administered							0.710
Yes	4	1348		0.46 (0.25-0.83)	13	59.9% (0.058)	
No	9	4477		0.45 (0.34-0.60)	18	0.0% (0.695)	
Placebo controlled or Not							0.047
Placebo controlled	5	3940		0.56 (0.36-0.88)	28	32.5% (0.205)	
No	8	1885		0.35 (0.26-0.49)	12	0.0% (0.953)	
Risk of CIAKI							0.583
High-risk (CKD or ACS patient)	9	5262		0.45 (0.33- 0.61)	14	34.1% (0.145)	
Low-risk (Others)	4	563		0.35 (0.16-0.75)	19	0.0% (0.932)	

0.1   1   10

Favours High-dose Statin   Favours Control

Figure 4. Subgroup analyses according to the study protocols. The forest plot shows relative risks (by random effects model) for the incidence of contrast-induced acute kidney injury associated with high-dose statin pre-treatment, compared with control group (low-dose statin or placebo), stratified according to (1) type of intervention, (2) type of contrast agent, (3) mean age of the patients, (4) underlying chronic kidney disease, (5) acute coronary syndrome, (6) N-acetylcystein as concomitant prophylactic measure, and (7) placebo controlled trial or not. Abbreviations: ACS, acute coronary syndrome; CI, confidence intervals; CKD, chronic kidney disease; RR, relative risks.

390 in high-dose statin versus 391 in control group. [33] In the present meta-analysis we evaluated over 5,800 patients from 13 RCTs, the benefit of high-dose statin was consistently observed in both overall population and various subgroups including patients with chronic kidney disease (RR 0.55, 95% CI 0.31–0.96, p = 0.036). The limited sample size of the pooled analysis and larger chance of type II error would explain the negative result of Li et al.

Previous studies have suggested that statin protects CIAKI through its pleotropic effect rather than its lipid lowering effect. The pleotropic effect includes enhancement of nitric oxide production, anti-inflammatory, and antioxidative effect. [34,35] These pleotropic effects could decrease renal cell injury after iodinated contrast exposure. In the NAPLES II trial, high-dose atorvastatin reduced contrast-induced JNK activation and p53 phosphorylation which is the key steps of oxidative stress induced intrinsic apoptosis. [13] Also, statin may modulate the kidney hypoperfusion after radio-contrast exposure by down-regulation of angiotensin receptors and by decrease of endothelin-1 synthesis.

[36] Lastly, anti-inflammatory effect of statin may prevent renal cell damage through decrease of pro-inflammatory cytokines which induce tissue factor expression by macrophage and activate nuclear factor-kappa B [37].

Although high-dose statin showed clear beneficial effect in preventing CIAKI, the risk of high-dose statin should be considered. Among the 13 RCTs, only 2 trials reported adverse events related with high-dose statin treatment. [14,28] Wei Li et al. reported that the rates of hepatotoxicity (defined as>3 times of upper normal limits of alanine aminotransferase within 1 month of the procedure) were 3.85% in high-dose statin group and 1.20% in control group (p = 0.57). In TRACK-D trial, they described that the rates of muscle pain, liver function abnormality, gastrointestinal disorders, edema or rash were not statistically different between high-dose statin and control group without presentation of actual numbers of the complications. Since limited data of adverse events in the included trials, the hazard of high-dose statin pre-treatment could not be evaluated in this meta-analysis. Previous meta-analysis of 35 RCTs comparing statin versus placebo, which was not a meta-analysis for CIAKI, reported that the absolute risk differences (RD) of most frequent adverse drug reactions were as follows; transaminase elevation (RD 4.2%, 95% CI 1.5 to 6.9%), myalgia (RD 2.7%, 95% CI −3.2 to 8.7%), rhabdomyolysis (RD 0.4%, 95% CI −0.1 to 0.9%), and discontinuation due to any adverse drug reaction (RD −0.5%, 95% CI −4.3 to 3.3%). [38] According to this report, the number needed to harm of statin treatment regarding adverse drug reaction are from 24 (hepatotoxicity) to 250 (rhabdomyolysis, defined as creatinine kinase elevations ≥10 times upper normal limit). Considering substantially lower NNT of 16 in this meta-analysis for reducing CIAKI and the clinical importance of CIAKI, high-dose statin pre-treatment before CAG with or without PCI could be considered as an effective prophylactic measure to prevent CIAKI.

Limitations

Several important limitations of the study should not be ignored. First, this meta-analysis included clinically- and method-ologically-diverse studies. Although we included only RCTs to the final analysis and assured statistically insignificant heterogeneity, there were some differences in the enrollment criteria (some studies exclusively enrolled patients with chronic kidney disease or diabetes mellitus), definition of the CIAKI, medication or hydration protocols. Also, basically this meta-analysis comprising 13 RCTs inherently shares the limitations of each trial. Second, variations in the type, dose, and duration of statin pretreatment among the included trials might have potential effects to our results, since all statins may not be equivalent to each other in their pleotropic and nephroprotective effects. Finally, as this study was a study-level meta-analysis, individual patient data were not included in the analysis, and therefore, we could not adjust for patient-level confounders.

Conclusion

High-dose statin pre-treatment significantly reduced the incidence of CIAKI in patients undergoing CAG. Considering prognostic importance of CIAKI and clear beneficial effect of statin in this meta-analysis, high-dose statin pre-treatment may be more actively employed as an effective prophylactic measure to prevent CIAKI.

Supporting Information

File S1 Supporting information files. Method S1, Search Strategy on Medline, EMBASE and Cochran Central. Method S2, Characteristics of the Excluded Study. Table S1, The Cochrane Collaboration's tool for assessing risk of bias. Figure S1, Risk of bias assessment graph. Risk of bias of each included trial was assessed with the Cochrane Collaboration's tool. This 'risk of bias graph' illustrates the proportion of studies with each of the judgments for each entry in the tool. Green represents 'Yes (low risk of bias)'; yellow, 'Unclear'; red, 'No (high risk of bias)'. Figure S2, Risk of bias assessment summary. Risk of bias of each included trial was assessed with the Cochrane Collaboration's tool. This 'risk of bias summary' figure presents all of the judgments in a cross-tabulation of study by entry. Green represents 'Yes (low risk of bias)'; yellow, 'Unclear'; red, 'No (high risk of bias)'. Figure S3,

The effect of High-dose statin on the incidence of contrast-induced nephropathy by fixed effects model. Forest plot with relative risks for the incidence of contrast-induced nephropathy associated with high-dose statin versus low-dose statin or placebo for individual trials and the pooled population. The squares and the horizontal lines indicate the relative risks (by fixed effects model) and the 95% confidence intervals (CI) for each trial included; the size of each square is proportional to the statistical weight of a trial in the frequentist meta-analysis; diamond indicates the effect estimate derived from meta-analysis, with the center indicating the point estimate and the left and the right ends the 95% CI. Abbreviations: CI, confidence intervals; RR, relative risks. Figure S4, The effect of High-dose statin on mean change of post-procedural serum creatinine. Forest plot with standardized mean difference (SMD) for the mean change of post-procedural serum creatinine from the baseline value associated with high-dose statin versus low-dose statin or placebo for individual trials and the pooled population. The squares and the horizontal lines indicate the SMD (by random effects model) and the 95% confidence intervals (CI) for each trial included; the size of each square is proportional to the statistical weight of a trial in the frequentist meta-analysis; diamond indicates the effect estimate derived from meta-analysis, with the center indicating the point estimate and the left and the right ends the 95% CI. Abbreviations: CI, confidence intervals; SD, standard deviation; SMD, standardized mean difference. Figure S5, Funnel plot for evaluation of publication and small study bias. Figure S6, Influence of individual studies Abbreviations: CI, confidence intervals; RR, relative risks. Figure S7, Cumulative Meta-analysis of high-dose statin on the incidence of contrast-induced nephropathy. The first row shows the effect of one study, the second row shows the cumulative pooled estimates based on the two studies, and so on. The squares and the horizontal lines indicate the cumulative relative risks (by random effects model) and the 95% confidence intervals (CI) for each trial included. Abbreviations: CI, confidence intervals; RR, relative risks. Figure S8, The effect of High-dose statin on the incidence of contrast-induced nephropathy, stratified according to the type of contrast. The squares and the horizontal lines indicate the relative risks (by random effects model) and the 95% confidence intervals (CI) for each trial included; the size of each square is proportional to the statistical weight of a trial in the meta-analysis; diamond indicates the effect estimate derived from meta-analysis, with the center indicating the point estimate and the left and the right ends the 95% CI. Abbreviations: CI, confidence intervals; RR, relative risks. Figure S9, The effect of High-dose statin on the incidence of contrast-induced nephropathy, stratified according to the mean age of the patients. The squares and the horizontal lines indicate the relative risks (by random effects model) and the 95% confidence intervals (CI) for each trial included; the size of each square is proportional to the statistical weight of a trial in the meta-analysis; diamond indicates the effect estimate derived from meta-analysis, with the center indicating the point estimate and the left and the right ends the 95% CI. Abbreviations: CI, confidence intervals; RR, relative risks. Figure S10, The effect of High-dose statin on the incidence of contrast-induced nephropathy, stratified according to the underlying chronic kidney disease. The squares and the horizontal lines indicate the relative risks (by random effects model) and the 95% confidence intervals (CI) for each trial included; the size of each square is proportional to the statistical weight of a trial in the meta-analysis; diamond indicates the effect estimate derived from meta-analysis, with the center indicating the point estimate and the left and the right ends the 95% CI. Abbreviations: CI, confidence intervals; CKD, chronic kidney disease; eGFR, estimated glomerular filtration rates; RR, relative risks. Figure S11, The effect of High-dose statin on the incidence of contrast-induced nephropathy, stratified according to the acute coronary syndrome. The squares and the horizontal lines indicate the relative risks (by random effects model) and the 95% confidence intervals (CI) for each trial included; the size of each square is proportional to the statistical weight of a trial in the meta-analysis; diamond indicates the effect estimate derived from meta-analysis, with the center indicating the point estimate and the left and the right ends the 95% CI. Abbreviations: CI, confidence intervals; RR, relative risks. Figure S12, The effect of High-dose statin on the incidence of contrast-induced nephropathy, stratified according to the concomitant treatment of N-acetylcystein. The squares and the horizontal lines indicate the relative risks (by random effects model) and the 95% confidence intervals (CI) for each trial included; the size of each square is proportional to the statistical weight of a trial in the meta-analysis; diamond indicates the effect estimate derived from meta-analysis, with the center indicating the point estimate and the left and the right ends the 95% CI. Abbreviations: CI, confidence intervals; RR, relative risks.

Author Contributions

Conceived and designed the experiments: JML JP HSK. Analyzed the data: JML JP KHJ JHJ SEL JKH HLK HMY KWP HJK BKK SHJ HSK. Contributed reagents/materials/analysis tools: JHJ SEL JKH HLK HMY KWP HJK BKK SHJ. Wrote the paper: JML JP.

References

1. McCullough PA (2008) Contrast-induced acute kidney injury. J Am Coll Cardiol 51: 1419–1428.
2. McCullough PA, Adam A, Becker CR, Davidson C, Lameire N, et al. (2006) Epidemiology and prognostic implications of contrast-induced nephropathy. Am J Cardiol 98: 5K–13K.
3. Klein LW, Sheldon MW, Brinker J, Mixon TA, Skelding K, et al. (2009) The use of radiographic contrast media during PCI: a focused review: a position statement of the Society of Cardiovascular Angiography and Interventions. Catheter Cardiovasc Interv 74: 728–746.
4. Kelly AM, Dwamena B, Cronin P, Bernstein SJ, Carlos RC (2008) Meta-analysis: effectiveness of drugs for preventing contrast-induced nephropathy. Ann Intern Med 148: 284–294.
5. Kitzler TM, Jaberi A, Sendlhofer G, Rehak P, Binder C, et al. (2012) Efficacy of vitamin E and N-acetylcysteine in the prevention of contrast induced kidney injury in patients with chronic kidney disease: a double blind, randomized controlled trial. Wien Klin Wochenschr 124: 312–319.
6. O'Gara PT, Kushner FG, Ascheim DD, Casey DE Jr, Chung MK, et al. (2013) 2013 ACCF/AHA guideline for the management of ST-elevation myocardial infarction: executive summary: a report of the American College of Cardiology Foundation/American Heart Association Task Force on Practice Guidelines: developed in collaboration with the American College of Emergency Physicians and Society for Cardiovascular Angiography and Interventions. Catheter Cardiovasc Interv 82: E1–27.
7. Task Force on Myocardial Revascularization of the European Society of C, the European Association for Cardio-Thoracic S, European Association for Percutaneous Cardiovascular I, Wijns W, Kolh P, et al. (2010) Guidelines on myocardial revascularization. Eur Heart J 31: 2501–2555.
8. Attallah N, Yassine L, Musial J, Yee J, Fisher K (2004) The potential role of statins in contrast nephropathy. Clin Nephrol 62: 273–278.
9. Khanal S, Attallah N, Smith DE, Kline-Rogers E, Share D, et al. (2005) Statin therapy reduces contrast-induced nephropathy: an analysis of contemporary percutaneous interventions. Am J Med 118: 843–849.
10. Pappy R, Stavrakis S, Hennebry TA, Abu-Fadel MS (2011) Effect of statin therapy on contrast-induced nephropathy after coronary angiography: a meta-analysis. Int J Cardiol 151: 348–353.
11. Jo SH, Koo BK, Park JS, Kang HJ, Cho YS, et al. (2008) Prevention of radiocontrast medium-induced nephropathy using short-term high-dose simvastatin in patients with renal insufficiency undergoing coronary angiography (PROMISS) trial—a randomized controlled study. Am Heart J 155: 499 e491–498.
12. Toso A, Maioli M, Leoncini M, Gallopin M, Tedeschi D, et al. (2010) Usefulness of atorvastatin (80 mg) in prevention of contrast-induced nephropathy in patients with chronic renal disease. Am J Cardiol 105: 288–292.
13. Quintavalle C, Fiore D, De Micco F, Visconti G, Focaccio A, et al. (2012) Impact of a high loading dose of atorvastatin on contrast-induced acute kidney injury. Circulation 126: 3008–3016.
14. Han Y, Zhu G, Han L, Hou F, Huang W, et al. (2014) Short-term rosuvastatin therapy for prevention of contrast-induced acute kidney injury in patients with diabetes and chronic kidney disease. J Am Coll Cardiol 63: 62–70.
15. Leoncini M, Toso A, Maioli M, Tropeano F, Villani S, et al. (2014) Early high-dose rosuvastatin for contrast-induced nephropathy prevention in acute coronary syndrome: Results from the PRATO-ACS Study (Protective Effect of Rosuvastatin and Antiplatelet Therapy On contrast-induced acute kidney injury and myocardial damage in patients with Acute Coronary Syndrome). J Am Coll Cardiol 63: 71–79.
16. Lee JM, Bae W, Lee YJ, Cho YJ (2014) The efficacy and safety of prone positional ventilation in acute respiratory distress syndrome: updated study-level meta-analysis of 11 randomized controlled trials. Crit Care Med 42: 1252–1262.
17. Jadad AR, Moore RA, Carroll D, Jenkinson C, Reynolds DJ, et al. (1996) Assessing the quality of reports of randomized clinical trials: is blinding necessary? Control Clin Trials 17: 1–12.
18. DerSimonian R, Laird N (1986) Meta-analysis in clinical trials. Control Clin Trials 7: 177–188.
19. Higgins JP, Thompson SG, Deeks JJ, Altman DG (2003) Measuring inconsistency in meta-analyses. BMJ 327: 557–560.
20. Moher D, Liberati A, Tetzlaff J, Altman DG (2009) Preferred reporting items for systematic reviews and meta-analyses: the PRISMA statement. Ann Intern Med 151: 264–269, W264.
21. Xinwei J, Xianghua F, Jing Z, Xinshun G, Ling X, et al. (2009) Comparison of usefulness of simvastatin 20 mg versus 80 mg in preventing contrast-induced nephropathy in patients with acute coronary syndrome undergoing percutaneous coronary intervention. Am J Cardiol 104: 519–524.
22. Zhou X, Jin YZ, Wang Q, Min R, Zhang XY (2009) [Efficacy of high dose atorvastatin on preventing contrast induced nephropathy in patients underwent coronary angiography]. Zhonghua Xin Xue Guan Bing Za Zhi 37: 394–396.
23. Acikel S, Muderrisoglu H, Yildirir A, Aydinalp A, Sade E, et al. (2010) Prevention of contrast-induced impairment of renal function by short-term or long-term statin therapy in patients undergoing elective coronary angiography. Blood Coagul Fibrinolysis 21: 750–757.
24. Ozhan H, Erden I, Ordu S, Aydin M, Caglar O, et al. (2010) Efficacy of short-term high-dose atorvastatin for prevention of contrast-induced nephropathy in patients undergoing coronary angiography. Angiology 61: 711–714.
25. X-p H, R-x W, Y Y, Zheng C, Bin C (2010) Prevention of contrast-induced nephropathy using high-dose atorvastatin in patients with coronary heart disease undergoing elective percutaneous coronary intervention] [in Chinese. Milit Med J South China 24: 448–451.
26. Patti G, Ricottini E, Nusca A, Colonna G, Pasceri V, et al. (2011) Short-term, high-dose Atorvastatin pretreatment to prevent contrast-induced nephropathy in patients with acute coronary syndromes undergoing percutaneous coronary intervention (from the ARMYDA-CIN [atorvastatin for reduction of myocardial damage during angioplasty—contrast-induced nephropathy] trial. Am J Cardiol 108: 1–7.
27. Cao S, Wang P, Cui K, Zhang L, Hou Y (2012) [Atorvastatin prevents contrast agent-induced renal injury in patients undergoing coronary angiography by inhibiting oxidative stress]. Nan Fang Yi Ke Da Xue Xue Bao 32: 1600–1602.
28. Li W, Fu X, Wang Y, Li X, Yang Z, et al. (2012) Beneficial effects of high-dose atorvastatin pretreatment on renal function in patients with acute ST-segment elevation myocardial infarction undergoing emergency percutaneous coronary intervention. Cardiology 122: 195–202.
29. Takagi H, Umemoto T (2011) A meta-analysis of randomized trials for effects of periprocedural atorvastatin on contrast-induced nephropathy. Int J Cardiol 153: 323–325.
30. Zhang BC, Li WM, Xu YW (2011) High-dose statin pretreatment for the prevention of contrast-induced nephropathy: a meta-analysis. Can J Cardiol 27: 851–858.
31. Zhang L, Zhang L, Lu Y, Wu B, Zhang S, et al. (2011) Efficacy of statin pretreatment for the prevention of contrast-induced nephropathy: a meta-analysis of randomised controlled trials. Int J Clin Pract 65: 624–630.
32. Zhang T, Shen LH, Hu LH, He B (2011) Statins for the prevention of contrast-induced nephropathy: a systematic review and meta-analysis. Am J Nephrol 33: 344–351.
33. Li Y, Liu Y, Fu L, Mei C, Dai B (2012) Efficacy of short-term high-dose statin in preventing contrast-induced nephropathy: a meta-analysis of seven randomized controlled trials. PLoS One 7: e34450.
34. John S, Schneider MP, Delles C, Jacobi J, Schmieder RE (2005) Lipid-independent effects of statins on endothelial function and bioavailability of nitric oxide in hypercholesterolemic patients. Am Heart J 149: 473.

35. Ridker PM, Rifai N, Clearfield M, Downs JR, Weis SE, et al. (2001) Measurement of C-reactive protein for the targeting of statin therapy in the primary prevention of acute coronary events. N Engl J Med 344: 1959–1965.

36. Ichiki T, Takeda K, Tokunou T, Iino N, Egashira K, et al. (2001) Downregulation of angiotensin II type 1 receptor by hydrophobic 3-hydroxy-3-methylglutaryl coenzyme A reductase inhibitors in vascular smooth muscle cells. Arterioscler Thromb Vasc Biol 21: 1896–1901.

37. Bonetti PO, Lerman LO, Napoli C, Lerman A (2003) Statin effects beyond lipid lowering—are they clinically relevant? Eur Heart J 24: 225–248.

38. Kashani A, Phillips CO, Foody JM, Wang Y, Mangalmurti S, et al. (2006) Risks associated with statin therapy: a systematic overview of randomized clinical trials. Circulation 114: 2788–2797.

11

Myxomavirus Anti-Inflammatory Chemokine Binding Protein Reduces the Increased Plaque Growth Induced by Chronic *Porphyromonas gingivalis* Oral Infection after Balloon Angioplasty Aortic Injury in Mice

Alexandra R. Lucas[1]*, Raj K. Verma[2], Erbin Dai[1], Liying Liu[1], Hao Chen[1], Sheela Kesavalu[2], Mercedes Rivera[2], Irina Velsko[2], Sriram Ambadapadi[1], Sasanka Chukkapalli[2], Lakshmyya Kesavalu[2,3]*

1 Division of Cardiovascular Medicine, Departments of Medicine and Molecular Genetics & Microbiology, College of Medicine, University of Florida, Gainesville, Florida, United States of America, 2 Department of Periodontology, College of Dentistry, University of Florida, Gainesville, Florida, United States of America, 3 Department of Oral Biology, College of Dentistry, University of Florida, Gainesville, Florida, United States of America

Abstract

Thrombotic occlusion of inflammatory plaque in coronary arteries causes myocardial infarction. Treatment with emergent balloon angioplasty (BA) and stent implant improves survival, but restenosis (regrowth) can occur. Periodontal bacteremia is closely associated with inflammation and native arterial atherosclerosis, with potential to increase restenosis. Two virus-derived anti-inflammatory proteins, M-T7 and Serp-1, reduce inflammation and plaque growth after BA and transplant in animal models through separate pathways. M-T7 is a broad spectrum C, CC and CXC chemokine-binding protein. Serp-1 is a *serine protease inhibitor* (*serpin*) inhibiting thrombotic and thrombolytic pathways. Serp-1 also reduces arterial inflammation and improves survival in a mouse herpes virus (MHV68) model of lethal vasculitis. In addition, Serp-1 demonstrated safety and efficacy in patients with unstable coronary disease and stent implant, reducing markers of myocardial damage. We investigate here the effects of *Porphyromonas gingivalis*, a periodontal pathogen, on restenosis after BA and the effects of blocking chemokine and protease pathways with M-T7 and Serp-1. ApoE$^{-/-}$ mice had aortic BA and oral *P. gingivalis* infection. Arterial plaque growth was examined at 24 weeks with and without anti-inflammatory protein treatment. Dental plaques from mice infected with *P. gingivalis* tested positive for infection. Neither Serp-1 nor M-T7 treatment reduced infection, but IgG antibody levels in mice treated with Serp-1 and M-T7 were reduced. *P. gingivalis* significantly increased monocyte invasion and arterial plaque growth after BA (P<0.025). Monocyte invasion and plaque growth were blocked by M-T7 treatment (P<0.023), whereas Serp-1 produced only a trend toward reductions. Both proteins modified expression of TLR4 and MyD88. In conclusion, aortic plaque growth in ApoE$^{-/-}$ mice increased after angioplasty in mice with chronic oral *P. gingivalis* infection. Blockade of chemokines, but not serine proteases significantly reduced arterial plaque growth, suggesting a central role for chemokine-mediated inflammation after BA in *P. gingivalis* infected mice.

Editor: Salomon Amar, Boston University, United States of America

Funding: This work was supported by USPHS research grant U24 DE016509 from National Institute of Dental, Craniofacial Research (NIH/NIDCR), NIH grants R01DE015720-01, DE020820-01, and 1RC1HL100202-01, and the University of Florida Research Opportunity seed fund. The funders had no role in study design, data collection and analysis, decision to publish, or preparation of the manuscript.

Competing Interests: The authors have declared that no competing interests exist.

* Email: alexandra.lucas@medicine.ufl.edu (AL); kesavalu@dental.ufl.edu (LK)

Introduction

Atherosclerotic plaque growth is accelerated by hyperlipidemia, hypertension, and diabetes which cause arterial injury. Percutaneous intervention (PCI) with either balloon angioplasty (BA) or stent implant, is associated with a rapid recurrent plaque growth, termed restenosis, that is characterized by endothelial cell dysfunction, smooth muscle cell migration into the intima, and inflammatory macrophage and T cell activation [1,2]. While acute thrombosis at sites of angioplasty and stent implant is well controlled with anti-platelet agents such as aspirin and clopidogrel, the causes for restenosis are only partially understood [1–3]. Prevention of restenosis is limited to the use of bare metal stents,

which reduce restenosis from 30–50% after BA alone to 20–30%, and drug eluting stents which further reduce restenosis to 3–10%. Inflammatory macrophage and T cell invasion can drive both early and late unstable atherosclerotic plaque progression, and can also induce restenosis. While restenosis is considered a specialized form of rapid arterial plaque growth, it is, by definition, formed at sites of already developed atheroma and thus is influenced both by angioplasty injury and the underlying atherosclerotic plaque.

Periodontal disease (PD) is a multispecies, subgingival, biofilm-mediated disease and an estimated 5–20% of the world's population suffer from chronic periodontitis [4]. Periodontitis is also believed to contribute to systemic diseases, including atherosclerotic vascular disease, diabetes mellitus, rheumatoid arthritis, and Alzheimer's disease [5–7]. *P. gingivalis,* the most common oral pathogen, is reported to increase plaque growth after wire-induced femoral arterial injury in mice upon systemic infection with subcutaneous bacterial inoculations [8]. *Streptococcus mutans* similarly increases plaque after BA [9]. Prior studies with oral *P. gingivalis* infection in ApoE$^{-/-}$ mice have demonstrated both periodontal disease and atherosclerosis [8,10,11] and genomic DNA from *P. gingivalis* has been detected in atherosclerotic plaque [12]. Apolipoprotein E (ApoE) is a ligand for receptors that clear remnants of chylomicrons and very low density lipoproteins. Lack of ApoE is, therefore, expected to cause accumulation in plasma of cholesterol-rich remnants whose prolonged circulation should be atherogenic. Apo E-deficient mice generated by gene targeting were used as a model to test this hypothesis and are known to for developing spontaneous atherosclerosis that is increased with balloon angioplasty [13,14]. Macrophage and T cell invasion, as well as expression of Toll-like receptors (TLRs) 2 and 4, pro-inflammatory cytokines interleukin-6 (IL-6) and vascular cell adhesion molecule-1 (VCAM-1) were also detected after *P. gingivalis* infection [8,15–18].

Viruses have developed potent anti-inflammatory proteins over millions of years of evolution that protect them from host immune defenses [19–26]. M-T7 and Serp-1 proteins increase viral pathogenesis in myxomaviral infection in European rabbits at picomolar concentrations, by blocking select steps in host inflammatory responses. M-T7 binds and inhibits C, CC, and CXC class chemokines through interfering with chemokine: glycosamnoglycan (GAG) interactions [19,20] and Serp-1 is a *serine protease inhibitor* (*serpin*) that blocks tissue- and urokinase-type plasminogen activators (tPA, uPA, respectively), plasmin, and factor Xa (fXa) [21–24]. Infusion of purified M-T7 or Serp-1 proteins markedly reduces inflammatory cell invasion and arterial plaque in animal models of atherosclerosis, restenosis, and transplant [19–24]. Serp-1 has also been tested in a clinical trial in patients with unstable coronary syndromes and coronary stent implant. Serp-1 treatment was safe with significant reductions in troponin and creatinine kinase MB (CKMB), biomarkers of myocardial damage [24,25]. Periodontal disease is predicted to increase inflammation and plaque growth, but anti-inflammatory treatment has not been tested for the capacity to reduce restenosis during active chronic periodontal bacterial infections. Both thrombotic and thrombolytic serine protease cascades as well as chemokines are upregulated at sites of arterial injury often initiating cellular invasion and even activation. Further it is not as yet known whether activation of serine protease coagulation pathways and/or chemokine: GAG interactions have central roles in Pg induced plaque growth after BA, nor if targeted inhibition of these selected pathways can alter plaque growth after Pg infection.

We investigate here the potential for chronic oral *P. gingivalis* infection to modify balloon angioplasty (BA)-induced plaque growth in hyperlipidemic ApoE$^{-/-}$ mice and examine the capacity of purified anti-inflammatory viral proteins alone, M-T7 and Serp-1, without antibiotic treatment, to reduce plaque growth after BA during *P. gingivalis* infection.

Methods

Microbial inocula

P. gingivalis FDC 381 (ATCC Manassas, VA, USA) was cultured both in mycoplasma broth and blood agar plates and grown anaerobically at $37°C$, as described [26,27]. Cells were harvested and mixed equally with sterile 4% (w/v) low viscosity carboxymethylcellulose (CMC; Sigma-Aldrich, St. Louis, MO) in

phosphate buffered saline (PBS) and used for oral lavage and infection (5×10^9 bacteria per mL) [27].

Anti-inflammatory protein source and purification

Serp-1 protein was provided by Viron Therapeutics Inc. (London, ON, Canada) and was purified from recombinant Chinese hamster ovary (CHO) cell supernatants $\geq$99% by sequential column chromatographic separation [21–25,28–30] as previously described. A baculovirus expression system in *Spodoptera frugiperda*, Sf 21 (Invitrogen) and *Trichoplusia ni*, High Five (Invitrogen) cells were used, as previously described, for the expression of M-T7. In brief, the N-terminal His-tagged M-T7 protein was purified by Co-NTA (Nickel-Nitrilo-triacetic acid, Sigma) column chromatography and purity verified by SDS-PAGE, Coomassie/Silver staining and western blot analysis [19,20,31,32].

Mouse aortic angioplasty model

All animal studies were approved by the University of Florida Institutional Animal Care and Use Committee (IACUC Protocol #F173) and conform to the Guide for the Care and Use of Laboratory Animals (United States National Institutes of Health). The right iliac artery of twenty five eight week old ApoE$^{-/-}$ mice (The Jackson Laboratory, Bar Harbor, ME, U.S.A.) under general anesthesia was exposed by laparotomy and a 0.62-mm caliber microcatheter balloon (1.5 mm$\times$6 mm (MED PLUS perfecseal, Inc., Oshkosh, WI) inserted using a surgical microscope [23–26]. The balloon was inflated, advanced retrograde to the thoracic aorta and pulled back 3 times, inducing endothelial disruption and inflammation and simulating restenosis. Anti-inflammatory proteins, Serp-1 (15 µg) or M-T7 (6 µg), or control sterile saline were injected intravenously immediately post-BA.

P. gingivalis infection and oral plaque sampling

Monomicrobial oral infection and plaque sampling methodology are described elsewhere [26,27,33]. ApoE$^{-/-}$ mice used to examine the role of oral pathogens in atherosclerotic plaque growth [5,6,27] were housed in microisolator cages and fed standard chow and water *ad libitum*. Mice were randomized into five groups after BA (Gr I = Sham-infected control + BA; Gr II = *P. gingivalis*; Gr III = *P. gingivalis* + BA; Gr IV = *P. gingivalis* + BA + Serp-1; Gr V = *P. gingivalis* + BA + M-T7) and infected as per the diagram (Figure 1A). Mice were administered kanamycin and ampicillin daily for 10 days in the drinking water and the oral cavity lavaged with 0.12% chlorhexidine gluconate (Peridex: 3 M ESPE Dental Products, St. Paul, MN) mouth rinse [27,33] to decrease endogenous flora and to enhance *P. gingivalis* colonization [27]. 10^9 cells in 0.2 ml per mouse were administered orally for 4 consecutive days per week, every 3 weeks (8 infection periods) to mimic chronic exposure during 24 weeks (Fig. 1A). Sham-infected mice (n = 5) received vehicle (sterile 4% CMC) only. Oral dental plaque samples from isoflurane anesthetized mice were collected post-infection as described [26,27]. In order to monitor the oral infection with minimal disruption of biofilms, a total of 2 post-infection oral plaque samples (following the 5th and 7th infections) were collected from infected mice (Figure. 1A).

Following 24 weeks of infection, mice were euthanized and blood, jaws, aorta, heart, spleen, liver, and kidneys were collected for analysis. Sera were stored at $-20°C$ for immunoglobulin G (IgG) antibody analysis [26,27,33]. The maxillar and mandibular regions were resected, autoclaved, and mechanically defleshed for analysis of horizontal alveolar bone loss. Maxillae were also resected and fixed in 10% buffered formalin and decalcified with

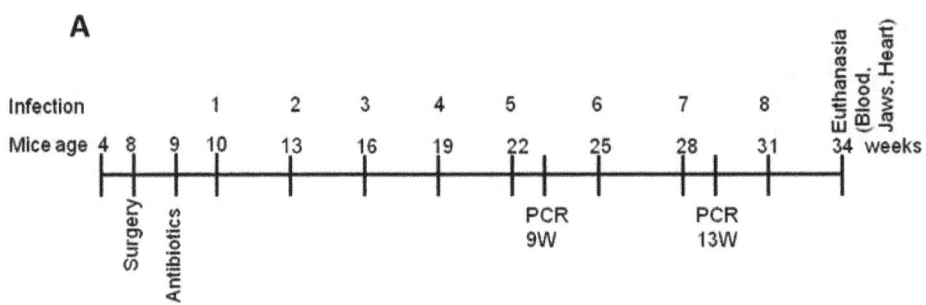

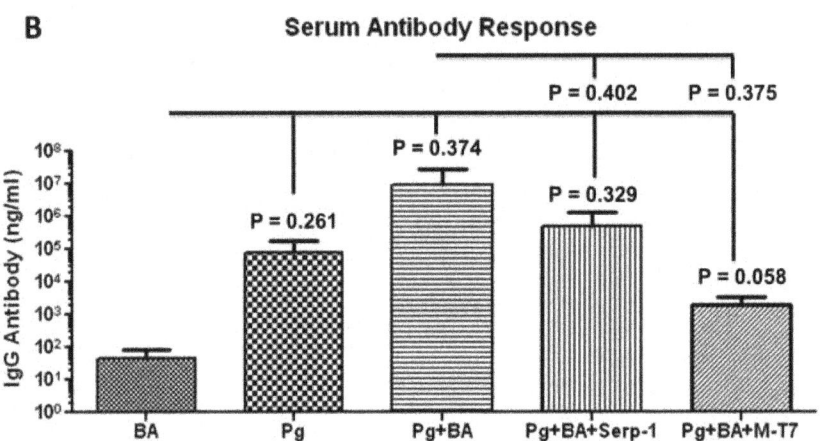

Figure 1. Experimental scheme and serum IgG levels in mice. (A) Schematic diagram illustrating experimental design and time course. (B) Serum *P. gingivalis* IgG antibody levels in ApoE$^{-/-}$ mice following 24 weeks oral infection (n = 3–5). Bar graphs show the mean ± SD IgG levels in serum from mice infected with *P. gingivalis* alone, *P. gingivalis* + BA with Serp-1 or M-T7, or from BA mice (P = 0.34 and 0.37, respectively). *Pg* - *P. gingivalis*; BA - balloon angioplasty.

Immunocal (Decal Chemical Corporation, Tallman, NY) for 28 days at 4°C for histologic analysis.

Detection of *P. gingivalis* genomic DNA in oral plaque

Genomic DNA was isolated from mouse oral plaque using the Wizard Genomic DNA Purification Kit (Promega, Madison, WI) following manufacturer's protocol [27,28]. PCR was performed with a Bio-Rad thermal cycler using 16S rRNA gene species-specific oligonucleotide primers: 5'-TGTAGATGACTGATGGT-GAAAACC-3' (forward), 5'-ACGTCATCCCCACCTTCCTC-3' (reverse). Genomic DNA extracted from *P. gingivalis* FDC 381

served as positive and PCR without template DNA served as negative controls. PCR products were separated by 1.5% agarose gel electrophoresis and bands visualized using BioRad Gel Doc XR/Chemidoc Gel Documentation System (BioRad, CA, USA).

Serum IgG antibody analysis

Diluted mouse sera (1:100 for IgG) were reacted with whole *P. gingivalis* coated with 0.5% formalin in buffered saline for 2 h at room temperature and subsequently goat anti-mouse IgG, conjugated to alkaline phosphatase (1:5000) (Bethyl Laboratories, Montgomery, TX) and *p*-Nitrophenyl phosphate (Sigma-Aldrich).

Table 1. Morphometric evaluation of horizontal area alveolar bone resorption induced by *P. gingivalis*.

Groups/Infection/Balloon angioplasty/Serpin	Maxilla		Mandible	
	Buccal	Lingual	Buccal	Lingual
I Sham-infected + BA	0.30±0.09*	0.57±0.05	0.28±0.09	0.66±0.01
II *P. gingivalis*	0.30±0.04	0.58±0.05	0.40±0.12	0.67±0.07
III *P. gingivalis* + BA	0.34±0.12	0.61±0.16	0.31±0.09	0.70±0.08
IV *P. gingivalis* + BA + Serp-1	0.36±0.78	0.71±0.01	0.37±0.01	0.89±0.04
V *P. gingivalis* + BA + M-T7	0.52±0.14	0.72±0.10	0.37±0.02	0.81±0.06

Alveolar bone resorption (ABR) area measured between cementoenamel junction (CEJ) to the alveolar bone crest (ABC) on the buccal and palatal surfaces of the roots of all molars in mice (mean value in mm^2± SD).
*Mean value in mm^2 and standard deviation from 3–5 mice per group measured using AxioVision line tool software. Mice jaw images captured at 10 x magnification and measured between CEJ to the ABC on the buccal and palatal surfaces of the roots of all molars.

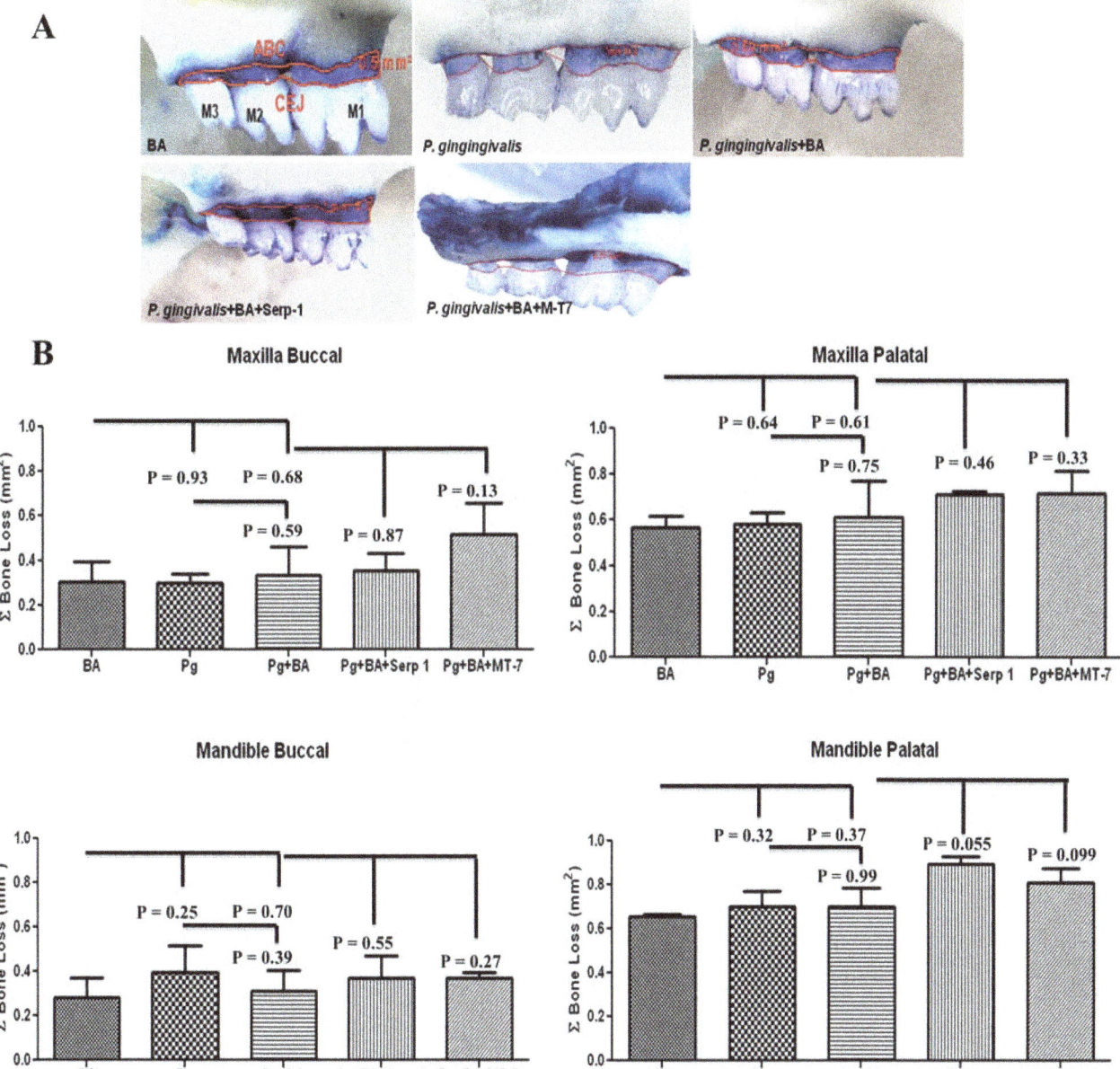

Figure 2. Morphometric evaluation of horizontal alveolar bone loss. (A) Representative ApoE$^{-/-}$ mouse left maxilla with BA showing palatal horizontal bone loss area by morphometry (n = 3–5, magnification-10X). The outline represents the area of horizontal alveolar bone resorption (mm^2). M1, M2, M3 are molars. (B) Bar graphs depicting bone loss in each of four quadrants; Maxilla (buccal and palatal) and mandible (buccal and palatal) (n = 3–5). No significant differences (P≤0.05) were observed between the treatment groups.

Reactions were stopped by 3 M NaOH and absorbance analyzed at OD$_{405}$ using a Bio-Rad Microplate Reader. Mouse serum IgG antibody levels were calculated using a gravimetric standard curve, consisting of 8 mouse IgG concentrations (Sigma-Aldrich) coated onto microtiter plates.

Morphometric analysis

Mouse jaws were immersed in 3% (v/v) hydrogen peroxide overnight, air dried and stained with 0.1% (w/v) aqueous methylene blue to delineate the cemento-enamel junction (CEJ) [34]. Digital images of mouse buccal and lingual root surfaces of molar teeth were captured under a 10X stereo dissecting microscope (SteReo Discovery V8; Carl Zeiss Microimaging,

Inc, Thornwood, NY), after superimposition of buccal and lingual cusps to ensure reproducibility. Horizontal alveolar bone loss was measured from CEJ to alveolar bone crest (ABC) using the calibrated line tool (AxioVision LE 29A software version 4.6.3.). Means of duplicate measurements performed by two blinded individual examiners are reported.

Paraffin-embedded 5 μm cross-sections were Hematoxylin and eosin stained and the aortic plaque measured using an Olympus system with Olympus DP7 color video camera attached to an Olympus BX51 microscope with the ImagePro MC 6.0 software program standardized to microscopic objective (Olympus America, Center Valley, PA) [19–23,29–31,33,35,36]. The mean cross-sectional intimal area or intimal thickness normalized to medial

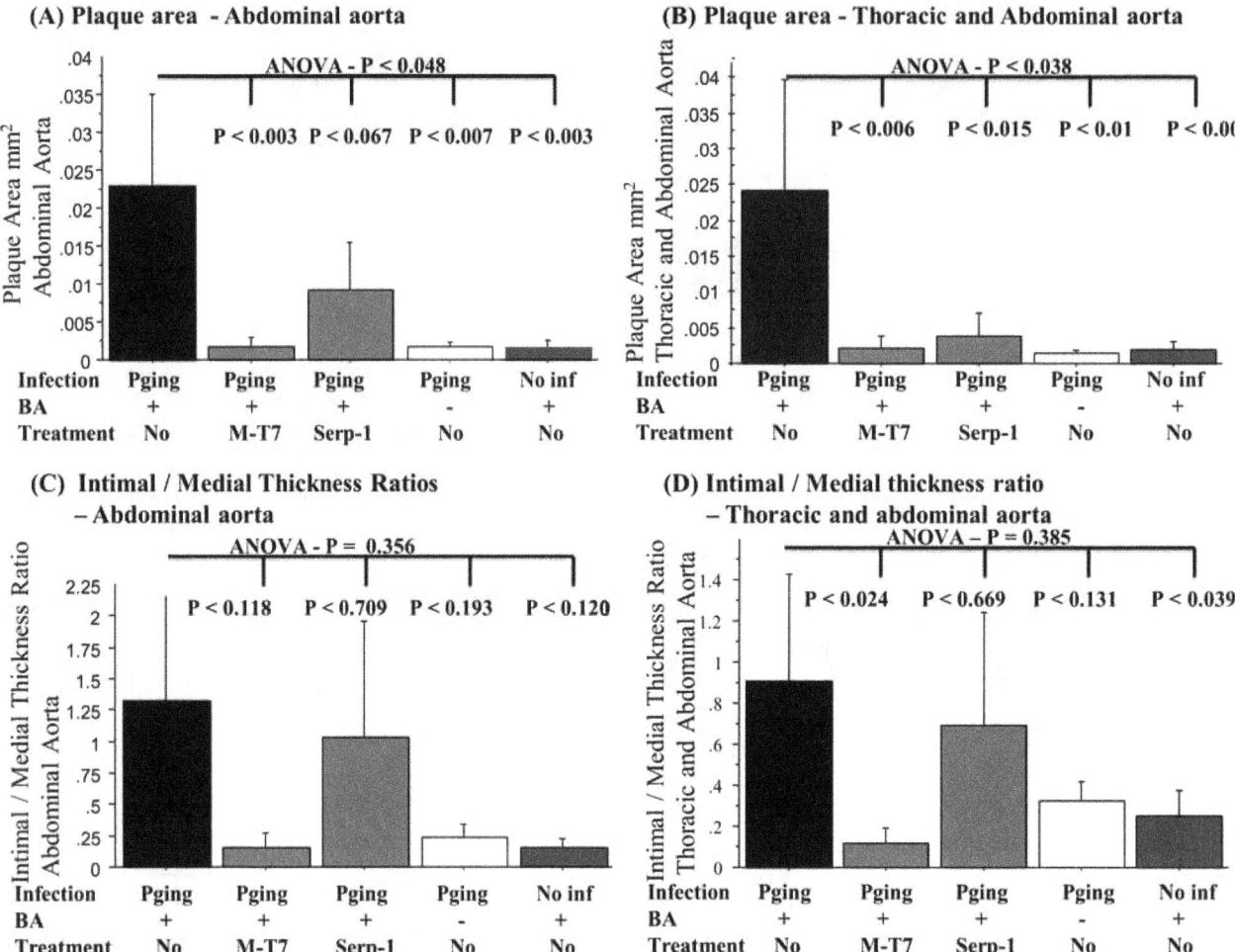

Figure 3. Plaque area and thickness in *P. gingivalis* infection. *P. gingivalis* infection increased plaque area significantly in ApoE$^{-/-}$ mice after BA (A and B, P<0.006) with a trend toward increased plaque thickness (C and D, P≤0.385). Bar graphs of combined thoracic and abdominal aortic plaque area at 24 weeks (A) or abdominal aortic data alone (B) and intimal/medial thickness ratios for combined thoracic and abdominal aorta (C) or abdominal aorta alone (D) (N = 3–5 mice per group). Pg - *P. gingivalis*, Serp-1, M-T7 - anti-inflammatory protein treatments, BA - balloon angioplasty.

thickness for each aortic section (ascending, thoracic, or abdominal aorta) or for combined data for all aortic specimens was used for statistical analyses.

Immunohistochemistry

Aortic specimens were stained for macrophage, TLR4 and MyD88 (Myeloid differentiation marker 88) [37]. Formalin fixed tissue sections were labeled using an ABC kit (Vector Laboratories, Burlingame, USA) per manufacturer's protocol. Blocked tissue sections were labeled using a 1:100 dilution of specific primary antibodies [(macrophage: rat monoclonal anti-mouse CD11b to macrophage: ab56297 and secondary antibody: rat IgG (Biotin) ab6733) (TLR: rabbit polyclonal anti-mouse to TLR4: ab47093 and secondary antibody: rabbit IgG (Biotin) ab6720) (MyD88: rabbit polyclonal anti-mouse to MyD88: (HFL-296): sc-11356 (Santa Cruz Biotechnology INC., CA, U.S.A)] (Abcam Inc, Cambridge, MA) overnight followed by 1:250 dilution of biotin-conjugated secondary antibodies [28–31,34,35]. Diaminobenzi-dine (Sigma-Aldrich, St. Louis, USA) was used for detection with hematoxylin counterstain. Specificity of staining was determined by omission of primary antibody or irrelevant primary antibody [29–31,35,36]. Positively stained cells were counted in three high

power fields (HPF, 100X) in intimal, medial and adventitial layers of each aortic section, and mean numbers of cells calculated.

Statistical analysis

All data is presented as mean ± SD or ± SE (Prism 4, GraphPad software, San Diego, CA or Statview software) with *P* values calculated using Kruskal Walis ANOVA with Dunn's correction for multiple comparisons and Mann-Whitney Student *t* test [19–23,26,28–31,35,36]. *P* value less than 0.05 were considered significant.

Results

Detection of *P. gingivalis* after oral infection

Oral dental plaques collected post-5th infection demonstrated that all the mice were positive for *P. gingivalis* in *Pg*, *Pg* + BA and *Pg* + BA + Serp-1 groups and 4 out of 5 mice in the *P. gingivalis* + BA + M-T7 group were positive. At post-7 weeks infection, all mice were positive for *P. gingivalis*. Neither anti-inflammatory protein treatment significantly reduced detectable *P. gingivalis* in the oral cavity. No sham-infected mice were positive for *P. gingivalis* at the two time points examined.

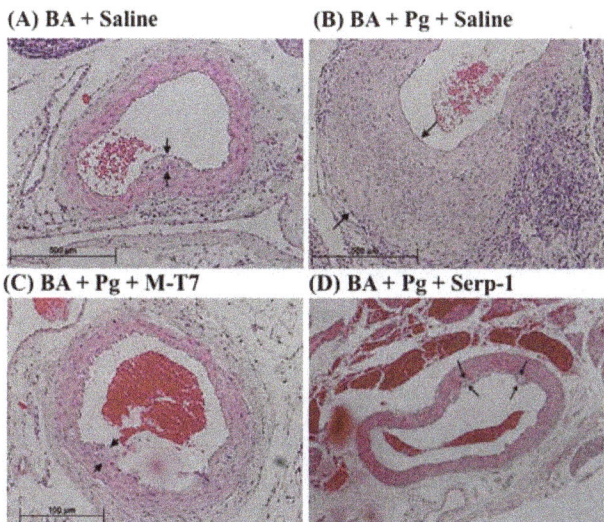

Figure 4. Histology of aortic plaque with *P. gingivalis* infection. Hematoxylin and eosin stained cross sections of abdominal aorta from ApoE$^{-/-}$ mice 24 weeks after BA. *P. gingivalis* induced increase plaque thickness is significantly reduced by M-T7, with Serp-1 showing a trend towards reduction. BA with saline treatment and no *P. gingivalis* infection (A). BA with saline treatment and *P. gingivalis* infection (B). M-T7 treatment with BA and *P. gingivalis* (C). Serp-1 treatment with BA and *P. gingivalis* (D). Arrows indicate margins of intimal plaque. Arrow heads point to inflammatory mononuclear cell invasion. Magnification 200X.

Antibody response to oral *P. gingivalis* is detected during infection

When evaluated for up to 24 weeks, all mice in the *P. gingivalis* + BA group developed elevated IgG antibody to *P. gingivalis* compared to sham-infected mice with BA, but this did not reach significance (P = 0.34) (Figure 1B). The IgG antibody levels in mice treated with Serp-1 and M-T7 with BA were lower than in untreated mice with *P. gingivalis*-infection (P = 0.37) (Figure 1B). Further, IgG antibody levels in mice treated with Serp-1 were

higher than with M-T7 treatment, suggesting differing immune responses after each specific treatment.

P. gingivalis infection induced alveolar bone resorption

Progression of PD resulting from *P. gingivalis* infection was examined by measuring alveolar bone resorption (ABR) (Table 1; Figure 2A and 2B). Higher horizontal ABR was detected in both the mandible and maxilla of the palatal surface than the buccal surface of all *P. gingivalis* infected mice and sham-infected mice and BA. No observable differences in ABR were found between Serp-1 or M-T7 treated mice compared to sham infected mice (P>0.05).

Balloon angioplasty induced aortic plaque is increased with *P. gingivalis* infection

Following 24 weeks of chronic oral *P. gingivalis* infection with BA, mean plaque area increased markedly throughout the aorta (P≤0.025) at all aortic sites from the ascending aorta to the thoracic and abdominal aortic sections, when compared to sham-infected controls with BA. Mean intimal/medial thickness ratios also increased with *P. gingivalis* infection in mice after BA (P≤ 0.039) when compared to uninfected mice. When analyzing data from the thoracic and abdominal aortic sections alone, areas of the aorta that had direct BA injury, the increase in plaque area was more pronounced as expected (Figure 3B, P≤0.01). Analysis of plaque area in the abdominal aorta alone, where the greatest direct BA injury occurred, demonstrated the same marked increase in plaque area in *P. gingivalis* + BA mice (Figure 3A, Figure 4A and 4B; P≤0.007). Analysis of intimal to medial thickness ratios, a measure of normalized thickness of aortic cross-sectional areas, did not reach significance, but demonstrated similar trends for increased plaque in the combined data for the thoracic and abdominal aorta (Figure 3D, P = 0.385 by ANOVA) and for the abdominal aorta data alone (Figure 3C, P = 0.356 by ANOVA).

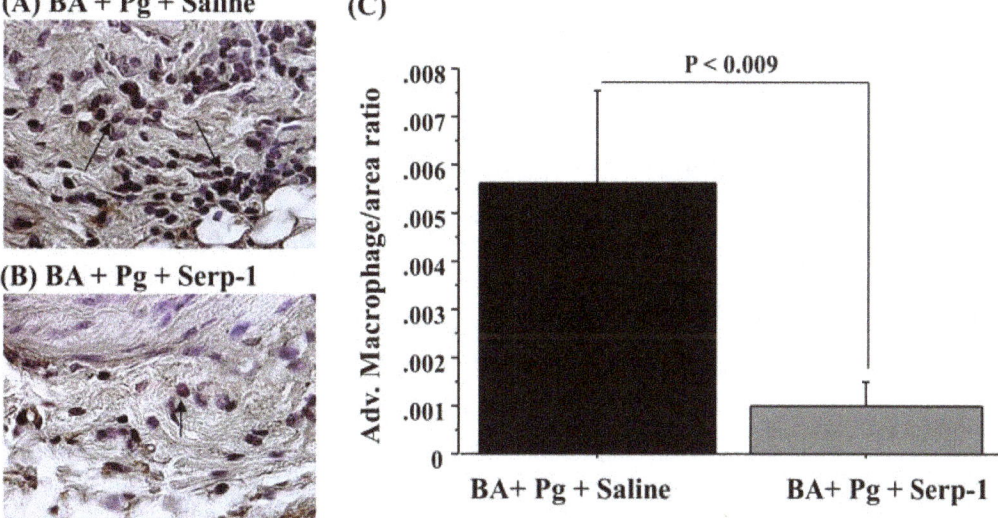

Figure 5. Immunohistochemistry of adventitial layer in abdominal aorta from ApoE$^{-/-}$ mice with *P. gingivalis* infection. (A) Saline treated mouse tissue (B) demonstrates reduced macrophage invasion with Serp-1 treatment. (C) Bar graph demonstrates significantly reduced counts of positively stained macrophage in the aortic adventitia in Serp-1 treated mice with *P. gingivalis* infection + BA (C; P≤0.009).

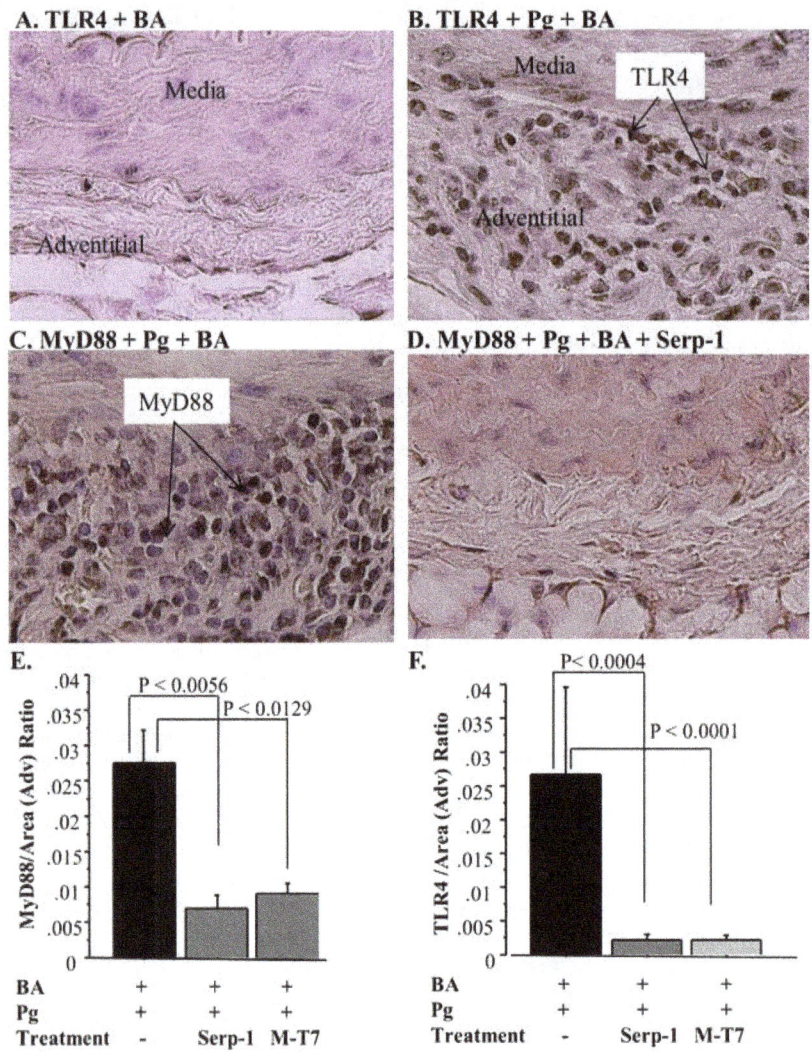

Figure 6. Anti-inflammatory protein treatment reduced TLR4 and MyD88 staining in mice after *P. gingivalis* infection + BA. (A) Immunohistochemical staining of TLR4 in sham-infected mice (left). (B) Increased TLR4 staining in mice infected with *P. gingivalis* + BA injury. (C) Increased MyD88 staining in mice infected with *P. gingivalis* + BA injury. (D) Decreased MyD88 staining in mice with *P. gingivalis* + BA after Serp-1 treatment. (E) Bar graph of MyD88 expression showing increased MyD88 in aortic adventitia in *P. gingivalis* infected mice + BA (24 weeks) compared to *P. gingivalis* + BA with Serp-1 ($P \leq 0.056$) or M-T7 treatment ($P \leq 0.013$). (F) Bar graph of TLR4 expression showing increased TLR4 in abdominal aortic adventitial in *P. gingivalis* + BA (24 weeks) compared to *P. gingivalis* + BA in Serp-1 ($P = 0.0004$) and in M-T7 treated mice ($P \leq 0.0001$).

Anti-inflammatory protein treatment reduced plaque growth after balloon angioplasty during active *P. gingivalis* infection

In the presence of active *P. gingivalis* oral infection and BA injury, anti-inflammatory M-T7 protein treatment significantly decreased aortic plaque area when compared to saline controls in combined analysis of all aortic sections (ascending, thoracic, and abdominal areas) ($P \leq 0.0227$) and also in areas with direct BA injury (thoracic and abdominal aorta, $P \leq 0.006$) or for abdominal aorta alone (Figure 3A, Figure 3C; $P \leq 0.003$). In contrast, Serp-1 treatment did not significantly reduce plaque area in *P. gingivalis* infected mice when analyzing mean data from all aortic sections ($P = 0.243$), although demonstrating a trend toward reduced plaque. When analyzing only combined thoracic and abdominal aortic data, where there was direct BA injury, Serp-1 treatment did significantly reduce plaque area (Figure 3B, Figure 4D, Figure 5C; $P \leq 0.015$). When analyzing the abdominal aorta alone

a similar, non-significant trend toward reduced plaque was detected for Serp-1 treatment (Figure 3A, $P = 0.067$). Intimal/medial thickness ratios demonstrated a significant reduction with M-T7 treatment when combined data for all aortic areas ($P \leq 0.024$) were analyzed, but not with Serp-1 treatment ($P = 0.669$). Analysis of combined intimal to medial ratio data from areas of BA damage in the thoracic and abdominal aorta did not reach significance, but demonstrated similar trends (Figure 3C and 3D).

Immunohistochemical Analysis demonstrates reduced inflammatory mononuclear cell invasion after BA with anti-inflammatory protein treatment

Both M-T7 and Serp-1 (Figure 5B and 5C; $P \leq 0.010$; Serp-1 shown) treatments significantly decreased inflammatory macrophage infiltration in the intimal and adventitial layers of the aorta after BA during active *P. gingivalis* infection, as compared to saline control-treated mice with active *P. gingivalis* + BA (Figure 5A and 5C).

Immunohistochemistry of the aortic adventitial layers detected increased TLR4 expression in ApoE$^{-/-}$ mice with *P. gingivalis* infection after BA (Figure 6A and B). Treatment with M-T7 ($P \le 0.0001$) or Serp-1 ($P \le 0.0004$) significantly reduced TLR4 (Figure 6F). With Serp-1 treatment in *P. gingivalis* infection + BA, MyD88 expression was decreased (Figure 6D) when compared to the control, saline-treated mice with *P. gingivalis* + BA (Figure 6C). On quantitative analysis of inflammatory cells staining positively for TLR signaling adaptor protein MyD88 expression, M-T7 ($P \le 0.013$) and Serp-1 ($P \le 0.006$), both significantly down-regulated MyD88 (Figure 6E) in the adventitia in mice with *P. gingivalis* infection + BA when compared to saline-treated *P. gingivalis* infected mice (Figure 6).

Discussion

Numerous epidemiological studies report associations between periodontal disease and atherosclerosis [2,37]. Recent research has revealed profound effects of the microbiome on host immune responses and any process leading to increased inflammation at sites of BA vascular injury is postulated to increase the risk of restenosis [1–3]. Among known oral pathogens, *P. gingivalis* is recognized as one of the leading causative agents for periodontal disease [37,38], a chronic inflammatory disease of the tissue, alveolar bone, and periodontal ligaments around teeth. Prior studies examined subcutaneous, *P. gingivalis* infections together with wire injury in rodent models [15], but did not assess effects of a true physiological model of chronic periodontal infection on BA-induced arterial plaque growth. Systemic infection with subcutaneous or intravenous inoculums of bacterial infection may not reproduce the effects of an ongoing oral infection on inflammation and plaque growth at remote arterial sites. The current study employed a physiological model of periodontal disease and BA to more accurately reproduce chronic and focal inflammatory states in the arterial wall. We have previously reported that Pg infection alone without BA injury can accelerate aortic plaque in hyperlipidemic ApoE$^{-/-}$ mice [11]. Wild type C57Bl/6 mice with normal ApoE expression do not have hyperlipidemia and have minimal plaque growth. Studies are ongoing examining the effects of Pg oral infections alone on atherosclerotic plaque growth, but have not as yet been reported. Here we have focused on the rapid plaque growth seen in ApoE^{null} hyperlipidemic mice after balloon angioplasty injury with Pg infections. Further, we have used two anti-inflammatory agents that selectively block chemokine and serine protease pathways to examine the role of these two differing innate immune pathways in the accelerated plaque growth produced by BA during oral *P. gingivalis* infection.

Myxomavirus, a poxvirus lagomorph pathogen, encodes a plethora of anti-immune proteins, that target different aspects of the host immune response that are activated by viral infection, acting as a viral defense system against the host immune response to viral infections. Serp-1 is a secreted glycoprotein that inhibits the early host animal inflammatory responses to myxomavirus infection [39,40] and is a member of the serpin superfamily inhibiting thrombotic and thrombolytic cascade proteases [40,41]. M-T7 exhibits rabbit-species specific inhibition for interferon-γ (IFN-γ) and non-species selective chemokine-glycosaminoglycan binding in a wide range of C, CC, and CXC chemokines. Our previous work has demonstrated that M-T7 and Serp-1 inhibit BA-induced plaque growth and arterial inflammatory cell invasion after balloon injury in rodent and rabbit models [19,31,32].

P. gingivalis successfully colonized the hyperlipidemic mice upon oral infection for 24 weeks and the high IgG titer seen in infected ApoE$^{-/-}$ mice demonstrated a specific host immune response against *P. gingivalis*. The mice also demonstrated increased alveolar bone resorption indicating development of periodontal disease and providing a model to examine infection-associated inflammation in the host artery. Markedly increased aortic plaque growth was detected after 24 weeks of infection in *P. gingivalis* infected mice with BA when compared to sham-infected controls. Treatment with viral anti-inflammatory protein M-T7 reduced plaque and inflammatory macrophage invasion after BA during *P. gingivalis* infection when compared to saline treatment, while Serp-1 also displayed similar but less effective inhibition of macrophage invasion and aortic plaque.

The reduction in recurrent plaque growth by the two anti-inflammatory proteins was not associated with a reduction in *P. gingivalis* infection suggesting that simple blockade of innate immune responses, without inhibition of bacterial proliferation can reduce plaque growth after BA during chronic oral bacterial infection. This observation is consistent with studies demonstrating reduced plaque growth in dexamethasone coated stent implants and further emphasizes the impact of the innate immune response in plaque growth after BA or with chronic *P. gingivalis* infection in periodontal disease [42,43]. Increased expression of TLR4 and MyD88 receptors was also detected with *P. gingivalis* infection in areas of increased plaque. It has been observed that innate immune signaling occupies a prominent role in cardiovascular diseases through systemic and local effects along with attendant acquired immune responses [7]. Significant decrease in expression of TLRs by M-T7 and Serp-1 reported here supports the role of innate immune signaling in restenosis.

The greater reduction of plaque growth observed in *P. gingivalis* infected and BA injured ApoE$^{-/-}$ mice after treatment with M-T7 treatment suggests that chemokines have a central role in early activation of the inflammatory response after angioplasty in mice with chronic *P gingivalis* oral infection. In contrast Serp-1 treatment, which inhibits cellular serine proteinases, such as plasmin or uPA, that activate matrix metalloproteinase after BA, was less effective and suggests a lesser role for the protease pathways in driving plaque growth in *P. gingivalis* infected mice after BA [28,35]. While the chemokine–chemokine receptor interaction as well as uPA, tPA and thrombin are associated with up-regulation of inflammatory responses after arterial injury whether with BA or transplant, the relative role or impact each pathway after BA injury or in *P. gingivalis* infections has not been previously examined. We have recently reported that prolonged treatment with Serp-1 improved survival in two differing lethal viral infections in mice with associated reduction in vasculitis and arterial inflammation, further supporting the potential for use of virus-derived anti-inflammatory proteins to block arterial inflammation and plaque growth [25] The effectiveness of the anti-inflammatory compounds at reducing aortic plaque growth, in particular M-T7, even in the presence of chronic infection with a periodontal pathogen, highlights the potential therapeutic benefit of immune modulators for treatment and prevention of restenosis in patients with chronic periodontal infections. However, work with animal models with angioplasty or stent implant at sites of already developed plaque growth is necessary to fully demonstrate whether true restenosis is induced by chronic periodontal infections and/or prevented by anti-inflammatory agents.

In conclusion, chronic oral bacterial infections can accelerate plaque growth after balloon angioplasty (BA) with associated increases in inflammation. Treatment with one anti-inflammatory protein selectively targeting chemokine: GAG interactions reduced recurrent plaque growth after BA during chronic oral *P. gingivalis* infection, without associated reductions in the level of oral bacteria.

References

1. Chaabane C, Otsuka F, Virmani R, Bochaton-Piallat ML (2013) Biological responses in stented arteries. Cardiovasc Res 99: 353–363.
2. Jukema JW, Verschuren JJ, Ahmed TA, Quax PH (2012) Restenosis after PCI. Part 1: pathophysiology and risk factors. Nat Rev Cardiol 9: 53–62.
3. Arora RR, Rai F (2009) Antiplatelet intervention in acute coronary syndrome. Am J Ther 16: e29–40.
4. Burt B, Research S, Therapy Committee of the American Academy of P (2005) Position paper: epidemiology of periodontal diseases. J Periodontol 76: 1406–1419.
5. Lockhart PB, Bolger AF, Papapanou PN, Osinbowale O, Trevisan M, et al. (2012) Periodontal disease and atherosclerotic vascular disease: does the evidence support an independent association?: a scientific statement from the American Heart Association. Circulation 125: 2520–2544.
6. Paquette DW, Brodala N, Nichols TC (2007) Cardiovascular disease, inflammation, and periodontal infection. Periodontol 2000 44: 113–126.
7. Mustapha IZ, Debrey S, Oladubu M, Ugarte R (2007) Markers of systemic bacterial exposure in periodontal disease and cardiovascular disease risk: a systematic review and meta-analysis. J Periodontol 78: 2289–2302.
8. Kobayashi N, Suzuki J, Ogawa M, Aoyama N, Hanatani T, et al. (2012) *Porphyromonas gingivalis* accelerates neointimal formation after arterial injury. J Vasc Res 49: 417–424.
9. Kesavalu L, Lucas AR, Verma RK, Liu L, Dai E, et al. (2012) Increased atherogenesis during *Streptococcus mutans* infection in ApoE-null mice. J Dent Res 91: 255–260.
10. Gibson FC 3rd, Hong C, Chou HH, Yumoto H, Chen J, et al. (2004) Innate immune recognition of invasive bacteria accelerates atherosclerosis in apolipoprotein E-deficient mice. Circulation 109: 2801–2806.
11. Velsko IM, Chukkapalli SS, Rivera MF, Lee JY, Chen H, et al. (2014) Active Invasion of Oral and Aortic Tissues by *Porphyromonas gingivalis* in Mice Causally Links Periodontitis and Atherosclerosis. Plos One 9.
12. Haraszthy VI, Zambon JJ, Trevisan M, Zeid M, Genco RJ (2000) Identification of periodontal pathogens in atheromatous plaques. J Periodontol 71: 1554–1560.
13. Zhang SH, Reddick RL, Piedrahita JA, Maeda N (1992) Spontaneous hypercholesterolemia and arterial lesions in mice lacking apolipoprotein E. Science 258: 468–471.
14. Bartee MY, Chen H, Dai E, Liu LY, Davids JA, et al. (2014) Defining the anti-inflammatory activity of a potent myxomaviral chemokine modulating protein, M-T7, through site directed mutagenesis. Cytokine 65: 79–87.
15. Kobayashi N, Suzuki J, Ogawa M, Aoyama N, Hanatani T, et al. (2012) *Porphyromonas gingivalis* accelerates neointimal formation after arterial injury. J Vasc Res 49: 417–424.
16. Yuan H, Zelka S, Burkatovskaya M, Gupte R, Leeman SE, et al. (2013) Pivotal role of NOD2 in inflammatory processes affecting atherosclerosis and periodontal bone loss. Proc Natl Acad Sci U S A 110: E5059–5068.
17. Madan M, Bishayi B, Hoge M, Messas E, Amar S (2007) Doxycycline affects diet- and bacteria-associated atherosclerosis in an ApoE heterozygote murine model: cytokine profiling implications. Atherosclerosis 190: 62–72.
18. Madan M, Bishayi B, Hoge M, Amar S (2008) Atheroprotective role of interleukin-6 in diet- and/or pathogen-associated atherosclerosis using an ApoE heterozygote murine model. Atherosclerosis 197: 504–514.
19. Liu L, Lalani A, Dai E, Seet B, Macauley C, et al. (2000) The viral anti-inflammatory chemokine-binding protein M-T7 reduces intimal hyperplasia after vascular injury. J Clin Invest 105: 1613–1621.
20. Dai E, Liu LY, Wang H, McIvor D, Sun YM, et al. (2010) Inhibition of chemokine-glycosaminoglycan interactions in donor tissue reduces mouse allograft vasculopathy and transplant rejection. PLoS One 5: e10510.
21. Viswanathan K, Richardson J, Togonu-Bickersteth B, Dai E, Liu L, et al. (2009) Myxoma viral serpin, Serp-1, inhibits human monocyte adhesion through regulation of actin-binding protein filamin B. J Leukoc Biol 85: 418–426.
22. Chen H, Zheng D, Davids J, Bartee MY, Dai E, et al. (2011) Viral serpin therapeutics from concept to clinic. Methods Enzymol 499: 301–329.
23. Tardif JC, L'Allier PL, Gregoire J, Ibrahim R, McFadden G, et al. (2010) A randomized controlled, phase 2 trial of the viral serpin Serp-1 in patients with acute coronary syndromes undergoing percutaneous coronary intervention. Circ Cardiovasc Interv 3: 543–548.
24. Lucas A, Liu L, Dai E, Bot I, Viswanathan K, et al. (2009) The serpin saga; development of a new class of virus derived anti-inflammatory protein immunotherapeutics. Adv Exp Med Biol 666: 132–156.
25. Chen H, Zheng D, Abbott J, Liu L, Bartee MY, et al. (2013) Myxomavirus-derived serpin prolongs survival and reduces inflammation and hemorrhage in an unrelated lethal mouse viral infection. Antimicrob Agents Chemother 57: 4114–4127.
26. Kesavalu L, Sathishkumar S, Bakthavatchalu V, Matthews C, Dawson D, et al. (2007) Rat model of polymicrobial infection, immunity, and alveolar bone resorption in periodontal disease. Infect Immun 75: 1704–1712.
27. Rivera MF, Lee JY, Aneja M, Goswami V, Liu L, et al. (2013) Polymicrobial infection with major periodontal pathogens induced periodontal disease and aortic atherosclerosis in hyperlipidemic ApoE(null) mice. PLoS One 8: e57178.
28. Dai E, Viswanathan K, Sun YM, Li X, Liu LY, et al. (2006) Identification of myxomaviral serpin reactive site loop sequences that regulate innate immune responses. J Biol Chem 281: 8041–8050.
29. Lucas A, Liu L, Macen J, Nash P, Dai E, et al. (1996) Virus-encoded serine proteinase inhibitor SERP-1 inhibits atherosclerotic plaque development after balloon angioplasty. Circulation 94: 2890–2900.
30. Bot I, von der Thusen JH, Donners MM, Lucas A, Fekkes ML, et al. (2003) Serine protease inhibitor Serp-1 strongly impairs atherosclerotic lesion formation and induces a stable plaque phenotype in ApoE−/−mice. Circ Res 93: 464–471.
31. Bartee MY, Dai E, Liu L, Munuswamy-Ramanujam G, Macaulay C, et al. (2009) 10 M-T7: measuring chemokine-modulating activity. Methods Enzymol 460: 209–228.
32. Liu L, Dai E, Miller L, Seet B, Lalani A, et al. (2004) Viral chemokine-binding proteins inhibit inflammatory responses and aortic allograft transplant vasculopathy in rat models. Transplantation 77: 1652–1660.
33. Bainbridge B, Verma RK, Eastman C, Yehia B, Rivera M, et al. (2010) Role of *Porphyromonas gingivalis* phosphoserine phosphatase enzyme SerB in inflammation, immune response, and induction of alveolar bone resorption in rats. Infect Immun 78: 4560–4569.
34. Jiang J, Arp J, Kubelik D, Zassoko R, Liu W, et al. (2007) Induction of indefinite cardiac allograft survival correlates with toll-like receptor 2 and 4 downregulation after serine protease inhibitor-1 (Serp-1) treatment. Transplantation 84: 1158–1167.
35. Dai E, Guan H, Liu L, Little S, McFadden G, et al. (2003) Serp-1, a viral anti-inflammatory serpin, regulates cellular serine proteinase and serpin responses to vascular injury. J Biol Chem 278: 18563–18572.
36. Petrov L, Laurila H, Hayry P, Vamvakopoulos JE (2005) A mouse model of aortic angioplasty for genomic studies of neointimal hyperplasia. J Vasc Res 42: 292–300.
37. Humphrey LL, Fu R, Buckley DI, Freeman M, Helfand M (2008) Periodontal disease and coronary heart disease incidence: a systematic review and meta-analysis. J Gen Intern Med 23: 2079–2086.
38. Holt SC, Kesavalu L, Walker S, Genco CA (1999) Virulence factors of *Porphyromonas gingivalis*. Periodontol 2000 20: 168–238.
39. Upton C, Macen JL, Wishart DS, McFadden G (1990) Myxoma virus and malignant rabbit fibroma virus encode a serpin-like protein important for virus virulence. Virology 179: 618–631.
40. Macen JL, Upton C, Nation N, McFadden G (1993) SERP1, a serine proteinase inhibitor encoded by myxoma virus, is a secreted glycoprotein that interferes with inflammation. Virology 195: 348–363.
41. Turner PC, Moyer RW (1995) Orthopoxvirus fusion inhibitor glycoprotein SPI-3 (open reading frame K2L) contains motifs characteristic of serine proteinase inhibitors that are not required for control of cell fusion. J Virol 69: 5978–5987.
42. Hamalainen M, Nieminen R, Uurto I, Salenius JP, Kellomaki M, et al. (2013) Dexamethasone-eluting vascular stents. Basic Clin Pharmacol Toxicol 112: 296–301.
43. Scott NA (2006) Restenosis following implantation of bare metal coronary stents: pathophysiology and pathways involved in the vascular response to injury. Adv Drug Deliv Rev 58: 358–376.

Author Contributions

Conceived and designed the experiments: AL LK. Performed the experiments: RV ED LL HC SK MR IV SA SC. Analyzed the data: AL RV ED LL HC SK MR IV SA SC LK. Contributed reagents/materials/analysis tools: AL LK. Contributed to the writing of the manuscript: AL RV ED LL HC SK MR IV SA SC LK.

12

Relationship of Glycated Hemoglobin Levels with Myocardial Injury following Elective Percutaneous Coronary Intervention in Patients with Type 2 Diabetes Mellitus

Xiao-Lin Li, Jian-Jun Li*, Yuan-Lin Guo, Cheng-Gang Zhu, Rui-Xia Xu, Sha Li, Ping Qing, Na-Qiong Wu, Li-Xin Jiang, Bo Xu, Run-Lin Gao

Division of Dyslipidemia, State Key Laboratory of Cardiovascular Disease, Fu Wai Hospital, National Center for Cardiovascular Diseases, Chinese Academy of Medical Sciences and Peking Union Medical College, XiCheng District, Beijing, China

Abstract

Background: Glycated hemoglobin (HbA1c) predicts clinical cardiovascular disease or cardiovascular mortality. However, the relationship between HbA1c and myocardial injury following elective percutaneous coronary intervention (PCI) in patients with type 2 diabetes mellitus (DM) has not been investigated.

Objectives: The study sought to assess the relationship between HbA1c and myocardial injury following elective PCI in patients with type 2 DM.

Methods: We studied a cohort of consecutive 994 diabetic patients with coronary artery disease (CAD) undergoing elective PCI. Periprocedural myocardial injury was evaluated by analysis of troponin I (cTnI). The association between preprocedural HbA1c levels and the peak values of cTnI within 24 hours after PCI was evaluated.

Results: Peak postprocedural cTnI >1×upper limit of normal (ULN), >3×ULN and >5×ULN were detected in 543 (54.6%), 337 (33.9%) and 245 (24.6%) respectively. In the multivariate model, higher HbA1c levels were associated with less risk of postprocedural cTnI >1×ULN (odds ratio [OR], 0.85; 95% confidence interval [CI], 0.76–0.95; P=0.005). There was a trend that higher HbA1c levels were associated with less risk of postprocedural cTnI >3×ULN (OR, 0.90; 95% CI, 0.81–1.02; P=0.088). HbA1c was not associated with the risk of postprocedural cTnI elevation above 5×ULN (OR, 0.95; 95% CI, 0.84–1.08; P=0.411).

Conclusions: The present study provided the first line of evidence that higher preprocedural HbA1c levels were associated with less risk of myocardial injury following elective PCI in diabetic patients.

Editor: Victor Sanchez-Margalet, Virgen Macarena University Hospital, School of Medicine, University of Seville, Spain

Funding: This study is partly supported by National Natural Scientific Foundation (81070171, 81241121), Specialized Research Fund for the Doctoral Program of Higher Education of China (20111106110013), Capital Special Foundation of Clinical Application Research (Z121107001012015), Capital Health Development Fund (2011400302), and Beijing Natural Science Foundation (7131014) awarded to Dr. Jian-Jun Li, MD, PhD. The funders had no role in study design, data collection and analysis, decision to publish, or preparation of the manuscript.

Competing Interests: The authors have declared that no competing interests exist.

* Email: lijianjun938@yahoo.com

Introduction

Glycated hemoglobin (HbA1c) is an index of metabolic control of diabetes, and reflects average blood glucose levels over the previous 2–3 months, including postprandial increases in the blood glucose level [1,2]. There was compelling evidence suggested that the level of HbA1c predicted clinical cardiovascular disease or cardiovascular mortality [3–6]. However, the optimal glycemic control of diabetic patients with cardiovascular diseases was not well characterized. ADA, coupled with AHA and ACC just recommend less stringent HbA1c goals for diabetic patients with advanced macrovascular complications [7]. With the introduction of drug-eluting stents, the proportion of diabetic patients with

coronary artery disease (CAD) who received percutaneous coronary intervention (PCI) is increasing. However, PCI is frequently accompanied with cardiac marker elevation after procedure or known as myocardial injury or infarction related to PCI [8,9]. To date, we are not aware of any studies elucidating the impact of preprocedural glycemic control on periprocedural myocardial injury or infarction in patients with type 2 DM who underwent elective PCI. Thus, the aim of this study was to characterize the relation between HbA1c and periprocedural myocardial injury or infarction in patients with type 2 DM undergoing elective PCI.

Methods

Study population

The study complied with the Declaration of Helsinki, and was approved by the hospital ethnic review board (Fu Wai Hospital & National Center for Cardiovascular Diseases, Beijing, China). Informed written consent was obtained from all patients included in this study.

Between December 2010 and December 2012, 1032 consecutive diabetic patients with normal levels of cardiac troponin I (cTnI) and creatine kinase-MB (CK-MB) and without acute myocardial infarction in the past 4 weeks who attempt to undergo elective PCI at our center were eligible for this study. Of these patients, 33 patients were excluded because a total or subtotal chronic occlusion could not be crossed with a wire, 2 patients were excluded because a severely calcified or tortuous lesion could not be crossed with a balloon, 3 patients were excluded because treated with atheroablative, distal protection devices or aspiration thrombectomy. None of the patients died in the hospital. Thus, 994 patients were effectively included in the present study.

Adult patients with type 2 diabetes were identified based on recorded type 2 diabetes diagnosis or a prescription for oral hypoglycemic medication or insulin. Angiographic success of PCI was defined as residual stenosis less than 20% with stenting and residual stenosis less than 50% with balloon angioplasty only by visual estimation. Unstable angina was defined as rest angina, new-onset severe angina and increasing angina within 2 months. Periprocedural myocardial injury was defined as postprocedural cTnI >1×ULN. Secondly, postprocedural cTnI >3×ULN which was the diagnosis criteria of periprocedural myocardial infarction published in 2007 and postprocedural cTnI >5×ULN which was a requirement in the arbitrarily revised diagnosis criteria published in 2012 were also examined in this study [10,11].

Percutaneous coronary intervention

The indication for PCI was based on the ACC/AHA recommendations and was performed by experienced interventional cardiologists. Before the procedure, all patients without contraindications received aspirin 100 mg daily or a loading dose of 300 mg depending on whether already taken daily aspirin therapy, and received clopidogrel 75 mg daily or a loading dose of 300 mg depending on whether already taken daily long-term clopidogrel therapy prior to intervention. All patients received either 5000 U or 70 U/kg bolus of unfractionated heparin just before procedure and an additional bolus of 2,000 to 3,000 U were given every hour if the procedure lasted for more than an hour. Vascular access and PCI type (angioplasty only, angioplasty and stenting, or primary stenting) were determined by the interventional cardiologist according to patients' characteristics. Total balloon inflation times and inflation pressures were determined by the interventional cardiologist according to the technical properties of the balloon and the stent. After the procedure, all patients continued with aspirin and clopidogrel therapy daily. Use of glycoprotein IIb/IIIa receptor antagonists or anticoagulants was at the discretion of the interventional cardiologist.

Electrocardiogram monitoring

All patients received a 12-lead Electrocardiogram record before, immediately after PCI, and in the case of the occurrence of symptoms which were interpreted as postprocedural ischaemic events. All patients received continuous Electrocardiogram monitoring using wireless technology after PCI during hospitalization.

Biochemical measurements

Fasting venous blood samples were obtained immediately before intervention for measurement of fasting glucose levels, HbA1c, CK-MB activity and lipid profile. Plasma HbA1C and glucose was determined with conventional standard techniques. Cardiac troponin I (cTnI) levels were determined in venous blood samples before PCI, 24 hours after PCI, and in the event of the occurrence of symptoms or signs suggestive of myocardial ischemia. cTnI was analyzed by an immunochemiluminometric assay (Access AccuTnI, Beckman Coulter, California). The upper limit of normal (ULN) was defined as the 99th percentile of normal population with a total imprecision of <10%. The ULN of this test was 0.04 ng/ml. The peak value of cTnI within 24 hours after procedure was used for statistical analysis.

Statistics

The baseline characteristics are presented according to the quartiles of HbA1c. Data are presented as mean ± SD, median with interquartile ranges, or frequencies with percentages, as appropriate. Comparisons among the HbA1c quartiles were made with analysis of variance, chi-square test, Fisher's exact test, Kruskal–Wallis test or Friedman test as appropriate. Univariate linear regression analyses were performed to determine the relation between clinical parameters and postprocedural cTnI levels. Variables with a P value <0.2 in the univariate linear regression were entered into a stepwise multivariable linear model to determine the independent predictive value of clinical parameters for postprocedural cTnI levels. Successful normalization of cTnI after log-transformation was evaluated using Kolmogorov-Smirnov test.

Logistic regression analyses were performed to determine the relationship of HbA1c with the occurrence of postprocedural cTnI elevations above various multiples of ULN. Logistic models were adjusted for variables independently associated with postprocedural cTnI levels. HbA1c was examined in quartiles and as continuous variables. A 2-tailed P value of <0.05 was considered statistically significant. All analyses were performed using SPSS version19.0 software (Chicago,Illinois,USA).

Results

Baseline characteristics according to quartiles of HbA1c

Baseline clinical characteristics according to quartiles of HbA1c were shown in Table 1. Fasting glucose, low-density lipoprotein cholesterol, C-reactive protein and triglycerides increased across the quartiles of HbA1c. Current smoking was more frequent in subjects with high HbA1c. There were no significant differences in distribution of sex, body mass index, hypertension, dyslipidemia, family history of CAD, unstable angina, prior MI, prior PCI, prior coronary artery bypass graft, high-density lipoprotein cholesterol, NT-proBNP, hemoglobin, preprocedural cTnI and medications at study entry among quartiles of HbA1c. Fasting glucose was highly correlated with HbA1c (r = 0.543, P<0.001). Higher quartiles of HbA1c were associated with less incidence of fasting glucose below 5 mmol/L (21.7%, 14.3%, 6.6% and 6.5% respectively; P< 0.001).

Procedural characteristics according to quartiles of HbA1c were shown in Table 2. Patients with higher HbA1c levels were more likely to receive more postdilatation. There were no significant differences in vascular access, target vessel, target lesion site and target lesion type among quartiles of HbA1c. There were also no significant differences in number of stents, total stent length, predilation times, maximum inflation pressure and maximum inflation time among quartiles of HbA1c.

Table 1. Baseline clinical characteristics.

Variable	HbA1c at baseline				
	Quartile 1 (n = 258)	Quartile 2 (n = 245)	Quartile 3 (n = 259)	Quartile 4 (n = 232)	P value
HbA1c, %	6.17±0.34	6.74±0.12	7.38±0.29	9.13±1.01	<0.001
Glucose, mmol/L	5.74±1.16	6.09±1.08	6.83±1.42	8.76±2.95	<0.001
Age, years	59.39±9.49	60.84±9.34	59.56±8.65	58.49±8.31	0.039
Male, n (%)	186 (72.1)	166 (67.8)	181 (69.9)	163 (70.3)	0.769
BMI, kg/m2	26.15±3.09	26.65±2.95	26.79±3.32	26.76±3.30	0.080
Hypertension, n (%)	193 (74.8)	175 (71.4)	187 (72.2)	157 (67.7)	0.374
Dyslipidemia, n (%)	227 (88.0)	211 (86.1)	218 (84.2)	198 (85.3)	0.651
Current smoker, n (%)	59 (22.9)	79 (32.2)	78 (30.1)	79 (34.1)	0.034
FH, n (%)	63 (24.4)	57 (23.3)	62 (23.9)	40 (17.2)	0.202
UA, n (%)	136 (52.7)	144 (58.8)	136 (52.5)	125 (53.9)	0.460
Prior MI, n (%)	61 (23.6)	60 (24.5)	57 (22.0)	57 (24.6)	0.898
Prior PCI, n (%)	80 (31.0)	69 (28.2)	76 (29.3)	72 (31.0)	0.877
Prior CABG, n (%)	8 (3.1)	9 (3.7)	7 (2.7)	6 (2.6)	0.896
LDL-C, mg/dl	89.78±31.61	92.92±29.47	94.85±31.18	100.12±33.83	0.003
HDL-C, mg/dl	40.36±9.77	40.74±9.18	41.42±11.97	39.59±8.61	0.234
Triglyceride, mg/dl	132.0 (92.8–177.1)	140.8 (107.2–178.5)	138.2 (98.3–199.3)	143.0 (109.8–207.9)	0.024
hs-CRP, mg/L	1.42 (0.83–2.66)	1.76 (1.07–3.92)	1.76 (0.97–2.96)	2.26 (1.14–4.09)	<0.001
NT-proBNP, fmol/ml	515.1 (410.0–683.3)	533.9 (424.5–699.7)	513.9 (413.5–683.7)	564.8 (461.3–732.7)	0.053
Hemoglobin, g/L	138.96±15.01	138.25±14.65	138.81±14.56	140.71±14.47	0.295
cTnI, ng/ml	0.005 (0.002–0.009)	0.004 (0.002–0.009)	0.005 (0.002–0.009)	0.006 (0.002–0.010)	0.097
Medications					
Statins, n (%)	256 (99.2)	242 (98.8)	254 (98.1)	228 (98.3)	0.687
Aspirin, n (%)	256 (99.2)	243 (99.2)	259 (100.0)	232 (100.0)	0.270
Clopidogrel, n (%)	258 (100.0)	245 (100.0)	259 (100.0)	232 (100.0)	-
β-Blockers, n (%)	229 (88.8)	218 (89.0)	224 (86.5)	209 (90.1)	0.641
Nitrates, n (%)	244 (94.6)	240 (98.0)	249 (96.1)	224 (96.6)	0.252
CCBs, n (%)	138 (53.5)	135 (55.1)	133 (51.4)	114 (49.1)	0.585
ACEIs, n (%)	79 (30.6)	78 (31.8)	82 (31.7)	75 (32.3)	0.981
ARBs, n (%)	87 (33.7)	81 (33.1)	88 (34.0)	85 (36.6)	0.854
Trimetazidine, n (%)	60 (23.38)	67 (27.3)	76 (29.3)	56 (24.1)	0.368

Values are expressed as mean ± SD, median with interquartile range or n (%).
LDL-C = low-density lipoprotein cholesterol; MI = myocardial infarcton; PCI = percutaneous coronary intervention; CABG = coronary artery bypass graft; CAD = coronary artery disease; HDL-C = high-density lipoprotein cholesterol; hs-CRP = high-sensitivity C-reactive protein; NT-proBNP = N-terminal pro-brain natriuretic peptide; cTnI = cardiac troponin I; CCBs = calcium channel blockers; ACE = angiotensin-converting enzyme; ARBs = angiotensin receptor blockers.

Association between HbA1c levels and postprocedural cTnI levels

There was a similar trend that lower preprocedural HbA1c and fasting glucose levels were associated with higher postprocedural cTnI levels in the simple regression analysis (Table 3). Simple regression analyses revealed that age, prior MI, NT-proBNP, creatinine, preprocedural cTnI, number of target vessels, number of B2/C type lesions, number of bifurcation lesions, number of predilation, number of postdilation, use of kissing balloon, maximum inflation pressure, number of stents and total stent length were positively associated with postprocedural cTnI levels, whereas high hemoglobin levels were associated with low postprocedural cTnI levels.

Stepwise multivariable analysis revealed that factors independently associated with postprocedural cTnI levels were age, prior myocardial infarction, NT-proBNP, preprocedural cTnI, number

of target vessels, number of postdilation and total stent length were positively associated with postprocedural cTnI levels, whereas HbA1c levels were inversely associated with postprocedural cTnI levels (Table 3).

Association between HbA1c levels and postprocedural cTnI elevation

Peak postprocedural cTnI >1×ULN, >3×ULN and >5×ULN were detected in 543 (54.6%), 337 (33.9%) and 245 (24.6%) respectively. Calculating HbA1c as a continuous variable, simple logistic regression showed that each increment of 1% in the HbA1c level was associated with less risk of postprocedural cTnI elevation above 1×ULN (Table 4). HbA1c was not significantly associated with postprocedural cTnI elevation above 3×ULN and 5×ULN. After adjusting for covariates, each increment of 1% in the HbA1c level was more strongly associated with less risk of

Table 2. Procedural characteristics.

Variable	HbA1c at baseline				P value
	Quartile 1 (n = 258)	Quartile 2 (n = 245)	Quartile 3 (n = 259)	Quartile 4 (n = 232)	
Transradial access, n (%)	234 (90.7)	220 (89.8)	237 (91.5)	216 (93.1)	0.622
Target vessel					0.748
LM	9	16	13	7	
LAD	138	141	153	128	
LCX	90	75	79	76	
RCA	98	103	99	98	
Grafts	0	2	1	1	
Lesion location					0.268
Proximal	130	147	151	151	
Middle	195	175	201	173	
Distal	82	79	69	75	
branch	78	56	82	58	
Lesion classification					0.365
ACC/AHA type A/B1	84	73	66	69	
ACC/AHA type B2/C	290	288	315	266	
Bifurcation lesions, n (%)	108 (41.9)	97 (39.6)	117 (45.2)	97 (41.8)	0.648
Use with kissing balloon, n (%)	14 (5.4)	22 (9.0)	23 (8.9)	20 (8.6)	0.384
Occlusion lesions, n (%)	32 (12.4)	36 (14.7)	51 (19.7)	28 (12.1)	0.058
In-stent restenosis, n (%)	16 (6.2)	11 (4.5)	14 (5.4)	10 (4.3)	0.759
Number of stents implanted	1.88±1.01	2.05±1.05	2.04±1.07	2.03±1.03	0.178
Total stent length, mm	40.89±27.20	45.99±24.97	46.88±29.08	46.00±27.09	0.051
Maximum pressure, atm	17.60±3.69	18.26±3.89	17.76±3.46	17.95±3.66	0.215
Maximum inflation time, s	10.58±4.04	10.29±4.74	10.13±3.65	10.03±3.51	0.443
Number of predilation	2 (1–4)	2 (1–5)	3 (1–6)	3 (2–5)	0.054
Number of postdilatation	3 (2–6)	4 (2–6)	4 (2–6)	4 (2–7)	0.042
Postprocedural medication					
LMWH, n (%)	170 (65.9)	167 (68.2)	176 (68.0)	159 (68.5)	0.922
GPI, n (%)	44 (17.1)	44 (18.0)	31 (12.0)	34 (14.7)	0.239

Values are expressed as n (%), mean ± SD or median with interquartile range.
HbA1c = glycated hemoglobin; LM = left main; LAD = left anterior descending; LCX = left circumflex; RCA = right coronary artery; LMWH = low molecular weight heparin; GPI = glycoprotein inhibitors.

postprocedural cTnI elevation above 1×ULN (Table 4, Figure 1). There was a trend that each increment of 1% in the HbA1c level was associated with less risk of postprocedural cTnI elevation above 3×ULN, but this did not reach a statistical significance (Table 4, Figure 2). HbA1c was not significantly associated with postprocedural cTnI elevation above 5×ULN (Table 4, Figure 3).

Association between HbA1c quartiles and postprocedural cTnI levels

The interquartile ranges of postprocedural cTnI levels for each quartile of HbA1c were 0.052 (0.018–0.203), 0.063 (0.021–0.184), 0.049 (0.015–0.217) and 0.041 (0.012–0.198) respectively. There is a linear trend that higher quartiles of HbA1c were associated with lower postprocedural cTnI levels. After multivariate adjustment for other factors which were independently associated with postprocedural cTnI levels, higher quartiles of HbA1c were significantly associated with lower postprocedural cTnI levels (Table 5). And higher quartiles of HbA1c were associated with less risk of postprocedural cTnI elevation above 1×ULN. There was a

trend that higher quartiles of HbA1c were associated with less risk of postprocedural cTnI elevation above 3×ULN, but this did not reach a statistical significance. The quartiles of HbA1c were not associated with the risk of postprocedural cTnI elevation above 5×ULN (Table 6).

Discussion

The present study provided the first line of evidence that higher preprocedural HbA1c levels were associated with less risk of myocardial injury following elective PCI in diabetic patients. Thus, our study provided the novel finding regarding the relationship between preprocedural HbA1c and periprocedural myocardial injury.

PCI has become an important strategy for patients with CAD. Patients with type 2 diabetes mellitus (DM) have a higher prevalence of CAD than the general population. Because of poor outcome, PCI in diabetic patients have been recognized as a complex procedure. With advances in PCI techniques and medications, especially with introduction of drug-eluting stents,

Table 3. Analysis of factors related to postprocedural cTnI levels (log-transformed).

Variable	Simple Regression		Multiple Regression	
	Standard coefficient	P value	Standard coefficient	P value
Age	0.125	<0.001	0.117	<0.001
Male	-0.023	0.473		
Unstable angina	-0.058	0.065		
Prior MI	0.095	0.003	0.076	0.012
Prior PCI	-0.015	0.640		
Prior CABG	0.008	0.791		
Hypertension	0.030	0.346		
Current smoking	0.011	0.739		
Family history of CAD	0.021	0.517		
HbA1C	-0.053	0.097	-0.071	0.018
Glucose	-0.053	0.095		
LDL-C	0.043	0.177		
HDL-C	0.005	0.866		
Triglyceride	0.007	0.833		
hs-CRP	-0.014	0.664		
NT-proBNP	0.117	<0.001	0.080	0.009
Creatinine	0.069	0.030		
Hemoglobin	-0.064	0.043		
Preprocedural cTnI	0.124	<0.001	0.086	0.005
Number of target vessels	0.220	<0.001	0.131	<0.001
Number of B2/C type lesions	0.201	<0.001		
Number of bifurcation lesions	0.132	<0.001		
Number of occlusion lesions	0.013	0.680		
Number of in-stent restenosis	-0.022	0.485		
Number of predilation	0.182	<0.001		
Number of postdilatation	0.201	<0.001	0.075	0.043
Use of kissing balloon	0.089	0.005		
Maximum inflation pressure	0.075	0.018		
Maximum inflation time	0.045	0.157		
Number of stents	0.248	<0.001		
Total stent length	0.252	<0.001	0.152	<0.001

MI = myocardial infarcton; PCI = percutaneous coronary intervention; CABG = coronary artery bypass graft; CAD = coronary artery disease; LDL-C = low-density lipoprotein cholesterol; HDL-C = high-density lipoprotein cholesterol; hs-CRP = high-sensitivity C-reactive protein; NT-proBNP = N-terminal pro-brain natriuretic peptide; cTnI, cardiac troponin I.

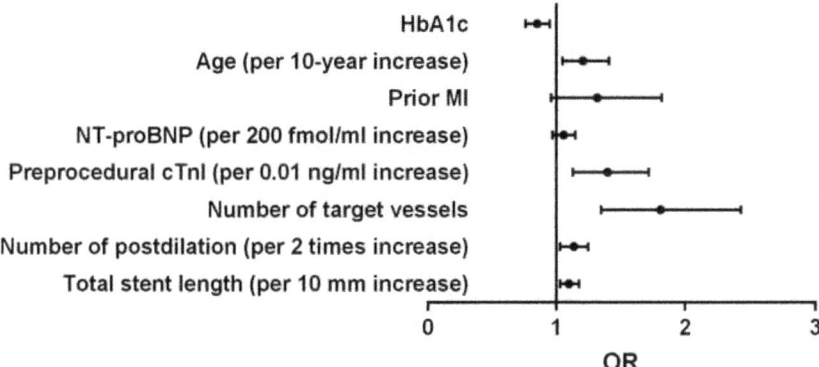

Figure 1. Odds ratio for postprocedural cTnI elevation above 1×ULN. HbA1c =glycated hemoglobin; cTnI = cardiac troponin I; OR = odds ratio; ULN = upper limit of normal; MI = myocardial infarcton; NT-proBNP = N-terminal pro-brain natriuretic peptide.

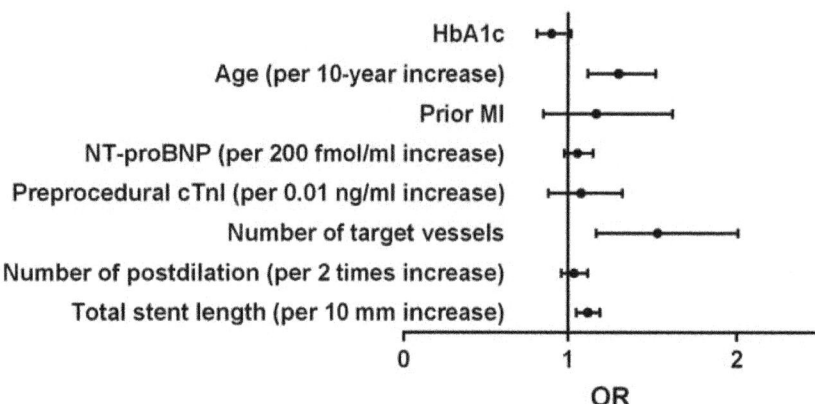

Figure 2. Odds ratio for postprocedural cTnI elevation above 3×ULN. HbA1c =glycated hemoglobin; cTnI = cardiac troponin I; OR = odds ratio; ULN = upper limit of normal; MI = myocardial infarcton; NT-proBNP = N-terminal pro-brain natriuretic peptide.

more and more diabetic patients receive PCI. However, PCI was still frequently companied with postprocedural cardiac marker elevation. There was a large body of data correlating troponin elevation after elective PCI with adverse clinical outcomes [12–15]. Third universal definition of myocardial infarction has raised the diagnostic threshold of PCI-related myocardial infarction from the elevation of troponin above 3 times ULN to the elevation of troponin above 5 times ULN, and suggested that this threshold was arbitrarily chosen, based on clinical judgement and societal implications of the label of PCI-related myocardial infarction. Myocardial injury is used for postprocedural cTn value is > 1×ULN and ≤5×ULN [16]. So, we used many different cTnI cut points. Although a number of studies have investigated the risk factors associated with periprocedural myocardial infarction or injury [9,17,18], less of them focused on diabetic patients or the impact of glycemic control on periprocedural myocardial infarction or injury in diabetic patients. And elevated HbA1c or poor glycemic control is associated with increased risk of cardiovascular events in diabetic patients [4–6], but whether elevated HbA1c is still associated with increased risk of myocardial infarction or injury following elective PCI in diabetic patients is still unknown.

In the present study, we included 994 diabetic patients undergoing elective PCI to determine the relation of preprocedural HbA1c levels with postprocedural cTnI elevation. Univariate analysis showed that some clinical and procedural characteristics were associated with postprocedural cTnI levels. There were almost identical pattern between the inverse associations of HbA1c and fasting glucose with postprocedural cTnI levels. However, after multivariate stepwise analysis, HbA1c was still in the model, but fasting glucose was not. HbA1c reflects both fasting and postprandial blood glucose levels over the previous 2–3 months, has less fluctuation individually than fasting blood glucose level, and can be measured in the nonfasting state. These characteristics may result that HbA1c outperform fasting glucose in prediction of periprocedural myocardial injury. Patients in the highest quartile of HbA1c were likely to receive more predilation and postdilation, and longer total stent length implanted. This maybe reflect high atherosclerotic burden in these patients with high HbA1c levels [19]. However, these patients experienced reduced risk of periprocedural myocardial injury. Regardless of calculating as quartiles or continuous variables, higher HbA1c levels were associated with less risk periprocedural myocardial injury. A U-shaped or J-shape association between HbA1c and periprocedural myocardial injury did not appear. Interestingly, there was also an inverse relationship between HbA1c levels and mortality in diabetic patients with advanced systolic heart failure [20].

The exact reasons for the relationship of lower HbA1c levels with periprocedural myocardial injury were unclear. There were some plausible explanations for this relationship. The energy supply of ischemic myocardium mainly dependents on anaerobic

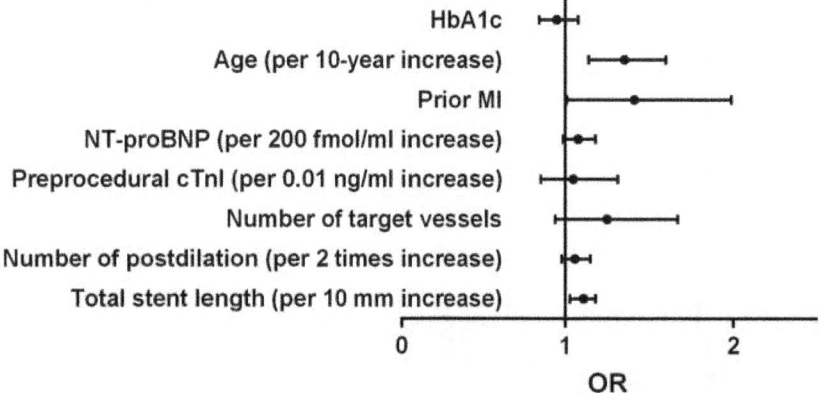

Figure 3. Odds ratio for postprocedural cTnI elevation above 5×ULN. HbA1c =glycated hemoglobin; cTnI = cardiac troponin I; OR = odds ratio; ULN = upper limit of normal; MI = myocardial infarcton; NT-proBNP = N-terminal pro-brain natriuretic peptide.

Table 4. Odds ratio for postprocedural cTnI elevation associated with 1% increment in the HbA1c.

Variable	cTnI elevation >1×ULN		cTnI elevation >3×ULN		cTnI elevation >5×ULN	
	OR (95%CI)	P	OR (95%CI)	P	OR (95%CI)	P
Unadjusted model						
HbA1C	0.90(0.81–0.99)	0.034	0.92(0.83–1.03)	0.151	0.96(0.85–1.09)	0.547
Adjusted model						
HbA1C	0.85(0.76–0.95)	0.004	0.90(0.81–1.02)	0.088	0.95(0.84–1.08)	0.411
Age	1.02(1.01–1.04)	0.011	1.03(1.01–1.04)	0.001	1.03(1.01–1.05)	0.001
Prior MI	1.32(0.96–1.82)	0.088	1.17(0.85–1.62)	0.344	1.41(1.01–1.99)	0.049
NT-proBNP	1.00(1.00–1.01)	0.192	1.00(1.00–1.01)	0.162	1.00(1.00–1.01)	0.075
Preprocedural cTnI	1.03(1.01–1.06)	0.002	1.01(0.99–1.03)	0.456	1.01(0.98–1.03)	0.632
Number of target vessels	1.81(1.35–2.43)	<0.001	1.53(1.17–2.01)	0.002	1.25(0.94–1.67)	0.128
Number of postdilatation	1.07(1.02–1.12)	0.008	1.02(0.98–1.06)	0.383	1.03(0.99–1.07)	0.180
Total stent length	1.01(1.00–1.02)	0.005	1.01(1.00–1.02)	0.001	1.01(1.00–1.02)	0.004

HbA1c = glycated hemoglobin; cTnI = cardiac troponin I; OR = odds ratio; ULN = upper limit of normal; MI = myocardial infarcton; NT-proBNP = N-terminal pro-brain natriuretic peptide.

pathways and carbohydrate substrates [21]. Patients with lower HbA1c may have less energy supply for ischemic myocardium during or after procedure. The present study showed that HbA1c was highly correlated with fasting glucose. Libby and colleagues have showed that hypoglycemia increased myocardial damage during acute experimental coronary artery occlusion in dogs [22]. The study by Nusca et al showed that preprocedural glucose levels were inversely associated with periprocedural myocardial infarction in 572 patients of which 198 was diabetic [23]. The study by Madani et al showed that low preprocedural glucose levels were associated with increased incidence of periprocedural myocardial injury in 1012 patients undergoing elective PCI of which 260 was diabetic [24]. Unlike these studies, we examined the relation of fasting glucose and HbA1c with periprocedural myocardial injury in diabetic patients undergoing elective PCI, and found the superiority of HbA1c over fasting glucose for prediction of periprocedural myocardial injury. This was consistent with the study by Nicholls which showed a stronger correlation between plaque characteristics and glycated hemoglobin than fasting glucose [25]. Although high levels of HbA1c were associated with large plaque volume [19], higher HbA1c levels were still associated with less risk of periprocedural myocardial injury in our study. The positive association between HbA1c and glucose might partly

explain the inverse relationship between HbA1c and periprocedural myocardial injury. The energy supply of ischemic myocardium mainly dependents on anaerobic pathways with carbohydrate substrates. Patients with hypoglycemia may be under greater energy stress and have less energy supply.

There were also some other reasons accounted for the inverse relationship between HbA1c and periprocedural myocardial injury in diabetic patients. Diabetic patients with high levels of HbA1c have increased coronary plaque calcification despite of large plaque volume [19,26]. Calcified and hard plaques were difficult to be dilated and less likely to be crushed to debris during balloon dilation. The negative or unexpected results of several clinical trials which were designed to determine the effect of achieving a low HbA1c level on cardiovascular events, could also partly explain our results. Because of increased mortality in participants randomized to intensive glucose control to achieve an HbA1c level below 6%, Action to Control Cardiovascular Risk in Diabetes (ACCORD) was terminated early [27]. Both Action in Diabetes and Vascular Disease–Preterax and Diamicron Modified Release Controlled Evaluation (ADVANCE) and the Veterans Affairs Diabetes Trial (VADT) showed no significant reduction in cardiovascular events with intensive glucose control by which a mean HbA1c level of 6.3% and 6.9% were achieved respectively

Table 5. Distribution of post-PCI cardiac troponin I.

Variable	HbA1c at baseline				β	P for trend
	Quartile 1 (n = 258)	Quartile 2 (n = 245)	Quartile 3 (n = 259)	Quartile 4 (n = 232)		
Post-PCI cTnI, ng/ml	0.052(0.018–0.203)	0.063(0.021–0.184)	0.049(0.015–0.217)	0.041 (0.012–0.198)	−0.073	0.014
Post-PCI cTnI elevation						
>1×ULN, n (%)	147 (57.0)	140 (57.1)	139 (53.7)	117 (50.4)	−0.145	0.018
>3×ULN, n (%)	91 (35.3)	87 (35.5)	86 (33.2)	73 (31.5)	−0.088	0.166
>5×ULN, n (%)	66 (25.6)	56 (22.9)	65 (25.1)	58 (25.0)	−0.019	0.785

Values were expressed as median with interquartile ranges or n (%). The analyses were adjusted for age, prior myocardial infarction, NT-proBNP, preprocedural cTnI, number of target vessels and total stent length.

Table 6. Unadjusted and adjusted OR for periprocedural myocardial injury according to quartiles of HbA1c.

Variable	cTnI elevation >1×ULN		cTnI elevation >3×ULN		cTnI elevation >5×ULN	
	OR (95%CI)	P	OR (95%CI)	P	OR (95%CI)	P
Unadjusted model						
Quartile 1 (reference)						
Quartile 2	1.01(0.71–1.43)	0.970	1.01(0.70–1.46)	0.955	0.86(0.57–1.30)	0.476
Quartile 3	0.88(0.62–1.24)	0.449	0.91(0.63–1.31)	0.621	0.98(0.66–1.45)	0.899
Quartile 4	0.77(0.54–1.10)	0.147	0.84(0.58–1.23)	0.373	0.97(0.65–1.46)	0.883
Adjusted model						
Quartile 1 (reference)						
Quartile 2	0.86(0.59–1.25)	0.437	0.88(0.60–1.28)	0.490	0.74(0.49–1.13)	0.167
Quartile 3	0.74(0.52–1.08)	0.116	0.82(0.56–1.19)	0.293	0.88(0.59–1.33)	0.549
Quartile 4	0.65(0.44–0.95)	0.025	0.77(0.52–1.14)	0.184	0.90(0.59–1.37)	0.610
Age	1.02(1.01–1.04)	0.009	1.03(1.01–1.04)	0.001	1.03(1.01–1.05)	<0.001
Prior MI	1.31(0.95–1.80)	0.099	1.16(0.84–1.61)	0.362	1.42(1.01–2.00)	0.047
NT-proBNP	1.00(1.00–1.01)	0.201	1.00(1.00–1.01)	0.170	1.00(1.00–1.01)	0.082
Preprocedural cTnI	1.03(1.01–1.06)	0.002	1.01(0.99–1.03)	0.471	1.01(0.98–1.03)	0.682
Number of target vessels	1.79(1.34–2.41)	<0.001	1.53(1.17–2.00)	0.002	1.26(0.95–1.68)	0.114
Number of postdilatation	1.06(1.02–1.12)	0.009	1.02(0.98–1.06)	0.381	1.03(0.99–1.07)	0.183
Total stent length	1.01(1.00–1.02)	0.004	1.01(1.00–1.02)	0.001	1.01(1.00–1.02)	0.004

HbA1c = glycated hemoglobin; cTnI = cardiac troponin I; OR = odds ratio; ULN = upper limit of normal; MI = myocardial infarcton; NT-proBNP = N-terminal pro-brain natriuretic peptide.

[28,29]. To date, the optimal HbA1C target in diabetic patients with coronary artery disease is still a subject of ongoing controversy.

Despite the detailed data collection in this study, we acknowledged several potential limitations of our study. First, although we attempted to adjust for potential confounders, we can not exclude the possibility that unmeasured variables may have confounded results. Second, it has been suggested that CK-MB might have a better predictive value than troponins [30], but we did not measure the CK-MB levels after procedure due to insurance cost. However, troponins are more sensitive and specific biomarkers for myocardium than CK-MB activity and CK-MB mass, and the third universal definition of myocardial infarction has recommended troponin using for diagnosis of PCI-related myocardial infarction and injury. And there was also a large body of data demonstrated that postprocedural troponin elevation was associated with a worse clinical outcome [12–15]. Third, we conjectured that hypoglycemia might be one cause of periprocedural myocardial injury for patients with low HbA1c, but hypoglycemic episodes were not monitored in the current study. Fourth, the lack of a control (non-diabetic) group was also a limitation. Finally, a single center study may also be a limitation in our study. However, the present study has revealed a previously unrecognized relationship between HbA1c level and myocardial injury following elective PCI in diabetic patients.

Conclusions

In summary, our prospective study in a large cohort of consecutive diabetic patient with CAD, for the first time, demonstrated that higher preprocedural HbA1c concentrations were linked with less risk of myocardial injury following elective PCI in patients with diabetes mellitus. Further prospective studies are needed to identify whether less stringent HbA1c goals before procedure is appropriate for diabetic patients undergoing elective PCI.

Acknowledgments

The authors thank the staff of the Cardiac Catheterization Laboratory at Fuwai hospital for their assistance in performing the studies. The authors also thank all the study investigators, staff, and patients.

Author Contributions

Conceived and designed the experiments: XLL JJL. Performed the experiments: XLL JJL YLG CGZ RXX SL PQ NQW LXJ BX RLG. Analyzed the data: XLL JJL YLG CGZ RXX SL PQ NQW LXJ BX RLG. Contributed reagents/materials/analysis tools: XLL JJL YLG CGZ RXX SL PQ NQW LXJ BX RLG. Wrote the paper: XLL JJL.

References

1. American Diabetes A (2009) Standards of medical care in diabetes—2009. Diabetes Care 32 Suppl 1: S13-61.
2. Nathan DM, Kuenen J, Borg R, Zheng H, Schoenfeld D, et al. (2008) Translating the A1C assay into estimated average glucose values. Diabetes Care 31: 1473–1478.
3. Selvin E, Marinopoulos S, Berkenblit G, Rami T, Brancati FL, et al. (2004) Meta-analysis: glycosylated hemoglobin and cardiovascular disease in diabetes mellitus. Ann Intern Med 141: 421–431.
4. Colayco DC, Niu F, McCombs JS, Cheetham TC (2011) A1C and cardiovascular outcomes in type 2 diabetes: a nested case-control study. Diabetes Care 34: 77–83.
5. Stratton IM, Adler AI, Neil HA, Matthews DR, Manley SE, et al. (2000) Association of glycaemia with macrovascular and microvascular complications of type 2 diabetes (UKPDS 35): prospective observational study. BMJ 321: 405–412.

6. Zhao W, Katzmarzyk PT, Horswell R, Wang Y, Johnson J, et al. (2014) HbA1c and coronary heart disease risk among diabetic patients. Diabetes Care 37: 428–435.

7. Skyler JS, Bergenstal R, Bonow RO, Buse J, Deedwania P, et al. (2009) Intensive glycemic control and the prevention of cardiovascular events: implications of the ACCORD, ADVANCE, and VA diabetes trials: a position statement of the American Diabetes Association and a scientific statement of the American College of Cardiology Foundation and the American Heart Association. Circulation 119: 351–357.

8. Prasad A (2013) Slow but steady progress towards understanding peri-procedural myocardial infarction. Eur Heart J 34: 1615–1617.

9. Herrmann J (2005) Peri-procedural myocardial injury: 2005 update. Eur Heart J 26: 2493–2519.

10. Thygesen K, Alpert JS, White HD, Joint ESCAAHAWHFTFftRoMI (2007) Universal definition of myocardial infarction. Eur Heart J 28: 2525–2538.

11. Thygesen K, Alpert JS, Jaffe AS, Simoons ML, Chaitman BR, et al. (2012) Third universal definition of myocardial infarction. J Am Coll Cardiol 60: 1581–1598.

12. Feldman DN, Kim L, Rene AG, Minutello RM, Bergman G, et al. (2011) Prognostic value of cardiac troponin-I or troponin-T elevation following nonemergent percutaneous coronary intervention: a meta-analysis. Catheter Cardiovasc Interv 77: 1020–1030.

13. Nienhuis MB, Ottervanger JP, Bilo HJ, Dikkeschei BD, Zijlstra F (2008) Prognostic value of troponin after elective percutaneous coronary intervention: A meta-analysis. Catheter Cardiovasc Interv 71: 318–324.

14. Prasad A, Singh M, Lerman A, Lennon RJ, Holmes DR, Jr., et al. (2006) Isolated elevation in troponin T after percutaneous coronary intervention is associated with higher long-term mortality. J Am Coll Cardiol 48: 1765–1770.

15. Prasad A, Rihal CS, Lennon RJ, Singh M, Jaffe AS, et al. (2008) Significance of periprocedural myonecrosis on outcomes after percutaneous coronary intervention: an analysis of preintervention and postintervention troponin T levels in 5487 patients. Circ Cardiovasc Interv 1: 10–19.

16. Thygesen K, Alpert JS, Jaffe AS, Simoons ML, Chaitman BR, et al. (2012) Third universal definition of myocardial infarction. Circulation 126: 2020–2035.

17. Cai Q, Skelding KA, Armstrong AT, Jr., Desai D, Wood GC, et al. (2007) Predictors of periprocedural creatine kinase-myocardial band elevation complicating elective percutaneous coronary intervention. Am J Cardiol 99: 616–620.

18. Park DW, Kim YH, Yun SC, Ahn JM, Lee JY, et al. (2013) Frequency, causes, predictors, and clinical significance of peri-procedural myocardial infarction following percutaneous coronary intervention. Eur Heart J 34: 1662–1669.

19. Yang DJ, Lee MS, Kim WH, Park HW, Kim KH, et al. (2013) The impact of glucose control on coronary plaque composition in patients with diabetes mellitus. J Invasive Cardiol 25: 137–141.

20. Eshaghian S, Horwich TB, Fonarow GC (2006) An unexpected inverse relationship between HbA1c levels and mortality in patients with diabetes and advanced systolic heart failure. Am Heart J 151: 91.

21. Neely JR, Morgan HE (1974) Relationship between carbohydrate and lipid metabolism and the energy balance of heart muscle. Annu Rev Physiol 36: 413–459.

22. Libby P, Maroko PR, Braunwald E (1975) The effect of hypoglycemia on myocardial ischemic injury during acute experimental coronary artery occlusion. Circulation 51: 621–626.

23. Nusca A, Patti G, Marino F, Mangiacapra F, D'Ambrosio A, et al. (2012) Prognostic role of preprocedural glucose levels on short- and long-term outcome in patients undergoing percutaneous coronary revascularization. Catheter Cardiovasc Interv 80: 377–384.

24. Madani M, Alizadeh K, Ghazaee SP, Zavarehee A, Abdi S, et al. (2013) Elective percutaneous coronary intervention: the relationship between preprocedural blood glucose levels and periprocedural myocardial injury. Tex Heart Inst J 40: 410–417.

25. Nicholls SJ, Tuzcu EM, Kalidindi S, Wolski K, Moon KW, et al. (2008) Effect of diabetes on progression of coronary atherosclerosis and arterial remodeling: a pooled analysis of 5 intravascular ultrasound trials. J Am Coll Cardiol 52: 255–262.

26. Anand DV, Lim E, Darko D, Bassett P, Hopkins D, et al. (2007) Determinants of progression of coronary artery calcification in type 2 diabetes role of glycemic control and inflammatory/vascular calcification markers. J Am Coll Cardiol 50: 2218–2225.

27. Action to Control Cardiovascular Risk in Diabetes Study G, Gerstein HC, Miller ME, Byington RP, Goff DC, Jr., et al. (2008) Effects of intensive glucose lowering in type 2 diabetes. N Engl J Med 358: 2545–2559.

28. Group AC, Patel A, MacMahon S, Chalmers J, Neal B, et al. (2008) Intensive blood glucose control and vascular outcomes in patients with type 2 diabetes. N Engl J Med 358: 2560–2572.

29. Duckworth W, Abraira C, Moritz T, Reda D, Emanuele N, et al. (2009) Glucose control and vascular complications in veterans with type 2 diabetes. N Engl J Med 360: 129–139.

30. Moussa ID, Klein LW, Shah B, Mehran R, Mack MJ, et al. (2013) Consideration of a new definition of clinically relevant myocardial infarction after coronary revascularization: an expert consensus document from the Society for Cardiovascular Angiography and Interventions (SCAI). J Am Coll Cardiol 62: 1563–1570.

13

Safety and Feasibility of Coronary Stenting in Unprotected Left Main Coronary Artery Disease in the Real World Clinical Practice—A Single Center Experience

Wei-Chieh Lee[1]ᗧ, Tzu-Hsien Tsai[1]ᗧ, Yung-Lung Chen[1], Cheng-Hsu Yang[1], Shyh-Ming Chen[1], Chien-Jen Chen[1], Cheng-Jei Lin[1], Cheng-I Cheng[1], Chi-Ling Hang[1], Chiung-Jen Wu[1], Hon-Kan Yip[1,2,3]*

1 Division of Cardiology, Department of Internal Medicine, Kaohsiung Chang Gung Memorial Hospital and Chang Gung University College of Medicine, Kaohsiung, Taiwan, **2** Center for Translational Research in Biomedical Sciences, Kaohsiung Chang Gung Memorial Hospital and Chang Gung University College of Medicine, Kaohsiung, Taiwan, **3** Institute of Shock Wave Medicine and Tissue Engineering, Kaohsiung Chang Gung Memorial Hospital and Chang Gung University College of Medicine, Kaohsiung, Taiwan

Abstract

Background: This study evaluated the feasibility, safety, and prognostic outcome in patients with significant unprotected left main coronary artery (ULMCA) disease undergoing stenting.

Method and Results: Between January 2010 and December 2012, totally 309 patients, including those with stable angina [13.9% (43/309)], unstable angina [59.2% (183/309)], acute non-ST-segment elevation myocardial infarction (NSTEMI) [24.3% (75/309)], and post-STEMI angina (i.e., onset of STEMI<7 days) [2.6% (8/309)] with significant ULMCA disease (>50%) undergoing stenting using transradial arterial approach, were consecutively enrolled. The patients' mean age was 68.9 ± 10.8 yrs. Incidences of advance congestive heart failure (CHF) (defined as $\geq$ NYHA Fc 3) and multi-vessel disease were 16.5% (51/309) and 80.6% (249/309), respectively. Mechanical supports, including IABP for critical patients (defined as LVEF <35%, advanced CHF, or hemodynamically unstable) and extra-corporeal membrane oxygenator (ECMO) for hemodynamically collapsed patients, were utilized in 17.2% (53/309) and 2.6% (8/409) patients, respectively. Stent implantation was successfully performed in all patients. Thirty-day mortality rate was 4.5% (14/309) [cardiac death: 2.9% (9/309) vs. non-cardiac death: 1.6% (5/309)] without significant difference among four groups [2.3% (1) vs. 2.7% (5) vs. 9.3% (7) vs. 12.5% (1), $p = 0.071$]. Multivariate analysis identified acute kidney injury (AKI) as the strongest independent predictor of 30-day mortality ($p < 0.0001$), while body mass index (BMI) and white blood cell (WBC) count were independently predictive of 30-day mortality ($p = 0.003$ and 0.012, respectively).

Conclusion: Catheter-based LM stenting demonstrated high rates of procedural success and excellent 30-day clinical outcomes. AKI, BMI, and WBC count were significantly and independently predictive of 30-day mortality.

Editor: Alberto Aliseda, University of Washington, United States of America

Funding: The authors have no support or funding to report.

Competing Interests: The authors have declared that no competing interests exist.

* Email: han.gung@msa.hinet.net

ᗧ These authors contributed equally to this work.

Introduction

Previous studies have revealed that medically treated patients with significantly unprotected left main coronary artery (ULMCA) disease (i.e., >50% stensosis) have a 3-year mortality rate up to 50% [1,2]. Several clinical trials have shown a superior survival benefit of coronary bypass grafting (CABG) compared with medical treatment for significant ULMCA disease [3–6]. Based on the evidence of these trials [3–6], the current practice guideline still recommends CABG as the gold standard for the treatment of significant left main coronary artery (LM) disease [7,8]. However, several points have to be taken into consideration. Despite a well-established technique, CABG is a major surgical procedure associated with significant operative risk and up to 3.0% in-hospital mortality [9]. Moreover, CABG carries an especially high

risk or is not feasible in patients with 1) advanced age or critical internal medical co-morbidities, 2) short estimated life expectancy as in those with malignancies, 3) significant ULMCA disease with urgent requirement for major non-cardiovascular surgical intervention, 4) low willingness to receive CABG, or 5) unstable condition/hemodynamic collapse due to an acute LM occlusion. Another therapeutic option other than CABG or medical treatment, therefore, is of utmost importance to physicians.

Over the last 20 years, with the accumulation of operators' experience, refinement in instruments, and advance in pharmacological development of anti-platelet and anti-ischemic agents, percutaneous coronary intervention (PCI) has been widely accepted as one of the most popular methods for the treatment of atherosclerotic occlusive syndrome, especially for patients with ST-segment elevation myocardial infarction (STEMI) with or without cardiogenic shock [10,11]. These advances in PCI techniques and stent technology have allowed evaluation of the role of PCI in significant ULMCA disease [12,13], especially focusing on the safety and efficacy of stenting the LMCA to determine whether it does provide a true alternative to CABG [12–15]. Results from previous clinical trials comparing the efficacy and safety between PCIs with stenting and CABG have shown comparable results in terms of procedural success rates, safety, favorable early outcomes, and the need for repeated revascularization [12–19]. However, many data were from clinical trials with strict exclusion criteria for patient selection [12–15,17–19] rather than a real-world clinical practice [16] without patient exclusion. Of importance is that patients with unstable clinical presentation, hemodynamic compromise upon presentation, or patients in the setting of acute or early myocardial infarction were usually excluded from the trials [12–15,17–19]. Thus, further evidence-based information should be acquired to assess the lay the clinical foundation for the practice of LMCA stenting [18]. The issue is of particular importance in Asia where the majority of patients are unwilling to receive CABG due to a fear for chest surgery based on a traditional belief, making PCI the last resort for the treatment of significant LM disease. Accordingly, this study, based on the needs arising from our daily clinical practice for clarifying the safety, feasibility, and assessing the 30-day clinical outcome of patients with significant ULMCA disease undergoing PCI because of refusal of CABG or unsuitability for surgery, attempted to evaluate the benefit of mechanical-assisted procedure to patients in critical condition upon presentation.

Materials and Methods

Patient Population, Ethics, Enrollment and Exclusion Criteria

This study was approved by the Institutional Review Committee on Human Research of Chang Gung Memorial Hospital (No 102-0789B) and conducted at Kaohsiung Chang Gung Memorial Hospital for retrospective assessment of procedural success rate, safety, efficacy, and 30-day clinical outcomes in patients with significant ULMCA disease with clinical presentations as (1) stable angina pectoris (SAP) (group 1), (2) unstable angina pectoris (UAP) (group 2), (3) acute or recent (i.e., onset < day 7) non-ST elevation myocardial infarction (NSTEMI) (group 3), and (4) post-ST-segment elevation myocardial infarction (STEMI) angina (i.e., >12 h <7-day presentation of STEMI) (group 4). The participants provide their written informed consent to participate in this study. The ethics committees approve this consent procedure.

Our daily clinical practice in Kaohsiung Chang Gung Memorial Hospital is still according to the current guideline for treatment of significant ULMCA disease [7,8]. Accordingly, if patients with angiographic findings of significant ULCMA in the setting of STEMI, immediate primary PCI/stenting was done for the patients without hesitation, especially for those with unstable hemodynamics. Thus, patients experienced acute LM occlusion resulted from acute STEMI were excluded from the study. On the other hand, if patients with angiographic findings of significant ULCMA in the settings of SAP, UAP, STEMI and post-STEMI angina, we (i.e., both interventional cardiologist and surgeon) fully explained to patients and recommended CABG as the treatment of choice for the disease. However, PCI for significant ULMCA disease was performed in the following situations: 1) Patients refused to receive CABG treatment; 2) Advanced age or in patients with critical internal medical co-morbidities who were unwilling to receive CABG; 3) Estimated life expectancy is short as in those with known malignancy; 4) Treatment of significant ULMCA disease as a bridge to enable urgent non-cardiovascular major surgical intervention; 5) Patients in unstable condition/hemodynamic collapse during cardiac catheterization due to significant ULMCA disease, or post-CABG with occlusion of left internal mammary artery (LIMA) to left anterior descending artery (LAD) and multiple vessel disease.

Between January 2010 and December 2012, totally 342 patients, including those with SAP [13.9% (43/309)], UAP [59.2% (183/309)], NSTEMI [24.3% (75/309)], and post-STEMI angina (i.e., onset of STEMI <7 days) [2.6% (8/309)], undergoing PCI/stenting for the significant ULMCA disease were retrospectively enrolled in the current study. Informed consent was obtained from each study subject. The Institutional Review Committee on Human Research at our institution approved the study protocol.

Procedure and Protocol of Cardiac Catheterization Approach and Indications of Intra-Aortic Balloon Pump Support

For elective or primary PCI, a transradial artery approach using a 6-French arterial sheath is a routine procedure for patients at Kaohsiung Chang Gang Memorial Hospital unless Allen's test is positive on both sides. Routine trans-radial or trans-brachial arterial approach is also adopted in each patient for LM stenting/PCI using 6-French (F) or 7-F guiding catheter dependent on the LM lesion character and the strategy of stent implantation. Additionally, other vessels with significant obstruction that limited the blood flow were eligible for PCI at the same stage or during hospitalization. The detailed procedure and protocol have been reported in our previous studies [10,11,20,21].

Intra-aortic balloon pump (IABP) support was performed via right femoral arterial approach in patients experiencing advanced congestive heart failure (CHF) [defined as New York Heart Association Function classification (Fc)≧ Fc III], or acute pulmonary edema associated with unstable condition or hemodynamic instability. Moreover, elective IABP support (i.e., as a bridge of mechanical support) prior to LM PCI was performed for patients with severe left ventricular dysfunction [i.e., left ventricular ejection fraction (LVEF) <35%] without CHF. IABP was promptly removed in patients after LM PCI.

Definitions of Cardiogenic Shock and Profound Shock and Criteria for Extra-Corporeal Membrane Oxygenator Support

Definitions of cardiogenic shock and profound shock were based on our previous report [10,11,22]. Briefly, patients who experienced cardiogenic shock upon presentation or were observed at catheterization room met the following prospectively defined criteria for early cardiogenic shock: (1) Chest x-ray showing pulmonary edema with systolic blood pressure (SBP) <90 mmHg, or (2) Persistent hypotension with SBP<90 mmHg associated with low cardiac output and clear lung fields, not related to dysrhythmia, showing no response to adequate fluid supply, and requiring vasopressor agent infusion. In addition, profound shock was defined as SBP<75 mmHg despite intravenous inotropic agent administration and IABP support associated with altered mental status and respiratory failure.

Extra-corporeal membrane oxygenator (ECMO) was inserted at catheterization room for patients whose SBP could not be maintained above 75 mmHg after IABP support and intravenous administration of dopamine >20 g/kg/min.

Table 1. Baseline Characteristics of 309 Patients.

Variables	Group 1* (n = 43)	Group 2* (n = 183)	Group 3* (n = 75)	Group 4* (n = 8)	p-value
Age (yrs)	67.7±9.5[a]	67.5±10.5[a]	72.6±11.1[b]	71.1±14.5[a]	0.005
Male gender (%)	69.8% (30)	82% (150)	69.3% (52)	87.5% (7)	0.077
Body mass index (kg/m²)	25.4±3.6	24.8±3.6	25.0±4.1	24.9±3.5	0.850
Current smoking (%)	30.3% (13)	35.5% (65)	34.7% (26)	62.5% (5)	0.378
Diabetes mellitus (%)	51.2% (22)	46.4% (85)	42.7% (32)	75% (6)	0.333
Hypertension (%)	25.6% (11)[a]	18% (33)[a]	21.3% (16)[a]	50% (4)[b]	0.032
Total Cholesterol (mg/dL)[†]	156.9±53.6	162.9±48.7	161.8±39.4	147.3±30.5	0.732
LDL (mg/dL)[†]	91.6±40.9	90.1±41.7	96.2±35.9	85.3±23.1	0.699
HDL (mg/dL)[†]	48.0±16.7	45.9±16.5	44.7±13.7	43.8±13.5	0.724
Old myocardial infarction (%)	74.4% (32)	71% (130)	68% (51)	87.5% (7)	0.652
Previous CABG (%)	0% (0)	4.4% (8)	2.7% (2)	0% (0)	0.310
Previous PCI for LM (%)	11.6% (5)	11.5% (21)	2.7% (2)	0% (0)	0.104
History of COPD (%)	11.6% (5)	5.5% (10)	14.7% (11)	0% (0)	0.066
Symptomatic PAOD (%)	7% (3)[a]	4.4% (8)[a]	14.7% (11)[b]	12.5% (1)[b]	0.037
Old stroke (%)	7% (3)	11.5% (21)	20% (15)	12.5% (1)	0.170
ARB/ACEI (%)[‡]	48.8% (21)	48.1% (88)	36% (27)	37.5% (3)	0.308
Statin use (%)[‡]	51.2% (22)[a]	48.1% (88)[a]	30.7% (23)[b]	25% (2)[b]	0.033
Ac sugar (mg/dL)[†]	101.8±44.0[a]	112.4±56.7[a]	135.5±85.1[b]	106.1±22.9[a]	0.018
HBA1C (%)[†]	5.50±2.61	6.36±2.02	6.40±2.11	5.93±0.61	0.092
ESRD (%)	0% (0)[a]	8.7% (16)[b]	25.3% (19)[b]	0% (0)[a,b]	<0.001
Creatinine level (mg/dL)[†]	1.02±0.34[a]	1.92±2.60[a]	3.42±3.36[b]	1.86±2.23[a]	<0.001
White blood cell count[†]	7.2±2.6[a]	7.7±3.8[a]	9.7±3.4[b]	9.8±2.9[b]	<0.001
Troponin-I (ng/mL)[†]	0.3±0.9[a]	2.09±1.18[a]	45.3±183.1[b]	16.7±40.3[b]	0.001
CK-MB (unit/L)[†]	0.2±0.7[a]	0.39±2.3[a]	13.3±59.1[b]	7.43±20.6[b]	0.004
Troponin-I (after PCI) (ng/mL)	15.2±29.9[a]	15.2±40.6[a]	44.6±90.3[b]	44.1±60.2[b]	<0.001
CK-MB (after PCI) (unit/L)	3.16±7.13[a]	3.72±11.72[a]	18.9±37.4[b]	17.9±23.9[b]	<0.001

Data are expressed as % (n) or mean ± SD.

*Group 1 = angina pectoris, Group 2 = unstable angina, Group 3 = non ST-segment elevation myocardial infarction, Group 4 = post-ST-segment elevation myocardial infarction angina.

LDL = Low-density lipoprotein; HLD = high-density lipoprotein; CABG = coronary artery bypass surgery; LM = left main; PCI = percutaneous coronary intervention; COPD = chronic obstructive lung disease; PAOD = peripheral arterial obstructive disease; ARB/ACEI = angiotensin II type I receptor blcoker/angiotensin converting enzyme inhibitor; HBA1C = hemoglobin A1C; ESRD = end-stage renal disease; CK = Creatine phosphokinase.

[†]indicated measurement upon presentation.

[‡]indicated therapy ≥5 week prior to be recorded.

Letters ([a,b]) indicate significant difference (at 0.05 level) by Bonferroni multiple-comparison post hoc test.

Functional Assessment by Echocardiography

LV function was assessed using transthoracic echocardiography. With the patients in a supine position, left ventricular internal dimensions [i.e. end-systolic diameter (ESD) and end-diastolic diameter (EDD)] were measured according to the American Society of Echocardiography leading-edge method using at least 3 consecutives cardiac cycles. The LV ejection fraction (LVEF) was calculated as: LVEF (%) = $[(LVEDD^3 - LVEDS^3)/LVEDD^3] \times 100$.

Angiographic Analysis and Definitions

Quantitative angiographic analysis of the degree of coronary artery luminal stenosis and the reference lumen diameter was conducted using a digital edge-detection algorithm (DUQUE System) by selecting end-diastolic frames to demonstrate stenosis in its most severe and non-foreshortened projection [23]. With the contrast-filled guiding catheter serving as the calibration standard, the reference and minimal lumen diameters were determined before and after angioplasty. Single-vessel disease was defined as stenoses of >50% in 1 major epicardial coronary artery. Multi-vessel disease was defined as stenoses of >50% in ≥2 major epicardial coronary arteries. Body mass index (BMI) was defined as body weight in kilograms divided by the square of body height in meters (kg/m²).

Definitions

Procedure success was defined a final residual stenosis of less than 10% and normal blood flow was achieved in the LM coronary artery. The clinical success was defined as uneventful discharge within 30 days after the procedure. The feasibility was defined as failed procedure rate of less than 1.0%. Safety was defined as a rate of procedure-related major complication (i.e., failed procedure rate and procedure-related mortality) less than 1.0%.

Table 2. Clinical Presentation, Heart Function, Incidence of Mechanical Supports, and 30-Day Clinical Outcome among 309 Patients.

Variables	Group 1* (n = 43)	Group 2* (n = 183)	Group 3* (n = 75)	Group 4* (n = 8)	p-value
Advanced CHF (≥Fc III) (%)[†]	14% (6)[a]	11.5% (21)[a]	26.7% (20)[b]	50% (4)[b]	0.001
Mean severity of CHF (mean ± SD)	0.21±0.68[a]	0.77±1.21[a]	1.60±1.54[b]	1.25±1.76[b]	<0.001
Acute respiratory failure (%)	2.3% (1)[a]	4.9% (9)[a]	26.7% (20)[b]	25% (2)[b]	<0.001
Systolic blood pressure (mmHg)[‡]	132±23	134±24	134±26	138±21	0.917
Diastolic blood pressure (mmHg)[‡]	71±13	72±15	71±15	78±25	0.709
Vasopressin agent use (%)[§]	4.7% (2)[a]	6% (11)[a]	32% (24)[b]	37.5% (3)[b]	<0.001
IABP support (%)[¶]	4.7% (2)[a]	10.4% (19)[a]	37.3% (28)[b]	50% (4)[b]	<0.001
ECMO support (%)[ξ]	0% (0)	2.2% (4)	5.3% (4)	0% (0)	0.294
LVEF (%)[δ]	55.1±25.8	56.7±20.4	53.1±14.6	55.6±12.7	0.611
Acute ischemic stroke (%)	0% (0)	0.5% (1)	1.3% (1)	0% (0)	0.823
Acute renal injury (%)	2.3% (1)	6% (11)	10.7% (8)	12.5% (1)	0.293
30-day mortality (%)	2.3% (1)	2.7% (5)	9.3% (7)	12.5% (1)	0.071
Hospital days (mean ± SD)	6.3±6.6[a]	8.6±15.6[a]	23.1±34.3[b]	15.1±10.9[b]	0.001

Data are expressed as % (n) or mean ± SD.
*Group 1 = angina pectoris, Group 2 = unstable angina, Group 3 = non ST-segment elevation myocardial infarction, Group 4 = post-ST-segment elevation myocardial infarction angina.
[†]defined as congestive heart failure (CHF) ≥ New York Heart Association Functional Classification (Fc) III.
[‡]measured upon presentation.
[§]intra-aortic balloon pump (IABP) was used for hypotension/shock.
[¶]indication for poor left ventricular function [i.e., left ventricular function (LVEF) <35%], pulmonary edema, or hypotension/cardiogenic shock.
[ξ]extra-corporeal membrane oxygenator (ECMO) was used for profound cardiogenic shock.
[δ]indicated measurement of LVEF by transthoracic echocardiography.
Letters ([a,b]) indicate significant difference (at 0.05 level) by Bonferroni multiple-comparison post hoc test.

Acute renal injury was defined as an elevation in serum creatinine level more than 0.5 mg/dL within 24 h.

Medications

All patients received a loading dose of clopidogrel (600 mg orally) in the emergency room or at ward prior to cardiac catheterization, followed by a maintenance dose (75 mg/day orally once daily) for at least 9 months based on the current guideline after the procedure. Aspirin (100 mg orally once daily) was given indefinitely to each patient. Other commonly prescribed medications also included angiotensin-converting enzyme inhibitors, angiotensin II type I inhibitors, statins, beta-blockers, isonitrate, and diuretics.

Data Collection and the End Points

For the purpose of the current study, all patients undergoing ULMCA PCI were retrospectively identified. Detailed in-hospital and follow-up data including age, gender, coronary risk factors, clinical condition on admission and during hospitalization, cardiac enzyme and creatinine level, New York Heart Association Functional Classification, number of diseased vessels, in-hospital adverse events, and 30-day mortality were obtained. In our hospital, we have had a program for catheter-based coronary intervention, including that of the primary percutaneous coronary intervention (primary PCI) since 31 may, 1993, the data, including those of the present study were collected prospectively and entered into a digital database consistently. The primary end point of this study was defined as the safety and efficacy of PCI. Secondary end point was defined as the 30-day survival rate.

Statistical Analysis

Data were expressed as mean ± SD or % (number). Continue data which were expressed as mean ± SD were compared using one way ANOVA and followed by Bonferroni multiple-comparison post hoc test. Categorical data which were expressed as % (n) were analyzed by χ^2 test and followed by Bonferroni multiple-

Table 3. 30-Day Cardiac and Non-Cardiac Mortality among Four Groups.

Variables	Group 1	Group 2	Group 3	Group 4
30-day total mortality	1	5	7	1
Cardiac death	0	4	4	1
Non-cardiac death*	1	1	3	0

Group 1 = angina pectoris, Group 2 = unstable angina, Group 3 = non ST-segment elevation myocardial infarction, Group 4 = post-ST-segment elevation myocardial infarction angina.
*All non-cardiac death was due to sepsis.

Table 4. 30-Day Outcome of 8 Patients Supported by ECMO*.

Variables	Group 1	Group 2	Group 3	Group 4
No. of ECMO support patients	0	4	4	0
30-day total mortality	0	1	3	0
Cardiac death	0	1	2	0
Non-cardiac death[†]	0	0	1	0

ECMO = extra-corporeal membrane oxygenator.
*ECMO support for profound cardiogenic shock. These 8 patients also received intra-aortic balloon pump (IABP) support.
[†]death due to sepsis.

comparison post hoc test. Univariate and multiple stepwise logistic regression analysis were used for determining the predictors of 30-day mortality. Statistical analysis was performed using SAS statistical software for Windows version 8.2 (SAS institute, Cary, NC). A P value of <0.05 was considered statistically significant.

Results

Baseline Characteristics of Four Groups (Table 1)

Table 1 shows the baseline characteristics of group 1 (SAP), group 2 (UAP), group 3 (NSTEMI), and group 4 (post-STEMI angina). The age was significantly higher in group 3 than that in groups 1, 2, and 4. Besides, the incidence of hypertension was significantly higher in group 4 than that in groups 1 to 3, but it showed no difference among the latter three groups. Furthermore, there were no significant differences in terms of male gender, body mass index, incidence of current smoking, diabetes mellitus, and serum level of total cholesterol, low-density lipoprotein, and high-density lipoprotein among the four groups. Moreover, the incidence of old myocardial infarction, previous stroke, chronic obstructive lung disease, previous PCI, or previous PCI for left main coronary artery disease also did not differ among four groups. However, the incidence of significant peripheral arterial obstructive disease was remarkably higher in groups 3 and 4 than that in groups 1 and 2.

The incidence of the use of angiotensin II type I receptor blocker/angiotensin converting enzyme inhibitor (ARB/ACEI) was similar among the four groups. However, the incidence of stain use was significantly higher in groups 3 and 4 than in groups 1 and 2. Moreover, although the serum level of hemoglobin A1C (HBA1C) did not differ among the four groups, the plasma level of AC sugar was notably higher in group 3 than in groups 1, 2 and 4. Furthermore, the incidence of end stage renal disease (ESRD) was significantly higher in groups 2 and 3 than that in group 1. Moreover, the serum level of creatinine was markedly increased in group 3 than that in groups 1, 2, and 4.

The circulating levels of white blood cell (WBC) count, troponin-I, and creatine phosphokinase (CK)-MB upon admission or after PCI were significantly higher in groups 3 and 4 than those in groups 1 and 2.

Clinical Presentation, Mechanical Supports, Heart Function, and Clinical Outcomes (Table 2)

Table 2 shows the clinically relevant factors and 30-day outcome in patients undergoing ULMCA PCI. The mean severity of CHF, the incidences of advanced CHF and acute respiratory failure were significantly higher in groups 3 and 4 than those in groups 1 and 2.

The mean systolic and diastolic blood pressures upon presentation did not differ among the four groups. In addition, the incidence of utilization of ECMO for profound cardiogenic shock did not differ among the four groups. However, the incidences of IABP support and utilization of inotropic agent for unstable hemodynamics were significantly higher in groups 3 and 4 than those in groups 1 and 2.

In addition to similarity in LVEF, the incidence of acute ischemic stroke also did not differ among four groups. However, the incidence of acute renal injury was significantly higher in groups 3 and 4 than in groups 1 and 2. Furthermore, the mean length of hospitalization showed an identical pattern compared to that of acute renal injury among the four groups. The overall 30-day mortality rate was 4.1% (14/342). There was no significant difference in the 30-day mortality among the four groups.

Subgroup Analysis for the Cause of 30-Day Mortality, Comparison of BMI and Age between Survival and Dead Patients, and the Outcome of Mechanical Device Support (Table 3, Table 4 and Table 5)

To further elucidate the causes of 30-day mortality, the database was carefully analyzed and the results showed that cardiac-related and non-cardiac-related death was 2.9% (9/309)

Table 5. 30-Day Outcome of 45 Patients Supported by IABP*.

Variables	Group 1	Group 2	Group 3	Group 4
No of IABP support patients	2	15	24	4
30-day total mortality	0	3	4	1
Cardiac death	0	2	2	1
Non-cardiac death*	0	1	2	0

IABP = intra-aortic balloon pump.
*death due to sepsis.

Table 6. Angiographic Findings and PCI Results among 342 Patients.

Variables	Group 1* (n = 43)	Group 2* (n = 183)	Group 3* (n = 75)	Group 4* (n = 8)	p-value
Multiple vessel disease (%)	79.1% (34)	79.8% (146)	81.3% (61)	100% (8)	0.553
Pre-PCI LM stenosis (%)	64.1±16.2[a]	67.5±12.3[a]	72.5±13.2[b]	73.9±5.1[b]	0.002
LM obstructive level					
Ostial/proximal level (%)	25.6% (11)	23.5% (43)	29.3% (22)	12.5% (1)	0.581
Middle level (%)	4.7% (2)	18% (33)	16% (12)	37.5% (3)	0.156
Distal/bifurcation level (%)	69.7% (30)	58.5% (107)	54.7% (41)	50% (4)	0.785
Pre-MLD (mm)	0.26±0.44	0.23±0.42	0.29±0.43	0.13±0.35	0.652
Pre-RLD (mm)	3.38±0.67	3.47±0.76	3.47±0.46	3.41±0.73	0.870
Pre-PCI TIMI flow					0.201
≥TIMI-2 flow	4.7% (2)	2.2% (4)	6.7% (5)	12.5% (1)	
≤TIMI-1 flow	95.3% (41)	97.8% (179)	93.3% (70)	87.5% (7)	
Stent position					
LM shaft (%)	14% (6)	15.3% (28)	16% (12)	0% (0)	0.665
LM-LAD (%)	58.1% (25)	54.1% (99)	53.3% (40)	62.5% (5)	0.922
LM-LCX (%)	7% (3)	7.7% (14)	4% (3)	0% (0)	0.675
LM-LAD-LCX (%)	20.9% (9)	23% (42)	26.7% (20)	37.5% (3)	0.653
Post-PCI LM stenosis (%)	2.95±0.21	2.95±0.33	2.89±0.42	2.87±0.35	0.539
Post-PCI MLD (mm)	3.39±0.59	3.39±0.61	3.77±0.67	3.27±0.77	0.387
Post-PCI RLD (mm)	3.38±0.58	3.48±0.60	3.91±0.64	3.49±0.44	0.863
Post-PCI TIMI-3 flow	100% (43)	100% (183)	100% (75)	100% (0)	1
Procedural success (%)	100% (43)	100% (183)	100% (75)	100% (8)	1
Type of stent implantation					0.021
Drug eluting stent	81.4% (35)[a]	91.8% (168)[b]	80% (60)[a]	100% (8)[a,b]	
Bare metal stenting	18.6% (8)[a]	8.2% (15)[b]	20% (15)[a]	0% (0)[a,b]	
Post stent dilatation (%)	100.0% (43)	100.0% (183)	100.0% (75)	100% (8)	1.0
IVUS examination (%)	67.4% (29)[a]	73.8% (135)[a]	49.3% (37)[b]	75% (6)[a,b]	0.002
No. PCI vessel (mean ± SD)	2.67±0.71	2.62±0.66	2.53±0.81	2.50±0.53	0.671
No. of stenting (mean ± SD)	2.34±1.15	2.32±1.11	2.40±1.01	3.12±0.76	0.252

Data are expressed as % (n) or mean ± SD.
*Group 1 = angina pectoris, Group 2 = unstable angina, Group 3 = non ST-segment elevation myocardial infarction, Group 4 = post-ST-segment elevation myocardial infarction angina.
PCI = percutaneous coronary intervention; LM = left main; MLD = minimal lumen diameter; RLD = reference lumen diameter; TIMI = thrombolisis in myocardial infarction; LAD = left anterior descending artery; LCX = left circumflex.
IVUS = intra-vascular ultra-sound.
Letters ([a,b]) indicate significant difference (at 0.05 level) by Bonferroni multiple-comparison post hoc test.

Table 7. Univariate Analysis for the Predictors of 30-Day Mortality.

Variables	Odds Ratio	95% CI	p-value
Age >70	4.466	1.221–16.339	0.024
Female gender	3.683	1.246–10.888	0.018
Body mass index*	1.261	1.105–1.437	0.001
Ac sugar*	1.007	1.001–1.013	0.025
White blood cell count (x10³)*	1.169	1.050–1.301	0.004
Acute kidney injury	20.071	6.185–65.132	<0.0001
Acute ischemic stroke	22.615	1.339–382.050	0.031

CI = confidence interval.
*indicated data were used as continuity.

Table 8. Multivariate Analysis for Independent Predictors of 30-Day Mortality.

Variables	Odds Ratio	95% CI	p-value
Body mass index*	1.243	1.079–1.431	0.003
White blood cell count (x10^3)*	1.153	1.032–1.288	0.012
Acute kidney injury	16.040	3.667–70.162	<0.0001

CI = confidence interval.
*indicated data were used as continuity.

and 1.6% (5/309). All the non-cardiac death was found to be related to sepsis after PCI. Additionally, the sepsis was suspected due to the implantations of catheters and or mechanical supports in the patient's body. Further analysis revealed that the BMI (28.5±5.0 vs. 24.8±3.6, p<0.001) and the age (73.4±13.9 vs. 68.7±10.6, p = 0.016) was significantly increased in the 30-day dead patients compared to that in survival patients.

ECMO-assisted PCI was performed in 8 patients, including 4 patients in group 2 (i.e., UAP) and 4 patients in group 3 (i.e., NSTEMI), at cardiac catheterization room due to profound cardiogenic shock. The PCI procedure was successful in all 8 patients without procedure-related death. Four [50% (4/8)] patients with ECMO support were dead, including 1 in group 2 and 3 in group 3. Of these 4 fatalities, 3 were related to cardiac death and 1 was related to sepsis during hospitalization.

Isolated IABP support (i.e., without combined ECMO support) was given to 45 patients, including 2 in group 1, 15 in group 2, 24 in group 3, and 4 in group 4 at cardiac catheterization room due to poor LV function, hypotension/cardiogenic shock, advanced CHF, or acute pulmonary edema. The PCI procedure was successful in all 45 patients without procedure-related death. Mortality occurred in 4 patients [17.8% (8/45)] with IABP support, including 3 in group 2, 4 in group 3, and 1 in group 4. Of these 8 patients, cardiac death was implicated in 5 and 3 were related to sepsis during hospitalization.

In these IABP support patients, 14 of 45 patients (31.1%) of patients had received prophylactic IABP support for ULMCA stenting. The IABP support was promptly and successfully removed from all of the patients. All of these patients were uneventfully discharged from hospital.

Angiographic Findings and PCI Results among Four Groups (Table 6)

Table 4 shows angiographic and PCI results among the study patients. The percentage of LM stenosis prior to PCI was significantly higher in groups 3 and 4 than that in groups 1 and 2. On the other hand, the incidences of multi-vessel disease, pre-PCI TIMI flow, and obstructive level and stenting position, including ostial/proximal, middle and distal/bifurcation portions, were similar among four groups. Moreover, pre-PCI and post-PCI minimal lumen diameter (MLD), reference lumen diameter, and post PCI residual stenosis were also similar among the four groups.

The achievement of final TIMI-3 flow and the procedural success rate did not differ among the four groups. Around 80% of all patients had received drug eluting stent implantation. The reasons for those 20% who did not receive drug eluting stent implantation were due to either economic problem or an LM diameter greater than 4.5 mm. The incidence of drug eluting stent use was significantly higher in group 2 than that in groups 1 and 3, but it showed no difference between groups 2 and 4 or among groups 1, 3, and 4. In addition, the incidence of bare metal stent

implantation showed a reversed pattern compared to that of drug eluting stent implantation among the four groups. Furthermore, incidence of intra-vascular ultrasound (IVUS) utilization during the procedure showed a pattern identical to that of drug eluting stent use among the four groups. The overall utilization of the IVUS was only 60.5% (207/342) in the current study, mainly due to the economic problem. On the other hand, all of our patients had received high-pressure dilation after stent implantation. The number of PCI vessels and the number of stenting vessels did not differ among the four groups.

Univariate and Multiple Stepwise Logistic Regression Analysis for 30-Day Mortality (Tables 7 and 8)

Table 5 shows the results of univariate analysis of the relevant variables in Table 1, 2, and 4 for predictors of 30-day mortality. The analytical results demonstrated that acute kidney injury was the first and body mass index was the second significantly strong predictor of 30-day mortality. In addition, WBC count, age, female gender, AC sugar, and acute ischemic stroke were also significantly associated with 30-day mortality.

Multiple stepwise logistic regression analysis demonstrated that acute kidney injury was the strongest independent predictor of 30-day mortality. Additionally, WBC count and BMI were significantly independent predictors of 30-day mortality.

Discussion

This study which investigated the safety and feasibility of coronary stenting in patients with significant ULMCA stenosis yielded several striking clinical implications. First, the results of the present study demonstrated that catheter-based stenting for significant ULMCA disease was safe and feasible with very high procedural and clinical successful rates in real-world clinical practice. Second, in high-risk subgroup of patients and those patients with unstable condition, mechanical-assisted (i.e., IABP and ECMO) PCI for significant ULMCA disease offered an additional benefit with high rates of procedural success (i.e., 100%) and clinical success (95.5%). Third, in the relatively low-risk subgroups (i.e., SAP and UAP), the 30-day clinical outcome in the present study was not inferior to that previously reported for PCI or CABG clinical trials [6,12–18] in a similar clinical setting of ULMAC disease.

Real World Clinical Practice-Compliance to the Guideline and Flexible Utilization of Matured PCI Technique for Treating ULMCA disease

Despite clear recommendation of CABG as the gold standard in the treatment of significant ULMCA disease [7,8], daily clinical practice demonstrates patients' choice of PCI rather than CABG as the preferred strategy in the treatment of their significant ULMCA disease [9,12–19]. Of importance is that not only are the outcomes of these randomized or non-randomized clinical studies [9,12–19] consistent, the safety, feasibility, and profits of the use of PCI in this clinical setting are also notable. In fact, myriad reasons for patients with significant ULMCA disease to choose other management options other than CABG in the real word clinical practice have been reported [11,16,24,25].

One important finding in the present study is that more than 300 patients who did not receive CABG due to various reasons (please see the inclusion and exclusion enrollment criteria) were willing to receive PCI for the treatment of their significant ULMCA disease within a period of less than 3 years. This implies that PCI may be an alternative treatment strategy in the treatment of patients with significant ULMCA obstruction in our daily clinical service.

Another significant finding is that the outcomes of angiography were excellent (100% procedural success) in various clinical settings in the current study. Our findings, therefore, highlight the reliability of PCI as a safe and feasible therapeutic option for patients with significant ULMCA disease unsuitable for CABG.

Stenting to ULMCA Disease-Procedural and Clinical Success Rate in Low-Risk and High-Risk Patients

It is noteworthy that in the relatively low-risk subgroups (i.e., SAP and UAP), not only was the procedural success rate (100%) excellent, but the clinical success rate is also very promising (i.e., < 2.8% of 30-day death). Previous clinical trials have shown that PCI treatment for significant ULMCA disease was associated with a very high successful rate with a very low incidence of 30-day major adverse cardiac event [12–19,24,25]. In this way, our findings are consistent with those of previous studies [12–19,24,25].

The most important finding in the present study is that the use of prophylactic IABP support (i.e., as a bridge to stenting) for patients with significant ULMCA disease and poor heart function undergoing stenting provided excellent angiographic results (i.e., 100% procedural success) and good 30-day clinical success (i.e., 0% mortality). Our findings provide important clinical information and encourage the use of this approach in the setting of significant ULMCA disease in our real word clinical practice.

In the current study, the 30-day mortality rate in the non-STEMI (i.e., high-risk) subgroup was around 8% after ULMCA stenting. Interestingly, one previous study has revealed that the 30-day mortality rate was 12% in patients with non-STEMI and significant ULMCA disease after receiving CABG [26]. Additionally, our previous study has shown that the 30-day mortality was notably high (15% mortality) in the high-risk subgroup of STEMI even after primary PCI [27]. Taken together, our results were not inferior to those of previous studies [26]. Furthermore, another previous study has shown that the in-hospital mortality was found to be remarkably high (i.e., >19.0%) in the high-risk subgroups of acute coronary syndrome (ACS) undergoing emergency CABG [28]. In this way our result was superior to that of the previous study [28].

Stenting to ULMCA Disease-Procedural and Clinical Success Rate in Very High-Risk Patients

Of particular importance is that mechanical (i.e., IABP and/or ECMO)-assisted PCI for the high-risk patients showed 100% procedural success rate and acceptable 30-day clinical outcome [30-day mortality: 17.8% (8/45)]. Further analysis revealed that the 30-day cardiac-related death in this very high-risk patient subgroup was 11.1% (5/45). Therefore, the results of the present study were comparable to those of previous studies [27,28].

Stenting to ULMCA Disease-The 30-Day Cardiac-Associated Death and the Independent Predictors of 30-Day Mortality

The overall 30-day cardiac-related death was 2.9% (9/309) (Table 3-A). The acceptable lower 30-day mortality was in a similar clinical setting of ULMAC disease reported by the previously PCI or CABG clinical trials [6,12–18].

In concert with the results of the previous studies that identified impaired renal function and acute renal failure as the strong predictors of short-term and long-term clinical outcome in ACS patients undergoing PCI [29–32], multivariate analysis identified acute kidney injury as the most powerful independent predictor of 30-day mortality in the current study. Additionally, WBC count, an index of inflammation, and increased BMI rather than the angiographic findings were another two in independently predictive of 30-day mortality. These findings suggest that successful PCI to ULMCA disease is no more the critical role for the poor prognostic outcome.

Study Limitations

This study has limitations. First, the retrospective nature of this study cannot completely exclude the possibility of the presence of bias. Second, additional information on risk and prognostic stratification of ULMCA disease using PCI as a therapeutic option was not available without routine calculation of the SYNTAX score prior to or after PCI in our daily clinical practice. However, this study did not attempt to exclude any patient in our real world practice and in fact that our results were promising.

Conclusion

The study presents high rates of procedural success and excellent 30-day clinical outcomes, without making assertions about safety.

Author Contributions

Analyzed the data: WCL THT. Performed the experiments: THT YLC CHY SMC CJC CJL CIC CLH CJW HKY. Contributed to the writing of the manuscript: YHK LWC.

References

1. Cohen MV, Gorlin R (1975) Main left coronary artery disease. Clinical experience from 1964–1974. Circulation. 52: 275–85.
2. Taylor HA, Deumite NJ, Chaitman BR, Davis KB, Killip T, et al. (1989) Asymptomatic left main coronary artery disease in the Coronary Artery Surgery Study (CASS) registry. Circulation. 79: 1171–9.
3. Yusuf S, Zucker D, Peduzzi P, Fisher LD, Takaro T, et al. (1994) Effect of coronary artery bypass graft surgery on survival: overview of 10-year results from randomised trials by the Coronary Artery Bypass Graft Surgery Trialists Collaboration. Lancet. 344: 563–70.
4. Chaitman BR, Fisher LD, Bourassa MG, Davis K, Rogers WJ, et al. (1981) Effect of coronary bypass surgery on survival patterns in subsets of patients with left main coronary artery disease. Report of the Collaborative Study in Coronary Artery Surgery (CASS). The American journal of cardiology. 48: 765–77.
5. Takaro T, Peduzzi P, Detre KM, Hultgren HN, Murphy ML, et al. (1982) Survival in subgroups of patients with left main coronary artery disease. Veterans Administration Cooperative Study of Surgery for Coronary Arterial Occlusive Disease. Circulation. 66: 14–22.
6. Caracciolo EA, Davis KB, Sopko G, Kaiser GC, Corley SD, et al. (1995) Comparison of surgical and medical group survival in patients with left main equivalent coronary artery disease. Long-term CASS experience. Circulation. 91: 2335–44.
7. Eagle KA, Guyton RA, Davidoff R, Edwards FH, Ewy GA, et al. (2004) ACC/AHA 2004 guideline update for coronary artery bypass graft surgery: a report of

the American College of Cardiology/American Heart Association Task Force on Practice Guidelines (Committee to Update the 1999 Guidelines for Coronary Artery Bypass Graft Surgery). Circulation. 110: e340–437.

8. Smith SC Jr, Feldman TE, Hirshfeld JW Jr, Jacobs AK, Kern MJ, et al. (2006) ACC/AHA/SCAI 2005 guideline update for percutaneous coronary intervention: a report of the American College of Cardiology/American Heart Association Task Force on Practice Guidelines (ACC/AHA/SCAI Writing Committee to Update 2001 Guidelines for Percutaneous Coronary Intervention). Circulation. 113: e166–286.

9. Taggart DP, Kaul S, Boden WE, Ferguson TB Jr, Guyton RA, et al. (2008) Revascularization for unprotected left main stem coronary artery stenosis stenting or surgery. Journal of the American College of Cardiology. 51: 885–92.

10. Yip HK, Wu CJ, Chang HW, Fang CY, Yang CH, et al. (2003) Effect of the PercuSurge GuardWire device on the integrity of microvasculature and clinical outcomes during primary transradial coronary intervention in acute myocardial infarction. The American journal of cardiology. 92: 1331–5.

11. Sheu JJ, Tsai TH, Lee FY, Fang HY, Sun CK, et al. (2010) Early extracorporeal membrane oxygenator-assisted primary percutaneous coronary intervention improved 30-day clinical outcomes in patients with ST-segment elevation myocardial infarction complicated with profound cardiogenic shock. Critical care medicine. 38: 1810–7.

12. Park SJ, Park SW, Hong MK, Lee CW, Lee JH, et al. (2003) Long-term (three-year) outcomes after stenting of unprotected left main coronary artery stenosis in patients with normal left ventricular function. The American journal of cardiology. 91: 12–6.

13. Silvestri M, Barragan P, Sainsous J, Bayet G, Simeoni JB, et al. (2000) Unprotected left main coronary artery stenting: immediate and medium-term outcomes of 140 elective procedures. Journal of the American College of Cardiology. 35: 1543–50.

14. Buszman PE, Kiesz SR, Bochenek A, Peszek-Przybyla E, Szkrobka I, et al. (2008) Acute and late outcomes of unprotected left main stenting in comparison with surgical revascularization. Journal of the American College of Cardiology. 51: 538–45.

15. Rodes-Cabau J, Deblois J, Bertrand OF, Mohammadi S, Courtis J, et al. (2008) Nonrandomized comparison of coronary artery bypass surgery and percutaneous coronary intervention for the treatment of unprotected left main coronary artery disease in octogenarians. Circulation. 118: 2374–81.

16. Vaquerizo B, Lefevre T, Darremont O, Silvestri M, Louvard Y, et al. (2009) Unprotected left main stenting in the real world: two-year outcomes of the French left main taxus registry. Circulation. 2009; 119: 2349–56.

17. Kappetein AP, Feldman TE, Mack MJ, Morice MC, Holmes DR, et al. (2011) Comparison of coronary bypass surgery with drug-eluting stenting for the treatment of left main and/or three-vessel disease: 3-year follow-up of the SYNTAX trial. European heart journal.32: 2125–34.

18. Park SJ, Kim YH, Park DW, Yun SC, Ahn JM, et al. (2011) Randomized trial of stents versus bypass surgery for left main coronary artery disease. The New England journal of medicine. 364: 1718–27.

19. Fajadet J, Chieffo A (2012) Current management of left main coronary artery disease. European heart journal. 33: 36–50b.

20. Cheng CI, Lee FY, Chang JP, Hsueh SK, Hsieh YK, et al. (2009) Long-term outcomes of intervention for unprotected left main coronary artery stenosis:

21. coronary stenting vs coronary artery bypass grafting. Circulation journal: official journal of the Japanese Circulation Society. 73: 705–12.

21. Yip HK, Chung SY, Chai HT, Youssef AA, Bhasin A, et al. (2009) Safety and efficacy of transradial vs transfemoral arterial primary coronary angioplasty for acute myocardial infarction: single-center experience. Circulation journal: official journal of the Japanese Circulation Society. 73: 2050–5.

22. Chung SY, Sheu JJ, Lin YJ, Sun CK, Chang LT, et al. (2012) Outcome of patients with profound cardiogenic shock after cardiopulmonary resuscitation and prompt extracorporeal membrane oxygenation support. A single-center observational study. Circulation journal: official journal of the Japanese Circulation Society. 2012; 76: 1385–92.

23. Hermiller JB, Cusma JT, Spero LA, Fortin DF, Harding MB, et al. (1992) Quantitative and qualitative coronary angiographic analysis: review of methods, utility, and limitations. Catheterization and cardiovascular diagnosis. 1992;25: 110–31.

24. Carrie D, Eltchaninoff H, Lefevre T, Silvestri M, Levy G, et al. (2009) Twelve month clinical and angiographic outcome after stenting of unprotected left main coronary artery stenosis with paclitaxel-eluting stents–results of the multicentre FRIEND registry. EuroIntervention: journal of EuroPCR in collaboration with the Working Group on Interventional Cardiology of the European Society of Cardiology. 2009; 4: 449–56.

25. Chieffo A, Park SJ, Valgimigli M, Kim YH, Daemen J, et al. (2007) Favorable long-term outcome after drug-eluting stent implantation in nonbifurcation lesions that involve unprotected left main coronary artery: a multicenter registry. Circulation. 116: 158–62.

26. Buszman PP, Bochenek A, Konkolewska M, Trela B, Kiesz RS, et al. (2009) Early and long-term outcomes after surgical and percutaneous myocardial revascularization in patients with non-ST-elevation acute coronary syndromes and unprotected left main disease. The Journal of invasive cardiology. 21: 564–9.

27. Tsai TH, Chua S, Hussein H, Leu S, Wu CJ, et al. (2011) Outcomes of patients with Killip class III acute myocardial infarction after primary percutaneous coronary intervention. Critical care medicine. 39: 436–42.

28. Rastan AJ, Eckenstein JI, Hentschel B, Funkat AK, Gummert JF, et al. (2006) Emergency coronary artery bypass graft surgery for acute coronary syndrome: beating heart versus conventional cardioplegic cardiac arrest strategies. Circulation. 114: I477–85.

29. Tsai TH, Yeh KH, Sun CK, Yang CH, Chen SM, et al. (2013) Estimated glomerular filtration rate as a useful predictor of mortality in patients with acute myocardial infarction undergoing primary percutaneous coronary intervention. The American journal of the medical sciences. 345: 104–11.

30. Sadeghi HM, Stone GW, Grines CL, Mehran R, Dixon SR, et al. (2003) Impact of renal insufficiency in patients undergoing primary angioplasty for acute myocardial infarction. Circulation. 108: 2769–75.

31. Kragelund C, Hassager C, Hildebrandt P, Torp-Pedersen C, Kober L. (2008) Impact of obesity on long-term prognosis following acute myocardial infarction. International journal of cardiology. 2005; 98: 123–31.

32. Lee SH, Park JS, Kim W, Shin DG, Kim YJ, et al. (2008) Impact of body mass index and waist-to-hip ratio on clinical outcomes in patients with ST-segment elevation acute myocardial infarction (from the Korean Acute Myocardial Infarction Registry). The American journal of cardiology. 102: 957–65.

14

Serum Iron Concentration, but Not Hemoglobin, Correlates with TIMI Risk Score and 6-Month Left Ventricular Performance after Primary Angioplasty for Acute Myocardial Infarction

Ching-Hui Huang[1,2,9], Chia-Chu Chang[3,4,9], Chen-Ling Kuo[5], Ching-Shan Huang[5], Tzai-Wen Chiu[2], Chih-Sheng Lin[2]*, Chin-San Liu[5,6,7]*

1 Division of Cardiology, Department of Internal Medicine, Changhua Christian Hospital, Changhua, Taiwan, 2 Department of Biological Science and Technology, National Chiao Tung University, Hsinchu, Taiwan, 3 Division of Nephrology, Department of Internal Medicine, Changhua Christian Hospital, Changhua, Taiwan, 4 School of Medicine, Chung Shan Medical University, Taichung, Taiwan, 5 Vascular and Genomic Research Center, Changhua Christian Hospital, Changhua, Taiwan, 6 Department of Neurology, Changhua Christian Hospital, Changhua, Taiwan, 7 Graduate Institute of Integrative Medicine, China Medical University, Taichung, Taiwan

Abstract

Objective: Anemia is associated with high mortality and poor prognosis after acute coronary syndrome (ACS). Increased red cell distribution width (RDW) is a strong independent predictor for adverse outcomes in ACS. The common underlying mechanism for anemia and increased RDW value is iron deficiency. It is not clear whether serum iron deficiency without anemia affects left ventricular (LV) performance after primary angioplasty for acute myocardial infarction (AMI). We investigated the prognostic value of serum iron concentration on LV ejection fraction (EF) at 6 months and its relationship to thrombolysis in myocardial infarction (TIMI) risk score in post MI patients.

Methods: We recruited 55 patients who were scheduled to undergo primary coronary balloon angioplasty after AMI and 54 age- and sex-matched volunteers. Serum iron concentration and interleukin-6 levels were measured before primary angioplasty. LVEF was measured by echocardiography at baseline and after 6 months. TIMI risk score was calculated for risk stratification.

Results: Serum iron concentration was significantly lower in those in whom LVEF had not improved ≥10% from baseline (52.7±24.1 *versus* 80.8±50.8 μg/dl, *P* = 0.016) regardless of hemoglobin level, and was significantly lower in the AMI group than in the control group (62.5±37.7 *versus* 103.0±38.1 μg/dl, *P*<0.001). Trend analysis revealed that serum iron concentration decreased as TIMI risk score increased (*P* = 0.002). In addition, lower serum iron concentrations were associated with higher levels of inflammatory markers. Multiple linear regression showed that baseline serum iron concentration can predict LV systolic function 6 months after primary angioplasty for AMI even after adjusting for traditional prognostic factors.

Conclusion: Hypoferremia is not only a marker of inflammation but also a potential prognostic factor for LV systolic function after revascularization therapy for AMI, and may be a novel biomarker for therapeutic intervention.

Editor: Yiru Guo, University of Louisville, United States of America

Funding: The study was supported by a research grant of Changhua Christian hospital (100-CCH-IRP-08). The funders had no role in study design, data collection and analysis, decision to publish, or preparation of the manuscript.

Competing Interests: The authors have declared that no competing interests exist.

* Email: lincs@mail.nctu.edu.tw (C-S Lin); liu48111@gmail.com (C-S Liu)

❾ These authors contributed equally to this work.

Introduction

Functional iron deficiency is associated with impaired left ventricular (LV) performance in patients with chronic heart failure (CHF) [1]. Treatment with intravenous iron can improve the symptoms of CHF in patients with reduced LV ejection fraction even in the absence of anemia [2]. In heart failure, systemic and myocardial iron stores are depleted [3], which raises the possibility that iron deficiency rather than lack of hemoglobin (Hb) might be

of primary concern in heart failure [4]. Red cell distribution width (RDW) represents the variability in the size of circulating erythrocytes [5]. Most recently, increased RDW was shown to be a strong independent predictor of increased morbidity and mortality in patients with acute coronary syndrome even in nonanemic patients [6–8]. The common underlying mechanism for anemia and increased RDW value is iron deficiency. RDW values are increased in iron deficiency anemia. Iron deficiency is a common cause of anemia; nevertheless Hb concentration may be normal in the presence of iron deficiency. Iron is essential to many biological processes, particularly in mitochondria, where it catalyzes enzymatic reactions and is involved in the regulation of oxidative stress. Heart tissue is rich in mitochondria, making iron of particular importance to cardiac function [9]. Several strands of evidence have shown that anemic patients have a worse outcome after acute myocardial infarction (AMI) [10–12]. Few studies, however, have fully explored whether iron status changes during the course of AMI, and whether serum iron concentration affects LV performance after primary angioplasty.

Longitudinal studies have demonstrated that Interleukin 6 (IL-6) is a better predictor of CHF after acute coronary syndrome (ACS) than C-reactive protein (CRP) [13], and that it is also an independent predictor of cardiovascular mortality [14]. To the best of our knowledge, however, no studies have analyzed the relation between IL-6 concentration and serum iron concentration in patients with acute ST-segment elevation myocardial infarction (STEMI).

In this study, we examined whether baseline serum iron concentration measured at the time of primary angioplasty is predictive of LV function 6 months after STEMI. We also examined whether there were associations between serum iron concentration and factors traditionally associated with outcome after myocardial infarction, such as the concentrations of circulating inflammatory cytokines and the thrombolysis in myocardial infarction (TIMI) risk score, a validated clinical risk score that predicts short- and long-term mortality after STEMI [15,16].

Methods

Subjects and study protocol

In this prospective study we enrolled 55 consecutive patients with de novo acute STEMI who underwent primary PCI and thromboaspiration between January 2010 and January 2011. We also enrolled a control group of 54 healthy age- and sex-matched volunteers to compare changes in serum iron and inflammatory cytokine levels after STEMI.

Serum iron and IL-6 concentrations were measured from specimens of venous blood obtained prior to PCI. A second sample was taken after an 8-hour fast to evaluate the lipid profile and measure serum glucose. Diagnosis of STEMI was based on a universal definition of myocardial infarction [17]. Specifically, symptoms of ischemia, ST segment elevation >0.2 mV in ≥2 contiguous electrocardiogram (ECG) leads, and an increase in systemic cardiac biomarkers (for example, troponin I and creatinine kinase (CK) MB mass) with at least one value above the 99th percentile of the upper reference limit within 24 hours of the onset of pain were considered diagnostic of AMI. The culprit vessel was identified based on clinical, ECG and angiographic findings. All patients were administered aspirin and clopidogrel before PCI. Echocardiography was undertaken within the first 2 days after primary PCI and 6 months later. Change in heart function was calculated by subtracting the LV ejection fraction at baseline from ejection fraction at 6 months, divided by baseline ejection fraction. Improvement in heart function was defined as a change in LVEF ≥10%, according to the clinical study results by Ndrepepa et al [18]. Data collected from the subjects included age, sex, and the presence of risk factors (e.g., cigarette smoking, diabetes mellitus, hypertension, and hypercholesterolemia), clinical signs and current medication history. TIMI risk score for STEMI was calculated for each patient based on the description by Morrow et al. [15]. The protocol was approved by the Institutional

Review Board of the Changhua Christian Hospital, Taiwan, and all subjects gave written and informed consent to participate.

Measurement of serum iron and IL-6 concentrations

Serum iron concentration was measured by a timed-endpoint method using a commercially available kit (Synchron Systems FE/IBCT Calibrator Kit; Beckman Coulter, Fullerton, CA, USA), which measures iron bound to transferrin. Serum IL-6 concentration was determined by a commercially available ELISA kit (Human IL-6 ELISA Ready-SET-Go!; eBioscience, San Diego, CA, USA).

Angiographic assessments

Quantitative coronary angiographic measurements were taken by a cardiologist blinded to the results of other investigations. The TIMI flow [19] and myocardial blush [20] grades for assessing microvascular perfusion were also reviewed by the same cardiologist. Characteristic coronary lesions were classified according to the American College of Cardiologists/American Heart Association classification [21].

Echocardiographic assessments

We used a modified Simpson's method to calculate LV ejection fraction as described by the American Echocardiographic Society [22]. Diastolic function was evaluated using Pulsed-wave Doppler recordings. Pulsed wave Doppler measurements were obtained from the apical four-chamber view. Peak E and A wave velocities and E wave deceleration time (DT) were measured from the mitral leaflet tip according to American Society of Echocardiography guidelines [23]. Regional wall motion score index (WMSI) were calculated as the sum of wall motion scores divided by the number of visualized segments (from 17-segment model), where 1 indicates normal; 2, hypokinesis; 3, akinesis; and 4, dyskinesis [24]. After AMI extensive regional wall motion abnormalities may be present but when compensated by regional hyperkinesis of the normal segments, LVEF will be (almost) normal; in these patients, WMSI could more correctly reflect the magnitude of myocardial damage [25].

Statistical analysis

We performed a sample size calculation according to the results of our pilot study because no case-control trials using the same laboratory test method for serum iron have been reported. A sample size of 19 patients in each group was determined to be sufficient to detect differences in serum iron concentration between the STEMI group and control group, assuming a standard deviation of 37.3, using a two-sided test of the difference between means, a type I error of 5%, and a power of 90%. We expended the sample size to 55 patients in the STEMI group and 54 subjects in the control group to enhance the reliability of the study. Based on current sample size, we had a mean of 62.5 μg/dl of serum iron and a standard deviation of 37.7 μg/dl in the STEMI group, and a mean of 103.0 μg/dl of serum iron and a standard deviation of 38.1 μg/dl in the control group, and then we have a power of 99.99%. We calculated the power from a reliable, freely available website is: http://www.stat.uiowa.edu/~rlenth/Power/index.html [26].

The Mann–Whitney U test was used to examine differences in serum iron concentration between patients whose LV ejection fraction had improved ≥10% over 6 months and those in whom ejection fraction improved <10%. A Spearman's rho correlation was used to analyze the relationships between serum iron concentration and patient characteristics. A general linear model

Table 1. Characteristics of patients grouped by change in left ventricular ejection fraction 6 months after percutaneous coronary interventions for acute myocardial infarction.

	Improvement in ejection fraction ≥10% (n = 19)	No improvement in ejection fraction (n = 36)	P value
Sex (M/F)	14/5	33/3	0.853
Age, years	53.3±14.7	59.1±8.9	0.124
BMI, kg/m^2	26.2±3.7	25.3±3.6	0.441
CPK, μ/l (Maximal)	2101±1817	2410±2140	0.862
CKMB, ng/ml (Maximal)	190±173	249±192	0.353
Troponin I, ng/ml	4.08±10.58	6.18±18.56	0.928
Fasting glucose, mg/dl	146±74	159±93	0.600
HBA1C, %	6.0±1.0	6.6±1.8	0.246
Cholesterol, mg/dl	193±51	194±46	0.894
HDL-C, mg/dl	38.9±9.5	42.9±9.7	0.098
LDL-C, mg/dl	134.8±40.9	138.0±39.9	0.614
Creatinine, mg/dl	1.01±0.24	1.01±0.36	0.537
hsCRP, mg/l	0.56±0.62	0.42±0.73	0.578
IL-6, pg/ml	19.8±9.8	16.1±8.5	0.993
Fibrinogen, mg/dl	439±102	449±89	0.452
Serum iron, μg/dl	80.8±50.8	52.7±24.1	0.016*
Statin used, %	80	89	0.324
TIMI risk score	2.53±1.20	2.91±1.07	0.191
LVMI, g/m^2	113.3±26.9	109.0±23.9	0.839
LV EF at baseline, %	57.8±11.3	62.2±10.3	0.135
LVEF at 6 M, %	67.9±10.1	59.8±11.4	0.005*
E/A ratio at baseline	1.07±0.46	1.05±0.46	0.866
DT at baseline, ms	162.5±44.3	187.7±53.2	0.104
E/A ratio at 6 M	1.08±0.50	0.93±0.32	0.252
DT at 6 M, ms	199.9±66.7	201.6±52.5	0.422
EDV at baseline, ml	80.9±26.4	73.2±17.9	0.396
ESV at baseline, ml	35.1±17.4	27.7±11.7	0.222
WMSI	1.29±0.21	1.26±0.19	0.730
Hb, g/dl	14.7±1.5	14.4±1.5	0.449
Hb at 6 M, g/dl	13.9±2.0	13.8±1.5	0.602
Hematocrit, %	42.7±4.4	53.5±7.7	0.410
Hematocrit at 6 M, %	40.5±6.0	40.9±3.9	0.759
RDW, %	13.58±0.74	13.79±0.84	0.416
RDW at 6 M, %	13.56±0.74	14.20±1.17	0.102
Culprit lesion	LAD (10)	LAD (20)	0.992
	LCX (3)	LCX (3)	
	RCA (6)	RCA (13)	
D2B time, minutes	85.5±38.4	84.3±38.0	0.916
Myocardial brush grade	2.10±0.87	2.00±0.93	0.693
Lesion length (mm)	19.8±7.9	19.1±5.8	0.726
Pre-PCI TIMI flow grade	0.35±0.79	0.88±1.20	0.079
Post-PCI TIMI flow grade	2.97±0.18	3.00±0.00	0.384
Lesion calcification	0.26±0.57	0.13±0.44	0.355
Lesion complexity	1.03±0.40	0.88±6.12	0.284

*P<0.05, Mann–Whitney U test.
6 M, six months; BMI, body mass index; CPK, creatine- phosphor-kinase; CKMB, creatine phosphokinase-MB; HbA1C, glycohemoglobin; HDL-C, high density lipoprotein cholesterol; LDL-C, low density lipoprotein cholesterol; hsCRP, high sensitivity C reactive protein; IL-6, interleukin 6; WMSI, wall motion score index; TIMI, thrombolysis in myocardial infarction; LVMI, left ventricular mass index; LVEF, left ventricular ejection fraction; E/A ratio, the ratio of the peak velocities of early (E wave) and late (A wave) diastolic filling; DT, the deceleration time of the E wave; EDV, left ventricular end diastolic volume; ESV, left ventricular end systolic volume; Hb, hemoglobin; RDW, red blood cell distribution width; LAD, left anterior descending artery; RCA, right coronary artery; LCX, left circumflex artery; D2B, door to balloon; PCI, percutaneous coronary interventions; TIMI, thrombolysis in myocardial infarction.

technique and linear regression were used to evaluate independent associations between serum iron and IL-6 concentrations. The Jonckheere-Terpstra test was used to analyze the association between the serum iron concentration and TIMI risk scores. Trend analysis for IL-6 concentrations after they had been divided into tertile groups was undertaken using the Jonckheere-Terpstra test, which was also used to analyze the association between IL-6 concentrations and serum iron concentrations. The Jonckheere-Terpstra test is similar to the Kruskal-Wallis test but is applied to samples with *a priori* ordering, such as TIMI risk scores, when it has greater statistical power. Parameters showing significant correlations in the univariate analyses were then included in multiple linear regression model to test for significant predictors of improvement in LV ejection fraction 6 months after primary angioplasty. A *P* value<0.05 was considered statistically significant. All statistical analyses were performed on a personal computer with the statistical package SPSS for Windows (Version 15.0, SPSS, Chicago, IL, USA).

Results

Baseline serum iron concentration was significantly lower in patients who did not show improvement in LV performance at 6-month follow-up

At 6-month follow-up after PCI, all of 55 AMI patients were alive and there were no adverse cardiac events. We divided the patients into two groups according to the LV performance at 6-month follow-up after PCI. Biochemical and physiological examinations of the patients were summarized in **Table 1**. There were no significant differences between the improvement and non-improvement groups in infarct-related artery location, lesion calcification, lesion complexity, maximal cardiac muscle enzyme concentrations-CKMB, troponin I concentrations, baseline Hb concentrations and 6 month follow-up Hb concentrations, baseline RDW values and 6 month follow-up RDW values, baseline LV ejection fraction, reperfusion quality-post PCI TIMI flow grade, myocardial brush grade and inflammatory marker-IL6. However, serum iron concentration was significantly lower in the non-improvement subgroup (80.8±50.8 *versus* 52.7±24.1 µg/dl, *P* = 0.016).

Factors correlated with serum iron concentration after AMI

Hb concentration, hematocrit, lymphocyte counts, the proportion of patients taking statins, and LV ejection fraction at 6 months were positively correlated with serum iron concentration (**Table 2**); however, TIMI risk score was negatively correlated with serum iron concentration.

Serum iron concentration significantly decreased as TIMI risk score increased after primary angioplasty

We divided AMI patients into four subgroups according to TIMI risk score for STEMI: group 1, TIMI risk score 1 (n = 8); group 2, risk score 2 (n = 15); group 3, risk score 3 (n = 19); and group 4, risk score ≥4 (n = 13). Trend analysis found that serum iron concentration significantly decreased as TIMI risk score rose (**Figure 1**; Jonckheere-Terpstra test, *P* = 0.002).

The relationship between serum iron and interleukin-6 levels in all study subjects

Serum iron concentration in the AMI group was significantly lower than in the control group (62.5±37.7 *vs.* 103.0±38.1 µg/dl, *P*<0.001) and IL-6 concentration was significantly higher in the AMI group than in the control group (17.80±13.19 *vs.* 6.98±8.26 pg/ml, *P*<0.001). Linear regression model was used to evaluate the independent associations between serum iron and IL-6 concentrations in all enrolled subjects. We found that serum iron concentration was negatively correlated with circulating IL-6 concentration (**Figure 2**; Serum iron = 95.994 − 1.246 (IL-6), $R^2 = 0.133$, *P*<0.001). We found no correlation between IL-6 and Hb concentration in all study subjects. Furthermore, we found that serum iron concentration in the control group was, on average, 35.494 µg/dl higher than that in the AMI group. For every one unit increase in IL-6 concentration, there was a decrease of 0.625 units in serum iron concentration (**Table 3**).

Trend analysis showed serum iron concentration, not Hb, was inversely proportional to IL-6 concentration

We divided AMI patients into three subgroups according to circulating IL-6 concentration tertile: group 1, IL-6 concentration ≤10.48 pg/ml (n = 19); group 2, IL-6 concentration between 10.49–19.67 pg/ml (n = 20); group 3, IL-6 concentration ≥19.68 pg/ml (n = 16). Trend analysis found that serum iron concentration significantly decreased as serum IL-6 concentration rose (**Figure 3**; Jonckheere-Terpstra test, *P* = 0.043).

Table 2. Univariate correlation between serum iron concentration and patient characteristics after acute myocardial infarction.

Variable	*Rho* correlation coefficient	*P* value
Hemoglobin, g/dl	0.273	0.036*
Hematocrit, %	0.257	0.047*
Lymphocyte, %	0.276	0.035*
Statin used	0.273	0.028*
TIMI risk score	−0.346	0.009*
EF 6 M, %	0.301	0.025*

*P<0.05, Spearman's rho correlation. 6 M, six months; TIMI, thrombolysis in myocardial infarction; EF 6 M, left ventricular ejection fraction at 6–month follow-up.

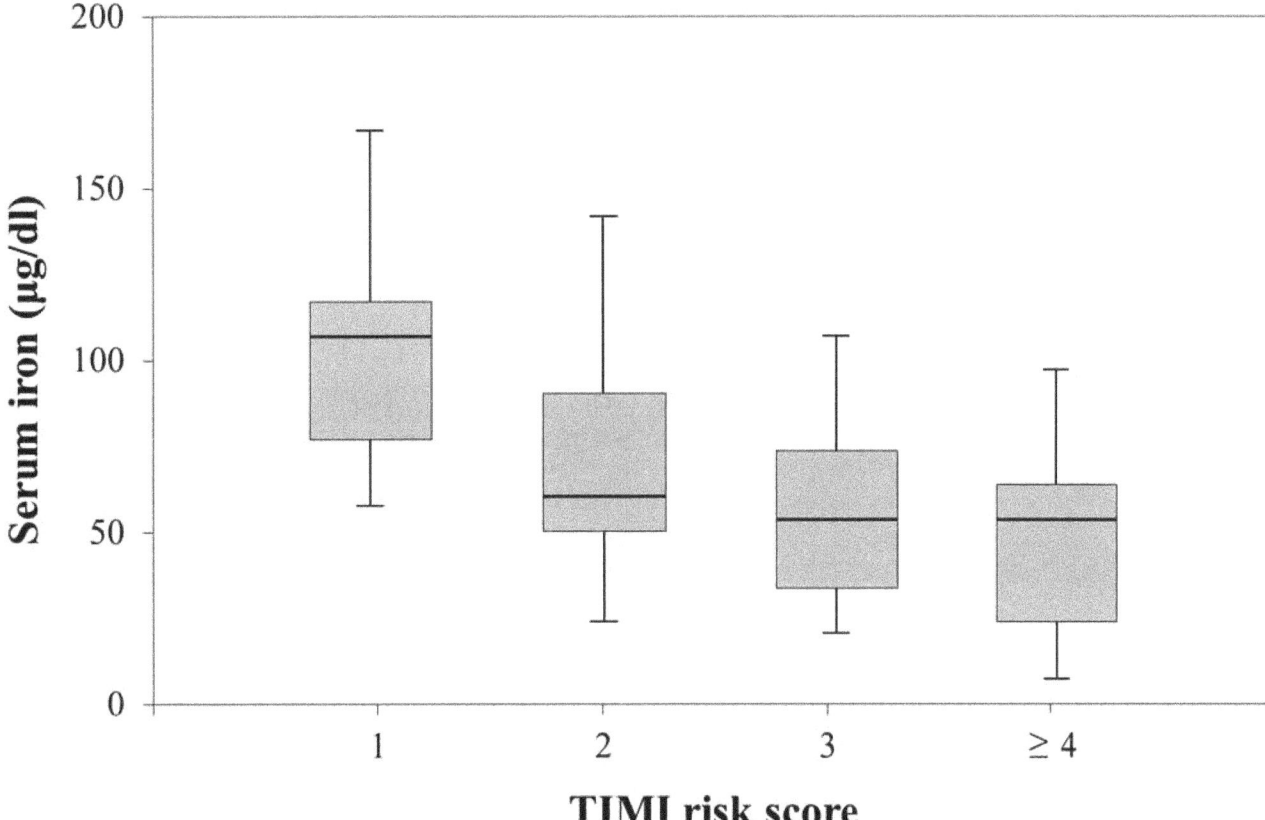

Figure 1. The relationships between serum iron concentration and TIMI risk scores after primary angioplasty for AMI. The AMI patients were divided into four subgroups according to TIMI risk score for STEMI: Group 1 (TIMI risk score 1, n = 8); Group 2 (TIMI risk score 2, n = 15); Group 3 (TIMI risk score 3, n = 19); and Group 4 (TIMI risk score ≥4, n = 13). Trend analysis with Jonckheere-Terpstra test found that serum iron concentration significantly decreased as TIMI risk score rose (P = 0.002).

Lower serum iron concentration is associated with higher TIMI risk score and has higher inflammatory markers after AMI

The patients in AMI group was divided into two subgroups, lower serum iron (<60 µg/dl) and higher serum iron (≥60 µg/dl), on the basis of the median serum iron concentration (**Table 4**). Patients in the lower serum iron subset had significantly higher concentrations of fibrinogen and IL-6 (P<0.05). Both fibrinogen and IL-6 are biomarkers of inflammation related with cardiovascular diseases. It is also noted that patients in the lower serum iron subset showed a higher TIMI risk score after AMI (P<0.05).

Baseline serum iron level predicts LV function 6 months after primary angioplasty for AMI

Multiple linear regression analysis of variables associated with LV performance 6 months after primary angioplasty was undertaken. The following variables were entered into the model: serum iron, IL-6, infarct related artery location, peak creatine kinase-MB and WMSI. It showed that serum iron concentration at the time of AMI could predict LV ejection fraction 6 months later, even when traditional prognostic factors such as LV wall motion score index, cardiac enzyme and IL-6 concentrations, and infarct locations were taken into account (**Table 5**). Baseline Hb concentrations, follow-up Hb concentrations, baseline RDW values and follow-up RDW values did not predict LV ejection fraction at 6 months when the same prognostic factors were considered.

Discussion

Our findings confirm the important role of serum iron in determining LV performance after STEMI. Furthermore, the recovery of LV function was impaired in those with lower serum iron concentration after revascularization. Anemia can be viewed as the net result of iron deficiency, but a normal Hb level does not necessarily mean that iron stores are adequate. An individual with normal body iron stores must lose a large portion of body iron before the Hb falls below the laboratory definition of anemia (generally, Hb<12 g/dl for women and Hb<13 g/dl for men). To investigate whether serum iron or Hb or RDW is the most important determinant of LV function after STEMI, multiple regression analyses were performed with serum iron or Hb concentration or RDW value as one of the covariates. In these analyses, serum iron concentrations were significantly predictive of LV systolic function after adjusting for possible confounding factors (such as infarct location, LV wall motion score index, and serum concentrations of cardiac enzymes and IL-6). Blood Hb concentrations and RDW values at baseline and at 6 months were found not to be significant predictors when the same prognostic factors were considered. These findings suggest that serum iron concentration is an independent predictor of LV systolic function after STEMI, rather than Hb level or RDW value. This conclusion is supported by a previous study that showed that the symptoms and signs of CHF can be ameliorated by the administration of intravenous iron regardless of whether the patient is anemic or not [2]. Furthermore, administration of an

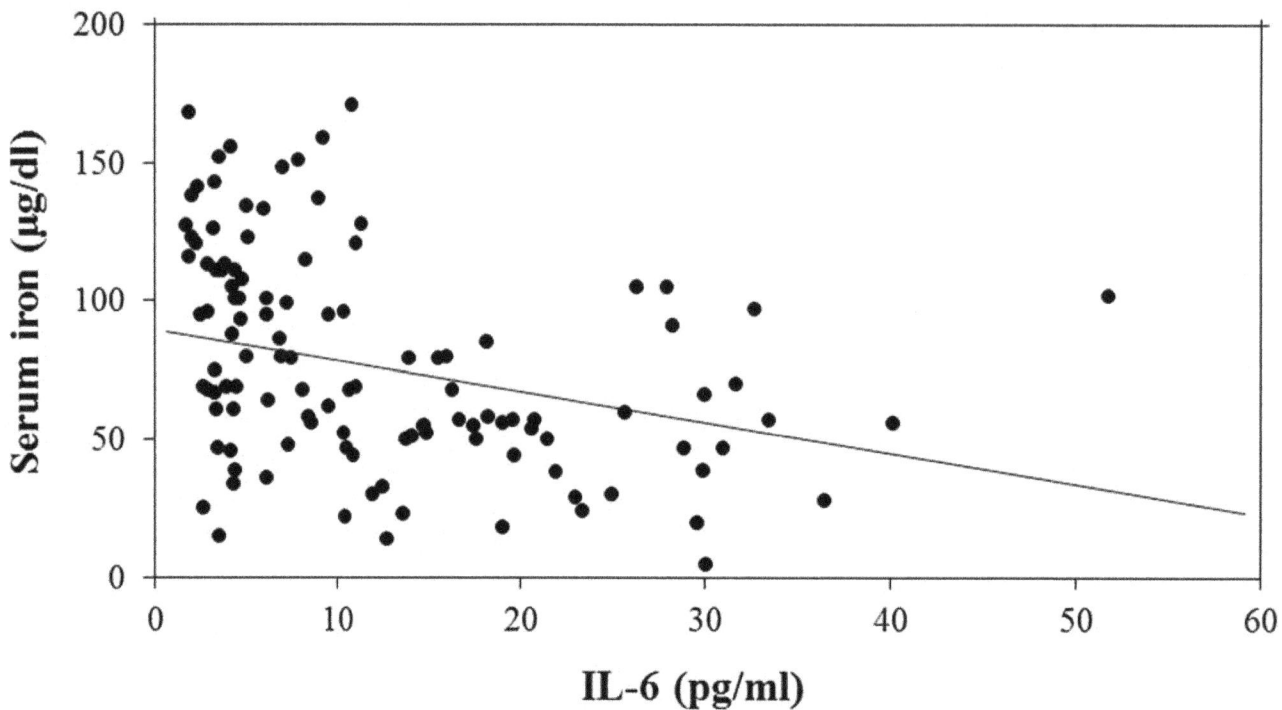

Figure 2. The relationship between serum iron concentration and IL-6 levels in all enrolled subjects. The result indicated that the serum iron concentration was negatively correlated with circulating IL-6 concentration in all study subjects. The linear relationship was well described by Serum iron = 95.994 − 1.246 (IL-6), R^2 = 0.133 and P < 0.001.

iron chelator after AMI but before PCI does not appear to get clinical benefit [27]. In addition, lower serum iron concentrations are associated with higher concentrations of proinflammatory markers and lower concentrations of the cardioprotectant insulin-like growth factor-1 in ischemic heart disease [28]. These data support the concept that serum ion is tightly regulated.

Iron is an essential micronutrient as it is required for satisfactory erythropoietic function, oxidative metabolism and cellular immune response. Functionally, iron exists in the body in two pools: utilized and stored [1]. Utilized iron consists of circulating and intracellular iron. Iron released into the circulation binds to transferrin and is transported to sites of use and storage [29]. The amount of transferrin-bound iron is around 4 mg, but this is the most important functional dynamic iron pool [29]. The vast majority of intracellular iron is in erythrocyte Hb and circulating reticulocytes. Iron pools interact with each other, and iron can be transferred between these compartments using tightly regulated mechanisms. A normal Hb level with a mean corpuscular Hb (MCH) in the lower limit of the normal range (28–35 pg) or an increased red cell distribution width (RDW, normal range 11–15%) indicates mild iron deficiency without anemia. Although a rising RDW may be an earliest indicator of iron deficiency, the main laboratory finding is a low serum ferritin concentration [1]. However, an RDW value within the reference interval can be used to exclude iron deficiency in those cases in which the serum ferritin concentration does not accurately reflect the iron stores owing to severe tissue damage, as in inflammation [30]. This is the reason why we did not check serum ferritin in STEMI. We also did not measure total iron-binding capacity (TIBC); hence, we were unable to determine participants' complete iron status. However, indirect data suggest that our subjects had normal iron stores, reflected in largely normal MCH and RDW values. Conceptually, a low serum iron concentration might be indicative of a diminished utilized iron pool. Cells with a high mitogenic potential (neoplastic, hematopoietic, immune) [31,32] and high-energy demand (hepatocytes, adipocytes, skeletal and cardiac myocytes, and renal cells) [33,34] are particularly sensitive to depleted iron supplies and/or abnormal iron utilization.

Table 3. The relationship between serum iron and interleukin-6 levels in all subjects.

Parameter	Estimate	SE	95% Confidence interval	P value
Intercept	71.872	6.984	58.040–85.704	<0.001**
Group (Control vs. AMI)	35.494	7.440	20.759–50.229	<0.001**
IL-6	−0.625	0.299	−1.218−−0.032	0.039*

(Dependent variable: serum iron concentration).
*P<0.05 and **P<0.001, general linear model. AMI, acute myocardial infarction; IL-6, interleukin 6; SE, standardized error. The intercept is the predicted value of serum iron concentration in AMI group. The predicted value is 71.872 µg/dl. The serum iron concentration in the control group was, on average, 35.494 µg/dl higher than that in the AMI group. For every one unit increase in IL-6 concentration, there was a decrease of 0.625 units in serum iron concentration.

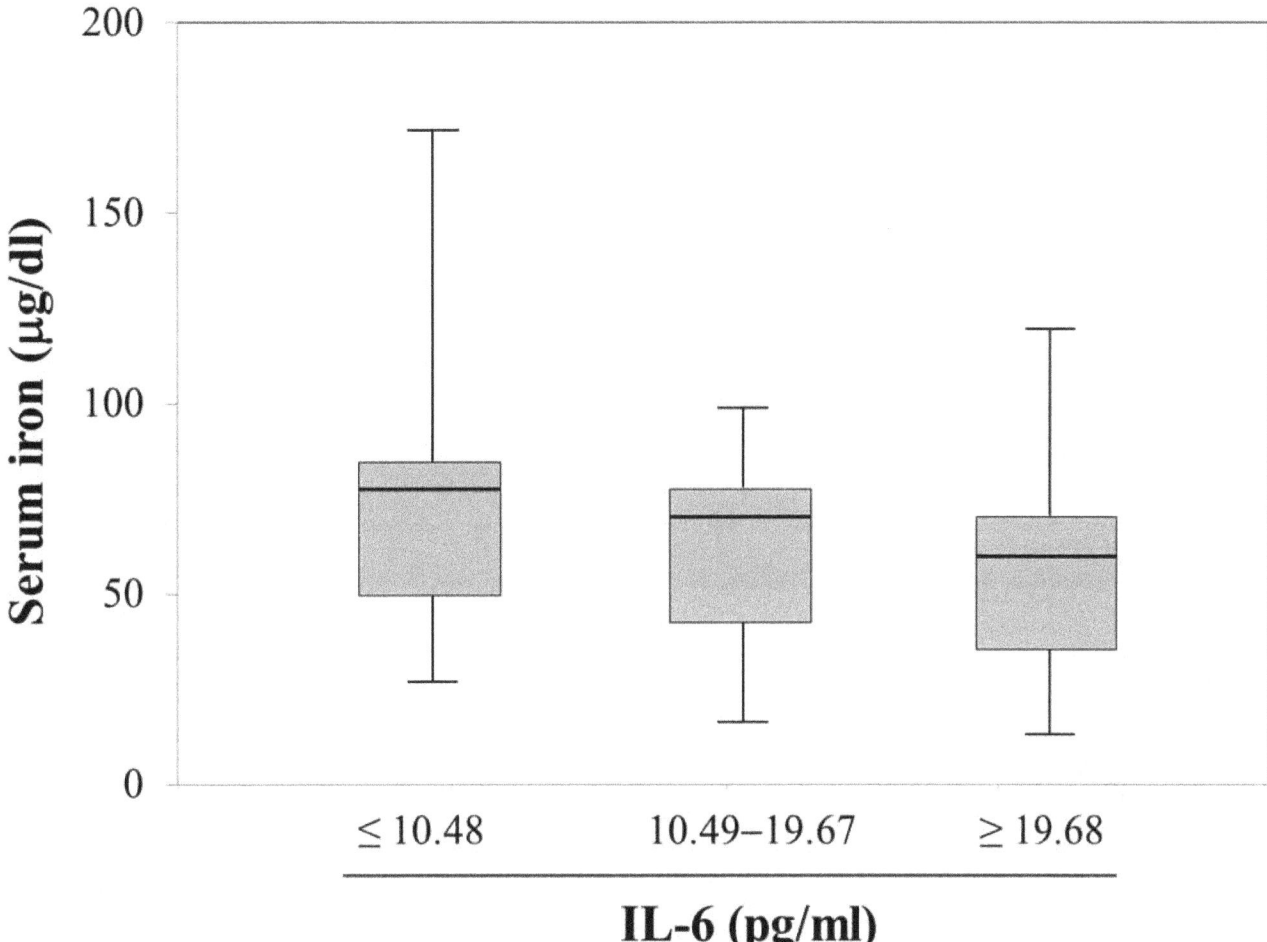

Figure 3. Trend analysis showed serum iron concentration was inversely proportional to IL-6 concentration in STEMI patients. AMI patients were divided into three subgroups according to circulating IL-6 concentration tertile: group 1, IL-6 concentration ≤10.48 pg/ml (n = 19); group 2, IL-6 concentration between 10.49–19.67 pg/ml (n = 20); group 3, IL-6 concentration ≥19.68 pg/ml (n = 16). Trend analysis showed serum iron concentration was inversely proportional to IL-6 concentration. (Jonckheere-Terpstra test, $P = 0.043$).

ACS is a disease characterized by inflammation-induced atherosclerotic plaque rupture, subsequent thrombus formation, coronary artery occlusion, and myocardial oxygen deficiency [35]. Hypoferremia is a common response to systemic infections or generalized inflammatory disorders. A recent longitudinal study demonstrated that IL-6 was a better predictor of CHF after ACS than CRP [13]. Our findings are in broad agreement with a previous report that elevated IL-6 concentrations immediately after AMI were negatively correlated with LV ejection fraction 6

months later [36]. We demonstrated clearly that serum iron concentration was inversely proportional to IL-6 concentration: For every one unit increase in IL-6 concentration, there was a decrease of 0.625 units in serum iron concentration. We also found that serum iron concentration in the control group was on average 35.494 µg/dl higher than that in the AMI group. However, there was no correlation between Hb concentrations and IL-6 concentration. One previous study conducted in human liver cell culture, mice and human volunteers reported that IL-6 was necessary and

Table 4. Lower serum iron concentration is associated with higher inflammatory markers and TIMI risk score after acute myocardial infarction.

	Lower serum iron (<60 µg/dl)	Higher serum iron (≥ 60 µg/dl)	P value
	n = 34	n = 21	
IL-6, pg/ml	19.8±14.6	14.2±9.4	0.042*
Fibrinogen, mg/dl	470±93	421±86	0.040*
TIMI risk score	3.10±1.00	2.43±1.27	0.025*

*$P < 0.05$, Mann–Whitney U test. TIMI, thrombolysis in myocardial infarction; IL-6, interleukin 6.

Table 5. Multiple linear regression analysis of variables associated with ejection fraction 6 months after primary angioplasty for acute myocardial infarction.

Explanatory variable	Unstandardized Coefficients		Standardized Coefficients	t	P value
	B	Std. error	Beta		
(Constant)	106.249	7.684		13.833	0.000
Serum iron	0.069	0.029	0.227	2.415	0.020*
CPK MB	−0.012	0.006	−0.200	−1.965	0.055
IL-6	−0.006	0.082	−0.007	−0.068	0.946
WMSI	−36.606	6.510	−0.631	−5.723	<0.001**
IRA (LAD *vs.* RCA)	0.943	2.670	0.041	0.353	0.725
IRA (LCX *vs.* RCA)	9.890	3.825	0.269	2.585	0.013*

(Dependent variable: ejection fraction at 6 months).
$R^2 = 0.620$.
*$P<0.05$ and **$P<0.001$.
CPK MB, creatine phosphokinase-MB; IL-6, interleukin 6; WMSI, wall motion score index; IRA, infarct related artery; LAD, left anterior descending artery; RCA, right coronary artery; LCX, left circumflex artery.

sufficient for the induction of hepcidin during inflammation, and that the IL-6–hepcidin axis was responsible for inflammation-induced hypoferremia [37]. In rodents [38] and humans [39], AMI was accompanied by increased circulating hepcidin, which subsequently subsided during recovery. These findings led us to postulate that after AMI, circulating IL-6 level increases, followed by elevation in hepcidin and a decrease in serum iron concentrations. However, reduced serum iron concentration represents depletion of the main functional iron pool, which could modulate LV function. Our hypothesis is also supported by the finding that after AMI, increased circulating IL-6 concentrations at baseline and after hospital discharge were associated with heart failure and impaired LV ejection fraction [40]. Low serum iron concentration may explain why activation of proinflammatory factors is believed to enhance myocardial damage, leading to dysfunction and heart failure.

The novelty of our study is that we analyzed the relationship between serum iron concentration and TIMI risk score for STEMI. In patients with ACS, risk scores are useful short- and long-term predictors of death and cardiovascular complications [15,16]. The score is calculated from patients' age, body mass, blood pressure and heart rate on admission and the Killip class. It was significantly higher in patients with low baseline serum iron concentration and *vice versa*, suggesting that serum iron has a protective effect on myocardial function.

The major limitation of the study is that it does not provide mechanistic insight. Other limitations include the relatively small size of the cohort, and the fact that iron status markers were only measured at baseline. Therefore, larger studies of patients with STEMI that measure serum iron concentration, total iron binding capacity and ferritin are needed to further confirm our hypothesis.

These might form the basis of intervention studies, to examine whether iron supplementation and/or control of serum IL-6 concentration might have a beneficial effect on the recovery of LV function after STEMI.

Conclusions

We found an association between lower serum iron concentration before PCI and impaired recovery of LV systolic function 6 months later. The circulating concentration of IL-6 was increased after STEMI and negatively correlated with serum iron concentration. Serum iron concentration was also negatively correlated with TIMI risk score. Our findings support the hypothesis that higher serum iron concentration is associated with a cardioprotective phenotype, and that it is a potential prognostic biomarker for complications after STEMI, and may be a novel biomarker that could therapeutic intervention.

Acknowledgments

We would like to thank Dr. Yu-Jun Chang for her contributions to the statistical analysis in the study.

Author Contributions

Conceived and designed the experiments: C-HH C-CC C-S Lin C-S Liu. Performed the experiments: C-LK C-SH. Analyzed the data: C-HH T-WC. Contributed reagents/materials/analysis tools: C-LK C-SH. Wrote the paper: C-HH C-CC. Performed the acquisition of data: C-HH. Contributed to the guidance of experiments: C-S Liu. Read the manuscript and revised it for important intellectual content: C-S Lin T-WC. Read and approved the final manuscript: C-S Lin C-HH C-CC C-LK C-SH T-WC C-S Liu.

References

1. Jankowska EA, von Haehling S, Anker SD, Macdougall IC, Ponikowski P (2013) Iron deficiency and heart failure: diagnostic dilemmas and therapeutic perspectives. European heart journal 34: 816–829.

2. Anker SD, Comin Colet J, Filippatos G, Willenheimer R, Dickstein K, et al. (2009) Ferric carboxymaltose in patients with heart failure and iron deficiency. New England Journal of Medicine 361: 2436–2448.

3. Maeder MT, Khammy O, dos Remedios C, Kaye DM (2011) Myocardial and Systemic Iron Depletion in Heart FailureImplications for Anemia Accompanying Heart Failure. Journal of the American College of Cardiology 58: 474–480.

4. McMurray J, Ponikowski P (2011) Heart FailureNot Enough Pump Iron? Journal of the American College of Cardiology 58: 481–482.

5. Simel DL, DeLong ER, Feussner JR, Weinberg JB, Crawford J (1988) Erythrocyte anisocytosis: visual inspection of blood films vs automated analysis of red blood cell distribution width. Archives of internal medicine 148: 822–824.

6. Uyarel H, Ergelen M, Cicek G, Kaya MG, Ayhan E, et al. (2011) Red cell distribution width as a novel prognostic marker in patients undergoing primary angioplasty for acute myocardial infarction. Coronary artery disease 22: 138–144.

7. Dabbah S, Hammerman H, Markiewicz W, Aronson D (2010) Relation between red cell distribution width and clinical outcomes after acute myocardial infarction. The American journal of cardiology 105: 312–317.

8. Ilhan E, Güvenç TS, Altay S, Çagdas M, Çalik AN, et al. (2012) Predictive value of red cell distribution width in intrahospital mortality and postintervention thrombolysis in myocardial infarction flow in patients with acute anterior myocardial infarction. Coronary artery disease 23: 450–454.

9. Rines AK, Ardehali H (2013) Transition metals and mitochondrial metabolism in the heart. Journal of molecular and cellular cardiology 55: 50–57.

10. Anker SD, Voors A, Okonko D, Clark AL, James MK, et al. (2009) Prevalence, incidence, and prognostic value of anaemia in patients after an acute myocardial infarction: data from the OPTIMAAL trial. European heart journal 30: 1331–1339.

11. Aronson D, Suleiman M, Agmon Y, Suleiman A, Blich M, et al. (2007) Changes in haemoglobin levels during hospital course and long-term outcome after acute myocardial infarction. European heart journal 28: 1289–1296.

12. Nikolsky E, Aymong ED, Halkin A, Grines CL, Cox DA, et al. (2004) Impact of anemia in patients with acute myocardial infarction undergoing primary percutaneous coronary interventionAnalysis from the controlled abciximab and device investigation to lower late angioplasty complications (cadillac) trial. Journal of the American College of Cardiology 44: 547–553.

13. Vasan RS, Sullivan LM, Roubenoff R, Dinarello CA, Harris T, et al. (2003) Inflammatory markers and risk of heart failure in elderly subjects without prior myocardial infarction the Framingham Heart Study. Circulation 107: 1486–1491.

14. Tan J, Hua Q, Li J, Fan Z (2009) Prognostic value of interleukin-6 during a 3-year follow-up in patients with acute ST-segment elevation myocardial infarction. Heart and vessels 24: 329–334.

15. Morrow DA, Antman EM, Charlesworth A, Cairns R, Murphy SA, et al. (2000) TIMI risk score for ST-elevation myocardial infarction: a convenient, bedside, clinical score for risk assessment at presentation an intravenous nPA for treatment of infarcting myocardium early II trial substudy. Circulation 102: 2031–2037.

16. Wiviott SD, Morrow DA, Frederick PD, Giugliano RP, Gibson CM, et al. (2004) Performance of the thrombolysis in myocardial infarction risk index in the National Registry of Myocardial Infarction-3 and-4A simple index that predicts mortality in ST-segment elevation myocardial infarction. Journal of the American College of Cardiology 44: 783–789.

17. Thygesen K, Alpert JS, White HD (2007) Universal definition of myocardial infarction. Journal of the American College of Cardiology 50: 2173–2195.

18. Ndrepepa G, Mehilli J, Martinoff S, Schwaiger M, Schömig A, et al. (2007) Evolution of left ventricular ejection fraction and its relationship to infarct size after acute myocardial infarction. Journal of the American College of Cardiology 50: 149–156.

19. Investigators GA (1993) The effects of tissue plasminogen activator, streptokinase, or both on coronary-artery patency, ventricular function, and survival after acute myocardial infarction. N Engl j Med 329: 1615–1622.

20. Gibson CM, Cannon CP, Murphy SA, Ryan KA, Mesley R, et al. (2000) Relationship of TIMI myocardial perfusion grade to mortality after administration of thrombolytic drugs. Circulation 101: 125–130.

21. Ellis SG, Vandormael MG, Cowley MJ, DiSciascio G, Deligonul U, et al. (1990) Coronary morphologic and clinical determinants of procedural outcome with angioplasty for multivessel coronary disease. Implications for patient selection. Multivessel Angioplasty Prognosis Study Group. Circulation 82: 1193–1202.

22. Schiller NB, Shah P, Crawford M, DeMaria A, Devereux R, et al. (1988) Recommendations for quantitation of the left ventricle by two-dimensional echocardiography. American Society of Echocardiography Committee on Standards, Subcommittee on Quantitation of Two-Dimensional Echocardiograms. Journal of the American Society of Echocardiography: official publication of the American Society of Echocardiography 2: 358–367.

23. Quiñones MA, Otto CM, Stoddard M, Waggoner A, Zoghbi WA (2002) Recommendations for quantification of Doppler echocardiography: a report from the Doppler Quantification Task Force of the Nomenclature and Standards Committee of the American Society of Echocardiography. Journal of the American Society of Echocardiography 15: 167–184.

24. Lang RM, Bierig M, Devereux RB, Flachskampf FA, Foster E, et al. (2005) Recommendations for chamber quantification: a report from the American Society of Echocardiography's Guidelines and Standards Committee and the Chamber Quantification Writing Group, developed in conjunction with the European Association of Echocardiography, a branch of the European Society of Cardiology. Journal of the American Society of Echocardiography 18: 1440–1463.

25. Feigenbaum H (1990) Role of echocardiography in acute myocardial infarction. The American journal of cardiology 66: H17–H22.

26. Lenth RV (2010) Java applets for power and sample size (computer software) 2006–9. Available: http://www.stat.uiowa.edu/~rlenth/Power. Accessed 2014 Jun 08.

27. Chan W, Taylor AJ, Ellims AH, Lefkovits L, Wong C, et al. (2012) Effect of Iron Chelation on Myocardial Infarct Size and Oxidative Stress in ST-Elevation–Myocardial Infarction. Circulation: Cardiovascular Interventions 5: 270–278.

28. Lee S-D, Huang C-Y, Shu W-T, Chen T-H, Lin JA, et al. (2006) Pro-inflammatory states and IGF-I level in ischemic heart disease with low or high serum iron. Clinica chimica acta 370: 50–56.

29. Muñoz M, García-Erce JA, Remacha ÁF (2011) Disorders of iron metabolism. Part 1: molecular basis of iron homoeostasis. Journal of clinical pathology 64: 281–286.

30. Zeben D, Bieger R, Wermeskerken RK, Castel A, Hermans J (1990) Evaluation of microcytosis using serum ferritin and red blood cell distribution width. European journal of haematology 44: 106–109.

31. Kell DB (2009) Iron behaving badly: inappropriate iron chelation as a major contributor to the aetiology of vascular and other progressive inflammatory and degenerative diseases. BMC medical genomics 2: 2.

32. Hower V, Mendes P, Torti FM, Laubenbacher R, Akman S, et al. (2009) A general map of iron metabolism and tissue-specific subnetworks. Molecular bioSystems 5: 422–443.

33. Cairo G, Bernuzzi F, Recalcati S (2006) A precious metal: Iron, an essential nutrient for all cells. Genes & nutrition 1: 25–39.

34. Beard JL (2001) Iron biology in immune function, muscle metabolism and neuronal functioning. The Journal of Nutrition 131: 568S–580S.

35. Libby P, Ridker PM, Maseri A (2002) Inflammation and atherosclerosis. Circulation 105: 1135–1143.

36. Karpiński L, Płaksej R, Kosmala W, Witkowska M (2008) Serum levels of interleukin-6, interleukin-10 and C-reactive protein in relation to left ventricular function in patients with myocardial infarction treated with primary angioplasty. Kardiologia polska 66: 1279–1285.

37. Nemeth E, Rivera S, Gabayan V, Keller C, Taudorf S, et al. (2004) IL-6 mediates hypoferremia of inflammation by inducing the synthesis of the iron regulatory hormone hepcidin. Journal of Clinical Investigation 113: 1271–1276.

38. Simonis G, Mueller K, Schwarz P, Wiedemann S, Adler G, et al. (2010) The iron-regulatory peptide hepcidin is upregulated in the ischemic and in the remote myocardium after myocardial infarction. Peptides 31: 1786–1790.

39. Suzuki H, Toba K, Kato K, Ozawa T, Tomosugi N, et al. (2009) Serum hepcidin-20 is elevated during the acute phase of myocardial infarction. Tohoku journal of experimental medicine 218.

40. Gabriel AS, Martinsson A, Wretlind B, Ahnve S (2004) IL-6 levels in acute and post myocardial infarction: their relation to CRP levels, infarction size, left ventricular systolic function, and heart failure. European Journal of Internal Medicine 15: 523–528.

15

Adjunctive Manual Thrombus Aspiration during ST-Segment Elevation Myocardial Infarction

Song-Bai Deng[1], Jing Wang[1], Jun Xiao[2], Ling Wu[1], Xiao-Dong Jing[1], Yu-Ling Yan[1], Jian-Lin Du[1], Ya-Jie Liu[1], Qiang She[1]*

1 Department of Cardiology, The Second Affiliated Hospital of Chongqing Medical University, Chongqing, China, 2 Department of Cardiology, The Medical Emergency Center of Chongqing, Chongqing, China

Abstract

Objective: The aim of this study was to synthesize evidence by examining the effects of manual thrombus aspiration on clinical outcomes in patients with ST-segment elevation myocardial infarction (STEMI).

Methods and Results: A total of 26 randomized controlled trials (RCTs), enrolling 11,780 patients, with 5,869 patients randomized to manual thrombus aspiration and 5,911 patients randomized to conventional percutaneous coronary intervention (PCI), were included in the meta-analysis. Separate clinical outcome analyses were based on different follow-up periods. There were no statistically reductions in the incidences of mortality (risk ratio [RR], 0.86 [95% confidence interval [CI]: 0.73 to 1.02]), reinfarction (RR, 0.62 [CI, 0.31 to 1.32]) or target vessel revascularization (RR, 0.89 [CI, 0.75 to 1.05]) in the manual thrombus aspiration arm at 12 to 24 months of follow-up. The composite major adverse cardiac events (MACEs) outcomes were significantly lower in the manual thrombus aspiration arm over the long-term follow-up (RR, 0.76 [CI, 0.63 to 0.91]). A lower incidence of reinfarction was observed in the hospital to 30 days (RR, 0.59 [CI, 0.37 to 0.92]).

Conclusion: The present meta-analysis suggested that there was no evidence that using manual thrombus aspiration in patients with STEMI could provide distinct benefits in long-term clinical outcomes.

Editor: Chiara Lazzeri, Azienda Ospedaliero-Universitaria Careggi, Italy

Funding: The authors have no support or funding to report.

Competing Interests: The authors have declared that no competing interests exist.

* Email: qshe98@hotmail.com

Introduction

Thrombus aspiration for ST-segment elevation myocardial infarction (STEMI) has been utilized for a long time and has received a level IIA endorsement according to the U.S. guidelines [1]. In the recent years, there has been increasing interest in manual thrombectomy devices, and the evidence to date has suggested that manual thrombus aspiration, but not mechanical aspiration, is beneficial in reducing major adverse cardiac events (MACEs), including mortality, compared with conventional percutaneous coronary intervention (PCI) alone [2–6]. In the largest randomized trial to date, the TASTE (Thrombus Aspiration in ST-Elevation myocardial infarction in Scandinavia) study suggested that routine manual thrombus aspiration before PCI provided no significant benefit to mortality over PCI alone in patients with STEMI at 30 days and 1 year of follow-up, settling the debate over the benefits of using manual thrombus aspiration in this setting [7,8]. Recently, thrombectomy was downgraded in the ESC/EACTS revascularization guidelines from a class IIa level of evidence B recommendation to a class IIb level of evidence A recommendation [9]. Despite two well-done updated meta-

analyses recently performed on this topic by Kumbhani DJ et al [5,6], controversy exists regarding the combination of outcome effects over different follow-up durations. Because additional studies and prolonged follow-ups of earlier trials have now been reported, we performed an updated meta-analysis of the reperfusion markers of STEMI patients undergoing PCI with manual thrombus aspiration devices, and we performed separate analyses of clinical outcomes based on different follow-up periods. Because the Rescue (Boston Scientific) and TVAC (Thrombus Vacuum Aspiration Catheter, Nipro) catheters, attached to aspiration pumps for vacuum creation, were defined inconsistently as manual or mechanical thrombectomy in previous published meta-analyses [2–6], these two catheters were classified as special thrombectomy devices in the present meta-analysis.

Methods

This study was performed in compliance with the quality of reporting for meta-analyses (PRISMA [Preferred Reporting Items for Systematic reviews and Meta-Analyses] statement) [10].

Data Sources and Searches

We performed a computerized literature search of the PubMed, Web of Science, and Central databases for relevant articles published until September 2014, using the Medical Subject Heading and keyword search terms myocardial infarction, ST-segment elevation myocardial infarction, STEMI, thrombus aspiration, thrombectomy, Diver, Pronto, Export, Thrombuster, Eliminate, Rescure, TVAC, revascularization, percutaneous coronary intervention, angioplasty and PCI. No restrictions were applied to the publication period of the articles. This search was supplemented with citation tracking of relevant review articles and prior meta-analyses. Furthermore, conference proceedings from the American College of Cardiology, American Heart Association, European Society of Cardiology, EuroPCR scientific sessions and Transcatheter Cardiovascular Therapeutics were scanned. Only English-language studies were included.

Study Selection

We selected studies in which patients with STEMI undergoing primary PCI or rescue PCI were randomly assigned either to manual thrombus aspiration followed by PCI or to PCI only. We only included studies that reported clinical outcome data and/or markers of post-procedure myocardial reperfusion. We excluded studies that performed thrombectomy only on saphenous vein grafts, studies that performed mechanical thrombectomy, studies of elective PCI and studies that compared one thrombectomy device to another.

Data Extraction and Quality Assessment

The data were independently abstracted by two reviewers (Song-Bai Deng, Ling Wu). Agreement between the reviewers was evaluated by Kappa statistics. Disagreements were resolved through discussion, and a third reviewer (Qiang She) was involved to achieve a consensus when necessary. The bias of the included studies was assessed by the Cochrane group's *Cochrane Handbook for Systematic Reviews of Interventions* [11].

Data Synthesis and Analysis

The primary clinical endpoint was all-cause mortality. The secondary endpoints were MACEs (composite of death, reinfarction, and target vessel revascularization), reinfarction, target vessel revascularization (TVR) and stent thrombosis. Angiographic and electrocardiographic outcomes that reflected post-procedure myocardial reperfusion included post-procedure myocardial blush grade (MBG) 3, thrombolysis and thrombin inhibition in myocardial infarction (TIMI) 3, and resolution of ST segment elevation (STR) >70%. We performed separate analyses of clinical outcomes based on different follow-up periods. The time frames were defined to reflect short-term (in hospital to 30 days), medium-term (6 to 9 months) and long-term (longer than or equal to 1 year) follow-ups, according to the different follow-up durations of the included studies. If manual and mechanical devices were both used in the same study, only data pertaining to manual aspiration thrombectomy were extracted. A subanalysis of the special thrombectomy devices (Rescue and TVAC) was performed. For all of the clinical outcomes, intention-to-treat analysis was utilized. The meta-analysis was performed using RevMan software, version 5.3 (Cochrane Collaboration). Summary risk ratios (RRs) and their corresponding 95% confidence intervals (CIs) were computed for each dichotomous outcome, using fixed or random effects models. For outcomes with significant heterogeneity (Chi^2 p<0.05 or I^2>50%), the random effects model is reported in the text and figures; for all of the other outcomes, the fixed effects models are reported. The random effects models were employed for sensitivity analysis when the fixed effects models produced positive results.

Outcome Quality Assessment

We evaluated the level of evidence using the GRADE (Grades of Recommendation, Assessment, Development and Evaluation) approach [12]. The GRADEpro software version 3.6 was used. We obtained our assessment by judging the designs of the studies, the risk of bias, inconsistency, and imprecision.

Results

Eligible studies

The initial search obtained 641 potentially relevant publications. After reading the abstracts and the full texts, 26 RCTs were finally included, enrolling 11,780 patients, with 5,869 patients randomized to manual thrombus aspiration and 5,911 patients randomized to conventional PCI (**Figure 1**). The follow-up periods varied between in-hospital and 5 years. Twelvetrials presented short-term follow-up results (in-hospital to 30 days) [9,13–22], 8 trials presented medium-term follow-up results (6 to 8 months) [23,29], and 2 trials presented long-term follow-up results (12 months) [30,31]. In addition, 5trials presented different follow-up periods: the TAPAS (The Thrombus Aspiration during Percutaneous Coronary Intervention in Acute Myocardial Infarction Study) [32,33] and INFUSE-AMI (Infuse–Acute Myocardial Infarction; An Optical Frequency Domain Imaging Study) [34,35] studies followed up from 30 days and then to up to 12 months, TASTE followed up from 30 days to 1 year [7,8], EXPIRA (The Thrombectomy With Export Catheter in Infarct-Related Artery During Primary Percutaneous Coronary Intervention Prospective, Randomized Trial) from 9 months and up to 24 months [36,37] and VAMPIRE (VAcuuM asPIration thrombus Removal trial) from 1 month to 5 years [38–41]. Kappa statistics showed good agreement between the reviewers in the selection and data extraction (Kappa = 0.85). Among 24 included studies, most of them did not explicitly describe random sequence generation or allocation, and few presented attrition or reporting bias. Because the participants and personnel could not be blinded to the trials, the vast majority of studies were only blinded to outcome assessment. The reviewers' judgments about each risk of bias item are presented in **Figure S1**. The baseline characteristics of the included patients are listed in **Table 1**.

Mortality

There was no significant mortality benefit from in hospital to 30 days (2.53% thrombus aspiration vs. 2.94% conventional PCI; RR = 0.87, 95% CI 0.69 to 1.09, p = 0.22; p for heterogeneity [phet] = 0.95, I^2 = 0%) or from 6 to 9 months of follow-up (1.43% vs. 1.78%; RR: 0.84, 95% CI: 0.39 to 1.80, p = 0.65; phet = 0.58, I^2 = 0%). We observed a decreased trend toward mortality in manual thrombus aspiration with long-term follow-up (longer than or equal to 1 year), but this trend was not statistically significant (5.04% vs. 5.83%; RR: 0.86, 95% CI: 0.73 to 1.02, p = 0.09; phet = 0.27, I^2 = 22%).A random-effects model yielded a similar result with long-term follow-up (RR: 0.80, 95% CI: 0.59 to 1.08, p = 0.14). Subgroup analysis of the different aspiration thrombectomy devices also showed similar results (**Figure 2**).

MACEs

Because the MACEs was not pre-defined, the TASTE trail could not be included in the meta-analysis in terms of MACE outcomes. The composite MACE outcomes were significantly

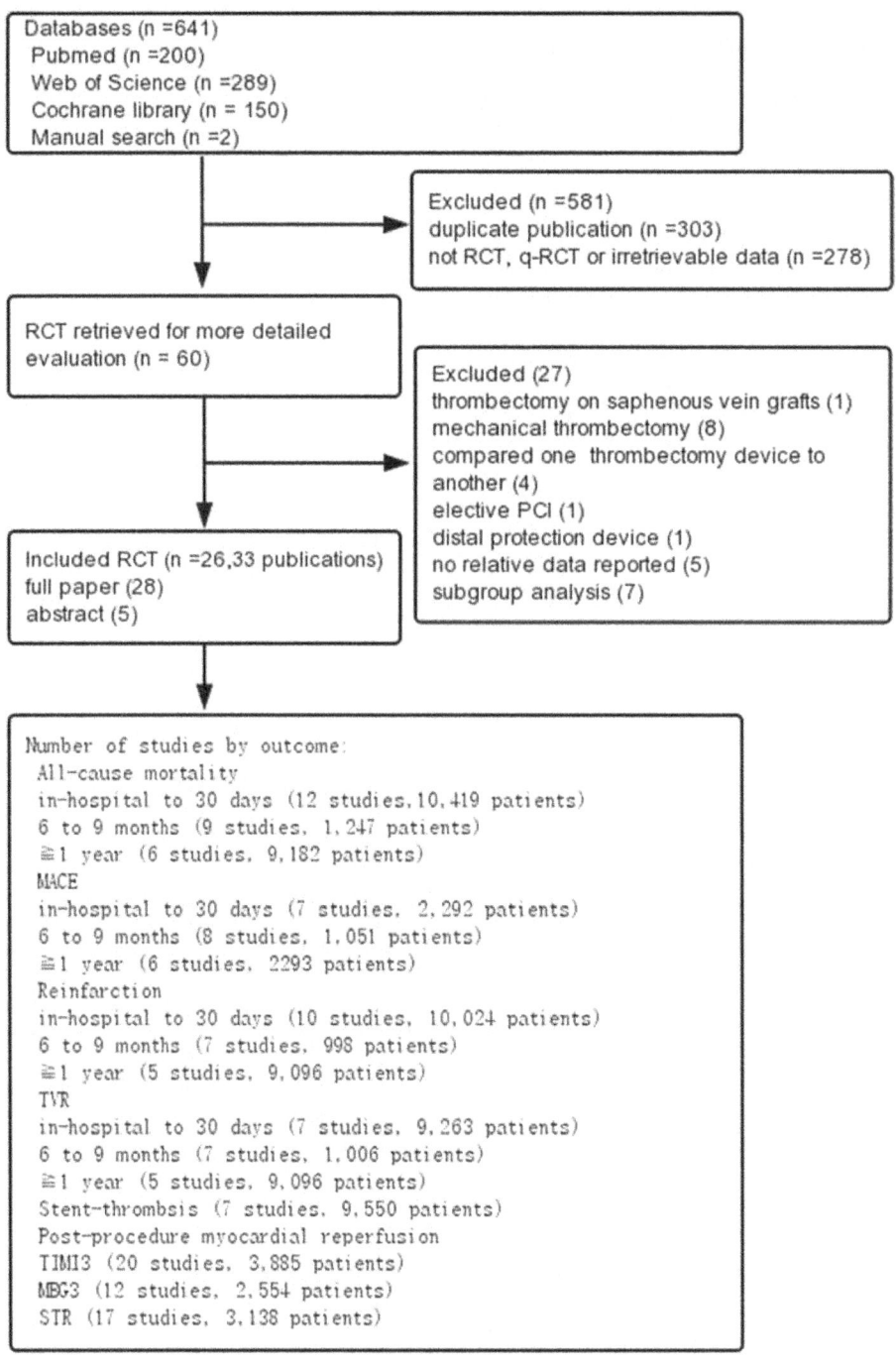

Figure 1. Flow diagram of the systematic overview process.

lower in the manual thrombus aspiration arm at 6 to 9 months (10.94% thrombus aspiration vs. 16.89% conventional PCI; RR: 0.65, 95% CI: 0.48 to 0.88, p = 0.005; phet = 0.94, I^2 = 0%) and with long-term (14.49% vs. 18.66%; RR: 0.76, 95% CI: 0.63 to 0.91, p = 0.003; phet = 0.73, I^2 = 0%) follow-up. A random-effects model yielded similar results (RR: 0.65, 95% CI: 0.48 to 0.88; RR: 0.76, 95% CI: 0.64 to 0.91, respectively). However, the composite MACEs were similar between the two arms from in hospital to 30 days of follow-up (4.34% vs. 6.75%; RR: 0.77, 95% CI: 0.56 to 1.07, p = 0.12; p_{het} = 0.98, I^2 = 0%) (**Figure 3**).

Reinfarction

The incidence of reinfarction was lower in the manual thrombus aspiration arm from in hospital to 30 days (0.56% thrombus aspiration vs. 0.98% conventional PCI; RR: 0.59, 95% CI: 0.37 to 0.92, p = 0.02; phet = 0.95, I^2 = 0%) but not at 6 to 9 months (3.38% vs. 5.35%; RR:0.62, 95% CI: 0.31to1.25, p = 0.18; phet = 0.81, I^2 = 0%) or with long-term (2.45% vs. 2.80%; RR:0.88, 95% CI: 0.68 to 1.13, p = 0.31; phet = 0.34, I^2 = 12%) follow-up (**Figure 4**). A random-effects model yielded similar results from in hospital to 30 days of follow-up (RR: 0.59, 95% CI:

Table 1. Baseline characteristics of trials included in the meta-analysis.

Study/Ref	Design	Device	Manual Thrombus Aspiration/Conventional Primary PCI						
			n	Mean Age, Yrs	Male,%	Baseline TIMI 0/1, %	Ischaemia time,h	GP IIb/IIIa inhibitor, %	Follow-Up time, months
TASTE [7,8]	multicenter	Eliminate/Pronto/Export	3621/3623	66.5/65.9	75.1/74.6	77.9/77.6	3.1/3.0†	15.4/17.4	1 m
REMEDIA [13]	single-center	Diver CE	50/49	61/60	90.0/77.6	86.0/89.8	4.6/5.0	68.0/63.3	1 m
Noel B et al [14]	single-center	Export	24/26	58/62	NA	NA	5.2/4.2	NA	H
DEAR-MI [15]	single-center	Pronto	74/74	57.3/58.9	84/76	81/73	3.4/3.3	100/100	H
EXPORT [16]	multicenter	Export	120/129	59.2/61.2	80.8/81.4	99.2/100	6.0/5.1	57.1/73.7	1 m
Lipiecki et al [17]	single-center	Export	20/24	59/59	60/75	100/96	7.1/7.4	5/12	H
Ciszewski et al [18]	single-center	Rescue/Diver CE	67/70	64.2/64.1	72/71	90/91	5.6/5.6	84/80	H
TROFI [19]	multicenter	Eliminate	71/70	61.1/60.9	75.7/69.1	48/46.4	NA	47.8/62.8	H
Dudek et al [20]	single-center	Rescue	40/32	57/59	NA	79/66	4.3/3.9	0/0	H
Kaltoft et al [21]	single-center	Rescue	108/107	65/11	76/80	68/69	4.0/3.5†	96/93	1 m
NONSOP [22]	multicenter	Rescue	129/129	64/65.9	79.8/79.8	NA	NA	NA	H
De Luca et al [23]	single-center	Diver CE	38/38	66.7/64.6	71.0/55.3	100/100	7.2/7.6	100/100	6 m
Chao et al [24]	single-center	Export	37/37	60/62	83.8/81.1	NA	5.6/5.9	19/32	6 m
Liistro et al [25]	single-center	Export	55/56	64/65	78/77	69/76	3.2/3.5	100/100	6 m
PIHRATE [26]	multicenter	Diver CE	100/96	60.8/58.8	80/81.7	96.7/97.9	NA	8/10.5	6 m
Bulum et al [27]	single-center	Export	30/30	54.3/58.5	83.3/73.3	NA	3.9/4.9	96.7/83.3	6 m
ITTI [28]	multicenter	Thrombuster II	52/48	60.5/56.5	90/81	83/92	2/8	54/52	6 m
Woo SI et al [29]	single-center	Export	33/30	55/53	84.8/100	78.8/83.3	4.4/4.7	0/0	6 m
MUSTELA [30]	multicenter	Export	50/104	62/63*	88.4/76*	91.3/77.9*	3.8/3.5*	100/100	12 m
Sim et al [31]	single-center	Thrombuster II	43/43	63/60	67.4/69.8	76.8/76.8	4.1/3.1†	30.2/46.5	12 m
TAPAS [32,33]	single-center	Export	535/536	63/63	67.9/73.1	54.8/59.5	3.2/3.1	93.4/89.9	1 m,12 m
INFUSE-AMI [34,35]	multicenter	Export	229/223	61/59	73.8/74	73.4/70	2.4/2.7	50.7/50.2	1 m,12 m
EXPIRA [36,37]	single-center	Export	88/87	66.7/64.6	57/48	100/100	6.2/6.1	100/100	9 m,24 m
VAMPIRE [38–41]	multicenter	TAVC	180/175	63.2/63.5	80.6/77.7	74.6/75.3	6.3/7.1	0/0	1 m,8 m,5years
Hamza et al [42]	single-center	Diver CE	25/25	53.7/56.2	88/96	NA	5.91‡	100/100	H
Shehata et al [43]	single-center	Export	50/50	60.3/59.4	62/66	NA	NA	100/100	8 m

REMEDIA = The Randomized Evaluation of the Effect of Mechanical Reduction of Distal Embolization by Thrombus-Aspiration in Primary and Rescue Angioplasty Trial; TASTE = Thrombus Aspiration in ST-Elevation myocardial infarction in Scandinavia; DEAR-MI = The Dethrombosis to Enhance Acute Reperfusion in Myocardial Infarction Study; EXPORT = A Multicentre Randomized Controlled Trial of The EXPORT Aspiration Catheter; TROFI = Randomized Study to Assess the Effect of ThRombus Aspiration on Flow Area in Patients with ST-Elevation Myocardial Infarction; NONSOP= Intracoronary Aspiration before coronary Stenting in Patients with Acute Myocardial Infarction; PIHRATE = the Polish-Italian-Hungarian RAndomized ThrombEctomy Trial; ITTI = The Initial Thrombosuction and Tirofiban Infusion trial; MUSTELA = MUltidevice Thrombectomy in Acute ST-Segment Elevation Acute Myocardial Infarction Trial; TAPAS = The Thrombus Aspiration during Percutaneous Coronary Intervention in Acute Myocardial Infarction Study; INFUSE-AMI = Infuse–Acute Myocardial Infarction; An Optical Frequency Domain Imaging Study; EXPIRA = The Thrombectomy With Export Catheter in Infarct-Related Artery During Primary Percutaneous Coronary Intervention Prospective, Randomized Trial; VAMPIRE = VAcuuM asPIration thrombus Removal trial;

*Values for all thrombectomy (manual and mechanical) vs. conventional PCI alone;
†Median;
‡mean ischaemia time of all patients;
NA: not available; H: In-hospital clinical outcomes.

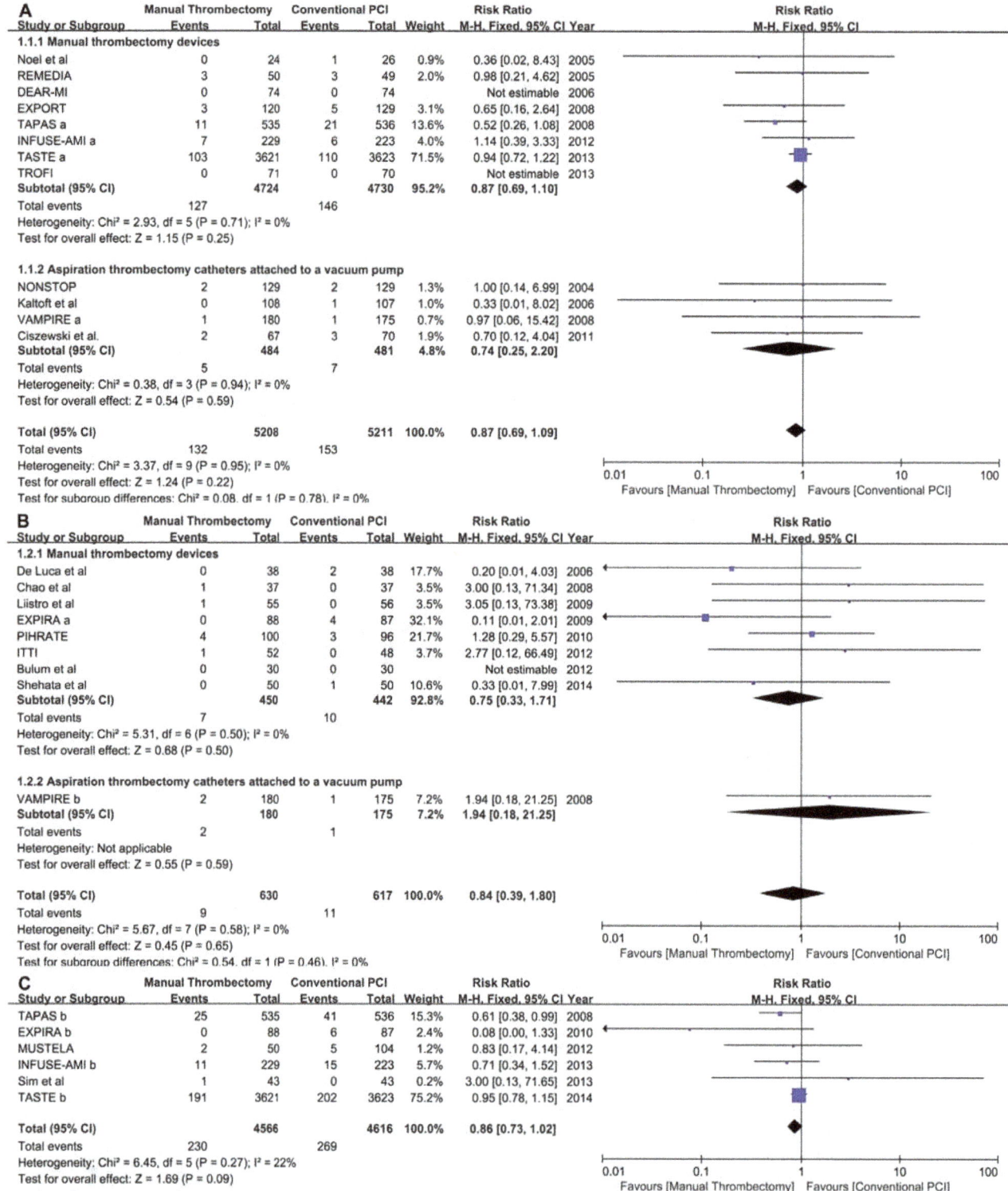

Figure 2. Forest plots for mortality in different follow-up periods. Footnote: A: short-term follow-up; B: medium-term follow-up; C: long-term follow-up; TAPAS a: 30-day of follow-up; TAPAS b: 12 months of follow-up; INFUSE-AMI a: 30-day of follow-up; INFUSE-AMI b: 12 months of follow-up; EXPIRA a: 6 months of follow-up; EXPIRA b: 24 months of follow-up; VAMPIRE a: 30-day of follow-up; VAMPIRE b: 8 months of follow-up. TASTE b, 1 year of follow-up.

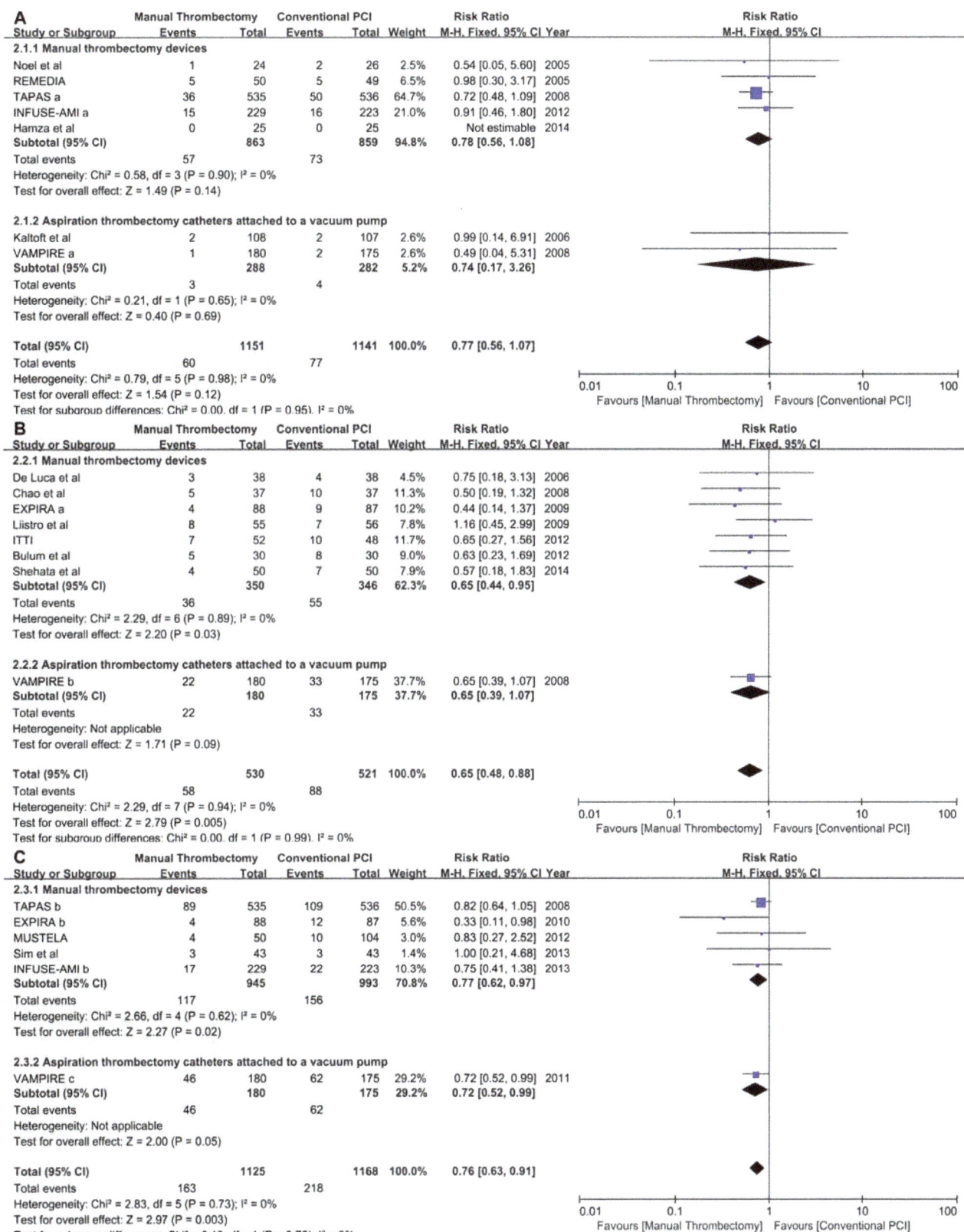

Figure 3. Forest plots for MACE in different follow-up periods. Footnote: A: short-term follow-up; B: medium-term follow-up; C: long-term follow-up; VAMPIRE c: 5 years of follow-up.

0.37 to 0.93, p = 0.02). Subgroup analysis suggested that the pure manual aspiration thrombectomy subgroup played a dominant role in the lower reinfarction incidence over short-term follow-up (**Figure 4**).

Target vessel revascularization

There were no differences between the two arms in the incidence of TVR from in hospital to 30 days (1.98% thrombus aspiration vs. 2.44% conventional PCI; RR: 0.82, 95% CI: 0.62 to 1.07, p = 0.14; p_{het} = 0.73, I^2 = 0%) or with long-term (5.13% vs. 5.75%; RR: 0.89, 95% CI: 0.75 to 1.05, p = 0.17; p_{het} = 1.00, I^2 = 0%) follow-up, but the incidence was significantly lower with manual thrombus aspiration from 6 to 9 months (7.54% vs. 11.55%; RR: 0.66, 95% CI: 0.45 to 0.96, p = 0.03; phet = 0.99, I^2 = 0%) (**Figure 5**). However, subgroup analysis showed that the positive results were dominated by the VAMPIRE study, in which a special thrombectomy device was used (TVAC). When we excluded this study, there were no differences between the two arms (RR: 0.69, 95% CI: 0.40 to 1.20, p = 0.19).

Stent thrombosis

Use of manual thrombus aspiration devices did not significantly reduce the incidence of total stent thrombosis (0.80% vs1.07%; RR: 0.75, 95% CI: 0.50 to 1.13, p = 0.17; p_{het} = 0.85, I^2 = 0%). A random-effects model yielded similar results (RR: 0.75, 95% CI: 0.49 to 1.14, p = 0.18) (**Figure 6**).

Markers of myocardial reperfusion

The use of manual thrombus aspiration devices was associated with significantly higher rates of post-procedure MBG 3 (RR: 1.43, 95% CI: 1.19 to 1.71, p<0.001; p_{het}<0.0001, I^2 = 73%), TIMI 3 flow (RR: 1.05, 95% CI: 1.02 to 1.09, p<0.001; p_{het} = 0.03, I^2 = 40%), and STR >70% (RR: 1.27, 95% CI: 1.12 to 1.45, p<0.001; p_{het}<0.0001, I^2 = 69%). There were still significant advantages of angiographic and electrocardiographic outcomes in the manual thrombus aspiration arm when individually excluding the included trials. Subgroup analysis showed that the benefits of TIMI3 and STR mainly derived from the pure manual thrombectomy devices subgroup but not from the Rescue and TAVC subgroup (see **Figures S2, S3 and S4**). There was no evidence of publication bias in the included studies in the meta-analysis of post-procedure TIMI 3 flow, as visually analyzed with a funnel plot (see **Figure S5**).

GRADE profile evidence

The GRADE system evidence for each outcome level and the reasons for upgrade and downgrade are shown in **Table 2**. According to the GRADE approach, the quality of evidence for the long-term follow-up of mortality, reinfarction and TVR was high, and the quality of evidence for stent thrombosis, long-term follow-up of MACEs and short-term follow-up of reinfarction was moderate.

Discussion

This meta-analysis performed separate analyses based on different follow-up periods to compare the clinical outcomes of manual thrombus aspiration with those of conventional PCI. The main findings of this meta-analysis were that the use of manual thrombus aspiration devices could significantly reduce the incidence of short-term reinfarction and long-term MACEs, but it did not result in lower rates of death, reinfarcion or TVR over long-term follow-up despite improved post-procedure myocardial reperfusion. These results were driven mainly by the TASTE trial.

There were some differences from the well-done updated meta-analysis on this topic performed recently by Kumbhani DJ et al [5,6]. First, we performed separate analyses of clinical outcomes based on different follow-up periods, and a subanalysis of the special thrombectomy devices (Rescue and TVAC) to avoid clinical heterogeneity as much as possible. Second, we included 6 additional studies and the results of the recent TASTE trial at the 1-year follow-up in this meta-analysis. Third, this meta-analysis presented fewer long-term clinical benefits of routine use of manual thrombus aspiration in patient with STEMI. Finally, we also assessed the level of evidence using the GRADE approach. The present meta-analysis showed that the composite MACE outcomes were significantly lower in the manual thrombus aspiration arm with long-term follow-up (RR: 0.76, 95% CI: 0.63 to 0.91). However, the number of included patients for this clinical outcome was far less than for the others because the TASTE trail could not be included due to MACEs not being pre-defined in this trail. In the TASTE trial, the composite incidence of death, rehospitalization for myocardial infarction, or stent thrombosis was 8.0% in the thrombus-aspiration group and 8.5% in the PCI-only group (hazard ratio, 0.94; 95% CI, 0.80 to 1.11; p = 0.48) [8]. Adding these factors together, we could not conclude that the use of manual thrombus aspiration devices could reduce the composite MACE outcomes.

In our meta-analysis, one trial warrants particular attention [7,8]. The TASTE trial, a registry-based RCT, was a prospective, multicenter, controlled trial that randomly allocated 7,244 patients to undergo manual thrombus aspiration followed by PCI or PCI alone. The sample size was larger than those of all previous studies combined, and the power to detect differences at well-defined end points was much higher. The TASTE study did not show any significant differences in the primary outcome of all-cause mortality, and it showed non-significant trends toward less myocardial infarction and stent thrombosis at 30 days and 1 year of follow-up. Additionally, the outcome of thrombus aspiration in candidate subjects not enrolled in TASTE failed to show an advantage of this adjunct, although this meta-analysis found that adjunctive manual thrombosis aspiration significantly reduced the incidence of reinfarction at 30 days of follow-up. Based on the rate of reinfarction with short-term follow-up (0.56% vs.0.98%, separately), 238 patients needed to be treated to prevent 1 reinfarction event. Given that the price of an average aspiration catheter is approximately €250,the potential clinicoeconomic effectiveness of the use of routine manual thrombosis aspiration is low.

Different inclusion criteria and different manual aspiration thrombectomy devices were used in the various trials, and it is not surprising that there was significant statistical heterogeneity in the results of post-procedure myocardial reperfusion. For example, myocardial reperfusion was not improved and infarct size was not reduced by manual aspiration thrombectomy in the INFUSE-AMI trial of patients with large anterior STEMI [34]. Post-procedure myocardial reperfusion improvements were observed despite the inclusion of the recent INFUSE-AMI trial. A random effects model was employed in the meta-analysis, and there were still significant advantages of angiographic and electrocardiographic outcomes in the manual thrombus aspiration arm when individually excluding the included trials.

In the real world, the benefits of using manual thrombus aspiration in patients with STEMI are also controversial. One study found that the routine use of thrombus aspiration was associated with reduced 12-month mortality in a large real-world patient cohort [42]. These data supported the observed survival benefit in the TAPAS trial. However, another study showed that

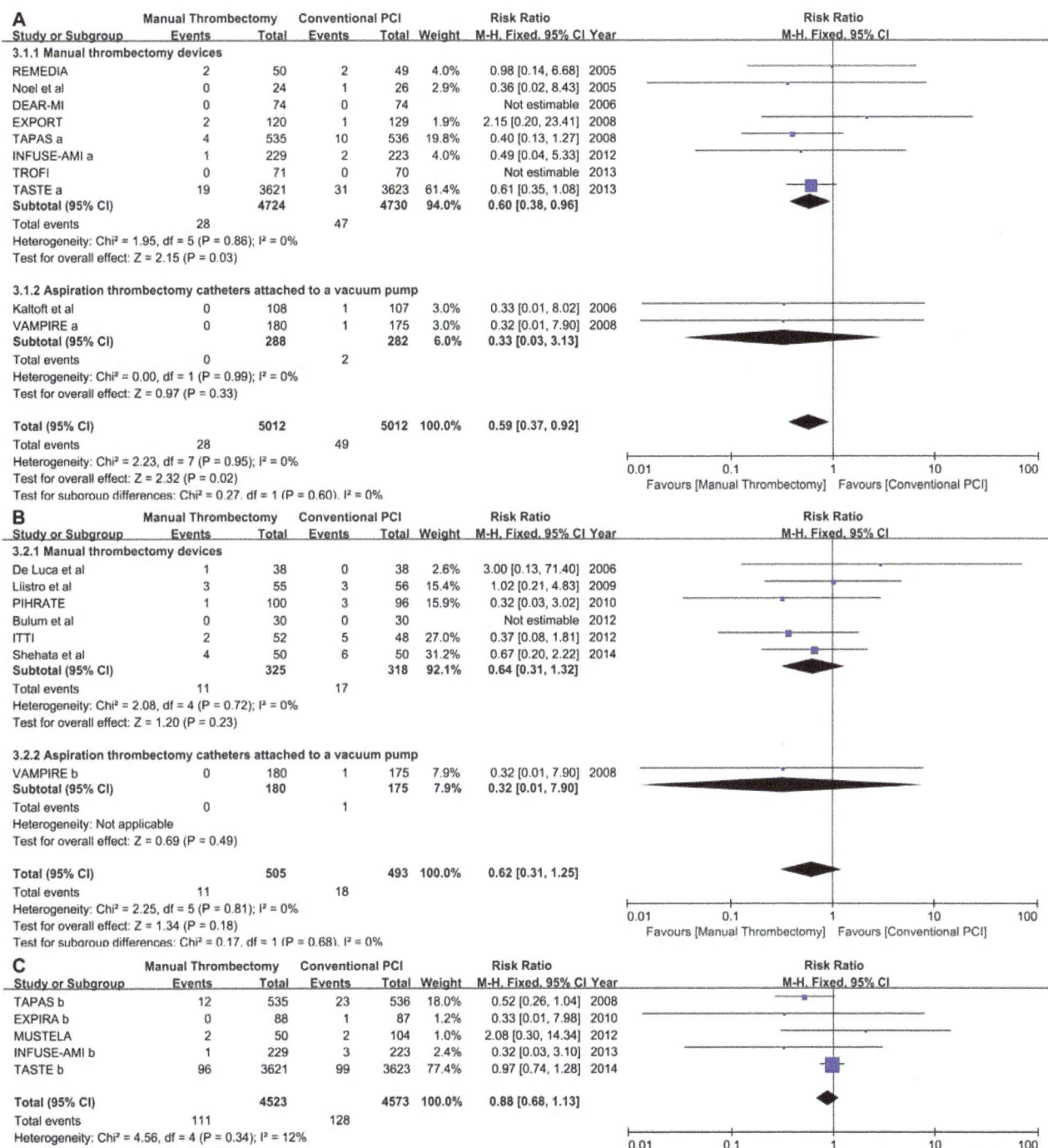

Figure 4. Forest plots for reinfarction in different follow-up periods. Footnote: A: short-term follow-up; B: medium-term follow-up; C: long-term follow-up.

one-year mortality was similar in both groups in a real-world STEMI population [43]. Recently, thrombectomy was downgraded in the ESC/EACTS revascularization guidelines from a class IIa level of evidence B recommendation to a class IIb level of evidence A recommendation. What will change in the U.S. STEMI guidelines is unknown. These results might have caused uncertainty in the minds of some cardiologists regarding the utility of adjunctive thrombus aspiration for primary PCI patients. Thus,

a subsequent analysis of the ongoing large-scale randomized trial (ClinicalTrials.gov number, NCT01149044) is imperative [44]. The TOTAL trial (A Randomized Trial of Routine Aspiration ThrOmbecTomy With PCI Versus PCI ALone in Patients With STEMI Undergoing Primary PCI) is an international, randomized, controlled, parallel-group study in which an estimated enrollment sample of 10,700 patients with STEMI will be allocated to manual aspiration thrombectomy with PCI or PCI

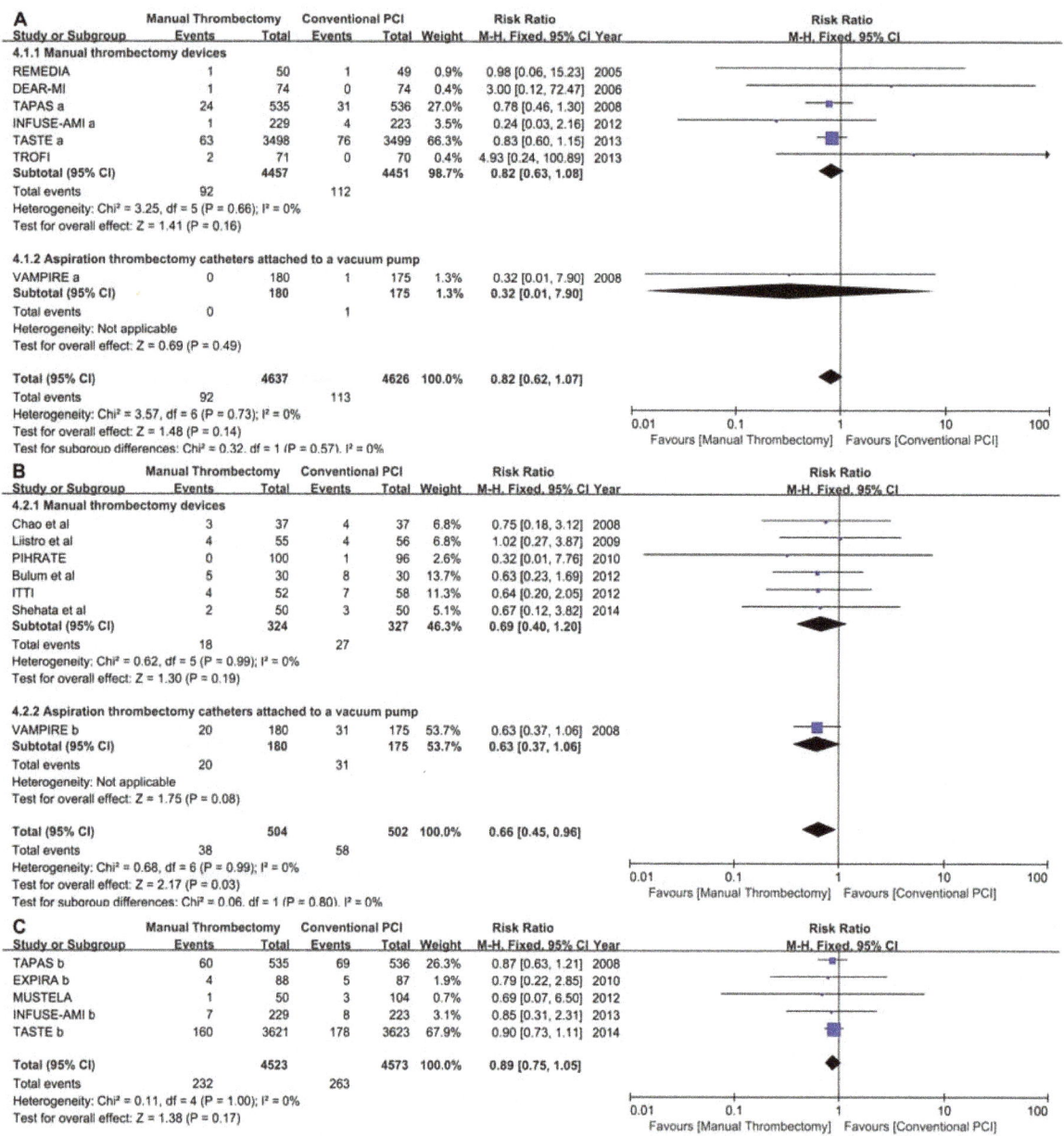

Figure 5. Forest plots for target vessel revascularization in different follow-up periods. Footnote: A: short-term follow-up; B: medium-term follow-up; C: long-term follow-up.

Figure 6. Forest plots for stent thrombosis.

Table 2. Summary of GRADE Evidence Profile of manual thrombectomy compared to conventional PCI for STEMI.

Outcomes	No of Participants (studies)	Quality of the evidence*	Relative effect	Anticipated absolute effects	
	Follow up	(GRADE)	(95% CI)	Risk with Conventional PCI	Risk difference with Manual thrombectomy (95% CI)
Long-term follow-up mortality	9182 (6 studies)	⊕⊕⊕⊕	RR 0.86	58 per 1000	8 fewer per 1000
	1 to 2 years	HIGH	(0.73 to 1.02)		(from 16 fewer to 1 more)
long-term follow-up MACEs	2293 (6 studies)	⊕⊕⊕⊖	RR 0.76	187 per 1000	45 fewer per 1000
	1 to 5 years	MODERATE1 due to imprecision	(0.63 to 0.91)		(from 17 fewer to 69 fewer)
Short-term follow-up reinfarction	10024 (10 studies)	⊕⊕⊕⊖	RR 0.59	10 per 1000	4 fewer per 1000
	in-hospital to 30 days	MODERATE2 due to imprecision	(0.37 to 0.92)		(from 1 fewer to 6 fewer)
long-term follow-up reinfarction	9096 (5 studies)	⊕⊕⊕⊕	RR 0.88	28 per 1000	3 fewer per 1000
	1 to 2 years	HIGH	(0.68 to 1.13)		(from 9 fewer to 4 more)
long-term follow-up TVR	9096 (5 studies)	⊕⊕⊕⊕	RR 0.89	58 per 1000	6 fewer per 1000
	1 to 2 years	HIGH	(0.75 to 1.15)		(from 14 fewer to 9 more)
Stent-thrombosis	9550 (7 studies)	⊕⊕⊕⊖	RR 0.75	11 per 1000	3 fewer per 1000
	in-hospital to 2 years	MODERATE3 due to risk of bias	(0.5 to 1.13)		(from 5 fewer to 1 more)

*The basis for the assumed risk (e.g. the median control group risk across studies) is provided in footnotes. The corresponding risk (and its 95% confidence interval) is based on the assumed risk in the comparison group and the relative effect of the intervention (and its 95% CI). CI: Confidence interval; RR: Risk ratio; 1 No enough optimal information size; 2 Risk ratio <0.75; 3 Different definition of stent thrombosis outcome.

alone, with follow-up of up to 180 days, and the primary end points are the first occurrence of cardiovascular death, recurrent myocardial infarction, cardiogenic shock, or new or worsening NYHA Class IV heart failure. In 2015 the results from the TOTAL trial are expected, and an updated meta-analysis including these data should be conducted. In clinical practice, thrombectomy catheters could be used to reduce thrombus burden by aspirating thrombi prior to stenting or balloon angiography; better reperfusion is predicted, and technically and procedurally using aspiration is also important. However, the use of thrombus aspiration during PCI in STEMI remains controversial

Our review had some limitations. First, this meta-analysis was not performed on individual patient data because complete data sets were not available. Second, only the TASTE trial was powered for mortality and the other clinical events reported, and the other included trials' sample sizes were small. Third, the number of screened subjects or percentages of included vs. candidate subjects in a number of included studies were not accounted for [13,15,20,21,24,26], which is an important limitation that confounds how we should interpret our selection and outcome results.

Conclusions

In summary, the present meta-analysis suggested that the use of manual thrombus aspiration devices could improve post-procedure myocardial reperfusion, but there was no evidence of a benefit in long-term clinical outcomes.

Supporting Information

Figure S1 Review authors' judgements about each risk of bias item presented as percentages across all included studies.

Figure S2 Forest plots for post-procedure MBG 3. Footnote: TAPAS a: 30-day of follow-up; VAMPIRE a: 30-day of follow-up.

Figure S3 Forest plots for post-procedure TIMI 3. Footnote: TAPAS a: 30-day of follow-up; INFUSE-AMI a: 30-day of follow-up; VAMPIRE a: 30-day of follow-up.

Figure S4 Forest plots for post-procedure STR. Footnote: TAPAS a: 30-day of follow-up; INFUSE-AMI a: 30-day of follow-up; EXPIRA a: 6 months of follow-up; VAMPIRE a: 30-day of follow-up.

Figure S5 Funnel plot of the included studies in meta-analysis of post-procedure TIMI 3 flow. Footnote: The inverted and symmetrical funnel aspect can be observed for the assessed end points, with 95% of the studies lying within the confidence limit lines. This suggests that publication bias is not present among the included studies for the meta-analysis.

Author Contributions

Conceived and designed the experiments: QS SBD. Performed the experiments: SBD JW JX LW XDJ YLY JLD YJL. Analyzed the data: SBD QS JW JX LW. Contributed reagents/materials/analysis tools: JX YLY XDJ YJL. Wrote the paper: SBD JW QS.

References

1. American College of Cardiology Foundation/American Heart Association Task Force on Practice Guidelines (2013) 2013 ACCF/AHA guideline for the management of ST-elevation myocardial infarction: a report of the American College of Cardiology Foundation/American Heart Association Task Force on Practice Guidelines. Circulation 127: 362–425.

2. De Luca G, Dudek D, Sardella G, Marino P, Chevalier B, et al. (2008) Adjunctive manual thrombectomy improves myocardial perfusion and mortality in patients undergoing primary percutaneous coronary intervention for ST-elevation myocardial infarction: a meta-analysis of randomized trials. Eur Heart J 29: 3002–10.

3. Bavry AA, Kumbhani DJ, Bhatt DL (2008) Role of adjunctive thrombectomy and embolic protection devices in acute myocardial infarction: A comprehensive meta-analysis of randomized trials. Eur Heart J 29: 2989–3001

4. Costopoulos C, Gorog DA, Di Mario C, Kukreja N (2013) Use of thrombectomy devices in primary percutaneous coronary intervention: a systematic review and meta-analysis. Int J Cardiol 163: 229–241.

5. Kumbhani DJ, Bavry AA, Desai MY, Bangalore S, Bhatt DL (2013) Role of aspiration and mechanical thrombectomy in patients with acute myocardial infarction undergoing primary angioplasty: an updated meta-analysis of randomized trials. J Am Coll Cardiol 62: 1409–1418.

6. Kumbhani DJ, Bavry AA, Desai MY, Bangalore S, Byrne RA, et al. (2014) Aspiration thrombectomy in patients undergoing primary angioplasty: Totality of data to 2013. Catheter Cardiovasc Interv. doi: 10.1002/ccd.25532. [Epub ahead of print]

7. Fröbert O, Lagerqvist B, Olivecrona GK, Omerovic E, Gudnason T, et al. (2013) Thrombus aspiration during ST-segment elevation myocardial infarction. N Engl J Med 369: 1587–1597.

8. Lagerqvist B, Fröbert O, Olivecrona GK, Gudnason T, Maeng M, et al. (2014) Outcomes 1 Year after Thrombus Aspiration for Myocardial Infarction. N Engl J Med. doi: 10.1056/NEJMoa1405707.[Epub ahead of print]

9. Authors/Task Force members, Windecker S, Kolh P, Alfonso F, Collet JP, et al. (2014) 2014 ESC/EACTS Guidelines on myocardial revascularization: The Task Force on Myocardial Revascularization of the European Society of Cardiology (ESC) and the European Association for Cardio-Thoracic Surgery (EACTS) Developed with the special contribution of the European Association of Percutaneous Cardiovascular Interventions (EAPCI). Eur Heart J. doi:10.1093/eurheartj/ehu278. [Epub ahead of print]

10. Liberati A, Altman DG, Tetzlaff J, Mulrow C, Gøtzsche PC, et al. (2009) The PRISMA statement for reporting systematic reviews and meta-analyses of studies that evaluate healthcare interventions: explanation and elaboration. BMJ 339:b2700.

11. Higgins J, Altman D, Gøtzsche P, Jüni P, Moher D, et al. (2011) Cochrane Bias Methods Group; Cochrane Statistical Methods Group. The Cochrane Collaboration's tool for assessing risk of bias in randomised trials BMJ 343: d5928.

12. Guyatt GH, Oxman AD, Vist GE, Kunz R, Falck-Ytter Y, et al. (2008) GRADE: an emerging consensus on rating quality of evidence and strength of recommendations. BMJ 336:924–926.

13. Burzotta F, Trani C, Romagnoli E, Mazzari MA, Rebuzzi AG, et al. (2005) Manual thrombus-aspiration improves myocardial reperfusion: The randomized evaluation of the effect of mechanical reduction of distal embolization by thrombus-aspiration in primary and rescue angioplasty (REMEDIA) trial. J Am Coll Cardiol 46: 371–376

14. Noel B, Morice MC, Lefevre T, Garot P, Tavolaro O, et al. (2005) Thromboaspiration in acute ST-elevation MI improves myocardial reperfusion. Circulation 112(Suppl 2): 579.

15. Silva-Orrego P, Colombo P, Bigi R, Gregori D, Delgado A, et al. (2006) Thrombus aspiration before primary angioplasty improves myocardial reperfusion in acute myocardial infarction: the DEAR-MI (Dethrombosis to Enhance Acute Reperfusion in Myocardial Infarction) study. J Am Coll Cardiol 48: 1552–1559.

16. Chevalier B, Gilard M, Lang I, Commeau P, Roosen J, et al. (2008) Systematic primary aspiration in acute myocardial percutaneous intervention: a multicentre randomised controlled trial of the export aspiration catheter. EuroIntervention 4: 222–228.

17. Lipiecki J, Monzy S, Durel N, Cachin F, Chabrot P, et al. (2008) Effect of thrombus aspiration on infarct size and left ventricular function in high-risk patients with acute myocardial infarction treated by percutaneous coronary intervention. Results of a prospective controlled pilot study. Am Heart J 157: 581–587.

18. Ciszewski M, Pregowski J, Teresinska A, Karcz M, Kalinczuk L, et al. (2011) Aspiration coronary thrombectomy for acute myocardial infarction increases myocardial salvage: single center randomized study. Catheter Cardiovasc Interv 78: 523–531.

19. Onuma Y, Thuesen L, van Geuns RJ, van der Ent M, Desch S, et al. (2013) Randomized study to assess the effect of thrombus aspiration on flow area in patients with ST-elevation myocardial infarction: an optical frequency domain imaging study–TROFI trial. Eur Heart J 34:1050–1060.

20. Dudek D, Mielecki W, Legutko J, Chyrchel M, Sorysz D, et al. (2004) Percutaneous thrombectomy with the RESCUE system in acute myocardial infarction. Kardiol Pol 61: 523–533.

21. Kaltoft A, Bøttcher M, Nielsen SS, Hansen HH, Terkelsen C, et al. (2006) Routine thrombectomy in percutaneous coronary intervention for acute ST-segment-elevation myocardial infarction: a randomized, controlled trial. Circulation 114: 40–47.

22. Kunii H, Kijima M, Araki T, Kenji T, Atsushi K, et al. (2004) Lack of benefit of intracoronary thrombus aspiration before coronary stenting in patients with acute myocardial infarction: a multicenter randomized trial. J Am Coll Cardiol 43: 245A.

23. De Luca L, Sardella G, Davidson CJ, De Persio G, Beraldi M, et al. (2006) Impact of intracoronary aspiration thrombectomy during primary angioplasty on left ventricular remodelling in patients with anterior ST elevation myocardial infarction. Heart 92: 951–957.

24. Chao CL, Hung CS, Lin YH, Lin MS, Lin LC, et al. (2008) Time-dependent benefit of initial thrombosuction on myocardial reperfusion in primary percutaneous coronary intervention. Int J Clin Pract 62: 555–561.

25. Liistro F, Grotti S, Angioli P, Falsini G, Ducci K, et al. (2009) Impact of thrombus aspiration on myocardial tissue reperfusion and left ventricular functional recovery and remodeling after primary angioplasty. Circ Cardiovasc Interv 2: 376–383.

26. Dudek D, Mielecki W, Burzotta F, Gasior M, Witkowski A, et al. (2010) Thrombus aspiration followed by direct stenting: a novel strategy of primary percutaneous coronary intervention in ST-segment elevation myocardial infarction. Results of the Polish-Italian-Hungarian RAndomized ThrombEctomy Trial (PIHRATE Trial). Am Heart J 160: 966–972.

27. Bulum J, Ernst A, Strozzi M (2012) The impact of successful manual thrombus aspiration on in-stent restenosis after primary PCI: angiographic and clinical follow-up. Coron Artery Dis 23: 487–491.

28. Liu CP, Lin MS, Chiu YW, Lee JK, Hsu CN, et al. (2012) Additive benefit of glycoprotein IIb/IIIa inhibition and adjunctive thrombus aspiration during primary coronary intervention: results of the Initial Thrombosuction and Tirofiban Infusion (ITTI) trial. Int J Cardiol 156: 174–179.

29. Woo SI, Park SD, Kim DH, Kwan J, Shin SH, et al. (2014) Thrombus aspiration during primary percutaneous coronary intervention for preserving the index of microcirculatory resistance: a randomised study. EuroIntervention 9: 1057–1062.

30. De Carlo M, Aquaro GD, Palmieri C, Guerra E, Misuraca L, et al. (2012) A prospective randomized trial of thrombectomy versus no thrombectomy in patients with ST-segment elevation myocardial infarction and thrombus-rich lesions: MUSTELA (MUltidevice Thrombectomy in Acute ST-Segment ELevation Acute Myocardial Infarction) trial. JACC Cardiovasc Interv 5: 1223–1230.

31. Sim DS, Ahn Y, Kim YH, Lee D, Seon HJ, et al. (2013) Effect of manual thrombus aspiration during primary percutaneous coronary intervention on infarct size: Evaluation with cardiac computed tomography. Int J Cardiol 168: 4328–4330.

32. Svilaas T, Vlaar PJ, van der Horst IC, Diercks GF, de Smet BJ, et al. (2008) Thrombus aspiration during primary percutaneous coronary intervention. N Engl J Med 358: 557–567.

33. Vlaar PJ, Svilaas T, van der Horst IC, Diercks GF, Fokkema ML, et al. (2008) Cardiac death and reinfarction after 1 year in the Thrombus Aspiration during Percutaneous coronary intervention in Acute myocardial infarction Study (TAPAS): a 1-year follow-up study. Lancet 371: 1915–1920.

34. Stone GW, Maehara A, Witzenbichler B, Godlewski J, Parise H, et al. (2012) Intracoronary abciximab and aspiration thrombectomy in patients with large anterior myocardial infarction: the INFUSE-AMI randomized trial. JAMA 307: 1817–1826.

35. Stone GW, Witzenbichler B, Godlewski J, Dambrink J-HE, Ochala A, et al. (2013) Intralesional Abciximab and Thrombus Aspiration in Patients With Large Anterior Myocardial Infarction: One-Year Results From the INFUSE-AMI Trial. Circulation Cardiovascular interventions 6: 527–534.

36. Sardella G, Mancone M, Bucciarelli-Ducci C, Agati L, Scardala R, et al. (2009) Thrombus aspiration during primary percutaneous coronary intervention improves myocardial reperfusion and reduces infarct size: the EXPIRA (thrombectomy with export catheter in infarct-related artery during primary percutaneous coronary intervention) prospective, randomized, trial. J Am Coll Cardiol 53: 309–315.

37. Sardella G, Mancone M, Canali E, Di Roma A, Benedetti G, et al. (2010) Impact of thrombectomy with EXPort Catheter in Infarct-Related Artery during Primary Percutaneous Coronary Intervention (EXPIRA Trial) on cardiac death. Am J Cardiol 106: 624–629.

38. Ikari Y, Sakurada M, Kozuma K, Kawano S, Katsuki T, et al. (2008) Upfront thrombus aspiration in primary coronary intervention for patients with ST-segment elevation acute myocardial infarction: report of the VAMPIRE (VAcuuM asPIration thrombus REmoval) trial. JACC Cardiovascular interventions 1: 424–431.

39. Ken Kozuma, Yuji Ikari, Masami Sakurada, Shigeo Kawano, Takaaki Katsuki, et al. (2007) Long-term clinical follow-up in ST elevation acute myocardial infarction (STEMI) patients with thrombus aspiration prior to coronary intervention, 2-year results of the Vampire study. Circulation 116(16 Suppl): 378.

40. Ken Kozuma, Yuji Ikari, Kenshi Fujii, Masami Sakurada, Hideki Hashimoto, et al. (2009) Three-year Clinical Follow-up of the Vampire Study in St Elevation Acute Myocardial Infarction (STEMI) Patients With Thrombus Aspiration Prior to Coronary Intervention. Circulation 120(18 Suppl): S985.

41. Kengo Tanabe, Ken Kozuma, Yuji Ikari, Kenshi Fujii, Masami Sakurada, et al. (2011) Five-Year Clinical Follow-Up of the Vampire Study in St Elevation Acute Myocardial Infarction (stemi) Patients With Thrombus Aspiration Prior to Coronary Intervention. Circulation 124(21 Suppl): A12838.

42. Kikkert WJ, Claessen BE, van Geloven N, Baan J Jr, Vis MM, et al. (2013) Adjunctive thrombus aspiration versus conventional percutaneous coronary intervention in ST-elevation myocardial infarction. Catheter Cardiovasc Interv 8: 922–929.

43. Kilic S, Ottervanger JP, Dambrink JH, Hoorntje JC, Koopmans PC, et al. (2013) The effect of thrombus aspiration during primary percutaneous coronary intervention on clinical outcome in daily clinical practice. Thromb Haemost 111: 165–171.

44. Jolly SS, Cairns J, Yusuf S, Meeks B, Shestakovska O, et al. (2014) Design and rationale of the TOTAL trial: a randomized trial of routine aspiration ThrOmbecTomy with percutaneous coronary intervention (PCI) versus PCI ALone in patients with ST-elevation myocardial infarction undergoing primary PCI. Am Heart J 167: 315–321.

16

Red Blood Cell Distribution Width and Long-Term Outcome in Patients Undergoing Percutaneous Coronary Intervention in the Drug-Eluting Stenting Era: A Two-Year Cohort Study

Hai-Mu Yao[1], Tong-Wen Sun[2]*, Xiao-Juan Zhang[2], De-Liang Shen[1], You-You Du[1], You-Dong Wan[2], Jin-Ying Zhang[1], Ling Li[1], Luo-Sha Zhao[1]

1 Department of Cardiology, the First Affiliated Hospital of Zhengzhou University, Zhengzhou, P. R. China, 2 Department of Integrated ICU, the First Affiliated Hospital of Zhengzhou University, Zhengzhou, P. R. China

Abstract

Background: Previous studies suggest the higher the red blood cell distribution width (RDW) the greater the risk of mortality in patients with coronary artery disease (CAD). However, the relationship between RDW and long-term outcome in CAD patients undergoing percutaneous coronary intervention (PCI) with a drug-eluting stent (DES) remains unclear. This study was designed to evaluate the long-term effect of RDW in patients treated with drug-eluting stent for CAD.

Methods: In total of 2169 non-anemic patients (1468 men, mean age 60.2 ± 10.9 years) with CAD who had undergone successful PCI and had at least one drug-eluting stent were included in this study. Patients were grouped according to their baseline RDW: Quartile 1 (RDW<12.27%), Quartile 2 ($12.27\% \leq$ RDW<13%), Quartile 3 ($13\% \leq$ RDW<13.5%), and Quartile 4 (RDW$\geq$13.5).

Results: The incidence of in-hospital mortality and death or myocardial infarction was significantly higher in Quartiles 3 and 4 compared with Quartile 1 (P<0.05). After a follow-up of 29 months, the incidence of all-cause death and stent thrombosis in Quartile 4 was higher than in Quartiles 1, 2, and 3 (P<0.05). The incidence of death/myocardial infarction/stroke and cardiac death in Quartile 4 was higher than in Quartiles 1 and 2 (P<0.05). Multivariate Cox regression analysis showed that RDW was an independent predictor of all-cause death (hazard ratio (HR) = 1.37, 95% confidence interval (CI) = 1.15–1.62, P<0.001) and outcomes of death/myocardial infarction/stroke (HR = 1.21, 95% CI = 1.04–1.39, P = 0.013). The cumulative survival rate of Quartile 4 was lower than that of Quartiles 1, 2, and 3 (P<0.05).

Conclusion: High RDW is an independent predictor of long-term adverse clinical outcomes in non-anemic patients with CAD treated with DES.

Editor: Michael Lipinski, Washington Hospital Center, United States of America

Funding: This study was supported by the National Natural Science Foundation of China (Grant No. 81370364), Program for Science and Technology Innovation of Henan Province (NO. 201203035), Innovative investigators project grant from the Health Bureau of Henan Province, Program Grant for Science & Technology Innovation Talents in Universities of Henan Province (2012HASTIT001), Henan Provincial Science and Technology Achievement Transformation Project (122102310581), Henan Province of Medical Scientific Province & Ministry Research Project (201301005), Henan Province of Medical Scientific Research Project (201203027), China. The funders had no role in study design, data collection and analysis, decision to publish, or preparation of the manuscript.

Competing Interests: The authors have declared that no competing interests exist.

* E-mail: suntongwen@163.com

Introduction

Red blood cell distribution width (RDW) is an objective measure of the heterogeneity in red blood cell (RBC) size (i.e., it is a coefficient of variability of RBC volume). RDW is obtained from RBC size distribution, and is commonly utilized in the differential diagnosis of anemia. A number of studies report that high levels of RDW are associated with increased mortality among patients with heart failure, myocardial infarction (MI), or coronary artery disease (CAD), and in those undergoing percutaneous coronary intervention (PCI) [1–6]. A high RDW is also associated with elevated cardiovascular biomarkers and cardiac enzymes [7].

Study of a Chinese population showed that elevated RDW predicts an increased risk of short-term adverse outcomes in patients with acute coronary syndrome [8].

The initial success rate of PCI is high; therefore, long-term follow-up results are most appropriate for evaluating the predictive value of RDW. However, the long-term prognostic value of RDW in patients with anemia is uncertain [6,9], since many studies did not exclude patients in the general population with anemia, thus affecting outcome. Previous studies of the prognostic value of RDW in patients undergoing PCI included those treated with drug-eluting stent (DES) or bare metal stent (BMS). While the clinical endpoints were the same regardless of choice of stent, DES was associated with a significantly reduced incidence of in-stent restenosis and need for revascularization of the target lesion. However, the potential for thrombosis following DES is a concern.

For the reasons outlined above we conducted a prospective observational cohort study to investigate the prognostic value of RDW in patients treated with DES.

Methods

Ethics Statement

The study was approved by the Ethics Committee of the first affiliated hospital of Zhengzhou University. All aspects of the study comply with the Declaration of Helsinki. Ethics Committee of the first affiliated hospital of Zhengzhou University specially approved that not informed consent was required because data were going to be analyzed anonymously.

Study Population

This study recruited consecutive patients without anemia who underwent PCI from July 2009 to August 2011 at a single large-volume PCI center. Qualitative and quantitative coronary angiographic analyses were carried out according to standard methods. PCI was performed using standard techniques. All patients were given loading doses of aspirin (300 mg) and clopidogrel (300 mg) before the coronary intervention, unless they had already received these antiplatelet medications. The treatment strategy, stenting techniques, selection of stent type, as well as use of glycoprotein IIb/IIIa receptor inhibitors or intravascular ultrasound were all left to the operator's discretion. Daily aspirin (100 mg) and clopidogrel (75 mg) were prescribed for at least the first 12 months after the procedure. Patients were excluded from analysis if they had been referred for urgent PCI following acute MI, if they had a history of blood transfusion or if they presented with cardiogenic shock

Definitions used in the study

Cardiovascular risk factors were assessed at the time of hospital admission. Patients ≥ 65 years old were defined as being elderly. A history of smoking was assumed if the patient had smoked within the last 10 years. Patients were classed as having diabetes mellitus if their fasting plasma glucose concentration was >6.1 mmol/L, their hemoglobin A1c (HbA1c) was $>6.5\%$, or if they were currently being treated with insulin or oral hypoglycemic agents. Patients were defined as having hypertension if their systolic blood pressure was ≥ 140 mmHg, their diastolic blood pressure was ≥ 90 mmHg, or if antihypertensive drugs were prescribed. Dyslipidemia was defined as low-density lipoprotein cholesterol > 140 mg/dL, high-density lipoprotein <40 mg/dL, or lipid-lowering drugs were prescribed. Anemia was defined as a hemoglobin level <12.0 g/dL in women and <13.0 g/dL in men, based on the World Health Organization definition [10]. Glomerular filtration rate was estimated by the Cockcroft-Gault formula [11]. Target vessel revascularization (TVR) was defined as a repeat procedure, either PCI or coronary artery bypass grafting (CABG) in the target vessel. Stent thrombosis (ST) was proven by angiography, or assumed as probable if an unexplained sudden death occurred within 30 days after stent implantation, or if a Q-wave MI was diagnosed in the distribution area of the stented artery. This classification was issued according to definitions proposed by the Academic Research Consortium (ARC): acute ($<$ 24 h), subacute (24 h to 30 days), late (1–12 months), and very late ($>$12 months) [12]. Major bleeding was defined using REPLACE-2 criteria [13], which include decreases in hematocrit of $\geq 12\%$,

and in hemoglobin of ≥ 4 g/dL, transfusion of ≥ 2 units of packed RBC and retroperitoneal, gastrointestinal or intracranial bleeding.

Classification of RDW

Patients were divided into four groups according to their baseline RDW: Quartile 1 (RDW$<12.27\%$), Quartile 2 ($12.27\%\leq$ RDW$<13\%$), Quartile 3 ($13\%\leq$RDW$<13.5\%$), and Quartile 4 (RDW$\geq 13.5\%$).

Clinical Outcomes and data collection

Prospective data were entered into a database that contained demographic, clinical, angiographic, and procedural information. Primary endpoints included all-cause death, occurrence of MI, stent thrombosis, and TVR. The composite endpoint was defined as MACCE, namely death/MI/stroke. Clinical follow-up was carried out through patient visits, telephone interview, and medical record review. Data were entered by independent research personnel and clinical events were adjudicated by physicians who were not involved in the procedures themselves. All deaths were considered to be cardiac unless an unequivocal noncardiac cause could be established. Cardiac deaths included all events related to a cardiac diagnosis, any complication of a procedure and treatment thereof, or any unexplained cause. Unexpected death, even in patients with a coexisting and potentially fatal noncardiac disease (e.g., cancer or infection), was classified as cardiac unless their history relating to the noncardiac diagnosis suggested death was imminent. Between July 2009 and August 2011, 2348 non-anemic patients in our hospital were treated with at least one DES. Data were collected from 2169 patients (92.4%) over a follow-up period of 29.1 ± 5.3 months (range 25.5–33.2months).

Statistics

Continuous variables were expressed as mean $\pm$ standard deviation (SD). Categorical variables were expressed as percentages. Normally distributed continuous variables were analyzed using one-way ANOVA test. Variables whose distribution could not be assumed to be normal were analyzed using the nonparametric Wilcoxon Rank-Sum tests. The Chi-square or Fisher's Exact test were used for categorical variables. Cumulative survival curves were constructed using the Kaplan–Meier method and comparisons made using log-rank tests. Cox regression analysis was performed to identify independent predictors of death and MACCE. All baseline, demographic, clinical, and angiographic variables were entered into the model. Results were reported as hazard ratios (HRs) and 95% confidence intervals (CIs). All statistical tests were 2-tailed, and p values were statistically significant at <0.05. All data were analyzed with SPSS 17.0 (SPSS Inc., Chicago, Illinois, USA)

Results

Baseline clinical characteristics

Demographic characteristics of the 2169 patients of the study are shown in Table 1. The mean age was 60.2 ± 10.9 years and 67.7% of the patients were men. RDW ranged from 9.3% to 23% (mean, $12.9\pm1.25\%$).

There were no significant differences among the groups with respect to body mass index, clinical presentation, medications at discharge, or hemoglobin level. The percentages of patients with prior revascularization, heart failure, or peripheral vessel disease, and the percentage of current smokers were similar in all four groups. However, patients with higher RDW values tended to be older and to have more cardiovascular risk factors and more

Table 1. Baseline characteristics of participants by Quartile of RDW.

	Quartile 1 (n = 539)	Quartile 2 (n = 578)	Quartile 3 (n = 546)	Quartile 4 (n = 506)	P value
RDW	11.36±0.65	12.65±0.23	13.23±0.18	14.39±1.13	0.000
Age, year	58.3±11.0	58.6±10.7	60.1±10.6	63.2±10.8	<0.001
Age>65 years	170(31.5)	181(31.3)	210(38.5)	243(48)	0.000
Male gender	383(71.1)	393(68)	377(69)	315(62.3)	0.018
BMI, kg/m^2	23.5±5.3	23.8±6.5	24.0±7.8	23.6±5.0	0.79
Prior PCI	40(7.4)	29(5.0)	42(7.7)	36(7.1)	0.32
Prior CABG	3(0.6)	7(1.2)	4(0.7)	4(0.8)	0.62
Prior myocardial infarction	35(6.5)	41(7.1)	64(11.7)	78(15.4)	0.000
Peripheral vessel disease	1(0.2)	1(0.2)	0(0)	2(0.4)	0.52
COPD	2(0.4)	7(1.2)	3(0.5)	7(1.4)	0.19
Heart Failure	42(7.8)	52(9.0)	43(7.9)	52(10.3)	0.29
Prior stroke	20(3.7)	26(4.5)	38(7.0)	38(7.5)	0.016
Risk factors					
Arterial hypertension	208(38.6)	224(38.8)	314(57.5)	348(68.8)	0.000
Dyslipidemia	294(54.5)	323(55.9)	299(54.8)	272(53.8)	0.92
Diabetes mellitus	89(16.5)	122(21.1)	125(22.9)	157(31)	0.000
Current smoker	175(32.5)	175(30.3)	202(37)	152(30)	0.052
GFR, ml·min^{-1}·1.73 m^{-2}	73.9±14.6	73.4±14.8	71.3±15.6	68.7±16.1	<0.001
Clinical presentation					
Stable angina	31(6.5)	32(5.5)	31(5.7)	38(7.5)	0.53
Unstable angina	355(65.9)	387(67)	378(69.2)	331(65.4)	0.55
Non-STEMI	8(1.5)	6(1.0)	6(1.1)	4(0.8)	0.76
STMI	128(23.7)	122(21.1)	110(20.1)	98(19.4)	0.32
Total cholesterol, mmol/L	4.24±1.01	4.24±1.06	4.31±1.05	4.31±1.14	0.56
Triglyceride, mmol/L	1.90±1.36	1.97±1.15	1.92±1.40	1.84±1.55	0.53
LDL-C, mmol/L	2.68±0.93	2.67±0.93	2.7±0.90	2.7±0.97	0.93
HDL-C, mmol/L	1.06±0.34	1.03±0.29	1.07±0.30	1.11±0.32	0.002
Glycemia, mmol/L	5.82±2.36	6.24±3.69	5.86±2.18	6.13±4.11	0.09
Haemoglobin, g/L	141.6±11.2	141.3±9.6	141.2±12.3	140.7±12.6	0.23
Medication at discharge					
Aspirin,	537(99.6)	568(98.3)	537(98.4)	499(98.6)	0.17
Clopidogrel	537(99.6)	576(99.7)	545(99.8)	505(99.8)	0.91
ACEI/ARB	286(53.1)	325(56.2)	297(54.4)	286(56.5)	0.63
Beta-blocker	380(70.5)	419(72.5)	397(72.7)	341(67.4)	0.20
Statins	507(94.1)	554(95.8)	511(93.6)	473(93.5)	0.28

Values are mean ± SD or n (%). RDW: red blood cell distribution width, PCI: percutaneous coronary intervention, CABG: coronary artery bypass graft, COPD: chronic obstructive pulmonary disease, GFR: glomerular filtration rate, STEMI: ST segment elevation myocardial infarction, Non-STEMI: Non-ST segment elevation myocardial infarction, LDL-C: Low density lipidprotein cholesterol, HDL-C: High density lipidprotein cholesterol, ACEI: Angiotensin-converting enzyme inhibitor, ARB: angiotensin recptor blocker.

cardiovascular diseases (prior MI and prior stroke) compared with patients with lower RDW values. Other factors that were independently associated with baseline RDW level are shown in Table 1.

Angiographic and procedural characteristic

The proportion of patients with a type B1 lesion was lower in Quartiles 3 and 4 than in Quartile 1 (p<0.001). Compared with quartile 1, the proportion of patients with a type B2 or type C lesion was significantly higher in quartile 4 (p<0.05). The left ventricular ejection fraction (LVEF) was significantly lower in quartile 4 than in Quartiles 1, 2, and 3 (p<0.05). By contrast, the location of the target lesion, the numbers of vessels treated and stents inserted, total stent length and stent diameter were not significantly different among the groups (Table 2).

Clinical Outcomes

The incidence of in-hospital death and of MACE (death/MI) was significantly higher in quartile 4 than in quartiles 1 and 2 (p< 0.05), but the incidence of any MI did not vary among the groups (p>0.05).

Table 2. Baseline angiographic and procedural characteristics of participants by Quartile of RDW.

	Quartile 1 (n = 539)	Quartile 2 (n = 578)	Quartile 3 (n = 546)	Quartile 4 (n = 506)	P value
Radial artery access[a]	528(98)	567(98.3)	532(97.4)	490(96.8)	0.35
Number of diseased vessels[a]					
1-vessel disease	222(41.2)	233(40.3)	203(37.2)	183(36.2)	0.29
2-vessel disease	196(36.4)	208(36)	214(39.2)	191(37.7)	0.69
3-vessel disease	120(22.3)	132(22.8)	129(23.2)	133(26.3)	0.44
Location of lesion[a]					
Left main stem	14(2.8)	16(2.8)	21(3.8)	18(3.6)	0.59
LAD	442(82)	485(83.9)	444(81.3)	408(80.6)	0.52
LCX	255(47.3)	265(45.8)	265(48.5)	269(53.2)	0.097
RCA	253(46.9)	273(47.2)	277(50.7)	256(50.6)	0.43
LVEF[b], (n = 1470)	61.2±7.5	61.2±7.1	61.4±6.3	59.4±8.6	0.005
LVEF<40%	3(0.6)	9(1.6)	8(1.5)	15(3.0)	0.021
Type of target lesion according to AHA/ACC[a] (n = 3426)					
A	83(10.1)	73(8.7)	75(8.5)	74(8.3)	0.58
B1	303(36.9)	276(33)	251(28.5)	227(25.6)	0.000
B2	241(29.3)	270(32.3)	311(35.3)	322(36.3)	0.01
C	195(23.5)	217(26)	244(27.7)	264(29.8)	0.035
Total chronic occlusion	40(7.4)	55(9.5)	47(8.4)	59(11.7)	0.11
Ostial lesions	53(9.8)	62(10.7)	57(10.4)	43(8.5)	0.63
Number of treated vessels[b]	1.51±0.67	1.5±0.65	1.53±0.65	1.51±0.66	0.92
Location of target lesions[a]					
Left main stem	16(3.0)	12(2.1)	17(3.1)	12(2.4)	0.67
LAD	389(72.2)	424(73.4)	390(71.4)	345(68.2)	0.28
LCX	209(38.8)	207(35.8)	203(37.2)	205(40.5)	0.42
RCA	201(37.3)	234(40.5)	223(40.8)	210(41.5)	0.51
NO. of stents per patient[b]	2.14±1.33	2.12±1.22	2.13±1.24	2.21±1.26	0.74
Total stent length per patient[b]	50.0±34.2	49.5±32.1	49.7±32.5	51.2±32.8	0.89
Stent Diameter (mm)[b]	3.01±0.44	3.12±0.43	3.06±0.43	3.04±0.45	0.57

RDW: red blood cell distribution width, LVEF: Left ventricular ejection fraction, LAD: left anterior descending artery, LCX: left circumflex artery, RCA: right coronary artery.
[a]: n(%),
[b]: mean ± SD.

During the mean follow-up of period 29 months, higher baseline levels of RDW were associated with an increased risk of all-cause death, cardiac death, MACCE, and stent thrombosis. When participants were grouped according their baseline RDW quartile the graded relationship between RDW and all-cause death, cardiac death and stent thrombosis remained. The incidence of cardiac death and MACCE was significantly higher in quartile 4 than in quartiles 1 and 2 (p<0.005). The incidence of all-cause death and stent thrombosis in quartile 4 was significantly higher than in quartiles 1, 2, and 3 (p<0.001). There were no significant differences among the groups with respect to the incidence of nonfatal MI, nonfatal stroke, any revascularization (PCI/CABG), or in-stent restenosis (Table 3).

Univariate and multivariate analysis

Results of univariate analyses for all-cause death are shown in Table 4, and for MACCE are shown in table 5. Multivariate Cox regression analysis was used to assess the predictors of all-cause death and MACCE. After adjusting for age, gender, diabetes mellitus, hypertension, peripheral vascular disease, number of vessels treated, multi-vessel disease, prior MI, GFR, LVEF, number of stents implanted, total stent length, and stent diameter, the continuous variable RDW was significantly associated with both an increased incidence of all-cause death (HR = 1.37, 95% CI = 1.15–1.62, P<0.001) and MACCE (HR = 1.21, 95% CI = 1.04–1.39, P = 0.013) (Table 6). The Kaplan–Meier curve revealed that the cumulative survival rate in quartiles 2, 3, and 4 was lower than in quartile1 (P<0.001, Figure 1) and the cumulative survival rate free from MACCE in quartiles 3 and 4 was lower than in quartiles 1 and 2 (p = 0.002, Figure 2)

Discussion

Variability in the size of circulating red cells (anisocytosis) is reflected by RDW, which is routinely reported by automated laboratory equipment for complete blood counts. Although its use has been limited to narrowing the differential diagnosis of anemia,

Table 3. Clinical events from PCI until discharge and end of follow up by Quartile of RDW.

	Quartile 1 (n = 539)	Quartile 2 (n = 578)	Quartile 3 (n = 546)	Quartile 4 (n = 506)	P value
In-hospital events, n (%)					
Death	1(0.2)	2(0.35)	5(0.9)	8(1.6)	0.047
Any MI	4(0.7)	2(0.35)	5(0.9)	5(1.0)	0.61
MACE(death or MI)	5(0.9)	4(0.7)	10(1.8)	13(2.6)	0.049
Follow-up(cumulated events), n (%)					
All cause death	11(2.0)	12(2.1)	14(2.6)	29(5.7)	0.001
Cardiac death	6(1.1)	9(1.6)	12(2.2)	19(3.8)	0.02
Nonfatal MI	6(1.1)	5(0.9)	9(1.6)	11(2.2)	0.31
Nonfatal stroke	6(1.1)	4(0.7)	11(2.0)	9 (1.8)	0.26
MACCE(death/MI/stroke)	21(3.9)	22(3.8)	30(5.5)	42(8.3)	0.004
Major bleeding	4(0.7)	3(0.5)	3(0.5)	6(1.2)	0.57
Any revascularization(PCI/CABG)	46(8.5)	42(7.3)	41(7.5)	41(8.1)	0.86
TVR	24(4.5)	21(3.6)	27(5.0)	22(4.3)	0.71
In-stent restenosis	35(6.5)	29(5.0)	35(6.4)	27 (5.3)	0.64
Stent thrombosis(definite/probable)	7(1.3)	8(1.4)	13(2.4)	27(5.3)	0.00

RDW: red blood cell distribution width, MACE: major adverse cardiac event, MI: myocardial infarction, PCI: percutaneous coronary intervention, CABG: coronary artery bypass graft, MACCE: major cardiovascular or cerebral adverse events, TVR: target vessel revascularization.

mounting evidence suggests that there are additional roles for this measurement.

The present study demonstrates that high RDW is an independent marker of a long-term adverse prognosis in non-anemic patients with CAD treated with DES. We found this association to be independent of multiple potential confounding factors, including age, renal insufficiency, diabetes mellitus, peripheral vascular disease, prior MI, and left ventricular dysfunction. Additionally, a higher RDW is also associated with a higher incidence of both cardiac death and stent thrombosis (definite/probable) during follow-up. The results suggest that RDW may be used to stratify patients treated with DES according to long term-risk. Therefore, particularly as no additional cost is incurred, closer evaluation of RDW is recommended.

Poludasu et al. [4] reported that RDW is an independent predictor of mortality in patients undergoing PCI; however, the association was only observed between RDW and mortality and their sample size was relatively small. In addition, their study included just those patients who had undergone bolus-only treatment with glycoprotein IIb/IIIa antagonists and excluded patients who had ST-segment elevation MI, some of whom may have been high risk, thus reducing the study's ability to demonstrate any relationship. Fatemi et al. [6] demonstrated the additive value of RDW in a larger cohort of patients undergoing coronary angiography. The cohort did not include consecutive patients and follow-up was limited to 1 year. Recently, in a larger cohort study, Arbel et al. [14] investigated the prognostic value of RDW in patients after PCI. They excluded patients with acute heart failure and did not analyze the association between RDW and in-hospital events. In addition, they did not collect data about bleeding events or stent thrombosis. Furthermore, all three studies included patients treated with either DES or BMS, and grouped anemic and non-anemic patients together in the analysis. Our study demonstrates the importance of RDW for both in-hospital and long-term clinical outcome in a large Chinese population treated with DES. Many studies have reported that the use of DES

is associated with improved prognosis after PCI [15,16], and DES is widely used in current clinical practice (over 98% of patients were treated with DES at our center). While DES and BMS share the same "hard" clinical endpoints, DES is associated with a significant reduction in both the incidence of in-stent restenosis and the need for revascularization of the target lesion. However, there is a concern over stent thrombosis after DES insertion, such that it is necessary to evaluate the prognostic value of RDW in patients treated with DES. Our data confirm and extend the prognostic significance of an elevated RDW in patients with heart failure [17], in patients post-MI without heart failure [1], and in those with chest pain referred to coronary angiography [5].

Anemia and hemoglobin levels are strong predictors for the development of CVD and mortality in a variety of populations [18–19]. A community cohort study [9] revealed that an elevated RDW is significantly associated with all-cause mortality in people without anemia, but that the mortality risks for patients with anemia are the same regardless of RDW. Furthermore, the association between high RDW and death not attributable to CVD was only significant in subjects without anemia. Recently, in a large community-based cohort study, Arbel et al. [20] found that, over a 5-year follow-up, elevated RDW levels were significantly associated with increased risk of cardiovascular morbidity and all-cause mortality in patients with and without anemia, the association being stronger in the latter group. The reasons for the differences between these studies were unclear; therefore, to exclude the effect of anemia on clinical outcome, our study only enrolled those patients without anemia. Our results show that elevated RDW is significantly associated with not only all-cause mortality and cardiac death but also the incidence of MACCE.

An interesting finding in our study was that higher RDW is also associated with an increased incidence of stent thrombosis, but not with major bleeding. Fatenmi et al. [21] reported that elevated RDW is an independent predictor of bleeding after PCI. In a study of 3845 adult outpatients, RDW was shown to have an

Table 4. Univariate Analysis for All-Cause death.

	HR	95%CI	P value
RDW (per 1%)	1.4	1.23–1.59	0.000
Age(years)	1.07	1.04–1.09	0.000
Gender(male)	0.857	0.52–1.41	0.55
Hypertension	1.07	0.66–1.72	0.79
Dyslipidemia	0.89	0.51–1.56	0.68
Total cholesterol	0.82	0.64–1.10	0.13
HDL-C	0.64	0.26–1.56	0.33
LDL-C	0.93	0.71–1.23	0.63
Triglyceride	0.82	0.63–1.08	0.16
Heart failure	0.96	0.45–2	0.9
Diabetes mellitus	1.8	1.08–3.0	0.024
Peripheral vascular disease	8.1	1.1–58	0.038
Prior myocardial infarction	1.88	0.99–3.59	0.055
Cerebral vascular disease	1.3	0.55–3.38	0.51
Number of treated vessels	1.16	0.89–1.60	0.371
number of stents implanted	1.16	0.97–1.48	0.11
total stent length	1.01	1.001–1.015	0.031
the stent diameter	0.72	0.41–1.26	0.69
STEMI	1.26	0.73–2.2	0.41
history of revascularization	2.38	0.68–11.4	0.22
GFR (ml·min^{-1}·1.73 m^{-2})	0.93	0.86–0.98	0.013
Multi-vessel disease	2.97	1.84–4.79	0.000
LVEF≤40%	3.09	2.11–4.52	0.000
DAPT	0.41	0.18–0.95	0.038
Use of ACEI/ARB	1.01	0.62–1.62	0.97
Use of β-blockers	0.66	0.40–1.07	0.96
Use of statins	0.75	0.30–1.86	0.53
Use of insulin	1	0.37–2.76	0.99

RDW: Red blood cell distribution width, HR: hazard ratio, CI: confidence interval, HDL-C: High density lipidprotein cholesterol, LDL-C: Low density lipidprotein cholesterol, STEMI: ST-segment elevation myocardial infarction, GFR: glomerular filtration rate, LVEF: Left ventricular ejection fraction, DAPT: dual antiplatelet therapy, ACEI: Angiotensin-converting enzyme inhibitor, ARB: angiotensin recptor blocker.

independent, graded relationship with high-sensitivity C-reactive protein (CRP) and erythrocyte sediment rate [22]. The relationship between inflammation, (which predisposes to thrombosis) and bleeding risk is a paradox whose cause may lie in the complex pathology of patients in poor health [23]. Frail, elderly patients have relatively higher levels of CRP, factor VIII, and D-dimer [24] and increased levels of activated factors VII, IX, and X [25], leading to an increased likelihood of thrombosis. Arbel et al. [14] reported that elevated RDW is associated with abnormal bone marrow function, which itself is related to increased platelet activation, aggregation and thrombus activation [26]. Further studies are required to confirm the association between RDW and major bleeding and to explore its underlying mechanisms of action.

It remains unclear how elevated RDW is associated with adverse cardiovascular outcomes. Chronic subclinical inflammation is the pathway most frequently hypothesized, as it is a well-established entity preceding de novo cardiovascular events and can adversely influence erythropoiesis by a variety of mechanisms, including direct myelosuppression of erythroid precursors, reduced renal erythropoietin production and iron bioavailability, increased erythropoietin resistance in erythroid precursor cell lines, the promotion of cell apoptosis, and RBC membrane deformability, all factors that might increase anisocytosis [27]. Recently, in a large cohort study included of 8513 adults participants (age>20 years) with no pre-existing cardiovascular disease, Veeranna et al. [28] found that RDW but not hs-CRP is associated with mortality from coronary heart disease. This suggests that mechanisms other than inflammation may be involved, for example oxidative stress, tissue hypoxia or endothelial dysfunction [29–30]. Furthermore, higher RDW may reflect enhanced erythropoiesis resulting from elevated circulating levels of neurohumoral mediators [2]. There is increasing evidence that the existence of a chronic inflammatory state and neurohumoral activation both contribute to adverse clinical outcomes in patients with acute coronary syndrome [5,31,32]. Additionally, an elevated RDW is often seen in patients with extensive comorbidities and therefore correlates with increased morbidity and mortality.

Our study also has some limitations that should be considered. First, this was a post-hoc observational analysis, and therefore we cannot rule out the possibility of residual confounding. However, the hypothesis that RDW levels are associated with adverse

Table 5. Univariate Analysis for MACCE.

	HR	95%CI	P value
RDW (per 1%)	1.27	1.13–1.42	0.000
Age(years)	1.056	1.04–1.08	0.000
Gender(male)	1.10	0.74–1.63	0.65
Hypertension	1.17	0.81–1.69	0.401
Dyslipidemia	1.034	0.66–1.62	0.88
Total cholesterol	0.97	0.81–1.16	0.75
HDL-C	0.83	0.44–1.56	0.56
LDL-C	1.034	0.85–1.26	0.74
Triglyceride	1.03	0.0.91–1.16	0.69
Heart failure	0.75	0.403–1.4	0.37
Diabetes mellitus	1.43	1.02–2.85	0.044
Peripheral vascular disease	5.01	0.699–35.86	0.075
Prior myocardial infarction	1.46	0.85–2.51	0.17
Cerebral vascular disease	0.913	0.401–2.08	0.83
Number of treated vessels	1.28	1.06–1.56	0.013
number of stents implanted	1.13	0.99–1.29	0.07
total stent length	1.01	1.001–1.011	0.25
the stent diameter	0.45	0.28–0.73	0.001
STEMI	1.204	0.79–1.84	0.39
history of revascularization	1.58	0.64–7.4	0.35
GFR(ml·min^{-1}·1.73 m^{-2})	0.94	0.81–0.99	0.021
Multi-vessel disease	2.29	1.58–3.33	0.000
LVEF≤40%	1.92	1.35–2.74	0.000
DAPT	0.54	0.21–0.86	0.035
Use of ACE-I/ARB	0.975	0.68–1.41	0.89
Use of β-blockers	0.644	0.44–0.94	0.021
Use of statins	0.57	0.31–1.06	0.076
Use of insulin	0.87	0.38–1.98	0.74

RDW: Red blood cell distribution width, HR: hazard ratio, CI: confidence interval, HDL-C: High density lipidprotein cholesterol, LDL-C: Low density lipidprotein cholesterol, STEMI: St-segment elevation myocardial infarction, GFR: glomerular filtration rate, LVEF: Left ventricular ejection fraction, DAPT: dual antiplatelet therapy, ACEI: Angiotensin-converting enzyme inhibitor, ARB: angiotensin recptor blocker.

Table 6. Multivariate analysis for All-Cause Mortality and MACCE.

	HR	95% CI	P value
All-Cause death			
RDW (per 1%)	1.37	1.15–1.62	0.000
Age(years)	1.064	1.03–1.1	0.000
GFR ml·min^{-1}·1.73 m^{-2})	0.91	0.78–0.96	0.037
Multi-vessel disease	2.15	1.19–3.85	0.011
LVEF≤40%	2.89	1.96–4.25	0.000
MACCE			
RDW (per 1%)	1.21	1.04–1.39	0.013
Age(years)	1.053	1.03–1.08	0.000
GFR(ml·min^{-1}·1.73 m^{-2})	0.94	0.86–0.98	0.005
LVEF≤40%	1.58	1.08–2.31	0.02

RDW: Red blood cell distribution width, HR: hazard ratio, CI: confidence interval, MACCE: Major cardiovascular or cerebral adverse events, GFR: glomerular filtration rate, LVEF: Left ventricular ejection fraction.

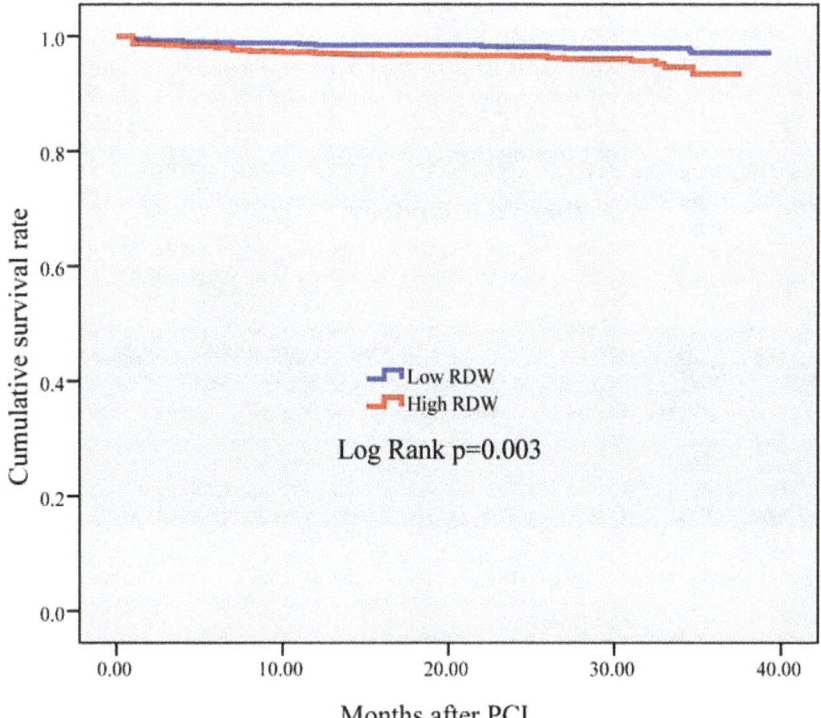

Figure 1. The Kaplan–Meier curve of all-cause mortality rate. It is significantly higher in quartiles 2, 3, and 4 than in quartile 1 (P<0.001).

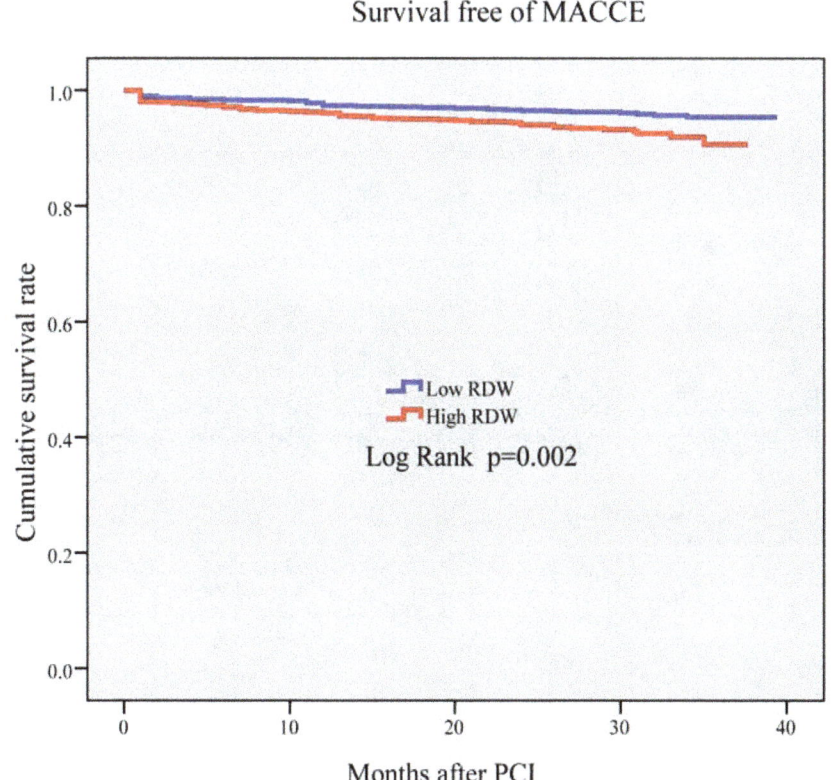

Figure 2. The Kaplan–Meier curve of MACCE rate. It is significantly higher in quartiles 3 and 4 than in quartiles 1 and 2 (p = 0.002).

outcomes was formulated before analyses began, reducing the risk of drawing spurious conclusions. Second, this was a single-center study. Patients who were referred for urgent PCI or who were in cardiogenic shock were excluded from this study, because their incidence of adverse outcomes is known to be high; therefore, there might be selection bias. Baseline characteristics across the RDW groups were reasonably consistent but adjustments had to be made for certain differences, in particular the increased prevalence of comorbidity in patients with a high RDW. Despite the adjustment for multiple variables, it is possible that residual unrecognized confounding variables influenced the observed differences in outcome between the groups. As with all analyses of observational data, this study cannot distinguish causality from association. Third, factors such as iron, vitamin B12, and folate were not measured in this study. Finally, because hs-CRP was not measured in most of patients, we were unable to analyze the relationship between RDW and hs-CRP.

Conclusion

In conclusion, our study demonstrates that elevated RDW predicts an increased risk of adverse clinical outcomes, both in hospital and over the long-term, in non-anemic patients with CAD treated with DES, and that RDW has the potential for use as a tool for risk stratification. Further studies are required to confirm the association between RDW and clinical outcomes and to elucidate its underlying mechanism.

Author Contributions

Conceived and designed the experiments: HMY TWS XJZ DLS YYD YDW JYZ LL LSZ. Performed the experiments: HMY TWS XJZ. Analyzed the data: HMY TWS XJZ DLS YYD YDW JYZ LL LSZ. Contributed reagents/materials/analysis tools: HMY TWS XJZ DLS YYD YDW JYZ LL LSZ. Wrote the paper: HMY YDW.

References

1. Tonelli M, Sacks F, Arnold M, Moye L, Davis B, et al. (2008) Relation Between Red Blood Cell Distribution Width and Cardiovascular Event Rate in People With Coronary Disease. Circulation 117: 163–168.
2. Allen LA, Felker GM, Mehra MR, Chiong JR, Dunlap SH, et al. (2010) Validation and potential mechanisms of red cell distribution width as a prognostic marker in heart failure. J Card Fail 16: 230–238.
3. Dabbah S, Hammerman H, Markiewicz W, Aronson D (2010) Relation between red cell distribution width and clinical outcomes after acute myocardial infarction. Am J Cardiol 105: 312–317.
4. Poludasu S, Marmur JD, Weedon J, Khan W, Cavusoglu E (2009) Red cell distribution width (RDW) as a predictor of long-term mortality in patients undergoing percutaneous coronary intervention. Thromb Haemost 102: 581–587.
5. Cavusoglu E, Chopra V, Gupta A, Battala VR, Poludasu S, et al. (2010) Relation between red blood cell distribution width (RDW) and all-cause mortality at two years in an unselected population referred for coronary angiography. Int J Cardiol 141: 141–146.
6. Fatemi O, Paranilam J, Rainow A, Kennedy K, Choi J, et al. (2013) Red cell distribution width is a predictor of mortality in patients undergoing percutaneous coronary intervention. J Thromb Thrombolysis 35: 57–64.
7. Lippi G, Filippozzi L, Montagnana M, Salvagno GL, Franchini M, et al. (2009) Clinical usefulness of measuring red blood cell distribution width on admission in patients with acute coronary syndrome. Clin Chem Lab Med 47: 353–357.
8. Wang YL, Hua Q, Bai CR, Tang Q (2011) Relationship between red cell distribution width and short-term outcomes in acute coronary syndrome in a Chinese population. Intern Med 50: 2941–2945.
9. Chen PC, Sung FC, Chien KL, Hsu HC, Su TC, et al. (2010) Red Blood Cell Distribution Width and Risk of Cardiovascular Events and Mortality in a Community Cohort in Taiwan. Am J Epidemiol 171: 214–220.
10. (1968) Nutritional anaemias. Report of a WHO scientific group. World Health Organ Tech Rep Ser 405: 5–37.
11. Cockcroft DW, Gault MH (1976) Prediction of creatinine clearance from serum creatinine. Nephron 16: 31–41.
12. (2007) Clinical End Points in Coronary Stent Trials: A Case for Standardized Definitions. Circulation 115: 2344–2351.
13. Lincoff AM, Bittl JA, Harrington RA, Feit F, Kleiman NS, et al. (2003) Bivalirudin and provisional. glycoprotein IIb/IIIa blockade compared with heparin and planned glycoprotein IIb/IIIa blockade during percutaneous coronary intervention: the REPLACE-2 randomized trial. JAMA 289: 853–63.
14. Arbel Y, Birati EY, Finkelstein A, Halkin A, Berliner S, et al. (2013) Red cell distribution width and 3-year outcome in patients undergoing cardiac catheterization. J Thromb Thrombolysis [Epub ahead of print]
15. Moses JW, Leon M B, Popma JJ,Fitzgerald PJ, Holmes DR, et al. (2008) Sirolimus -eluting stents versus standard stents in patients with stenosis in a native coronary artery. N Engl J Med 349: 1315–1323.
16. Stone GW, Ellis SG, Cox DA, Hermiller J, O'Shaughnessy C, et al. (2004) A polymer-based, paclitaxel-eluting stent inpatients with coronary artery disease. N Engl J Med. 350: 221–231.
17. Felker GM, Allen LA, Pocock SJ, Shaw LK, McMurray JJ, et al. (2007) Red cell distribution width as a novel prognostic marker in heart failure: data from the CHARM Program and the Duke Databank. J Am Coll Cardiol 50: 40–47.
18. Sabatine MS, Morrow DA, Giugliano RP, Burton PB, Murphy SA, et al. (2005) Association of hemoglobin levels with clinical outcomes in acute coronary syndromes. Circulation 111: 2042–2049.
19. Zakai NA, Katz R, Hirsch C, Shlipak MG, Chaves PH, et al. (2005) A prospective study of anemia status, hemoglobin concentration, and mortality in an elderly cohort: the Cardiovascular Health Study. Arch Intern Med 165: 2214–2220.
20. Arbel Y, Weitzman D, Raz R, Steinvil A, Zeltser D, et al. (2014) Red blood cell distribution width and the risk of cardiovascular morbidity and all-cause mortality. A population-based study. Thromb Haemost 111: 300–307.
21. Fatemi O, Torguson R, Chen F, Ahmad S, Badr S, et al. (2013) Red cell distribution width as a bleeding predictor after percutaneous coronary intervention. Am Heart J 166: 104–9.
22. Lippi G, Targher G, Montagnana M, Salvagno GL, Zoppini G, et al. (2008) Relation between red blood cell distribution width and inflammatory biomarkers in a large cohort of unselected outpatients. Arch Pathol Lab Med 133: 628–32.
23. Klein LW, Arrieta-Garcia C (2012) Is patient frailty the unmeasured confounder that connects subacute stent thrombosis with increased periprocedural bleeding and increased mortality? J Am Coll Cardiol 59: 1760–1762.
24. Walston J, McBurnie MA, Newman A, Tracy RP, Kop WJ, et al. (2002) Frailty and activation of the inflammation and coagulation systems with and without clinical comorbidities: results from the Cardiovascular Health Study. Arch Intern Med 162: 2333–2341.
25. Mari D, Mannucci PM, Coppola R, Bottasso B, Bauer KA, et al. (1995) Hypercoagulability in centenarians: the paradox of successful aging. Blood 85: 3144–3149.
26. Abou-Saleh H, Yacoub D, Theoret JF, Gillis MA, Neagoe PE, et al. (2009) Endothelial progenitor cells bind and inhibit platelet function and thrombus formation. Circulation 120: 2230–2239.
27. Weiss G, Goodnough LT (2005) Anemia of chronic disease. N Engl J Med 352: 1011–1023.
28. Veeranna V, Zalawadiya SK, Panaich S, Patel KV, Afonso L (2013) Comparative analysis of red cell distribution width and high sensitivity C-reactive protein for coronary heart disease mortality prediction in multi-ethnic population:Findings from the 1999–2004 NHANES. Int J Cardiol 168: 5156–5161
29. Minetti M, Agati L, Malorni W (2007) The microenvironment can shift erythrocytes from a friendly to a harmful behavior: pathogenetic implications for vascular diseases. Cardiovasc Res 75: 21–8.
30. Patel KV, Ferrucci L, Ershler WB, Longo DL, Guralnik JM (2009) Red blood cell distribution width and the risk of death in middle-aged and older adults. Arch Intern Med 169: 515–23.
31. Nabais S, Losa N, Gaspar A, Rocha S, Costa J, et al. (2009) Association between red blood cell distribution width and outcomes at six months in patients with acute coronary syndromes. Rev Port Cardiol 28: 905–924.
32. Ward MJ, Boyd JS, Harger NJ, Deledda JM, Smith CL, et al. (2012) An automated dispensing system for improving medication timing in the emergency department. World J Emerg Med 3: 102–107.

17

Deep Sea Water Prevents Balloon Angioplasty-Induced Hyperplasia through MMP-2: An *In Vitro* and *In Vivo* Study

Pei-Chuan Li[1], Chun-Hsu Pan[2], Ming-Jyh Sheu[1]*, Chin-Ching Wu[3], Wei-Fen Ma[4], Chieh-Hsi Wu[1,2,5]*

1 School of Pharmacy, China Medical University, Taichung, Taiwan, 2 College of Pharmacy, Taipei Medical University, Taipei, Taiwan, 3 Department of Public Health, China Medical University, Taichung, Taiwan, 4 School of Nursing, China Medical University, Taichung, Taiwan, 5 Department of Biological Science and Technology, China Medical University, Taichung, Taiwan

Abstract

Major facts about the development of restenosis include vascular smooth muscle cells (VSMCs) proliferation and migration. A previous study showed that in vitro treatment with magnesium chloride has the potential to affect the proliferation and migration of VSMCs. Magnesium is the major element in deep sea water (DSW) and is a biologically active mineral. It is unclear whether DSW intake can prevent abnormal proliferation and migration of VSMCs as well as balloon angioplasty-induced neointimal hyperplasia. Thus, we attempted to evaluate the anti-restenotic effects of DSW and its possible molecular mechanisms. Several concentrations of DSW, based on the dietary recommendations (RDA) for magnesium, were applied to a model of balloon angioplasty in SD rats. The results showed that DSW intake markedly increased magnesium content within the vascular wall and reduced the development of neointimal hyperplasia. The immunohistochemical analysis also showed that the expression of proteins associated with cell proliferation and migration were decreased in the balloon angioplasty groups with DSW supplement. Furthermore, in vitro treatment with DSW has a dose-dependent inhibitory effect on serum-stimulated proliferation and migration of VSMCs, whose effects might be mediated by modulation of mitogen-activated protein kinase (MAPK) signaling and of the activity of matrix metalloproteinase-2 (MMP-2). Our study suggested that DSW intake can help prevent neointimal hyperplasia (or restenosis), whose effects may be partially regulated by magnesium and other minerals.

Editor: Francis Miller Jr., University of Iowa, United States of America

Funding: This research was supported by a grant from China Medical University (CMU-10142624). The funders had no role in study design, data collection and analysis, decision to publish, or preparation of the manuscript.

Competing Interests: The authors have declared that no competing interests exist.

* E-mail: chhswu@mail.cmu.edu.tw (CHW); soybean13mtdtw@gmail.com (MJS)

Introduction

As a result of balloon injury-induced restenosis, VSMCs predominantly undergoes proliferation and migration [1].The restenotic process is initiated by balloon angioplasty-induced vascular injury, which stimulates VSMCs to migrate from the medial layer to the intimal layer of the vessel wall and eventually results in uncontrolled neointimal hyperplasia. Accordingly, to inhibit proliferation and migration of VSMCs is valuable of reducing balloon injury-induced angioplasty.

The major problem of mineral deficiencies caused by the recent westernization of lifestyles and eating habits has resulted in so-called lifestyle-related illnesses such as coronary heart disease, angina pectoris, myocardial infarct, stroke, cancer, and diabetes [2,3]. Moreover, Mg^{2+} is hypothesized to play an important role as a protective element of cardiovascular diseases. [4], And, intake of Mg^{2+} has been linked with reduction of blood pressure, triglyceride, and arrhythmia from congestive heart failure patients [5]. Recently, Sternberg *et al.* indicated that appropriate concentration of magnesium chloride has a potential in vitro effect to reduce cell viability of the primary VSMCs while increasing the viability of endothelial

cells isolated from human coronary artery [6]. Additionally, the experimental analysis from a cDNA microarray also demonstrated that numerous genes for growth factors and their receptors, as well as for cell cycle and apoptosis-related signaling cascades, have been markedly up- or down regulated within these magnesium-chloride-treated VSMCs compared to those of endothelial cells [6]. Mg^{2+} deficiency has been associated with hypertrophic vascular remodeling, however, this phenomenon could be attenuated by Mg^{2+} supplementation [7]. From abovementioned results, Mg^{2+} deficiency might attribute to the development of hypertension, atherosclerosis, and other cardiovascular diseases (CVD).

Recently, deep sea water (DSW) has received increasing attention for the treatment or prevention of various diseases, such as hyperlipidemia, atherosclerosis, hypertension, and dermatitis [8–11]. DSW is characteristically clear, sanitary, and plentiful in nutrients, being especially rich in Mg^{2+}, Ca^{2+} and K^+. [8,12]. In this study, we investigate if DSW is of beneficial to prevent balloon angioplasty-induced neointima hyperplasia and its possible pharmacological mechanisms.

Materials and Methods

Materials and DSW Preparation

The DSW was obtained from the Pacific Ocean (662 m in depth) and was then concentrated. This concentrated DSW (#LC-90K) with a hardness of 400,000 mg/L was supplied by Taiwan Yes Deep Ocean Water Co., Ltd. (Hualien, Taiwan) The DSW composition contained Mg^{2+}, K^+, Ca^{2+}, sodium (Na^{2+}), chloride (Cl^-), lithium (Li^+), and other trace elements. In this experiment, the Mg^{2+} content in DSW was 96,000 mg/L, as mentioned in our previous study [8].

Balloon Injury Animal Model

Male Sprague Dawley (SD) rats (250~300 g) were bought from BioLASCO Taiwan Co. Ltd (Taipei, Taiwan). Surgery was performed under zoletil anesthesia. The rats were randomly divided into six groups (n = 6/group): (A) sham control+water, (B) balloon angioplasty (BA)+water, (C) BA+37.2 mg Mg^{2+}/kg/day ($MgCl_2$), (D) BA+0.1x DSW (equivalent to 3.72 mg Mg^{2+}/kg/day), (E) BA+1x DSW (equivalent to 37.2 mg Mg^{2+}/kg/day), and (F) BA+2x DSW (equivalent to 74.4 mg Mg^{2+}/kg/day).Reverse osmotic (RO) water was considered as water administration in groups A and B. The magnesium RDA for adult males is 360 mg/day (6 mg/kg/day); thus, the dosage of Mg^{2+} for SD rats is 37.2 mg Mg^{2+}/kg/day conversed by using a U.S. FDA dose conversion table, human equivalent dose. The dosages of DSW applied in the present study were calculated as the equivalent content of Mg^{2+} RDA for rats. Therefore, 1x DSW was defined as water-diluted DSW containing 37.2 mg/kg of Mg^{2+}. The rats were given DSW for 4 weeks and performance angioplasty during the second week. Balloon injury-induced neointimal hyperplasia was carried out using a balloon embolectomy catheter as described previously [13] A Fogarty 2F (Becton-Dickinson, Franklin Lakes, NJ, USA) embolectomy balloon catheter was inserted into the left external carotid artery and inflated under the same pressure (1.3 kg/cm^2) for three consecutive three times. All animal care followed the institutional animal ethical guidelines of China Medical University. The experimental protocol was approved by the Committee on Animals Research, China Medical University (Permit Number: 100-49N).

Histopathological Analysis

The left carotid artery was excised and fixed in 4% paraformaldehyde solution for 24 h, processed for paraffin embedding, and cut into 7-mm transverse sections. The tissue sections were stained with a routine H&E staining. Five random sections of each studied sample were randomly selected and measured with image analysis software (Image J) to calculate the neointima-to-media area ratio (N/M ratio).

For immunohistochemical analysis, the DAKO system (#K0679; Dako LSAB+System-HRP, DAKO, Tokyo, Japan) was used. It employs a refined avidin-biotin technique in which a biotinylated secondary antibody reacts with several peroxidase-conjugated streptavidin molecules. The tissue sections were rehydrated and immersed in 3% H_2O_2 for 30 minutes to quench endogenous peroxidase, and then all sections were further incubated in 1% bovine serum albumin (BSA; Sigma Aldrich, USA) for 1 h at 25 °C. Next, the sections were incubated with a primary antibody against either matrix metalloproteinase-2 (MMP-2; #ab37150; Abcam, USA) or proliferating cell nuclear antigen (PCNA; #sc-56; Santa Cruz, USA) overnight at 4°C. Then, the sections were incubated for 30 min at room temperature with the biotinylated link antibody and peroxidase-labeled streptavidin. For signal detection, the sections were incubated with the ready-to-use DAB substrate-chromogen solution for 5 min according to the manufacturer's protocol and then washed with distilled water. Finally, sections were counterstained with hematoxylin for 3 min, followed by washing with distilled water and mounting with a hard-set media (Assistant-Histokitt, Germany). Negative controls consisted of primary antibody replaced with buffer-specific antibody absorbed with antigen. Photomicrographs were taken with a microscope (Olympus, Japan) at 200-fold magnification.

Blood Biochemical Assay

The serum was collected in non-heparinized tubes and centrifuged at 3000 rpm for 10 min at 4°C. The blood biochemical parameters including alanine aminotransferase (ALT), aspartate aminotransferase (AST), alkaline phosphatase (ALP), γ-glutamyltransferase (GGT), and the serum concentration of Mg^{2+} were measured by ChenChang Co., Ltd. (Taichung, Taiwan).

Measurement of Arterial Magnesium Content

The harvested arterial tissues were rinsed with deionized water and dried in 60°C for 24 h, followed by measuring tissue weight. Approximately 0.5 g of dried tissue was further digested with 5 mL of 65% HNO_3 (E. Merck, Darmstadt, Germany). The determine sample was diluted to 10 mL with deionized water. We measured the tissue Mg^{2+} levels with quadruple inductively coupled plasma mass spectrometry (ICP-MS) (Elan DRC II, Perkin Elmer, USA), which is capable of detecting metals and several non-metals at concentrations as low as one part per trillion (ppt). The sample is typically introduced into the ICP plasma as an aerosol, either by aspirating a liquid or by using a laser to directly convert solid samples into an aerosol, and the elements are converted into ions that are then brought into the mass spectrometer via the interface cones [14].

Cell Culture

VSMCs were prepared from thoracic aortas of 4–6-week old male SD rats. Cells at passages 3–6 were applied for the present study. The cells were cultured in Dulbecco's modified Eagle's medium (DMEM) with 10% FBS, 100 units/L penicillin, and 100 mg/L streptomycin. The cells were maintained at 37°C in a humidified 5% CO_2 incubator.

Cell Proliferation Assay (MTT Assay)

VSMCs were seeded and cultured in 96-well plates (8×10^3 cells/well) for 24 h. VSMCs were then treated with $MgCl_2$ or different concentration of DSW for 24 h. For in vitro experiments, $MgCl_2$ or different concentration of DSW were added to medium containing 15% FBS. MTT assay was used to determine VSMCs proliferation: 100 μl of 3-(4, 5-Dimethylthiazol-2-yl)-2, 5-Diphenyltetrazolium Bromide (MTT) (0.5 mg/ml) was added to each well and incubated at 37°C for 4 h, after which the supernatant was removed and replaced with DMSO (100 μl). The product was quantified by measuring absorbance at 590 nm. The cell viability was normalized to the values from the group that received 15% FBS alone.

Cell Migration Assay (Transwell Assay)

Cell migration of VSMCs (5×10^3 cells/well) was analyzed with wound-healing and transwell assays in 24-well multiwall plates (8.0 μm pore-size, Greiner bio-one, USA) for 24 h. The cell were loaded into the upper compartment and incubated for 18 h. Afterward, the cells were collected from the lower membrane and

Table 1. Effect of blood biochemical parameters of SD rats after 4-week treatment with sham + water, BA + water, BA + MgCl$_2$, and DSW.

Groups Parameters	Sham	BA	BA	BA	BA	BA
	water	water	MgCl$_2$	0.1x DSW	1x DSW	2x DSW
ALT	58.0±8.9	49.5±2.9	49.50±3.6	42.7±3.4	50.8±6.2	49.0±8.9
AST	152.7±51.2	123.3±19.1	103.8±12.5	114.8±23.6	115.0±9.2	104.8±20.4
ALP	573.3±36.8	877.2±17.9*	765.0±19.9*	506.3±45.6	657.8±11.9	778.5±19.4*
GGT	0.6±0.2	0.9±0.9	1.6±0.3	0.5±0.3	0.57±0.3	1.1±0.6
Initial Mg^{2+}	21.9±2.4	24.5±4.2	21.1±0.9	22.4±2.1	23.4±2.6	24.3±1.8
Final Mg^{2+}	23.1±2.0	22.5±2.7	23.0±1.2	20.7±1.8	20.7±1.4	20.0±2.5

Concentration unit: U/L. BA, balloon angioplasty; RDA, recommended dietary allowances; ALT, alanine aminotransferase; AST, aspartate aminotransferase; ALP, alkaline phosphatase; GGT, γ-glutamyltransferase. Mg^{2+}: serum Mg^{2+} concentration. Values are mean ± SEM, n = 6.
*$p < 0.05$ compared to sham + water.

fixed with 70% methanol. VSMCs were stained with Giemsa and hematoxylin solutions and then counted under a microscope (Olympus, Japan) in five randomly selected squares per well. The cell migration was normalized to the values of the 15% FBS group.

Western Blotting Assay

Cells were lysed in PRO-PREP protein extraction solution (iNtRON Biotechnology, Sungnam, South Korea). Protein samples (30 μg/well) were electrophoresed via 10% SDS-PAGE. Gels were transferred onto polyvinylidene difluoride (PVDF) membranes (BioTrace™, USA). Then, blotted membranes were blocked in 5% non-fat milk for 1 h and incubated overnight at 4°C with the primary antibodies against phospho-mitogen-activated protein kinase (p-MEK1/2) (#9121; Cell Signaling, UK.), extracellular signal-regulated kinase 1/2 (p-ERK 1/2) (#sc7383; Santa Cruz Biotechnology, U.S.A.), or matrix metalloproteinase-2 (MMP-2) (#ab37150; Abcam, U.S.A.). After incubation with appropriate secondary antibodies (Gene Tex, U.S.A.) for 1 h, blot were incubated with enhanced chemiluminescent (ECL) reagent, and the images were acquired using an ImageQuant LAS4000 gel imager (Fujifilm Life Science, Tokyo, Japan). Data were quantified by densitometry using Multi Gauge v 3.0 software (Fujifilm Life Science, Tokyo, Japan). The protein expression was normalized to β-actin and 15% FBS group was considered as 100%.

Gelatinase Zymography

The culture medium was harvested to examine gelatinase activity via 10% SDS–PAGE gel electrophoresis with 0.2% gelatin under non-reducing conditions. After electrophoresis, gelatinases were renatured by rinsing the gel in 2.5% Triton X-100 at 25°C for 30 min, and then activated in reaction buffer (2 M Tris-HCl, pH 8.0, 1 M CaCl$_2$, and 1% NaN$_3$) at 37°C for 24 h. The gels were stained with 0.25% Coomassie brilliant blue R250 for 90 min and destained with 10% acetic acid in 40% methanol. Gelatinase activity was evident as a clear band against the blue background of stained gelatin. Bands were quantified by densitometry using Multi Gauge v3.0 software. The MMP-2 activity was normalized to 15% FBS group.

Data Analysis

Experiments data were presented as the mean ± SEM. Data were analyzed using one-way ANOVA. Calculations were carried out using SPSS for Windows, version 18.0 (SPSS, Chicago, USA).Differences were considered significant at $P < 0.05$.

Results

Changes of Blood Biochemical Parameters and Body Weight

SD rats were grouped into six experimental conditions, as described in the Experimental Methods. All rats were weighed and blood samples were taken once a week during the 4-week study. Numerous blood biochemical parameters including ALT, AST, ALP, and GGT, and the serum concentration of Mg^{2+} were examined and shown in Table 1. Our data showed that ALP level was significantly increased on BA + water group, however, DSW-treated groups reversed the results (Table 1). Our results shown no dramatic change of the serum Mg^{2+} concentration between DSW-treated and sham + water group (Table 1). Furthermore, no significant differences were found between the DSW-treated (0.1x, 1x and 2x DSW) and control groups (sham + water or BA + water group) in body weights after 4-week study (Data not shown). Our results suggested the dosages of DSW had no marked toxic effects, such as hepatotoxicity.

Effect of DSW on Balloon Angioplasty-induced Neointimal Hyperplasia

The rat carotid arteries were harvested for examination of the histopathological changes in the arterial wall at the 14th day after balloon injury (Figure 1). The balloon angioplasty procedure (BA + water group; Figure 1B) induced significant induced neointimal hyperplasia compared to the sham control (Sham + water group; Figure 1A). The N/M ratio of the positive control (BA + water group) was increased more than 10-fold over that of the sham group (Figure 1G). However, the groups co-treated with DSW (Figure 1D–1F) possessed markedly less development of neointima formation, in a dose-dependent pattern (Figure 1G). Similarly, MgCl$_2$ treatment also reduced balloon injury-induced neointimal hyperplasia (Figures 1C and 1G). These results demonstrated that DSW intake exhibits an inhibitory effect on the prevention of neointimal hyperplasia, implying that ionic magnesium may participate in some of the mechanisms of DSW on prevention of neointima formation. The sections were also evaluated by immunohistochemistry to detect MMP 2 (MMP-2; Figure 1H), a cell migration and invasion-associated protein, and PCNA (PCNA; Figure 1I), a cell proliferation marker. MMP-2 expression was

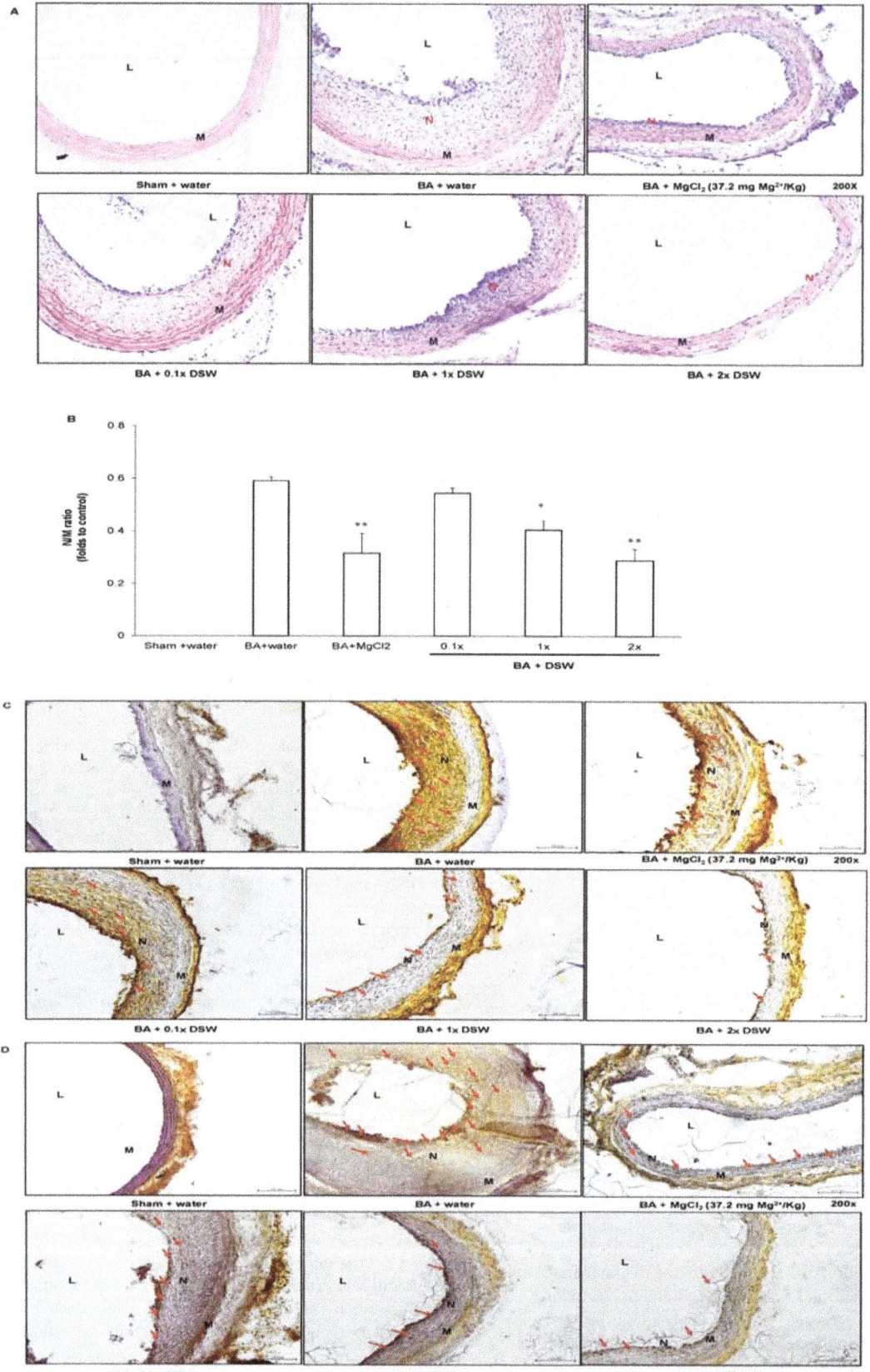

Figure 1. Inhibitory effect of DSW on balloon angioplasty-induced neointimal hyperplasia. Tissue sections from rat carotid arteries were further stained with hematoxylin-eosin to observe the thickness of neointimal layer of arterial wall (A–F). The expression levels of MMP-2 and PCNA proteins were detected with immunohistopathological analysis (H and I). The images were acquired by microscopy at 200-fold magnification. The

manifestation of vessel restenosis was presented as the ratio of neointima- to-media area (N/M ratio). L, lumen; N, neointima layer; M, media layer. Red arrow is protein experssion.*$P<0.05$, and **$P<$ compared with BA + water group, respectively.

visibly induced in the neointimal and media layers after balloon angioplasty, and pretreatment with DSW (1x and 2x DSW) and $MgCl_2$ could reduce the expression of MMP-2 within the vessel wall. A similar trend was visible for PCNA expression after supplementation with DSW or $MgCl_2$.

Magnesium Content of the Carotid Artery

The rat carotid arteries were harvested to examine the changes of Mg^{2+} content within arterial wall at the 14th day after balloon injury (Figure 2). Mg^{2+} content of the tissue samples were measured by quadruple ICP-MS. DSW intake clearly increased the magnesium content within balloon-injured arteries in a dose-dependent manner when compared to the BA + water group. However, the level of serum Mg^{2+} did not significantly change in any group in the present study (data not shown). Ma et al. showed a negative association between serum Mg^{2+} and average carotid wall thickness [15]. Pascal et al. have shown that Mg^{2+} deficiency modifies the mechanical properties of the common carotid artery, thereafter attribute to cardiovascular diseases (CVD) development in animal models [16]. They also indicated that long-term oral supplementation of magnesium improves blood lipid composition and suppresses the development of atherosclerotic lesions in rodents [17,18]. In contrast, Ferre et al. showed that low Mg^{2+} accelerated atherogenesis by stimulating inflammation and oxidative stress in endothelial cells, suggesting a possible mechanism linked to CVD [19]. Wolf et al. also reported that Mg^{2+} deficiency could be associated with inflammatory responses resulting into the increased cytokines levels, which cause an oxidative damage in endothelial cells [20]. Especially, low intracellular Mg^{2+} may be linked with the development of thrombus formation [21].

Effects of DSW on VSMC Proliferation and Migration

VSMCs isolated from rat thoracic aorta were used to determine the effects of DSW on cell proliferation and migration. First, magnesium chloride was applied, to verify that it inhibits VSMC growth. We found that 15% FBS can significantly stimulate cell proliferation of VSMCs when compared with the low serum

stimulation (0.5% FBS) group, and treatment of magnesium chloride can block half of the VSMC proliferation at the concentration of 6.62 mM (Figure 3A). Next, the effects of DSW on cell growth of VSMCs were examined. DSW treatment could markedly decrease cell viability in a dose-dependent manner (Figure 3B). The 1x DSW and $MgCl_2$ groups showed similar growth inhibition on VSMCs. However, treatment with 2x DSW was more inhibitory toward cell growth than was the $MgCl_2$ treatment ($P<0.05$).

The transwell assay was used to explore the effect of DSW treatment on VSMC migration (Figure 4). High serum stimulation (15% FBS) can induce cell migration of VSMCs (Figure 1B) compared with the 0.5% FBS group (Figure 1A), and this migration-promoting effect can be markedly attenuated by incubation with DSW, in a dose-dependent manner (Figure 1D–1F). Administration with magnesium chloride showed a similar reduction of serum-stimulated VSMC migration (Figure 1C).

DSW Inhibits Proliferation and Migration-associated Proteins on VSMCs

MAPK signaling pathways are associated with cardiovascular disease [22].The signaling of the MAPK pathway plays an important role in the regulation of VSMC proliferation [23]. The first member of this family was ERK1/2, which is activated after MEK1/2 phosphorylation. It has been reported that ERK1/2 activation is rapidly induced after arterial injury and might trigger a series of molecular events leading to neointima hyperplasia [24]. The inhibition of the ERK pathway by drugs or gene therapy has been demonstrated to reduce neointimal hyperplasia [25]. Phosphorylation MEK and ERK1/2 were both examined at multiple time points including 5 min., 10 min., and 20 min. And the levels of phosphorylation MEK and ERK1/2 showed obvious changes at 20 min (Figure 5A–5C). DSW inhibited ERK phosphorylation and MEK phosphorylation, which are associated with VSMC proliferation and migration (Figures 5A, 5B and 5C). Besides, MMPs is evident to regulate the migration activity of VSMCs in in vitro and in vivo studies [26]. The results from gelatin

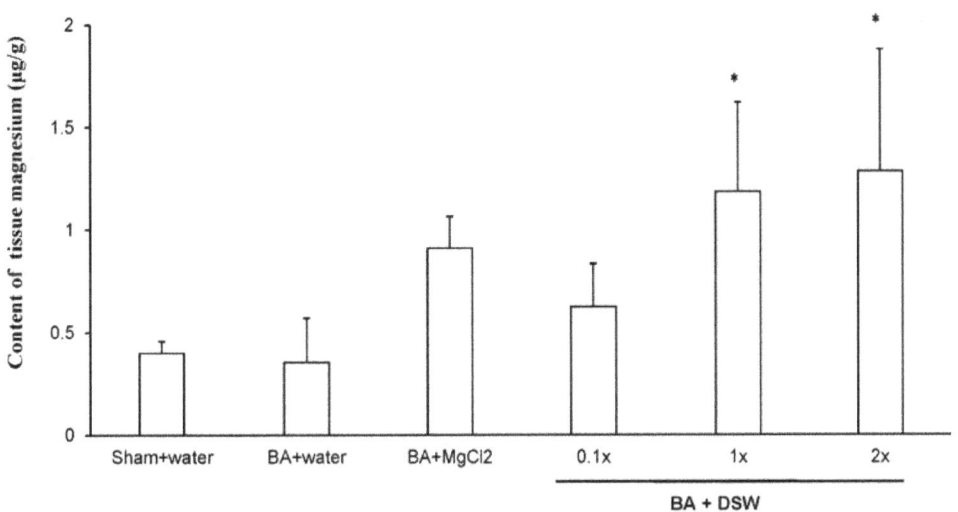

Figure 2. Differences in magnesium content in the balloon-injured carotid artery. *$P<0.05$ compared with BA + water group, respectively.

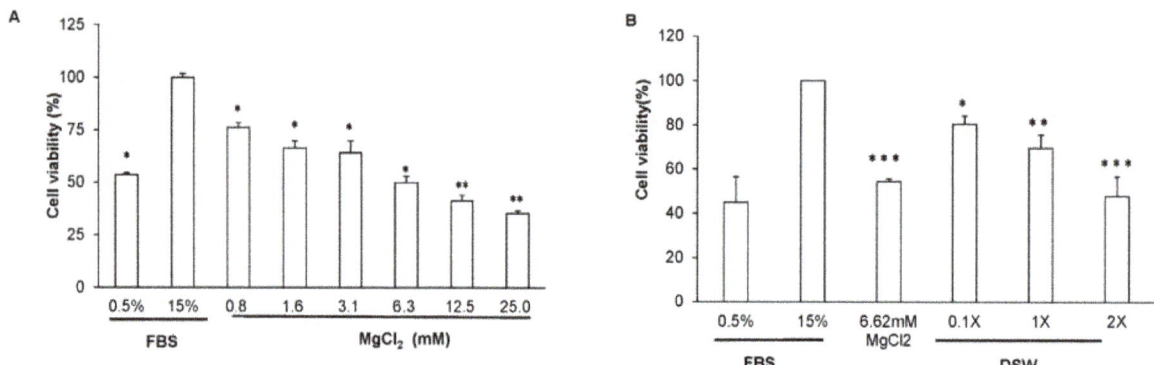

Figure 3. DSW-induced regulation of VSMC viability. Cell viability was analyzed with the MTT proliferation assay. One-fold (1x) DSW was defined as water-diluted DSW containing a level of magnesium equal to that of the magnesium chloride used in the present experiment. The results are shown as % of the control. *$P<0.05$, and **$P<0.01$ compared with the 15% FBS-treated group, respectively.

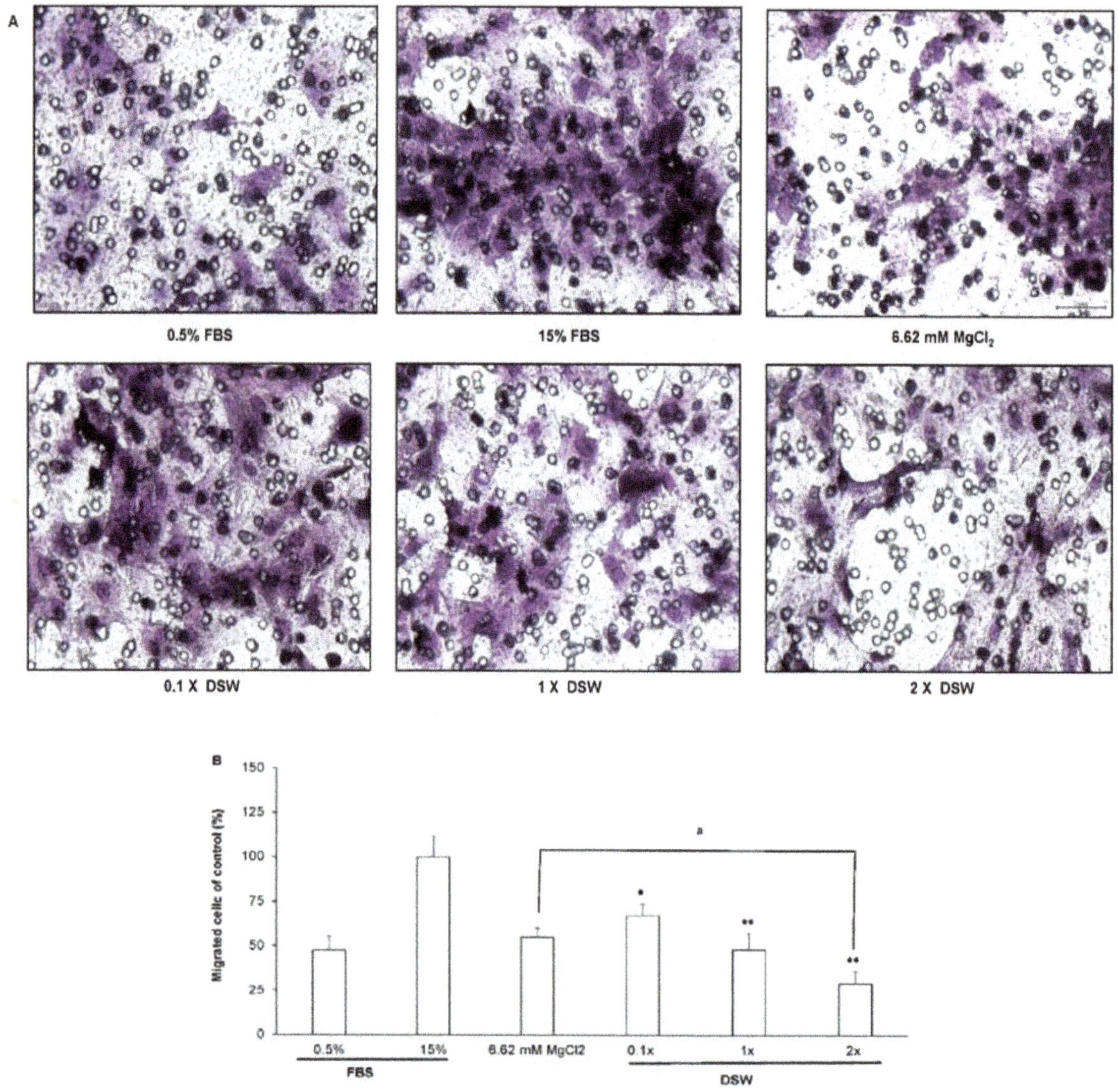

Figure 4. Effects of DSW on VSMC migration. Cell migration was analyzed with transwell assays. The images were taken at 400-fold magnification. The 1x DSW was defined as water-diluted DSW containing the same level of magnesium as the magnesium chloride used in the present experiment. The results are shown as % of the control (15% FBS).*$P<0.05$, and **$P<0.01$ compared with the 15% FBS-treated group, respectively. #$P<0.05$ compared with the MgCl$_2$-treated group.

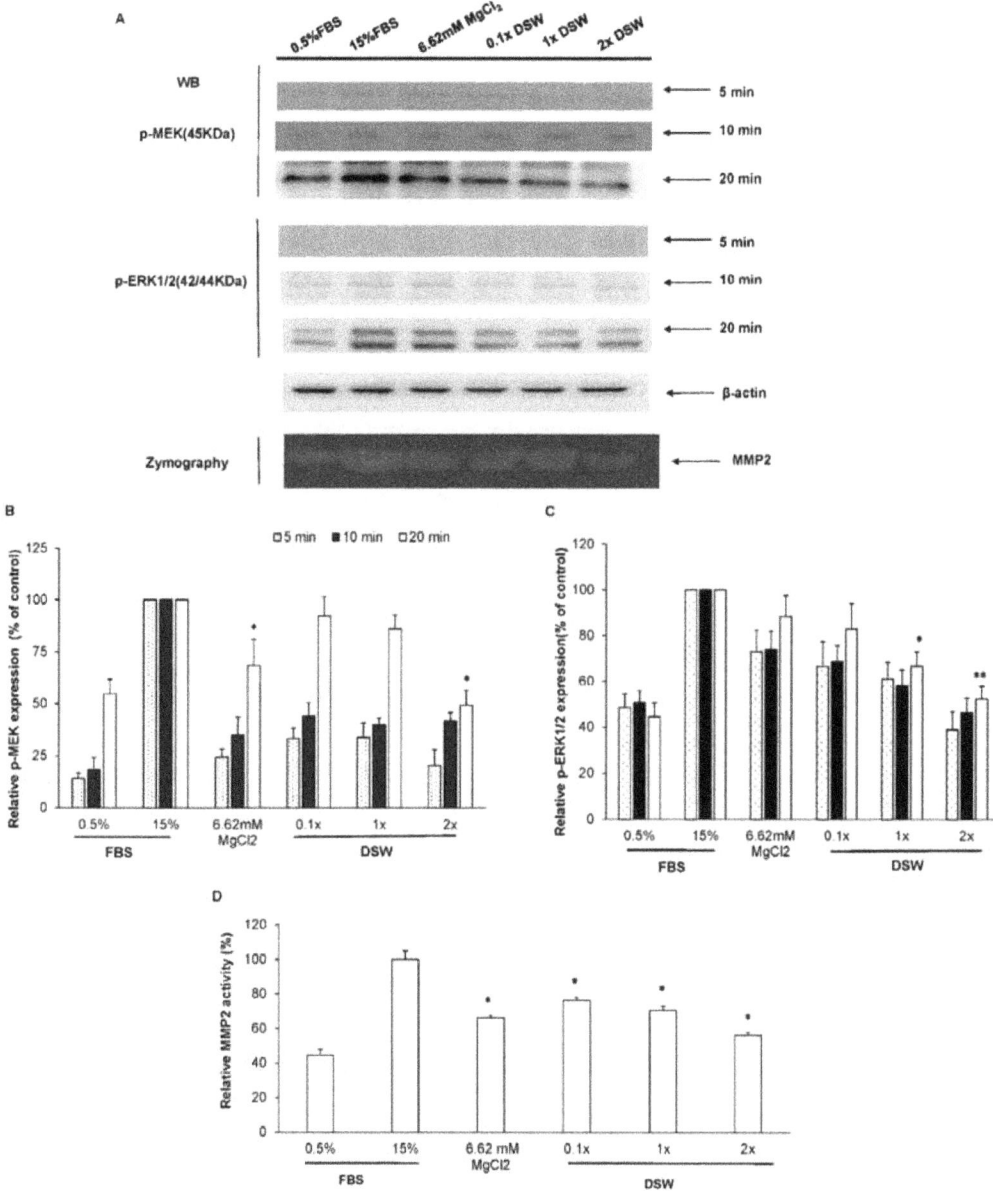

Figure 5. Molecular regulation by DSW of cell growth and migration of VSMCs. Inhibitory mechanisms of DSW on cell growth- and migration-associated proteins were analyzed by using the methods of Western blot (WB) and gelatin zymography. Beta-actin was used as internal control in Western blot. The results are shown as % of the control (15% FBS). The MMP-2 activity was normalized to the values of the 15% FBS group. *$P<0.05$, and **$P<0.01$ compared with the 15% FBS-treated group, respectively.

zymography suggested that high-dose DSW decreased MMP-2 activity by half compared with that from the 15% FBS group (Figures 5A and 5D), implying that the DSW-induced inhibitory effect on the migration of VSMCs may be partially mediated by decreased MMP-2 activity.

Our results shown that DSW intake inhibits VSMCs proliferation and migration in addition to its anti-restenosis effect in *in vivo* study.

Discussion and Conclusions

As a rich source of inorganic nutrients such as Mg^{2+}, Ca^{2+}, and other minerals (K^+, Cu^{2+}, Mn^{2+}, Zn^{2+}, B^-, and Li^+), DSW in particular hold the attention in CVD studies.

As a Ca^{2+} channel blocker, Mg^{2+} is a key role regulating the reduction of Ca^{2+} release and thus reduce vascular resistance [7]. Fruits and vegetables, diets rich in K^+, Mg^{2+}, and Ca^{2+} is associated with lower incidence of and mortality of CVD [27]. Moreover, Turgut *et al.* reported that supplementation of Mg^{2+} can efficiently reduce the carotid intimal hyperplasia [28]. Mg^{2+} has been found to have many effects, including improving hyperlipidemia and preventing the development of atherosclerosis [12,29]. Patients with hypertension or hyperlipidemia orally supplied with calcium or Mg^{2+} showed reductions in blood pressure and serum levels of total cholesterol [30].

DSW has shown an inhibitory effect on serum-stimulated proliferation and migration of VSMCs *via* inhibition of ERK1/2-MAPK signaling and MMP-2 activation (Figure 5). Based on our previous report [8]. Mg^{2+} is found to be the most abundant ingredient in DSW. Mg^{2+} regulates a MAPK signaling cascade, which is associated with VSMCs cell growth, cell division, migration, and proliferation [6,31]. Accordingly, our data showed no change on intracellular Mg^{2+} (Table 1); however, tissues Mg^{2+} concentration has been significantly increased after DSW supplementation (Figure 2). Touyz *et.al.* showing modulation of cell growth by Mg^{2+} was due to influx/efflux Mg^{2+} and regulation of MEK and ERK1/2 [32]. Intracellular Mg^{2+} is delicately regulated in the physiological condition and because Mg^{2+} plays important roles in multiple physiological reactions, even small changes in VSMCs, markedly affects intracellular signaling transduction regulating VSMCs [3,32].

Our data demonstrated that $MgCl_2$ only slightly regulated phosphorylation MEK, with no effects on phosphorylation ERK1/2 (Figure 5). However, DSW significantly affect the MAPK signaling molecules including MEK and ERK1/2 (Figure 5). Therefore, minerals other than $MgCl_2$ in DSW such as Cu^{2+}, Zn^{2+}, Li^+, B^- and Mn in DSW might have certain effects on VSMCs proliferation and migration *via* regulating MEK and ERK1/2. Cu/Zn-superoxide dismutase (SOD) and Mn-SOD were found to play important roles in scavenging of superoxide [33]. Zhuyao *et al.* also reported that lithium chloride inhibited VSMCs proliferation, migration and alleviated balloon injury-induced angioplasty [34]. Furthermore, Nielsen *et al.* reported that boron prevents Mg^{2+} loss in humans [19]. Therefore, Mg^{2+} may not be sole strategy of dealing injury from balloon angioplasty. However, DSW is a well-balanced mineral resource, and dietary supplementation with DSW provides more beneficial functions than magnesium chloride alone in the prevention of cardiovascular diseases, such as restenosis and atherogenesis.

As DSW will be applied for the nutrition supplement, therefore, the toxic effect has to be concerned. Our results showed that levels of ALT, and AST on DSW-treated groups had no significant change compared to Sham + water or BA + water groups (Table 1). Previously, Sheu *et.al.* reported that drinking DSW for a long period (56 days; 8 weeks) demonstrated no liver toxicity in rats and rabbits [8]. Fu *et.al.* showed that fed a 6 months DSW diet decreased serum total and low-density lipoprotein in a human study [35]. Based on the abovementioned, DSW could be a potential functional supplement to prevent balloon angioplasty-induced neointimal formation.

Acknowledgments

Specially appreciate from the Medical Research Core Facilities Center, Office of Research & Development at China medical University, Taichung, Taiwan, R.O.C. on data analysis. We are grateful to Taiwan Yes Deep Ocean Water Co., Ltd. (Hualien, Taiwan) for offering samples of the DSW mineral concentrate.

Author Contributions

Conceived and designed the experiments: PCL CHP CHW. Performed the experiments: PCL CCW CHP. Analyzed the data: PCL MJS WFM CHW. Wrote the paper: PCL.

References

1. Weintraub WS (2007) The pathophysiology and burden of restenosis. The American journal of cardiology 100: 3K–9K.

2. Ford ES, Mokdad AH (2003) Dietary magnesium intake in a national sample of US adults. J Nutr 133: 2879–2882.

3. Shechter M (2010) Magnesium and cardiovascular system. Magnes Res 23: 60–72.

4. Chakraborti S, Chakraborti T, Mandal M, Mandal A, Das S, et al. (2002) Protective role of magnesium in cardiovascular diseases: a review. Molecular and cellular biochemistry 238: 163–179.

5. Zhang W, Iso H, Ohira T, Date C, Tamakoshi A (2012) Associations of dietary magnesium intake with mortality from cardiovascular disease: the JACC study. Atherosclerosis 221: 587–595.

6. Sternberg K, Gratz M, Koeck K, Mosterz J, Begunk R, et al. (2012) Magnesium used in bioabsorbable stents controls smooth muscle cell proliferation and stimulates endothelial cells in vitro. Journal of biomedical materials research Part B, Applied biomaterials 100: 41–50.

7. Cunha AR, Umbelino B, Correia ML, Neves MF (2012) Magnesium and vascular changes in hypertension. International journal of hypertension 2012: 754250.

8. Sheu MJ, Chou PY, Lin WH, Pan CH, Chien YC, et al. (2013) Deep Sea Water Modulates Blood Pressure and Exhibits Hypolipidemic Effects via the AMPK-ACC Pathway: An in Vivo Study. Marine drugs 11: 2183–2202.

9. Katsuda S, Yasukawa T, Nakagawa K, Miyake M, Yamasaki M, et al. (2008) Deep-sea water improves cardiovascular hemodynamics in Kurosawa and Kusanagi-Hypercholesterolemic (KHC) rabbits. Biological & pharmaceutical bulletin 31: 38–44.

10. Hataguchi Y, Tai H, Nakajima H, Kimata H (2005) Drinking deep-sea water restores mineral imbalance in atopic eczema/dermatitis syndrome. European journal of clinical nutrition 59: 1093–1096.

11. Yoshioka S, Hamada A, Cui T, Yokota J, Yamamoto S, et al. (2003) Pharmacological activity of deep-sea water: examination of hyperlipemia prevention and medical treatment effect. Biological & pharmaceutical bulletin 26: 1552–1559.

12. Miyamura M, Yoshioka S, Hamada A, Takuma D, Yokota J, et al. (2004) Difference between deep seawater and surface seawater in the preventive effect of atherosclerosis. Biological & pharmaceutical bulletin 27: 1784–1787.

13. Chien YC, Huang GJ, Cheng HC, Wu CH, Sheu MJ (2012) Hispolon attenuates balloon-injured neointimal formation and modulates vascular smooth muscle cell migration via AKT and ERK phosphorylation. Journal of natural products 75: 1524–1533.

14. Murphy KE, Vetter TW (2013) Recognizing and overcoming analytical error in the use of ICP-MS for the determination of cadmium in breakfast cereal and dietary supplements. Analytical and bioanalytical chemistry 405: 4579–4588.

15. Ma J, Folsom AR, Melnick SL, Eckfeldt JH, Sharrett AR, et al. (1995) Associations of serum and dietary magnesium with cardiovascular disease, hypertension, diabetes, insulin, and carotid arterial wall thickness: the ARIC study. Atherosclerosis Risk in Communities Study. J Clin Epidemiol 48: 927–940.

16. Laurant P, Hayoz D, Brunner H, Berthelot A (2000) Dietary magnesium intake can affect mechanical properties of rat carotid artery. The British journal of nutrition 84: 757–764.

17. Rasmussen HS, Aurup P, Goldstein K, McNair P, Mortensen PB, et al. (1989) Influence of magnesium substitution therapy on blood lipid composition in patients with ischemic heart disease. A double-blind, placebo controlled study. Arch Intern Med 149: 1050–1053.

18. Saito N, Okada T, Moriki T, Nishiyama S, Matsubayashi K (1990) Long-Term Drinking of Mgcl2 Solution and Arterial Lesions in Female Shrsp. Annals of the New York Academy of Sciences 598: 527–529.

19. Ferre S, Mazur A, Maier JA (2007) Low-magnesium induces senescent features in cultured human endothelial cells. Magnes Res 20: 66–71.

20. Wolf FI, Trapani V, Simonacci M, Ferre S, Maier JA (2008) Magnesium deficiency and endothelial dysfunction: is oxidative stress involved? Magnes Res 21: 58–64.

21. Shechter M, Merz CN, Rude RK, Paul Labrador MJ, Meisel SR, et al. (2000) Low intracellular magnesium levels promote platelet-dependent thrombosis in patients with coronary artery disease. Am Heart J 140: 212–218.

22. Muslin AJ (2008) MAPK signalling in cardiovascular health and disease: molecular mechanisms and therapeutic targets. Clin Sci (Lond) 115: 203–218.

23. Indolfi C, Coppola C, Torella D, Arcucci O, Chiariello M (1999) Gene therapy for restenosis after balloon angioplasty and stenting. Cardiology in review 7: 324–331.

24. Lai K, Wang H, Lee WS, Jain MK, Lee ME, et al. (1996) Mitogen-activated protein kinase phosphatase-1 in rat arterial smooth muscle cell proliferation. The Journal of clinical investigation 98: 1560–1567.

25. Gennaro G, Menard C, Michaud SE, Deblois D, Rivard A (2004) Inhibition of vascular smooth muscle cell proliferation and neointimal formation in injured arteries by a novel, oral mitogen-activated protein kinase/extracellular signal-regulated kinase inhibitor. Circulation 110: 3367–3371.

26. Newby AC (2006) Matrix metalloproteinases regulate migration, proliferation, and death of vascular smooth muscle cells by degrading matrix and non-matrix substrates. Cardiovasc Res 69: 614–624.

27. Houston M (2011) The role of magnesium in hypertension and cardiovascular disease. Journal of clinical hypertension 13: 843–847.

28. Turgut F, Kanbay M, Metin MR, Uz E, Akcay A, et al. (2008) Magnesium supplementation helps to improve carotid intima media thickness in patients on hemodialysis. International urology and nephrology 40: 1075–1082.

29. Griendling KK, Rittenhouse SE, Brock TA, Ekstein LS, Gimbrone MA Jr, et al. (1986) Sustained diacylglycerol formation from inositol phospholipids in angiotensin II-stimulated vascular smooth muscle cells. The Journal of biological chemistry 261: 5901–5906.

30. Kawano Y, Yoshimi H, Matsuoka H, Takishita S, Omae T (1998) Calcium supplementation in patients with essential hypertension: assessment by office, home and ambulatory blood pressure. Journal of Hypertension 16: 1693–1699.

31. Ikari A, Atomi K, Kinjo K, Sasaki Y, Sugatani J (2010) Magnesium deprivation inhibits a MEK-ERK cascade and cell proliferation in renal epithelial Madin-Darby canine kidney cells. Life Sci 86: 766–773.

32. Touyz RM (2003) Role of magnesium in the pathogenesis of hypertension. Mol Aspects Med 24: 107–136.

33. McIntyre M, Bohr DF, Dominiczak AF (1999) Endothelial function in hypertension: the role of superoxide anion. Hypertension 34: 539–545.

34. Wang Z, Zhang X, Chen S, Wang D, Wu J, et al. (2013) Lithium chloride inhibits vascular smooth muscle cell proliferation and migration and alleviates injury-induced neointimal hyperplasia via induction of PGC-1alpha. PloS one 8: e55471.

35. Fu ZY, Yang FL, Hsu HW, Lu YF (2012) Drinking deep seawater decreases serum total and low-density lipoprotein-cholesterol in hypercholesterolemic subjects. J Med Food 15: 535–541.

18

The Incidence and Prevalence of Diabetes Mellitus and Related Atherosclerotic Complications in Korea: A National Health Insurance Database Study

Bo Kyung Koo[1,2], Chang-Hoon Lee[1], Bo Ram Yang[3,4], Seung-sik Hwang[5], Nam-Kyong Choi[3,6]*

1 Department of Internal Medicine, Seoul National University College of Medicine, Seoul, Republic of Korea, 2 Department of Internal Medicine, Boramae Medical Center, Seoul, Republic of Korea, 3 Division of Clinical Epidemiology, Medical Research Collaborating Center, Seoul National University College of Medicine, Seoul, Republic of Korea, 4 Department of Preventive Medicine, Seoul National University College of Medicine, Seoul, Republic of Korea, 5 Department of Social and Preventive Medicine, Inha University School of Medicine, Incheon, Republic of Korea, 6 Institute of Environmental Medicine, Seoul National University Medical Research Center, Seoul, Republic of Korea

Abstract

Aims/Introduction: The incidence and prevalence of type 2 diabetes mellitus (T2DM) and related macrovascular complications in Korea were estimated using the Health Insurance Review and Assessment (HIRA) database from 2007–2011, which covers the claim data of 97.0% of the Korean population.

Materials and Methods: T2DM, coronary artery disease (CAD), cerebrovascular disease (CVD), and peripheral artery disease (PAD) were defined according to ICD-10 codes. We used the Healthcare Common Procedure Coding System codes provided by HIRA to identify associated procedures or surgeries. When calculating incidence, we excluded cases with preexisting T2DM within two years before the index year. A Poisson distribution was assumed when calculating 95% confidence intervals for prevalence and incidence rates.

Results: The prevalence of T2DM in Korean adults aged 20–89 years was 6.1–6.9% and the annual incidence rates of T2DM ranged from 9.5–9.8/1,000 person-year (PY) during the study period. The incidence rates of T2DM in men and women aged 20–49 years showed decreasing patterns from 2009 to 2011 ($P<0.001$); by contrast, the incidence in subjects aged 70–79 years showed increased patterns from 2009 to 2011 ($P<0.001$). The incidence rates of CAD and CVD in patients newly diagnosed with T2DM were 18.84/1,000 PY and 11.32/1,000 PY, respectively, in the year of diagnosis. Among newly diagnosed individuals with T2DM who were undergoing treatment for PAD, 14.6% underwent angioplasty for CAD during the same period.

Conclusions: Our study measured the national incidences of T2DM, CAD, CVD, and PAD, which are of great concern for public health. We also confirmed the relatively higher risk of CAD and CVD newly detected T2DM patients compared to the general population in Korea.

Editor: Mohammad Ebrahim Khamseh, Institute of Endocrinology and Metabolism, Islamic Republic Of Iran

Funding: This study was supported by a grant from the Korean Diabetes Association (2012-228). The funders had no role in study design, data collection and analysis, decision to publish, or preparation of the manuscript.

Competing Interests: The authors have declared that no competing interests exist.

* Email: likei1@snu.ac.kr

Introduction

The International Diabetes Federation (IDF) estimated the global prevalence of diabetes to be 151 million in 2000 [1] and 285 million in 2010 [2]. The IDF reported that 366 million people had diabetes in 2011, and this prevalence is expected to rise to 552 million by 2030 [3].

From 1970 to 2000, the prevalence of diabetes in South Korea increased about threefold [4], and 9–10% of Korean adults aged ≥30 years were affected by the disease in the early 2000s according to the Korea National Health and Nutritional Examination Survey (KNHANES) [4,5]. The prevalence of diabetes is also increasing in other developing countries in Asia such as China [6–8] and India [9]. A recent meta-analysis reported that the prevalence of diabetes mellitus has significantly increased in China from 2.6% to 9.7% from 2000–2010 [10]. In developed countries such as Canada [11] and the US [12], the prevalence of diabetes has also continued to increase throughout the past decade. However, the prevalence in the Korean population remained stable over the same time period [13]. Furthermore, we recently reported that the prevalence of diabetes among women aged 30–59 years decreased trend from 2001 to

2010 [14]. It is important to investigate the incidence and prevalence of diabetes mellitus in the Korean population considering these trends in the occurrence of diabetes mellitus; however, current data are limited. In one community-based cohort study that included individuals in Korea between the ages of 40 and 79, the annual incidence of type 2 diabetes (T2DM) ranged from 1.33% to 5% [15].

The National Health Insurance (NHI) program in Korea was initiated in 1977 and achieved universal coverage of the population by 1989. The Health Insurance Review and Assessment (HIRA) service covers the claims of 97.0% of the population in Korea; those of the remaining 3% of the population are covered by the Medical Aid Program. Accordingly, the HIRA database contains information on almost the entirety of the insurance claims, including prescribed medications and procedures, for the Korean population of approximately 50 million [16]. The present study was performed to estimate the incidence and prevalence of T2DM and related macrovascular complications in the entire population of South Korea using the NHI claims database from 2007–2011.

Methods

Data collection

We used HIRA data recorded between 1 January 2007 and 31 December 2011. The HIRA database contains information on all insurance claims for about 97.0% of the population in Korea [16]. The HIRA service provided the data after de-identification, and the data included age, gender, diagnosis, date of hospital visits, drug prescriptions received during inpatient and outpatient visits, hospital admissions, medical procedures, and emergency department visits. Drug information included the brand name, generic name, prescription date, and duration and route of administration. Diagnoses were coded according to the International Classification of Disease (10th revision; ICD-10). The study was approved by the Boramae Medical Center Institutional Review Board.

Study population

The prevalence of T2DM patients aged 20–89 years from 2008 to 2010 was defined according to the following eligibility criteria: the presence of (1) at least two claims per year under ICD-10 codes E11–14 or (2) at least one claim per year for the prescription of anti-diabetic medication (under ICD-10 codes E11–14) [17]. Anti-diabetic medications included insulin, sulfonylureas, metformin, thiazolidinediones, α-glucosidase inhibitors, and meglitinides. We excluded patients with type 1 diabetes mellitus, defined as those who (i) were prescribed insulin without oral anti-diabetic agents and (ii) had at least one claim under the ICD-10 code E10, without the code E11, from 2007 to 2011 (**Figure 1**).

The incidence of T2DM from 2009 to 2011 was defined in individuals who met either of the selection criteria, (1) or (2), for estimating the prevalence of T2DM. We subsequently excluded those with preexisting diabetes two or more years before the study period, which included patients who were diagnosed with any type of diabetes mellitus (E10–14) or prescribed any anti-diabetic medications from 1 January 2007 to 31 December 2008 (**Figure 1**). Accordingly, the remaining cases had at least two years and up to five years of disease-free status before the index date and were regarded as the new cases of T2DM. The date of the earliest claim regarding T2DM on or after 1 January 2009 was defined as the index date. The index date was regarded as the incident time, and the patient was counted as a new case in that year.

Case definition of cardiovascular and cerebrovascular disease

To investigate the incidence and prevalence of macrovascular complications in subjects with T2DM, we constructed sub-cohorts of new cases of T2DM and pre-existing cases of T2DM in 2009 (**Figure 1**). The incidence and prevalence, from 2009 to 2011, of macrovascular diabetic complications such as coronary artery disease (CAD), cerebrovascular disease (CVD), and peripheral artery disease (PAD), and amputation were analyzed within the sub-cohorts. CAD and CVD were identified by the following criteria, respectively: (1) medical claim(s) (including all inpatient hospital, outpatient hospital, medical visit, and emergency room claims) with the corresponding disease as the principal diagnosis, or additional diagnosis with an ICD-10 diagnosis code, or procedure code (**Table S1** in File S1) and (2) medical claim(s) regarding any percutaneous intervention or surgery associated with the corresponding disease. We used the Healthcare Common Procedure Coding System codes provided by the HIRA service to identify the associated procedure or surgery (**Table S1** in File S1). Since previous studies showed that the current diagnostic coding system is less sensitive to and less specific for PAD-related illness and treatment than for CAD or CVD [18,19], we did not use ICD-10 diagnosis codes for defining PAD; instead, we defined PAD using claims regarding any percutaneous intervention or surgery associated with PAD (**Table S1** in File S1). Amputation of lower extremities was identified by the medical claim(s) that included an associated procedure or surgery code (**Table S1** in File S1). To detect new cases of CAD, CVD, and PAD in each cohort year, we eliminated all cases with a claim for each corresponding disease that occurred before the cohort year. Hospital admissions for CAD, CVD, and PAD were measured using inpatient claims with the principal diagnosis of the corresponding disease.

Statistical analysis

All data were analyzed using SAS software version 9.3 (SAS Institute, Inc., Cary, NC, USA). Age- and gender-specific annual prevalence rates of T2DM from 2008 to 2010 were calculated by dividing the number of T2DM patients by the Korean population from the 2010 Population and Housing Census (**Table S2** in File S1) [20]. The age- and gender-specific annual incidence rate (number of new cases in each year/number of individuals at risk), and the person-time incidence rate, for 2009–2011, were calculated. The number of individuals at risk in each year was calculated using the following equation [the total population from the 2010 Census − (number of pre-existing cases in the previous year + half of the number of new cases in the year)]; this equation which assumes that new cases developed in the middle of a year. A Poisson distribution was assumed for calculating 95% confidence intervals (CIs) for rates of prevalence and incidence. The annual trends in prevalence and incidence were tested using Poisson regression within age–gender strata. Additionally, Poisson regression was used to analyze the annual trends in prevalence and incidence, with adjustment for age and gender.

Results

Prevalence and incidence of type 2 diabetes mellitus

There were 2,224,876 cases in 2008, 2,368,587 cases in 2009, and 2,516,350 cases in 2010 that fulfilled the study criteria for T2DM and were included in the final analysis. The prevalence of T2DM was 6.1% in 2008, 6.5% in 2009 and 6.9% in 2010 (6.4–7.3% in men and 5.7–6.4% in women from 2008–2010) (**Table 1**). With adjustment for age and gender, annual preva-

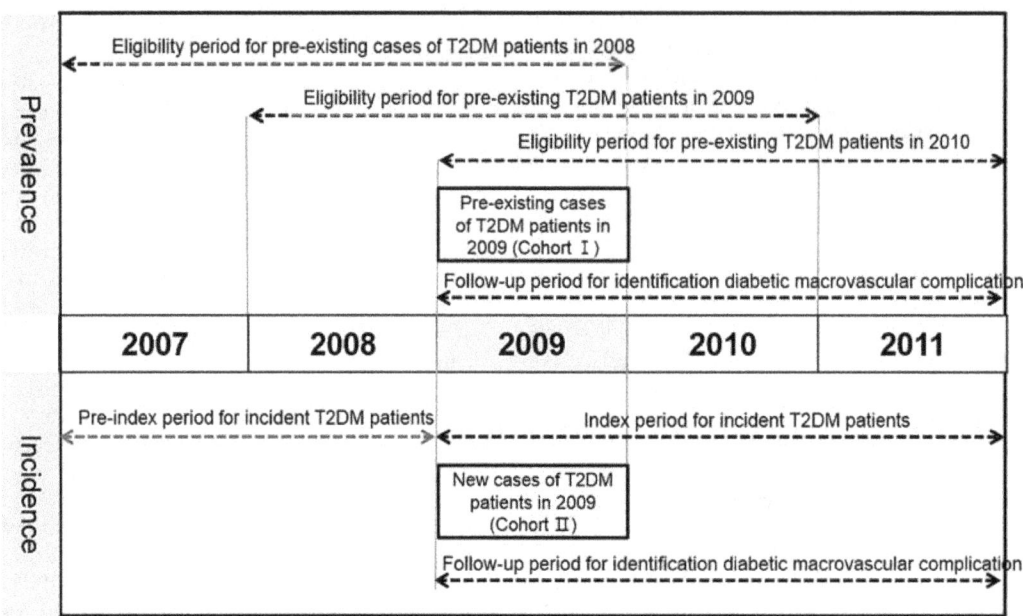

Figure 1. Schematic description of the study period.

lence increased from 2008 to 2010 (*P*<0.0001). In men aged 60–79, the prevalence of T2DM increased each year and reached 19.2–20.0% in 2010 (*P*<0.0001). In women, the prevalence of T2DM was substantially lower than in men of same age in subjects aged <60 years; notably, women aged 30–49 years were shown to have about half the prevalence of T2DM than men of the same age (**Table 1**).

The numbers of newly diagnosed T2DM patients in each year were 336,078, 331,387, and 321,966 in 2009, 2010, and 2011, respectively. The corresponding annual incidence rates of T2DM were 9.8, 9.7, and 9.5 per 1,000 person-years (PY), respectively (**Table 2**). The annual incidence of T2DM decreased after adjusting for age and gender (*P*<0.0001). We subsequently analyzed the annual incidence rate according to gender and age groups. The incidence rates per 1,000 PY were 10.7, 10.6, and 10.4 for men and 9.0, 8.9, and 8.5 for women (**Table 2**). Men and women aged 20–49 years showed a decreasing rate of incidence from 2009 to 2011; the incidence of diabetes in individuals aged 40–49 years decreased from 11.4 to 10.6 (per 1,000 PY) in men and from 6.0 to 5.2 (per 1,000 PY) in women (*P*<0.0001 in both).

Prevalence of macrovascular complication in the 2009 cohort

A total of 1,233,009 men and 1,135,578 women were defined as T2DM patients in 2009 (Cohort I). Among them, 177,999 men and 158,079 women were newly diagnosed as T2DM in that year (Cohort II). In Cohort I, the prevalence of CAD during the three-year period was 16.82%; among these individuals, 11.2% (N = 45,488, 1.92% of Cohort I) and 1.00% (N = 3,984, 0.17% of Cohort I) underwent percutaneous coronary intervention (PCI) and coronary artery bypass graft surgery (CABG), respectively (**Table 3**). As a marker of PAD incidence, 12,282 (0.52% of Cohort I) and 1,162 (0.05% of Cohort I) underwent percutaneous or open revascularization therapy, respectively, which corresponded to about 27% of the number of interventions for CAD during the same period. The amputation of lower extremities was

detected in 6,891 (0.29% of Cohort I). CVD was detected in 11.38% of Cohort I from 2009–2011.

In Cohort II, the prevalence of CAD and CVD from 2009–2011 was 14.05% and 8.75%, respectively, which were lower rates than those in Cohort I (**Table 3**). Percutaneous and open revascularization for PAD was performed in 772 (0.23% of Cohort II) and 126 (0.04% of Cohort II) subjects, respectively; and the amputation of lower extremities was detected in 512 (0.15%) subjects in Cohort II from 2009–2011.

Next, we analyzed the incidence of macrovascular complications in Cohort II. Among 336,078 subjects in Cohort II, 21,634 (mean days of follow-up ± standard deviation, 401±283 days) and 13,430 (408±280 days) subjects were newly diagnosed with CAD and CVD, respectively, from 2009–2011 (**Table 4**). Among these individuals, 6,107 and 4,510 were admitted for the management of CAD and CVD, respectively. The annual incidence rates of CAD per 1,000 PY in Cohort II were 18.84 in 2009, 25.71 in 2010, and 21.98 in 2011. About 30% of subjects diagnosed with CAD underwent admission for management of CAD (**Table 4**). The annual incidence rates of PCI for CAD per 1,000 PY in Cohort II were 1.58 in 2009, 2.43 in 2010, and 2.44 in 2011, while the annual incidence rates of percutaneous and open revascularization for PAD were 0.4, 0.6, and 0.7 during the same time period. From 2009–2011, 2,292 and 533 subjects in Cohort II underwent angioplasty for CAD and PAD, respectively. Among them, 78 subjects received angioplasty for both CAD and PAD. The annual incidence rates of admission for CVD per 1,000 PY were 3.83, 5.02, and 4.65 in 2009, 2010, and 2011, respectively.

Discussion

Our retrospective cohort study evaluated the incidence and prevalence of T2DM and associated macrovascular complications in Korea using the NHI HIRA database, which includes information for about 97% of Koreans. The prevalence of T2DM in Korean adults aged 20–89 years ranged from 6.1–6.9% from 2008–2010, and the annual incidence rate of T2DM ranged from 9.5–9.8/1,000 PY from 2009–2011. Women aged <

Table 1. The prevalence of type 2 diabetes mellitus in the Korean population aged 20–89 years.

		Year								P-value*
		2008		2009		2010		2008–2010		
		N	Prevalence % (95% CI)	N	Prevalence % (95% CI)	N	Prevalence % (95% CI)	N	Prevalence % (95% CI)	
Total		**2,224,876**	**6.1 (6.1–6.1)**	**2,368,587**	**6.5 (6.4–6.5)**	**2,516,350**	**6.9 (6.9–6.9)**	**3,079,126**	**8.4 (8.4–8.4)**	**<0.0001**
Men	Total	1,152,366	6.4 (6.4–6.4)	1,233,009	6.9 (6.9–6.9)	1,315,234	7.3 (7.3–7.3)	1,605,387	8.9 (8.9–9.0)	<0.0001
	20–29	8,379	0.2 (0.2–0.2)	8,592	0.3 (0.2–0.3)	8,382	0.2 (0.2–0.2)	14,936	0.4 (0.4–0.4)	0.982
	30–39	57,920	1.5 (1.5–1.5)	58,464	1.5 (1.5–1.5)	57,000	1.5 (1.4–1.5)	87,496	2.2 (2.2–2.2)	0.007
	40–49	220,675	5.4 (5.3–5.4)	229,411	5.6 (5.6–5.6)	228,034	5.5 (5.5–5.6)	308,762	7.5 (7.5–7.5)	<0.0001
	50–59	341,748	10.5 (10.5–10.6)	369,824	11.4 (11.3–11.4)	400,527	12.3 (12.3–12.4)	472,318	14.5 (14.5–14.6)	<0.0001
	60–69	321,544	17.0 (17.0–17.1)	341,361	18.1 (18.0–18.1)	363,451	19.2 (19.2–19.3)	429,228	22.7 (22.6–22.8)	<0.0001
	70–79	171,270	15.8 (15.7–15.9)	190,251	17.6 (17.5–17.6)	216,713	20.0 (19.9–20.1)	243,737	22.5 (22.4–22.6)	<0.0001
	80–89	30,830	11.9 (11.7–12.0)	35,106	13.5 (13.4–13.6)	41,127	15.8 (15.7–16.0)	48,910	18.8 (18.6–19.0)	<0.0001
Women	Total	1,072,510	5.7 (5.7–5.7)	1,135,578	6.1 (6.1–6.1)	1,201,116	6.4 (6.4–6.4)	1,473,739	7.9 (7.9–7.9)	<0.0001
	20–29	8,024	0.3 (0.2–0.3)	8,225	0.3 (0.3–0.3)	7,774	0.2 (0.2–0.3)	15,005	0.5 (0.5–0.5)	0.048
	30–39	30,799	0.8 (0.8–0.8)	30,816	0.8 (0.8–0.8)	30,974	0.8 (0.8–0.8)	50,097	1.3 (1.3–1.3)	0.481
	40–49	107,543	2.6 (2.6–2.6)	111,253	2.7 (2.7–2.7)	109,449	2.7 (2.7–2.7)	153,814	3.8 (3.7–3.8)	<0.0001
	50–59	230,093	6.9 (6.9–7.0)	243,840	7.4 (7.3–7.4)	256,632	7.7 (7.7–7.8)	318,061	9.6 (9.6–9.6)	<0.0001
	60–69	343,318	16.3 (16.3–16.4)	354,917	16.9 (16.8–16.9)	365,360	17.4 (17.3–17.4)	443,797	21.1 (21.0–21.2)	<0.0001
	70–79	281,703	18.0 (17.9–18.0)	304,826	19.5 (19.4–19.5)	334,111	21.3 (21.3–21.4)	382,547	24.4 (24.3–24.5)	<0.0001
	80–89	71,030	11.7 (11.6–11.8)	81,701	13.5 (13.4–13.6)	96,816	16.0 (15.9–16.1)	110,418	18.2 (18.1–18.3)	<0.0001

CI = confidence interval.
*P-values were obtained using Poisson regression.

Table 2. The incidence of type 2 diabetes mellitus in the Korean population aged 20–89 years.

		Year 2009		2010		2011		2009–2011		P-value*
		N	Incidence per 1,000 PY (95% CI)	N	Incidence per 1,000 PY (95% CI)	N	Incidence per 1,000 PY (95% CI)	N	Incidence per 1,000 PY (95% CI)	
Total		**336,078**	**9.8 (9.8–9.8)**	**331,387**	**9.7 (9.7–9.7)**	**321,966**	**9.5 (9.4–9.5)**	**989,431**	**9.7 (9.6–9.7)**	**<.0001**
Men	Total	177,999	10.7 (10.6–10.7)	175,808	10.6 (10.5–10.6)	172,967	10.4 (10.4–10.5)	526,774	10.6 (10.5–10.6)	<.0001
	20–29	2,931	0.9 (0.8–0.9)	2,748	0.8 (0.8–0.8)	2,622	0.8 (0.7–0.8)	8,301	0.8 (0.8–0.8)	<.0001
	30–39	16,609	4.3 (4.2–4.4)	15,445	4.0 (3.9–4.1)	15,216	3.9 (3.9–4.0)	47,270	4.1 (4.0–4.1)	<.0001
	40–49	44,215	11.4 (11.3–11.5)	41,628	10.8 (10.7–10.9)	40,838	10.6 (10.5–10.7)	126,681	10.9 (10.9–11.0)	<.0001
	50–59	52,070	18.1 (17.9–18.2)	52,952	18.6 (18.4–18.7)	53,702	19.0 (18.9–19.2)	158,724	18.6 (18.5–18.6)	<.0001
	60–69	38,778	25.0 (24.8–25.3)	38,627	25.3 (25.0–25.5)	36,400	24.1 (23.9–24.4)	113,805	24.8 (24.7–25.0)	<.0001
	70–79	19,482	21.6 (21.3–21.9)	20,331	23.0 (22.7–23.3)	20,104	23.5 (23.1–23.8)	59,917	22.7 (22.5–22.9)	0.002
	80–89	3,914	17.2 (16.7–17.8)	4,077	18.3 (17.7–18.8)	4,085	18.8 (18.3–19.4)	12,076	18.1 (17.8–18.4)	0.057
Women	Total	158,079	9.0 (9.0–9.0)	155,579	8.9 (8.8–8.9)	148,999	8.5 (8.5–8.6)	462,657	8.8 (8.8–8.8)	<.0001
	20–29	3,275	1.0 (1.0–1.1)	2,889	0.9 (0.9–0.9)	2,606	0.8 (0.8–0.9)	8,770	0.9 (0.9–0.9)	<.0001
	30–39	9,529	2.5 (2.4–2.5)	9,653	2.5 (2.5–2.6)	8,840	2.3 (2.3–2.4)	28,022	2.4 (2.4–2.5)	<.0001
	40–49	23,621	6.0 (5.9–6.0)	22,463	5.7 (5.6–5.7)	20,762	5.2 (5.2–5.3)	66,846	5.6 (5.6–5.7)	<.0001
	50–59	40,022	13.1 (12.9–13.2)	40,481	13.3 (13.1–13.4)	40,424	13.3 (13.2–13.4)	120,927	13.2 (13.1–13.3)	0.157
	60–69	42,119	24.2 (24.0–24.4)	40,756	23.6 (23.3–23.8)	37,756	22.0 (21.7–22.2)	120,631	23.2 (23.1–23.4)	<.0001
	70–79	30,783	24.2 (24.0–24.5)	30,587	24.5 (24.3–24.8)	29,938	24.6 (24.3–24.9)	91,308	24.5 (24.3–24.6)	0.001
	80–89	8,730	16.4 (16.1–16.8)	8,750	16.8 (16.5–17.2)	8,673	17.2 (16.8–17.5)	26,153	16.8 (16.6–17.0)	0.666

PY = person-years; CI = confidence interval.
* P-values were obtained using Poisson regression.

Table 3. The prevalence of diabetic macrovascular complications in patients with type 2 diabetes mellitus aged 20–89 years.

Year		N (%)							
		Pre-existing cases of T2DM in 2009 (N=2,368,587, Cohort I)				New cases of T2DM in 2009 (N=336,078, Cohort II)			
		2009	2010	2011	2009–2011	2009	2010	2011	2009–2011
CAD	Total*	241,924 (10.21)	244,348 (10.32)	244,988 (10.34)	398,389 (16.82)	29,365 (8.74)	26,444 (7.87)	26,067 (7.76)	47,211 (14.05)
	PCI	17,026 (0.72)	15,850 (0.67)	15,973 (0.67)	45,488 (1.92)	2,362 (0.70)	1,377 (0.41)	1,278 (0.38)	4,641 (1.38)
	Coronary bypass	1,583(0.07)	1,253 (0.05)	1,152 (0.05)	3,984 (0.17)	206 (0.06)	77 (0.02)	91 (0.03)	373 (0.11)
CVD	Total*	159,698 (6.74)	158,704 (6.70)	157,526 (6.65)	269,538 (11.38)	18,458 (5.49)	16,876 (5.02)	16,305 (4.85)	29,412 (8.75)
PAD	Percutaneous angioplasty	4,067 (0.17)	3,867 (0.16)	4,348 (0.18)	12,282 (0.52)	300 (0.09)	236 (0.07)	236 (0.07)	772 (0.23)
	Open revascularization	480 (0.02)	404 (0.02)	327 (0.01)	1,162 (0.05)	74 (0.02)	38 (0.01)	26 (0.01)	126 (0.04)
Amputation	Total	2,703 (0.11)	2,418 (0.10)	2,408 (0.10)	6,891 (0.29)	280 (0.08)	147 (0.04)	120 (0.04)	512 (0.15)
	Femur	147 (0.01)	131 (0.01)	118 (0.00)	386 (0.02)	26 (0.01)	15 (0.00)	12 (0.00)	53 (0.02)
	Below knee	729 (0.03)	645 (0.03)	603 (0.03)	1,914 (0.08)	71 (0.02)	39 (0.01)	22 (0.01)	131 (0.04)
	Foot	502 (0.02)	434 (0.02)	479 (0.02)	1,367 (0.06)	43 (0.01)	23 (0.01)	12 (0.00)	77 (0.02)
	Toe	1,722 (0.07)	1,550 (0.07)	1,579 (0.07)	4,529 (0.19)	175 (0.05)	90 (0.03)	84 (0.02)	329 (0.10)

T2DM = type 2 diabetes mellitus; CAD = coronary artery disease; CVD = cardiovascular disease; PAD = peripheral artery disease; PCI = percutaneous coronary intervention.
*Claim with an ICD-10 diagnosis code as the principal or additional diagnosis, or claims involving a procedure related to the corresponding disease.

Table 4. The incidence of diabetic macrovascular complications in Cohort II.

Year		Incidence, N (/1,000 person-year) (N = 336,078)					Mean days of follow-up (SD)
		2009		2010		2011	
						2009–2011	
CAD	Total*	6,274 (18.84)		8,373 (25.71)		6,987 (21.98)	21,634 (22.17)	400.8 (283.2)
	PCI	531 (1.58)		816 (2.43)		817 (2.44)	2,164 (2.15)	439.9 (287.6)
	Coronary bypass	37 (0.11)		45 (0.13)		63 (0.19)	145 (0.14)	463.5 (301.1)
	Admission†	1,725 (5.15)		2,293 (6.88)		2,089 (6.31)	6,107 (6.11)	409.4 (291.0)
CVD	Total*	3,782 (11.32)		5,189 (15.74)		4,459 (13.73)	13,430 (13.59)	408.3 (279.7)
	Admission†	1,286 (3.83)		1,677 (5.02)		1,547 (4.65)	4,510 (4.50)	414.9 (285.6)
PAD	Percutaneous angioplasty	108 (0.32)		183 (0.54)		205 (0.61)	496 (0.49)	453.0 (291.7)
	Open revascularization	24 (0.07)		19 (0.06)		14 (0.04)	57 (0.06)	320.1 (243.6)
Amputation	Total	160 (0.48)		126 (0.4)		102 (0.30)	388 (0.39)	340.3 (293.7)
	Femur	18 (0.05)		13 (0.04)		11 (0.03)	42 (0.04)	317.7 (270.1)
	Below knee	39 (0.12)		37 (0.11)		21 (0.06)	97 (0.10)	341.9 (286.2)
	Foot	26 (0.08)		23 (0.07)		11 (0.03)	60 (0.06)	303.8 (277.4)
	Toe	99 (0.29)		78 (0.23)		73 (0.22)	250 (0.25)	353.0 (304.1)

CAD = coronary artery disease; CVD = cardiovascular disease; PAD = peripheral artery disease; PCI = percutaneous coronary intervention; SD = standard deviation.
*Claim with an ICD-10 diagnosis code as the principal or additional diagnosis, or claims involving a procedure related to the corresponding disease.
†Hospital admissions were measured using inpatient claims with the principal diagnosis of corresponding disease.

60 years showed a lower prevalence of T2DM compared to men of the same age, and women between the ages of 30 and 49 years demonstrated about half the prevalence and incidence rate of men of the same age.

The incidence of T2DM in our study is similar to a previous report in Taiwan, that used diagnosis code-based claim data to show that the incidence was 7.8/1,000 PY in 2004. In Japan, a recent pooled analysis showed that the incidence rate of T2DM was 8.8/1,000 PY, which is also similar to our results [21]. Given that the populations of countries adjacent to Korea such as China and Japan have similar genetic backgrounds related to the risk of developing T2DM [22–24], and that such countries have similar T2DM prevalence [5,6,8,25], our results for the Korean population are reasonable.

However, claim-based diagnoses may underestimate the real prevalence or incidence of T2DM. The mean annual incidence rate of T2DM in a Korean community-based cohort was 21.5/1,000 PY in adults aged 40–69 years [15,26], which is higher than our results. The prevalence of T2DM in adults aged ≥30 years in 2010, according to the KNHANES 2010 was 10.1%, which is also higher than our result [13]. The consideration that only 73.0% of diabetic subjects were aware of their glucose disorder in 2008–2010 according to the KNHANES [13] may explain these differences explained. A previous national survey of diabetes in Korea based on 2003 HIRA data showed an incidence rate of diabetes of 5.7/1,000 PY, which is lower than our results [27]. As the proportion of diabetic subjects with a medical diagnosis of diabetes increased from 43% in 2001 and 66.5% in 2005 [28] to 73.0% in 2008–2010, according to the KNHANES [13], misclassification bias may account for a potential underestimation in the incidence of diabetes based on claims data in 2003 compared with data from 2009–2011.

Interestingly, the incidence of T2DM in men and women aged 20–49 years showed a decrease from 2009 to 2011, despite an increase in the prevalence of T2DM in the overall population. The incidence of diabetes in individuals aged 40–49 years decreased from 11.4 to 10.6/1,000 PY in men and from 6.0 to 5.2/1,000 PY in women, which corresponds to previous data from the KNHANES showing that the prevalence of diabetes among women aged 30–59 years decreased from 2001 to 2010 [14]. Lifestyle improvements such as decreasing total daily energy intake and performing regular exercise along with decreased rates of obesity in young adults in Korea, may be the causes of these trends [14]. In contrast, both the incidence and the prevalence of T2DM in individuals aged ≥70 years increased in our study. Korea is one of most rapidly aging countries, similar to Japan; the proportion of the elderly population aged ≥65 in Korea increased from 7.2% of the total population in 2000 to 11.0% in 2010 [29]. Our study showed that the incidence of T2DM in individuals aged 70–79 years was as high as that in individuals aged 60–69 years; furthermore, in women, individuals aged 70–79 years showed a higher incidence rate than those aged 60–69 years, which is worth noting. In general, the incidence of diabetes increases with age until about 65 years of age, after which both incidence and prevalence seem to decrease [30,31]. We cannot explain the cause of the relatively high incidence of newly detected T2DM in individuals aged ≥70 years; further studies characterizing the elderly population with incident T2DM should be performed because increasing rates of T2DM among these individuals may increase the economic burden in Korea.

The prevalence of CAD and CVD in diabetic subjects in our study ranged from 10.2–10.3% and 6.7%, respectively, which was more than 2 times higher than the general population. In the 2010 KNHANES, the prevalence of CAD and CVD in adults aged ≥30 years was 2.4% and 1.4%, respectively [13]. Previous studies based on the NHI system in the general Korean population also showed a lower prevalence of both CAD and CVD (2.5% and 2.4%, respectively) [32,33]. Comparing the newly diagnosed T2DM patients (Cohort II) with all T2DM patients (Cohort I), the prevalence of CAD and CVD was lower in Cohort II than in Cohort I. However, in Cohort II, up to 8.7% and 5.5% of Cohort II had CAD and CVD, respectively, in the year of T2DM diagnosis, which are still higher rates than those in the general Korean population.

The incidence of CAD and CVD in newly detected T2DM patients (Cohort II) was 18.84/1,000 PY and 11.32/1,000 PY in the year of T2DM diagnosis; these increased in subsequent years. The incidence of CAD was 25.71/1,000 PY in 2010 and 21.98/1,000 PY in 2011, and the incidence of CVD was 15.74/1,000 PY in 2010 and 13.73/1,000 PY in 2011. The incidence of ischemic stroke (resulting from CVD) in the general population of Korea was reported as 1.3/1,000 PY in 2004 [34].

The number of claims for PAD was relatively small compared to CAD and CVD. However, the finding that, among the 533 subjects in Cohort II who underwent angioplasty for PAD during study period, 78 (14.6%) of them experienced angioplasty for CAD during the same period emphasizes the importance of screening for CAD in T2DM patients with PAD considering the morbidity and mortality from CAD [35].

We confirmed the relatively higher risk of CAD and CVD in diabetic subjects compared to the general Korean population using nationwide health insurance claim data from HIRA. However, there are limitations regarding the accuracy of the diagnoses from claim data, since they were not based on clinical data. Furthermore, claims data provide limited information on disease severity, co-morbid conditions, past history, and specific treatment. As previously mentioned, the proportion of the population aware of their disease status may influence the estimation of prevalence or incidence of a disease in a claim study. In addition, three years of follow-up is a relatively short time period to evaluate trends in the incidence of T2DM. However, the usefulness of claim data in the nationwide survey for T2DM has been confirmed previously [36,37]. The accuracy of diagnosis of T2DM from claim data reached a sensitivity of 68–71% and positive predictive value of 85–88% for clinically diagnosed T2DM from health examinations [37]. In addition, we extensively reviewed two years of prior claim data to calculate the incidence of T2DM, which may result in reasonable incidence rates compared to those from adjacent Asian populations and previous reports in Korea.

In summary, in recent years, the prevalence of T2DM in Korean adults aged 20–89 years was 6.1–6.9% and the annual incidence rate of T2DM was 8.8–9.2/1,000 PY. The fact that the incidence of T2DM in the elderly population increased significantly in the opposite direction to that in young men and women in the same period may result in an increasing economic burden in Korea, and necessitates a call for public health planning for the elderly population. Even in newly detected T2DM subjects, the prevalence of CAD and CVD was much higher than that in the general population. Our extensive investigation of epidemiologic data from nationwide claim data should be invaluable for planning national public health strategies.

Author Contributions

Conceived and designed the experiments: BK CL NC. Performed the experiments: BY NC. Analyzed the data: BK BY SH NC. Contributed reagents/materials/analysis tools: BY NC. Wrote the paper: BK NC.

References

1. International Diabetes Federation (2000) IDF Diabetes Atlas. Brussels: International Diabetes Federation.
2. International Diabetes Federation (2009) IDF Diabetes Atlas. Brussels: International Diabetes Federation.
3. Whiting DR, Guariguata L, Weil C, Shaw J (2011) IDF diabetes atlas: global estimates of the prevalence of diabetes for 2011 and 2030. Diabetes Res Clin Pract 94: 311–321.
4. Kim DJ (2011) The epidemiology of diabetes in Korea. Diabetes Metab J 35: 303–308.
5. Choi YJ, Kim HC, Kim HM, Park SW, Kim J, et al. (2009) Prevalence and management of diabetes in Korean adults: Korea National Health and Nutrition Examination Surveys 1998–2005. Diabetes Care 32: 2016–2020.
6. Ning F, Pang ZC, Dong YH, Gao WG, Nan HR, et al. (2009) Risk factors associated with the dramatic increase in the prevalence of diabetes in the adult Chinese population in Qingdao, China. Diabet Med 26: 855–863.
7. Yang W, Lu J, Weng J, Jia W, Ji L, et al. (2010) Prevalence of diabetes among men and women in China. N Engl J Med 362: 1090–1101.
8. Shen J, Goyal A, Sperling L (2012) The emerging epidemic of obesity, diabetes, and the metabolic syndrome in china. Cardiol Res Pract 2012: 178675.
9. Ramachandran A, Snehalatha C, Vijay V (2002) Temporal changes in prevalence of type 2 diabetes and impaired glucose tolerance in urban southern India. Diabetes Res Clin Pract 58: 55–60.
10. Li H, Oldenburg B, Chamberlain C, O'Neil A, Xue B, et al. (2012) Diabetes prevalence and determinants in adults in China mainland from 2000 to 2010: A systematic review. Diabetes Res Clin Pract.98: 226–235.
11. Lipscombe LL, Hux JE (2007) Trends in diabetes prevalence, incidence, and mortality in Ontario, Canada 1995–2005: a population-based study. Lancet 369: 750–756.
12. Cowie CC, Rust KF, Ford ES, Eberhardt MS, Byrd-Holt DD, et al. (2009) Full accounting of diabetes and pre-diabetes in the U.S. population in 1988–1994 and 2005–2006. Diabetes Care 32: 287–294.
13. Korea Centers for Disease Control and Prevention (2010) The Korean National Health and Nutrition Examination Survey. Chungwon: Ministry of Health and Welfare.
14. Koo BK, Kim EK, Choi H, Park KS, Moon MK (2013) Decreasing trends of the prevalence of diabetes and obesity in korean women aged 30–59 years over the past decade: results from the korean national health and nutrition examination survey, 2001–2010. Diabetes Care 36: e95–96.
15. Cho NH (2010) The epidemiology of diabetes in Korea: from the economics to genetics. Korean Diabetes J 34: 10–15.
16. Choi NK, Chang Y, Choi YK, Hahn S, Park BJ (2010) Signal detection of rosuvastatin compared to other statins: data-mining study using national health insurance claims database. Pharmacoepidemiol Drug Saf 19: 238–246.
17. Sloan FA, Belsky D, Ruiz D, Jr., Lee P (2008) Changes in incidence of diabetes mellitus-related eye disease among US elderly persons, 1994–2005. Arch Ophthalmol 126: 1548–1553.
18. Hirsch AT, Hartman L, Town RJ, Virnig BA (2008) National health care costs of peripheral arterial disease in the Medicare population. Vasc Med 13: 209–215.
19. Margolis J, Barron JJ, Grochulski WD (2005) Health care resources and costs for treating peripheral artery disease in a managed care population: results from analysis of administrative claims data. J Manag Care Pharm 11: 727–734.
20. Statistics Korea (2010) 2010 Population and Housing Census. Daejeon: Statistics Korea.
21. Goto A, Goto M, Noda M, Tsugane S (2013) Incidence of type 2 diabetes in Japan: a systematic review and meta-analysis. PLoS One 8: e74699.
22. Ng MC, Tam CH, Lam VK, So WY, Ma RC, et al. (2007) Replication and identification of novel variants at TCF7L2 associated with type 2 diabetes in Hong Kong Chinese. J Clin Endocrinol Metab 92: 3733–3737.
23. Ng MC, Park KS, Oh B, Tam CH, Cho YM, et al. (2008) Implication of genetic variants near TCF7L2, SLC30A8, HHEX, CDKAL1, CDKN2A/B, IGF2BP2, and FTO in type 2 diabetes and obesity in 6,719 Asians. Diabetes 57: 2226–2233.
24. Miyake K, Horikawa Y, Hara K, Yasuda K, Osawa H, et al. (2008) Association of TCF7L2 polymorphisms with susceptibility to type 2 diabetes in 4,087 Japanese subjects. J Hum Genet 53: 174–180.
25. Ramachandran A, Snehalatha C, Kapur A, Vijay V, Mohan V, et al. (2001) High prevalence of diabetes and impaired glucose tolerance in India: National Urban Diabetes Survey. Diabetologia 44: 1094–1101.
26. Korea Centers for Disease Control and Prevention (2008) Results of the Second Follow-up Survey of Ansung and Ansan Cohort. Chungwon: Korea Centers for Disease Control and Prevention.
27. Task Force Team for Basic Statistical Study of Korean Diabetes Mellitus of Korean Diabetes A, Park Ie B, Kim J, Kim DJ, Chung CH, et al. (2013) Diabetes epidemics in Korea: reappraise nationwide survey of diabetes "diabetes in Korea 2007". Diabetes Metab J 37: 233–239.
28. Korea Centers for Disease Control and Prevention (2005) The Korean National Health and Nutrition Examination Survey. Chungwon: Korea Centers for Disease Control and Prevention
29. Statistics Korea (2011) Population Projections for Korea. Daejeon: Statistics Korea.
30. Selvin E, Coresh J, Brancati FL (2006) The burden and treatment of diabetes in elderly individuals in the u.s. Diabetes Care 29: 2415–2419.
31. Kirkman MS, Briscoe VJ, Clark N, Florez H, Haas LB, et al. (2012) Diabetes in older adults. Diabetes Care 35: 2650–2664.
32. Chang HS, Kim HJ, Nam CM, Lim SJ, Jang YH, et al. (2012) The socioeconomic burden of coronary heart disease in Korea. J Prev Med Public Health 45: 291–300.
33. Lim SJ, Kim HJ, Nam CM, Chang HS, Jang YH, et al. (2009) Socioeconomic costs of stroke in Korea: estimated from the Korea national health insurance claims database. J Prev Med Public Health 42: 251–260.
34. Hong KS, Kim J, Cho YJ, Seo SY, Hwang SI, et al. (2011) Burden of ischemic stroke in Korea: analysis of disability-adjusted life years lost. J Clin Neurol 7: 77–84.
35. Su Kyung Park M-KP, Ji Hye Su, Mi Kyung Kim, Yong Ki Kim, In Ju Kim, Yang Ho Kang, Kwang Jae Lee, Hyun Seung Lee, Chang Won Lee, Bo Hyun Kim, Kyung Il Lee, Mi Kyoung Kim, Duk Kyu Kim (2009) Cause-of-Death Trends for Diabetes Mellitus over 10 Years Korean Diabetes Journal 33: 65–72.
36. Ngo DL, Marshall LM, Howard RN, Woodward JA, Southwick K, et al. (2003) Agreement between self-reported information and medical claims data on diagnosed diabetes in Oregon's Medicaid population. J Public Health Manag Pract 9: 542–544.
37. Southern DA, Roberts B, Edwards A, Dean S, Norton P, et al. (2010) Validity of administrative data claim-based methods for identifying individuals with diabetes at a population level. Can J Public Health 101: 61–64.

19

An Agent-Based Model of the Response to Angioplasty and Bare-Metal Stent Deployment in an Atherosclerotic Blood Vessel

Antonia E. Curtin[1¤], Leming Zhou[1,2]*

1 Department of Bioengineering, University of Pittsburgh, Pittsburgh, Pennsylvania, United States of America, **2** Department of Health Information Management, University of Pittsburgh, Pittsburgh, Pennsylvania, United States of America

Abstract

Purpose: While animal models are widely used to investigate the development of restenosis in blood vessels following an intervention, computational models offer another means for investigating this phenomenon. A computational model of the response of a treated vessel would allow investigators to assess the effects of altering certain vessel- and stent-related variables. The authors aimed to develop a novel computational model of restenosis development following an angioplasty and bare-metal stent implantation in an atherosclerotic vessel using agent-based modeling techniques. The presented model is intended to demonstrate the body's response to the intervention and to explore how different vessel geometries or stent arrangements may affect restenosis development.

Methods: The model was created on a two-dimensional grid space. It utilizes the post-procedural vessel lumen diameter and stent information as its input parameters. The simulation starting point of the model is an atherosclerotic vessel after an angioplasty and stent implantation procedure. The model subsequently generates the final lumen diameter, percent change in lumen cross-sectional area, time to lumen diameter stabilization, and local concentrations of inflammatory cytokines upon simulation completion. Simulation results were directly compared with the results from serial imaging studies and cytokine levels studies in atherosclerotic patients from the relevant literature.

Results: The final lumen diameter results were all within one standard deviation of the mean lumen diameters reported in the comparison studies. The overlapping-stent simulations yielded results that matched published trends. The cytokine levels remained within the range of physiological levels throughout the simulations.

Conclusion: We developed a novel computational model that successfully simulated the development of restenosis in a blood vessel following an angioplasty and bare-metal stent deployment based on the characteristics of the vessel cross-section and stent. A further development of this model could ultimately be used as a predictive tool to depict patient outcomes and inform treatment options.

Editor: Timothy W. Secomb, University of Arizona, United States of America

Funding: This work is supported in part by a National Science Foundation Remove text grant to L.Z. (IIS-0938393). The funders had no role in study design, data collection and analysis, decision to publish, or preparation of the manuscript. No additional external funding received for this study.

Competing Interests: The authors have declared that no competing interests exist.

* E-mail: lmzhou@gmail.com

¤ Current address: Department of Biomedical Engineering, University of Minnesota, Minneapolis, Minnesota, United States of America

Introduction

In an atherosclerotic blood vessel, blood flow is restricted by the accumulation of plaque, which causes the walls of the vessel to become inflamed [1]. The subsequent narrowing of the lumen of the blood vessel by the plaque causes ischemia, and vascular intervention is usually required to compress the plaque and regain the lumen area to restore blood flow [2]. According to a report published recently, an estimated 492,000 patients underwent percutaneous coronary intervention (PCI) procedures in 2010 in the United States [3], and stents (drug-eluting stents and bare-metal stents) were deployed in 454,000 of these patients (or roughly 92% of all patients) during these PCI procedures [3]. Although the goal of a PCI intervention is to re-expand the lumen

of the target blood vessel, the body's natural wound healing response at the site of the intervention can cause a re-narrowing of the treated vessel, or restenosis, which often counteracts what would be an otherwise successful intervention [2,4]. Up to 60% of such PCI and similar interventions to treat ischemic lesions fail because of restenosis [2,5]. The ensuing target lesion revascularization caused by in-stent restenosis can be severe and detrimental to a patient's recovery [6]. Some studies have shown that as many as one-third of patients with in-stent restenosis developed subsequent myocardial infarctions or unstable angina that required the patient to be hospitalized [7].

Animal models such as rats, mice, rabbits, and pigs have been used extensively to investigate the progression of restenosis in stented arteries and have provided a wealth of insightful information about this complication in the past several decades [8,9]. Nevertheless, because computational models are useful for simulating situations that cannot be created in an animal and permit fast and precise perturbations of the simulation environment, they are conducive to identifying the major effectors of the process being simulated and present a viable alternative to animal models. Agent-based modeling is a computational modeling technique for simulating the actions and interactions of agents (such as cytokines, cells, tissues, and organs) in an environment of interest [10]. When agents interact with each other stochastically, their aggregate behavior leads to complex, emergent phenomena that represent the system as a whole. Agent-based models can provide both numerical values and overall *visual patterns* in the course of the simulations, which are typically very informative. The model presented in this article was developed with the NetLogo platform [11].

The rest of this article is broken into four sections: materials and methods, results, discussion, and conclusions. The materials and methods section presents the clinical events simulated, model construction procedure, model interface, outputs, parameter sensitivity analysis, and model validation procedures. The results section describes the results from various simulations for a single stent and overlapping stents, including quantitative values and visual outputs. The discussion section provides detailed explanation of the obtained results, limitations of the model, and plans for further development of the model. The conclusion section includes a brief summary of the model results and possible future directions.

Materials and Methods

A. Clinical Events Simulated

A normal coronary artery consists of three concentric layers, from the innermost to the outermost, called the intima, media, and adventitia. The intima is covered by a single layer of endothelial cells (**ECs**); the media comprises mainly smooth muscle cells (**SMCs**) and elastic tissues; and the adventitia is rich in fibroblasts and connective tissues [1,2]. In the course of an inflammatory reaction, **platelets**, **neutrophils**, and **macrophages** are activated and recruited to the wound site. These cell types can produce pro-inflammatory or anti-inflammatory cytokines, such as **TNF-α** (tumor necrosis factor alpha) and **TGF-β** (transforming growth factor beta) [1,12,13]. After an angioplasty and subsequent stent deployment procedure, **stent struts** become part of the artery and are therefore included in this model from the beginning of simulation. These are the major contributors to restenosis development and are represented by agents in this agent-based model.

In addition to these major components, an atherosclerotic coronary artery (the blood vessel simulated in this model) has a lipid-rich core called plaque [14] between the intimal and medial layers. At the interface of the intima and the plaque, SMCs and elastic tissues may also be present. Depending on the thickness and composition of this particular layer (sometimes referred to as a "fibrous cap" in the literature), the plaque can be stable or vulnerable to breaking (*plaque rupture*) during the angioplasty and stent-deployment procedure. Plaque rupture can lead to an intense inflammatory reactions and be accompanied by an acute thrombosis, and therefore requires a different therapeutic approach for controlling acute inflammatory reactions and thrombosis, such as administering anti-platelet drugs and anti-inflammatory drugs [15–19]. The behavior of cells that contribute to restenosis development is altered in the presence of such drugs and is dependent on drug type and dosage. Because the goal of the model is to elucidate how the cell types and cytokines of interest

contribute to in-stent restenosis development when drugs are not present, it is assumed that there is no plaque rupture during the angioplasty and stent procedure. The model solely simulates the vessel's and body's response to the injuries created by the angioplasty and stent procedure.

As a result, the processes simulated in the model are quite similar to the typical wound healing following tissue injury [20]. The first phase of the wound healing response involves the aggregation of platelets and the infiltration of inflammatory cells (such as macrophages and neutrophils), followed by proliferation and apoptosis of ECs and SMCs under the stimulation of inflammatory cytokines (such as TGF-β and TNF-α) [21–23]. Inter-patient differences in the extent and rate of wound healing are largely due to differences in physiological variables such as the cytokine-dependent SMCs and ECs proliferation rates.

A holistic summary of the processes simulated in the model is presented below. Prior to simulation initiation, SMCs and ECs are injured during the angioplasty and stent procedure. The result of this procedure is the starting point of the model simulation. **Step 1**: Exposure of the subendothelial matrix (SEM) and collagens as a result of the endothelial cell damage immediately activates circulating latent platelets [24]. Activated platelets aggregate to form a growing thrombus and activate circulating latent platelets upon contact [24]. **Step 2**: SMCs, ECs, and activated platelets release anti-inflammatory cytokines such as TGF-β [25,26]. **Step 3**: Sufficient amounts of TGF-β trigger the recruitment of monocytes and neutrophils to the wound site [27,28]. *In vivo*, this recruitment is actually performed by the SEM, which releases TGF-β and other chemoattractants to draw monocytes and neutrophils to the wound site [29–31]. Monocytes migrate through the thrombus [30] and mature into macrophages when they reach the tissue [26,32]. Neutrophils form contact-based aggregates with activated platelets and become integrated into the thrombus [30,31,33]. **Step 4**: Monocytes, neutrophils, and macrophages release pro-inflammatory cytokines such as TNF-α [34]. **Step 5**: Both pro- and anti-inflammatory cytokines (TNF-α and TGF-β) diffuse through the tissues adjacent to the site of their initial release. When the local concentration of TGF-β reaches a certain threshold, SMC and EC proliferation in that area will be triggered [35,36]. When the local concentration of TNF-α reaches a given threshold, SMCs and ECs apoptosis will be triggered [37]. This simplified description of the *in vivo* interactions among the major cell types and cytokines of interest in the development of restenosis is illustrated in Figure 1. In this figure, these cell types and cytokines are color-coded to make it consistent with the colors of agents used in the model.

It is important to note that the *in vivo* interactions are much more complicated than this simplified description. For instance, TGF-β can act as both a pro- and anti-inflammatory cytokine at different stages of restenosis development [38,39]. There are also many other cytokines and growth factors (e.g., interleukin 8, interleukin 6, platelet-derived growth factor, fibroblast growth factor, vascular endothelial growth factor, etc.) involved in the whole process [40]. In this model, TGF-β and TNF-α were used to represent anti-inflammatory cytokines and pro-inflammatory cytokines, respectively. The use of only a few cytokines in agent-based models of inflammatory-based healing responses is a frequently applied practice [41,42]. This simplification is necessary because the precise roles of these cytokines within the complex *in vivo* environment are not clear while the presence of anti-inflammatory and pro-inflammatory cytokines are vital to the dynamic interactions among the major contributors to restenosis development [5,40]. The major purpose of this work is to simulate the dynamic interactions among these major contributors and to

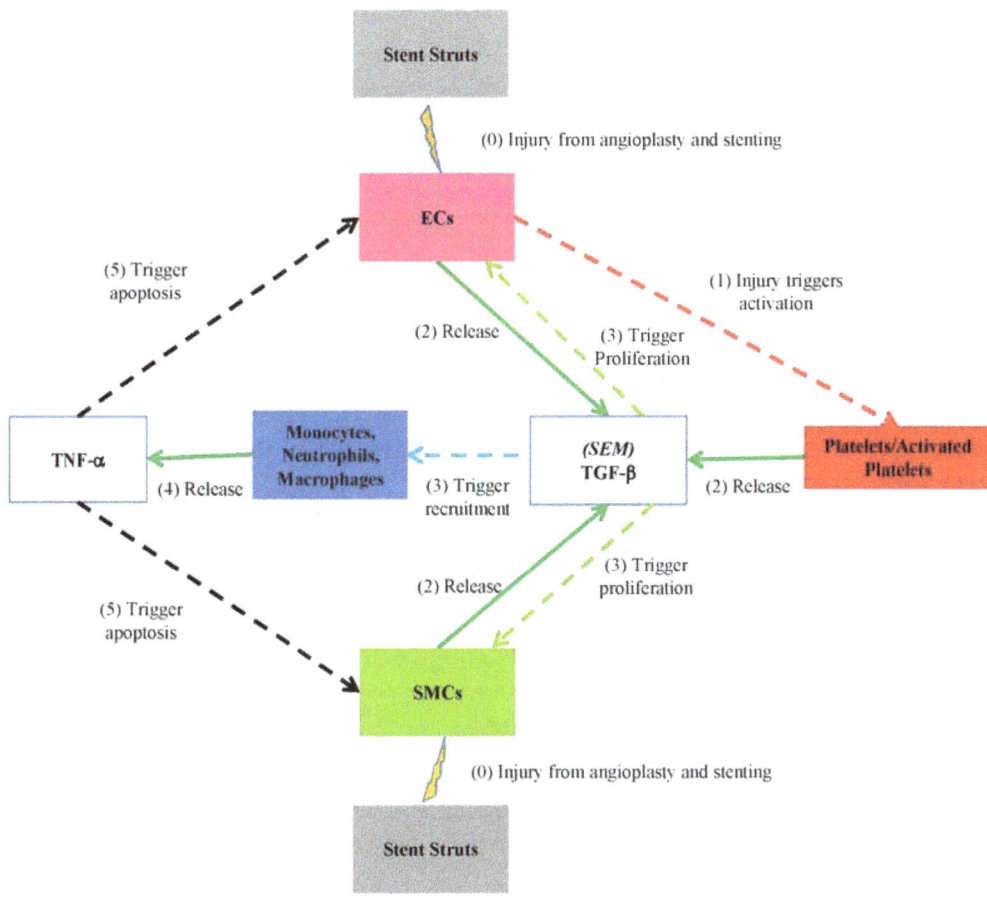

Figure 1. An interaction diagram for cells and cytokines represented in the model. The major players in the interaction are shown in boxes with colors. These colors are the same as the ones used in the visual output of the agent-based model. The solid green lines mean something is releasing and the dashed lines mean an event is being triggered. Here is the color code for events: light-green for proliferation, light-blue for recruitment, red for activation, and black for apoptosis. The numbers in the diagram indicate the order of those events at the beginning of a model simulation.

determine their roles in the development of restenosis. Without proper simplification, this model with detailed interactions among a large number of cytokines and growth factors would not produce any meaningful results.

B. Model Construction

i) Settings of the model. Corresponding to the structure of the coronary artery, the agent-based model developed in this work contains four major compartments in a simulated arterial cross-section: the **lumen**, **intima** or **neointima** layer (endothelial cells and some smooth muscle cells), the **media** layer (mainly smooth muscle cells), and the **adventitia** layer. The model also includes agents representing platelets, monocytes, neutrophils, and macrophages, along with cytokines such as TNF-α and TGF-β.

The environment of interest in the model is the treated blood vessel post-implantation of the stent. The simulated environment is a two-dimensional cross-section of the treated blood vessel. Although three-dimensional agent-based models can also be created, the use of a two-dimensional model is supported by the prevalence of the use of two-dimensional cross-sections in assessing vulnerable atherosclerotic plaques [43]. The cross-section with the smallest lumen diameter is the limiting factor for blood flow and is thus the case of greatest interest. The simulated results from this

two-dimensional model can also be directly compared with those obtained in published serial angiography or ultrasound studies.

The agent-based model is created on a 150×150 grid, which corresponds to 22,500 square patches in total. All the agents in the model are contained on these patches in the grid. In the NetLogo program, one distance unit is defined as the distance between the centers of two adjacent patches in the grid, which is also the side length of a patch. In this model, one distance unit represents 0.05 mm *in vivo*. The size of a patch is also used as a reference for agent sizes. For instance, if the size of an agent is 1.0 unit, the agent's diameter (for a circular agent) or side length (for a square agent) is the same as that of a patch side.

In this model, one time step represents 6 hours. In the agent-based model, each agent's behavior follows a list of *behavioral rules* (Table 1). These behavioral rules are implemented as functions in the model within the NetLogo platform. When the agent-based model is running, in each time step the model checks the agents' current situation and determines which function(s) should be executed and what input values should be utilized. If the current value of a variable is needed by a function, the model assesses the corresponding local environment to determine the correct value to use. Here an agent's *local environment* is defined as the patch with the desired agent on it, and its 8 immediately adjacent patches in the grid space (illustrated in Figure S1 in Text S1). For instance, if a

Table 1. A list of simplified rules of agents in the model.

Agent	Interaction rules
Platelets	Latent platelets move randomly in the lumen.
	When latent platelets meet injury sites or activated platelets, they are activated.
	Activated platelets aggregate together and lead to thrombus formation.
	Platelets die when they reach their given life-span.
TGF-β	Representing anti-inflammatory cytokines
	Activated platelets, SMCs, and ECs release TGF-β.
	A greater injury site triggers an increased release of TGF-β.
	A change in lumen area affects the release rate of TGF-β.
	Recruiting monocytes and neutrophils
	If the local concentration of TGF-β goes beyond a threshold, SMCs and ECs proliferation will be triggered.
TNF-α	Representing pro-inflammatory cytokines
	Monocytes, neutrophils, and macrophages release TNF-α in the same rate, and the release is triggered by a TGF-β gradient.
	If the local concentration of TNF-α goes beyond a threshold, SMCs and ECs apoptosis will be triggered.
Monocytes, neutrophils, macrophages	When the local TGF-β concentration in the intimal layer exceeds the femtomolar level, circulating neutrophil and monocytes appear in the lumen.
	The migration rate of these monocytes, neutrophils, and macrophages is 1μm/min. During the migration, if neutrophils meet activated platelets, neutrophils attach to the thrombus.
	Monocytes move through the thrombus and change into mature macrophages.
	Some macrophages stay with stent struts and simulate a foreign body response. Other macrophages are elsewhere and trigger typical inflammatory actions.
SMCs	Injured intimal SMCs replicate twice every proliferation cycle.
	Proliferating medial SMCs can migrate to the intimal layer and change to intimal SMCs.
	Each patch in the grid can only hold 15 SMC agents. Once this limit is reached, the extra SMCs are pushed to neighborhood patches in the direction of the lumen.
ECs	ECs always reside on patches adjacent and interior to the forward-most patches holding SMCs. When SMCs move toward the lumen, ECs move accordingly.

function requires the local TGF-β concentration, the model will count the number of TGF-β agents on the patches in the local environment and calculate the concentration value accordingly (counts/volume).

An agent-based model is advantageous in that the number of each type of agent can be tracked continuously in one run of a simulation. All these numbers of agents in different types are discrete values obtained by counting each type of agent on all the patches in the grid. In some cases, the numbers of agents themselves are sufficient for providing the desired information, for instance, the populations of ECs and SMCs. In other cases, these numbers of agents need to be compared with values reported in the literature, for instance, the concentrations of TNF-α and TGF-β. In the latter situation, the number of agents in the model collected during a simulation is converted to a value with the same unit as the ones measured in experiments. This conversion mechanism is set up when the model is initially constructed and is not changed in any subsequent simulations.

In the model, the coronary artery cross-section environment is populated by multiple types of agents. Some of these agents are initially bound to a specific location in the grid space and some of them freely circulate in the lumen. The agents initially assigned to a specific location are based on the *in vivo* makeup of the vessel wall layers. The intimal layer is chiefly populated by a small number of SMC agents and EC agents, representing the endothelial monolayer. The medial and adventitial layers are populated entirely by SMC agents. The other agent types present in the model prior to simulation initiation are platelet agents, latent

TGF-β agents, plaque agents, and stent strut agents. Stent strut agents (representing the struts in a bare-metal stent) are evenly placed around the initial lumen boundary and remain unchanged during the course of a simulation. Illustrations from Thim *et al.* were consulted during the creation of the visual environment of the model prior to the start of a simulation [14]. The plaque size and location are set prior to simulation initiation and are maintained throughout the simulation. Once a simulation starts, other types of agents, such as monocytes, neutrophils, macrophages, appear in the model in accordance with the behavioral rules described in the following section.

ii) Behavioral rules of agents in the model. In an agent-based model, the behaviors of agents are controlled by type-specific rules. In this model, the agents' behavioral rules control replication rates, responses to the presence of other agents, and interactions of agents with their environment. In certain cases, the type of agent can be changed and consequently, the corresponding behavioral rules of the new type would be applied to the agent. This transition is typically based on the agent's position, type, and the local environment. One example of an agent type reassignment is the transformation from latent platelets to activated platelets. When circulating latent platelets encounter the wound site, their agent type is changed to activated platelet to reflect the activation event that would take place *in vivo*. In the model, latent platelets and activated platelets are distinct agent types and they are associated with different colors, sizes, and behavioral rules.

The behavioral rules for agents in the model are compiled according to an extensive literature survey and are summarized in a list form in Table 1. These rules have been simplified in order that they may be presented in the table. Further explanation of these rules and the corresponding supporting evidence are provided in Text S1.

iii) Parameters. The second main component of an agent-based model is the parameters associated with different types of agents. In this model, the parameters that are associated with the different cell types were set to the correct relative proportions based on data from the literature. Each agent is associated with multiple parameters that govern its behavior. The size and color of each agent were selected so that the simulation output is similar to a real situation and easy to understand. The parameters for each agent type in the model are presented in Table 2. Further details about how these parameters were chosen and implemented in the model are explained in Text S1.

C. Model Interface, Outputs, and Parameter Sensitivity

i) Modifiable parameters in the model interface. The model interface consists of modifiable parameters and quantitative and visual outputs. These modifiable input parameters include the lumen diameter (in mm) following angioplasty and stent implantation, the stent length (in mm), the number of stents, and the arrangement of the stent struts in the vessel cross-section. All of these parameters have default values. Prior to the initiation of the model in each simulation, these parameters can be set to desired values according to the purpose of the simulation.

Some input parameters were incorporated into the model due to the increasing interest in overlapping-stent cases and the effects of novel stent designs. Parameters specifically relevant to these topics are the number of stents in the simulated cross-section, the number of struts per stent, and the spacing of the stent struts, all of which can be manipulated in the model interface. When simulating an overlapping-stent scenario, the same input parameters are applied to both stents. In the model interface, there are two options for the two stent strut arrangement: aligned and staggered. In the aligned arrangement, the struts of the interior

stent are placed right above the ones of the exterior stent. In the staggered placement, each of the struts on the interior stent is placed at the center of two adjacent struts on the exterior stent.

For both single- and multi-stent simulations, the size of the stent struts and either the number of stent struts or the spacing between two adjacent struts (in mm) can be set at the beginning of the simulations. The default stent strut size is 0.1 mm [44], and the default number of struts per stent is 20 in the vessel cross section [45,46]. For any designated number of struts in the stent(s), those struts are always evenly spaced around the post-stenting boundary of the lumen. For any given spacing between two adjacent struts, an appropriate number of struts is determined by dividing the post-stenting lumen circumference by the selected spacing and rounding to the nearest integer value.

An additional modifiable parameter is the vessel wall thickness. This parameter does not appear in the model interface, but its value is calculated based on the initial lumen diameter. Since the vessel thickness is typically not reported in experimental studies, in this model the default wall thickness is defined as being equal to the given lumen radius, based on the observation that the typical ratio between the lumen radius and the vessel wall is roughly 1:1 [47].

ii) Simulation outputs: value measurement protocols. The agent-based model can produce both numerical and visual outputs in the user interface. The quantitative outputs are the final lumen diameter, the days to reach a stable lumen diameter (the time to lumen diameter stabilization), the percent change in lumen area, and the local and serum concentrations of TGF-β and TNF-α (both in ng/ml, or nanogram/milliliter, or 10^{-6} kg/m^3). In this model, one of the visual outputs is a plot that tracks the population of SMC and EC agents during a simulation. The other visual output is a color-coordinated diagram of the blood vessel cross-section, which is continuously updated during each simulation to illustrate the positions of different types of agents in the model and the changes to the lumen area. In this model, a few variable measurement protocols were implemented to obtain the information for all these valuable outputs.

Table 2. Summary of parameter values governing release rates, cytokine sensitivities, migration rates, proliferation rates, color, size, and lifespans of agents in the model.

Agent (color, size)	Parameter	Parameter Value of Reference	Source
TGF-β (invisible, 0.0002)	Release rate	0.02 pg/10 hours/cell	[74]
TNF-α (invisible, 0.0002)	Release rate	0.02 pg/10 hours/cell	[74]
SMCs (green, 0.6)	TGF-β sensitivity	3 ng/ml	[49]
	Migration rate	20 µm/hour	[75]
	Proliferation rate	Population doubles every 30 hours	[76]
Monocytes, neutrophils, and macrophages	TGF-β sensitivity	1 fmole	[28]
ECs (pink, 0.42) and SMCs	TNF-α sensitivity	4 ng/ml	[37]
	Maximum apoptosis rate following TNF-α exposure	15% of the population	[77]
Platelets (red, activated: 0.4, latent: 0.3)	Lifespan	5–10 days	[78]
Monocytes (blue, 0.54)	Migration rate	1 µm/min	[79]
	Lifespan	3 days	[80]
Macrophages (cyan, 0.54)	Lifespan	45 days	[81]
Neutrophils (light blue, 0.54)	Lifespan	5 days	[82]
Stent struts (gray, 2.7)	Default size	0.1 mm	[44]
	Default number of struts per stent	20	[45,46]
Plaque (violet, 0.7)	Lifespan	No limit	

To measure the changes in the lumen cross-sectional area, the model used the location of intimal EC agents as the reference points for the boundary of the new lumen. This lumen diameter measurement method was utilized to ensure that the model monitors the worst-case lumen obstruction, which is considered to be most clinically significant. Consequently, percent change in lumen area was calculated according to the equation below:

$$\Delta S = \frac{L_i - L_2}{L_2} \times 100$$

where ΔS is the percent change in lumen area, L_i is the initial lumen area (in mm^2) prior to the start of a simulation and L_2 is the new lumen area (in mm^2) based on the minimum lumen diameter (in mm).

In the numerical outputs of the model, the concentrations of TGF-β and TNF-α are reported as values comparable to the ones reported in the literature (in ng/ml). The local cytokine concentrations are calculated by counting the numbers of these cytokine agents on a patch of interest and its adjacent 8 patches (the local environment), and then dividing this count by the volume for the chosen patch set. For any patch of interest, the corresponding volume of the local environment is defined as V = C×AP, where V is the volume, C is a constant for the thickness of the patch, and AP is the area of 9 patches. In the numerical output in the model interface, the reported cytokine concentrations include both the local and serum concentrations of the cytokines. The local cytokine concentrations directly affect the proliferative and apoptotic behavior of those cell agents within the measurement perimeter according to the behavioral rules. The serum concentration of the cytokines does not affect the behavior of any cells in the model but rather serves as a checkpoint to ensure that the net cytokine release does not exceed normal physiological ranges. Acceptable serum TNF-α values were determined to be between 0 and 10 ng/ml, based on *in vivo* studies [37], and the same range was considered to be acceptable for the serum TGF-β concentrations [48,49].

The model constantly reports the simulated days post-intervention in the model interface. In each simulation, the number of days from the beginning of the simulation to the end of TGF-β release is used as the lumen diameter stabilization time (in days). After this point, data are recorded for an additional 60 simulated days to confirm that the lumen diameter had become static.

iii) Simulation outputs: examples of visual lumen area changes. The visual outputs for the blood vessel cross-section from both single-stent and overlap-stent simulations using the initial parameters from [50] are shown in Figures 2A–2H. These visual outputs were randomly selected from simulations. Figures 2A–2F are the results from single-stent simulations while Figures 2G and 2H are the results from an overlapping-stent simulation. Figures 2A–2D are all from one individual simulation while Figures 2E–2G are from different simulations. Figure 2A illustrates the initial setting of the vessel cross-section right after the initiation of the simulation, which represents the status of the vessel immediately following the angioplasty and stent implantation procedure. Visible agents at this stage include platelets (red) in the lumen, stent struts (gray squares), ECs (pink), SMCs (green), and plaque (violet, bottom-left corner). Figure 2B presents the vessel cross-section 15 simulated days after the stent procedure. Monocytes (blue), neutrophils (light blue), and macrophages (cyan) were present in the model by this time point. The population of SMC agents (green) increased significantly during the 15 days. Figure 2C shows the status of the blood vessel 59 days after the procedure. Figure 2C clearly reflects the proliferation of EC and

SMC agents and migration of SMC agents towards the lumen. Figure 2D illustrates the ultimate results of this simulation. The lumen diameter was stable after 84 simulated days and 45.52% of the original lumen area was occupied by the neointima. In this particular case, the neointima did become thicker, however, it did not reach the point of restenosis (greater than 50% lumen area loss [51]). In other simulations, the SMCs and ECs keep proliferating and migrating towards the lumen. The neointima may then occupy a large portion of the lumen (≥50% of the lumen area). This phenomenon is demonstrated in Figure 2E, which is the result from a different simulation from Figure 2D. The lumen was stabilized after 88 days and the neointima occupied 77.67% of the original lumen area. The result depicted in Figure 2F, which is from yet another separate simulation, represents the worst-case result. In this instance, the neointima advanced to such an extent that it occupied the entirety of the lumen space, which occurred 69 days after the intervention. In the cases of both Figures 2E and 2F, restenosis would have been developed in the simulated artery since the neointima occupied more than 50% of the original lumen area. Figures 2G and 2H display the initial setting and the final result of an overlapping-stent simulation, respectively. A staggered stent strut arrangement was selected for this simulation, which is illustrated in Figure 2G.

iv) Parameter sensitivity analysis. The purpose of the parameter sensitivity analysis was to identify any parameters for which a small change in the parameter value resulted in a *significant alteration* in the behavior of the model. Sometimes, the model's sensitivity to a particular parameter does not have an obvious connection to *in vivo* events based on the literature. The sensitivity analysis was also meant to check the *reasonableness of the model results* when small perturbations were made to model parameters. Any physiologically impossible or implausible results stemming from minor alterations to model parameters would highlight a potential weakness in the model construction. As exhibited by the results of the sensitivity analysis, no such weaknesses were identified during the course of the testing on this model.

A few hundred simulations were performed to confirm the consistency of the simulation results. No irregularities (i.e., a simulation reaching completion within a timeframe of only a few simulated days, dramatic/unexpected changes of simulated behavior in the middle of a simulation, or failure to reach lumen diameter stabilization, etc.) were observed in these test simulations. For each given set of initial parameters, the final lumen diameters obtained from those simulations were consistent. A simple test was conducted using one set of input parameters to demonstrate the consistency of the results. The test procedure and results are presented in Text S1. This simple test indicates that the average values of two groups with the same input parameters and 10 random runs are highly consistent. Therefore, it is sufficient to have 10 runs per simulation for data reporting. In the rest of this article, all of the reported results are the average values of 10 random runs of the simulation with the indicated parameters.

The results of the sensitivity analysis for functions with direct physiological meaning are presented in Tables S1 and S2 in Text S1. After all simulations for one alteration were completed, the model was run in its normal configuration for two simulations to confirm all changes had been reversed prior to performing the next alteration. The results presented in Tables S1 and S2 in Text S1 indicate that the model is extremely sensitive to functions related to intimal and medial apoptosis and proliferation, inflammatory cell adherence and migration, and TNF-α. The influence of intimal and medial apoptosis and proliferation functions on the final results of the model is expected based on the *in vivo* pathogenesis of restenosis, and the significance of the

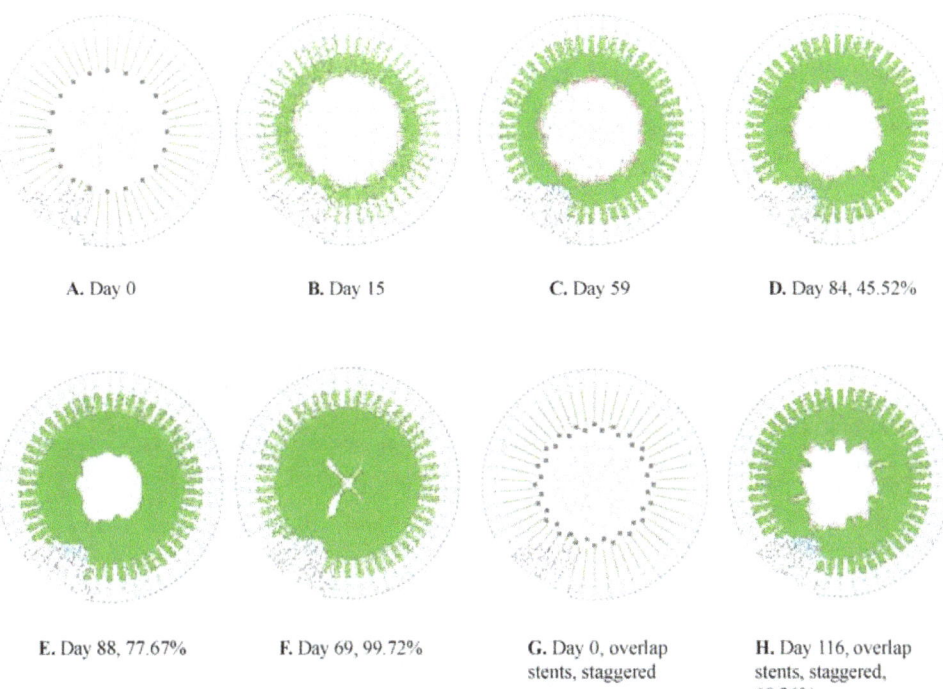

A. Day 0   B. Day 15   C. Day 59   D. Day 84, 45.52%

E. Day 88, 77.67%   F. Day 69, 99.72%   G. Day 0, overlap
stents, staggered   H. Day 116, overlap
stents, staggered,
60.26%

Figure 2. Visual outputs from single-stent and overlapping-stent simulations. Simulations utilized the initial vessel parameters from Kimura et al. [50]. 2A–2D: Snapshots from a single-stent simulation at different days (days 0, 15, 59, and 84). 2E–2F: Final results from two single-stent simulations with different levels of restenosis. 2G–2H: The initial and final images from one overlapping-stent simulation.

inflammatory cells (monocytes, neutrophils, and macrophages in this model) is because they release cytokines in their local environment. The adventitial SMCs' apoptotic and proliferative functions do not have a significant impact on model outcomes because adventitial SMCs do not migrate to other layers of the vessel wall and thus changes in the adventitial SMC population do not contribute to the development of neointima. As noted in Table S2 in Text S1, the endothelial proliferation functions do not contribute to increases in neointima thickness due to the single layer feature of ECs in the neointima layer. The locations of ECs are, however, crucial to the *measurement* of the lumen diameter.

D. Model Validation and Overlapping-stent Simulation Procedures

The goal of the model validation testing was to assess the integrity of the model's quantitative outputs. To this end, simulations were performed using vessel parameters from three serial imaging studies [50,52,53]. These three imaging studies were selected specifically because these studies reported both initial and final lumen diameters and had extended follow-up times and high participant retention rates. For each comparison, 10 runs of each simulation were performed with the parameters of the corresponding imaging study as the input parameters of the model. The average final lumen diameter and average time to lumen diameter stabilization (± standard deviation) from these 10 runs of each simulation were then reported. The time to lumen diameter stabilization was rounded to the nearest day. The outer diameters of the imaged vessels were not given in any of these three imaging studies, and therefore the default vessel thickness (the same as the given lumen radius) was used in these simulations.

The plaque in the model was placed at the bottom left corner of the simulated cross section across all simulations. Because the vessel's cross-section is a circle, repositioning the plaque along the circumference should not affect the simulation results. The plaque size in the model was also preset at a specific value, described by four boundary values (x_1, x_2, y_1, y_2). The location and size of the plaque can be manipulated by modifying these four boundary values within the code of the model. However, because there was no information about the position and size of the plaque in the targeted vessels imaged in the comparison studies, the plaque location and size were maintained at the model's default configuration. If the location and size of the plaque need to be changed, the new boundary of the plaque should not protrude into the lumen or distort the stent. This is required by the innate assumption that the blood vessel's cross-section is a circle after the angioplasty and stenting procedure. In all other respects, the consequences of plaque rupture should be taken into account in the model. As indicated at the beginning of the Materials and Methods section, this model does not incorporate the contribution of a ruptured plaque to the inflammatory reactions in the process of restenosis development.

For the overlapping-stent simulations, the expected result was an increase in lumen cross-sectional area loss as a consequence of the increased vessel wall damage inflicted by the second set of stent struts and the corresponding increased intimal hyperplasia [10]. Overlapping-stent simulations were run using the initial post-implantation vessel parameters from Kimura et al. [50]. This study was chosen after the completion of the model validation simulations due to the closeness of the model's results with the results reported in the comparison study. Ten runs of each overlapping-stent simulation were conducted to make sure that the obtained results were stable.

Results

A. Single-stent Simulations for Model Validation

i) Final lumen diameter. The average final lumen diameter and the average time to lumen diameter stabilization for each comparison simulation are given in Table 3. Across all three sets of validation simulations, the average values of the final lumen diameters generated by the model were all within one standard deviation of the means reported in the corresponding serial imaging studies from which the input model parameters were taken. The results from the simulation using the parameters from Chamié et al. differed more from the reported mean diameter than the results for the other two sets of simulations [52]. This discrepancy is likely due to the size of the vessels investigated in the Chamié et al study. Chamié et al specifically evaluated stent patency in smaller vessels. A smaller diameter atherosclerotic blood vessel may undergo stress-induced remodeling, resulting in a different lumen radius to vessel wall thickness ratio [54]. However, because no vessel wall thickness values were reported in the study by Chamié et al., the validation simulations were conducted with the default 1:1 ratio between lumen radius and vessel wall thickness. If accurate values of vessel thickness were available, the accuracy of the model predictions would likely increase.

ii) Time to lumen diameter stabilization. The average time to lumen diameter stabilization from the model validation testing is also presented in Table 3. The time to lumen diameter stabilization generated by the model paralleled the study follow-up times for all three studies, in spite of the inter-study variation in follow-up periods. It is pertinent to note, however, that these investigator-determined follow-up periods may not reflect the actual time needed for lumen diameter stabilization *in vivo*.

iii) Percent change in lumen area. Due to wide variations in the method of calculation for percent change in lumen cross-sectional area reported in the literature, the values of percent change in lumen area from the model were not compared with the values reported in the literature. Instead, the average percent change in lumen area over time generated from model simulations was compared across the three sets of validation simulations. Figure 3 displays the simulated percent change in lumen area over time.

While the initial parameters, final lumen diameter, and time to lumen diameter stabilization varied according to input parameters, the curves in Figure 3 show that the percent change in lumen diameter followed the same trajectory across all three sets of simulations from simulation initiation to lumen diameter stabilization. The consistent nature of these curves reflects consistent cell and cytokine positive- and negative-feedback interactions across simulations and reinforces the validity of the numerical results presented in Table 3. If the path to lumen diameter stabilization varied significantly when different input parameters were used, it would indicate that the cell and cytokine interactions were not the main effectors of the lumen diameter change over time and the model results were artificially affected by the input parameters.

iv) Comparison of local cytokine levels. As discussed earlier in the Materials and Methods section, the serum cytokine concentration does not affect the behavior of any agents in the model. The serum concentrations of TGF-β and TNF-α serve as a checkpoint to ensure that the cytokine release does not exceed normal physiological ranges. As noted earlier, TGF-β and TNF-α concentrations are between 0 and 10 ng/ml. In all three sets of validation simulations, the serum cytokine concentrations remained within the normal range.

Local cytokine concentrations, however, are critically important to the functionality of the model as the local cytokine concentrations dictate the changes in the SMC and EC populations. For all validation simulations, the local cytokine levels for both TGF-β and TNF-α were within the expected ranges, which was the same as the normal serum range defined above. The maximum local TGF-β concentration experienced in the 30 runs of validation simulations was approximately 6 ng/ml, and the maximum local concentration for TNF-α was approximately 9 ng/ml.

B. Overlapping-stent Simulations

The average final lumen diameter for the overlapping-stent simulations (using the Kimura et al. parameters [50]) was $1.79\pm.02$ mm^2, and the average time to lumen diameter stabilization was 112 ± 8 days. These results represent a 14.5% decrease in average final lumen diameter and a 25.6% increase in the average time to lumen diameter stabilization from the single stent simulation results that used the same input parameters.

The overlapping-stent simulations exhibited an increase in lumen area loss and in time to lumen diameter stabilization. Both of these findings were expected based on the literature. The increased damage to the vessel wall caused by the additional stent resulted in increased apoptosis at the time of the intervention. The increased cytokine release also recruited more inflammatory cells, which released more TNF-α, requiring a prolonged vessel recovery time. The increased damage also triggered a chain reaction of increased cytokine release and subsequent increased cell proliferation and migration, which created amplified intimal hyperplasia. This reasonable explanation may indicate the qualitative expectation based on the literature, however, it cannot provide quantitative results when some specific input parameters are given. The simulations conducted in this agent-based model can provide the desired quantitative values.

C. Comparison between Single-stent and Overlapping-stent Simulation Outcomes

i) Percent change in lumen area. Figure 4 presents the average percent change in lumen area over time from the single-stent simulations (solid line) and the overlapping-stent simulations

Table 3. Initial parameters and final results from serial imaging studies used for comparison by Kimura et al. [50], Hoffman et al. [53], and Chamié et al. [52] and model final lumen diameter and time-to-stabilization results.

Comparison Study	Measurement method	Study initial LD* (mm)	Study final LD (mm)	Study follow-up time (months)	Model final LD (mm)	Model time to LD stabilization (days)
Kimura et al.	Angiography	2.9±.04	2.2±.6	3–6	2.13±.02	89±7
Hoffman et al.	Intravascular ultrasound	3.19±.51	2.12±.82	5.4±3.8	2.34±.02	82±16
Chamié et al.	Intravascular ultrasound	2.39±.13	1.28±.74	7.2±1.0	1.75±.05	93±15

*LD=lumen diameter.

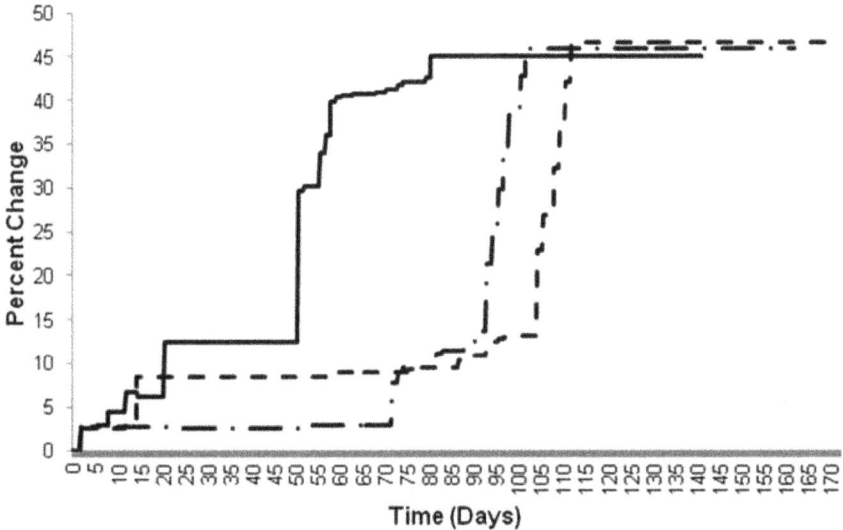

Figure 3. Percent change in lumen area in single-stent simulations from each set of validation simulations. Simulation using Kimura et al. parameters = solid; Hoffman et al. parameters = dash-dot; Chamié et al. parameters = dashed.

(dashed line). Both sets of simulations utilized the initial parameters from Kimura *et al.* [50]. The differences between the two curves in Figure 4 illustrate the effects of altered hyperplasia-apoptosis balance. Although the trajectory of the overlapping-stent simulation curve is similar to the results for the single-stent simulations in Figure 3, the curve of the overlapping-stent simulation (dashed line) exhibits a phase delay with respect to the single-stent case (solid line). This delay is likely due to the increase in initial levels of apoptotic cell death, caused by the presence of the second stent. The lower initial SMC population in the case of overlapping-stent likely contributed to the delayed re-growth of the intima. However, the increased vessel wall injury also triggered an increase in the number of cells releasing the anti-inflammatory cytokine TGF-β. Thus, once the concentration of TGF-β reached a certain level, the change in lumen diameter was accelerated with respect to that in the single-stent simulation. This is reflected in the slope and magnitude of the curve for overlapping-stent simulations following the phase delay.

ii) Local cytokine concentrations. Overall, the concentrations of local TNF-α and TGF-β were higher in the overlapping-stent simulations than in the single-stent simulations. While the TNF-α levels were only higher by approximately 1 ng/ml, the increase in the TGF-β levels was more significant, >2 ng/ml, which represents a 33% increase. Notably, neither increase in local cytokine concentrations elevated the total concentrations beyond the physiologically appropriate limit (≤10 ng/ml).

The increased local cytokine concentrations seen in the overlapping-stent simulations provide support for the proposed mechanisms behind the differences between the single- and overlapping-stent simulations. Specifically, the altered local cytokine levels coincide with the changes seen in the lumen diameter data and in the percent change in lumen diameter curve. The increased TGF-β levels are a reflection of the increased hyperplasia, and the increased TNF-α levels are due to the increase in the number of recruited inflammatory cells (monocytes, neutrophils, and macrophages) drawn to the wound sites by the increased TGF-β levels.

iii) Cell population changes. One set of results for the percent change in the SMC population and the EC population over time from the single-stent and overlapping-stent simulations

utilizing the initial parameters from Kimura *et al.* [50] are plotted in Figures 5 and 6, respectively.

The effects of the altered cytokine concentrations in the overlapping-stent simulations are reflected mainly in the SMC population. The SMC population curve for the overlapping-stent simulation displays the same phase delay coupled with a slope and magnitude increase seen in the percent change in lumen diameter graph for the overlapping-stent simulations.

In contrast, the effects of the altered cytokine concentrations on the EC population appear to predominantly affect the initial population and did not significantly alter the rate or magnitude of the subsequent population growth. This disparity in the behavior of the SMC and EC populations is likely due to the reduced aggregate population of ECs in the model compared to SMCs. There are more than twice as many SMCs as there are ECs present in the model by the time of lumen diameter stabilization in a number of simulations, and the effects of the altered cytokine levels were more readily apparent on the larger scale.

Discussion

By utilizing the developed behavioral rules and the vessel's post-intervention parameters, the agent-based model described in this article successfully simulated the response of an atherosclerotic blood vessel to an angioplasty and bare-metal stent deployment procedure as described in the literature. In addition, the model was capable of accurately simulating the effects of overlapping-stent deployment.

Simulations with three sets of parameters from imaging studies verified the correctness and robustness of the model. The reported results indicate that the model can reproduce the results observed in the serial imaging studies by using the input parameters obtained from these studies. Based on these results, it is obvious that this model can be used to perform simulations with different input parameters and produce correct predictions without any alterations to the model's mechanisms. The reasonableness of the percent change in lumen area and time for lumen stabilization results obtained from these simulations clearly demonstrate the accuracy of the model.

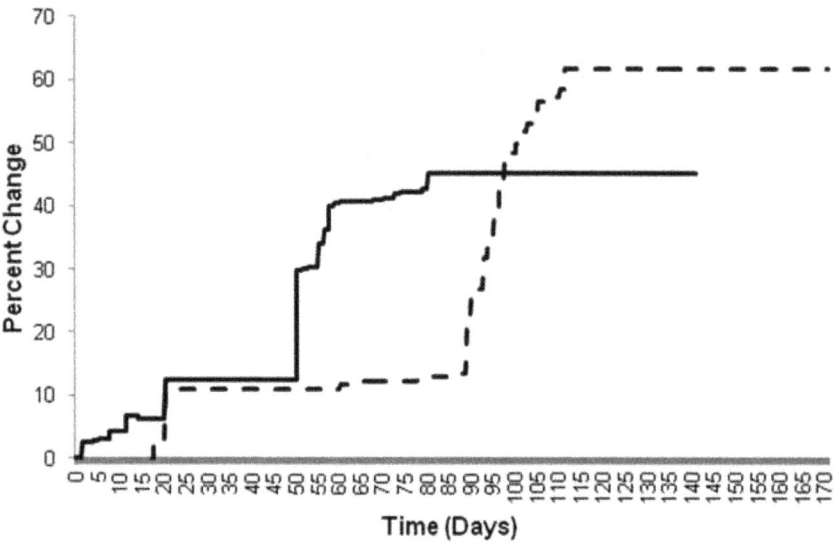

Figure 4. Comparison of percent change in lumen diameter in single-stent and overlapping-stent simulations. Single-stent simulations = solid and overlapping-stent simulations = dashed, all simulations using parameters from Kimura et al. [50].

The results from the overlapping-stent simulations can also be used as a prediction of the *in vivo* response to multi-stent deployment. In a clinical setting, rather than in experiments, two overlapping stents would not be placed concurrently. The second stent is usually implanted after the restenosis in the first stent has developed to a serious stage. This is one limitation of the model in overlapping-stent simulations.

In the simulation for lumen area change in the case of a single stent implantation, the simulated time to lumen diameter stabilization was similar across all three compared imaging studies (Table 3). However, since the follow-up periods for the study were predetermined by the respective investigators in those studies, they may not reflect the actual time point at which the lumen diameter

was stabilized. In addition, the variability in the simulation time course is constrained by the effects of using a default vessel thickness and assumed uniformity of the cell behaviors in the model.

All model parameters were based on values for human cells and cytokines reported in the literature. However, the exact regulation mechanism for many of these processes, including growth factor- and injury-regulated cell proliferation, has yet to be fully delineated. The necessary assumption was that the adopted model parameters held true for all cells of a given type in the simulated environment when, in fact, the behavior of cells *in vivo* is not uniform. Induced randomness in the model functions and using *in vivo* measurements for the vessel thickness would likely further

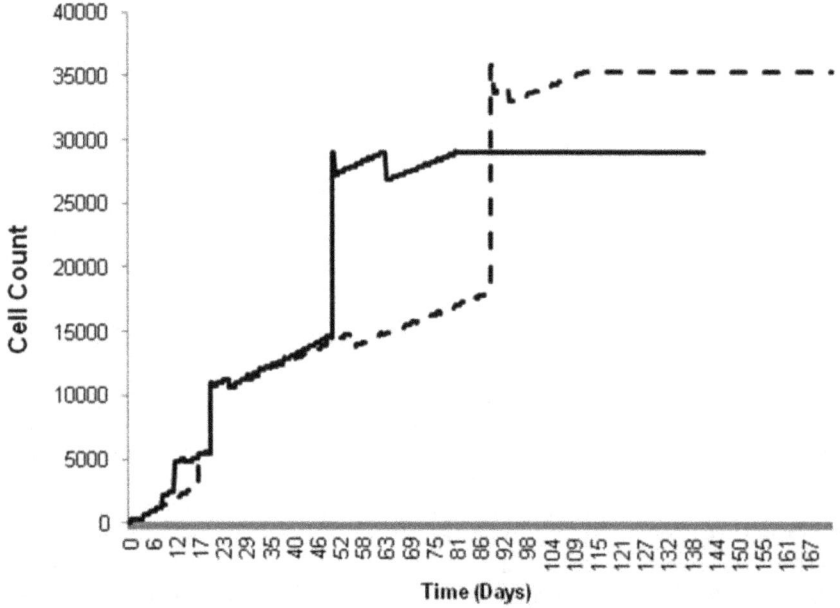

Figure 5. Comparison of the time course of SMC population changes in single-stent and overlapping-stent simulations. Single-stent simulations = solid and overlapping-stent simulations = dashed, all simulations using parameters from Kimura et al. [50].

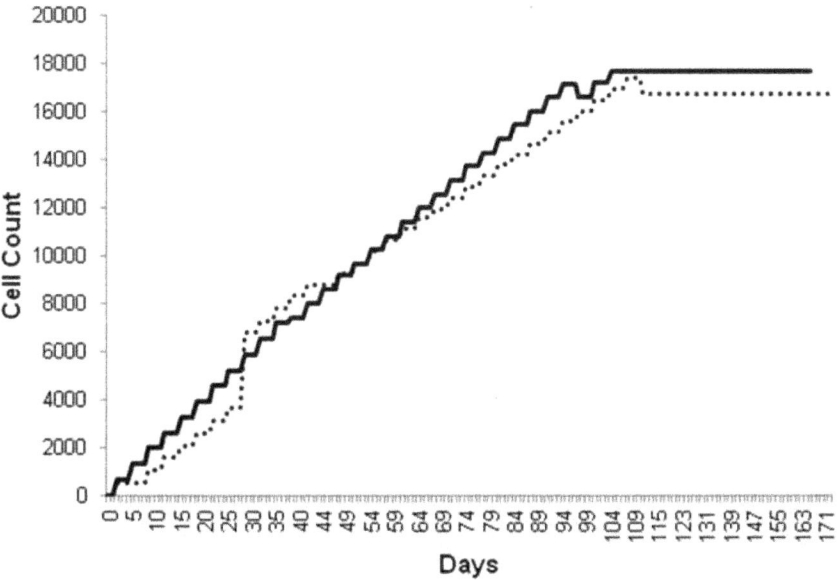

Figure 6. Comparison of the time course of EC population changes in single-stent and overlapping-stent simulations. Single-stent simulations = solid and overlapping-stent simulations = dashed, all simulations using parameters from Kimura et al. [50].

increase the accuracy of the simulation. The use of different values for vessel wall thickness would impact simulation results since the subsequent alterations to the TGF-β release parameter is influenced by hoop stress, which is directly related to the vessel wall thickness and lumen radius (More details about hoop stress and its effect on TGF-β release rate can be found in Text S1).

The limitations of the model stem from the nature of computational modeling itself. The size constraints imposed on the model by the computing power of the NetLogo modeling environment negatively affected the scale the model could simulate by limiting the total number of agents that could be tracked within the simulation. While there are more powerful modeling environments that would partially alleviate this problem, attempting to simulate all the cells present in even a small cross-sectional area of a human blood vessel would be an unwieldy undertaking for any computational modeling environment.

In addition, it is difficult to recreate the precise natural variations seen in the behavior of cells and cytokines in the body. For instance, it is known that TGF-β has different behavioral patterns at different stages of disease development [38], and subsequently varies in its impacts on the behavior of other cells and cytokines. In the model, TGF-β was treated as a single-modality cytokine. One motivation for this type of simplification was that the properties of those cells and cytokines are not yet well-understood by investigators in the field. Thus, in order to recreate those variations seen *in vivo*, modelers would have to make many assumptions which might be random in nature and lack supporting evidence in the literature. The other motivation for the chosen simplification was that there are a large number of cell and cytokine types involved in the process of restenosis development. Attempting to include all of these cells and cytokines in the model would introduce a number of unknown or not-well-defined parameters into the model. Simplifications are a critical component in the construction of effective and rigorous models and can help investigators to concentrate on a limited number of essential components in the simulated system [55]. This approach may sacrifice the power of simulating the subtle differences of different

cytokines but yield a much clearer understanding of the critical components that lead to in-stent restenosis.

However, the model created with these simplifications is fully capable of simulating the variations in cell and cytokine effects on a larger scale. As mentioned earlier in the Materials and Methods section, the visual outputs of multiple random model runs for simulations with the same set of input parameters produced different results. In some model simulation runs (roughly 40% of all runs), there was neointima layer thickening, but it did not reach the point of clinically-defined restenosis [51]. In other model runs, in-stent restenosis developed at different severity levels. This result reflects the variation seen in the clinical manifestation of in-stent restenosis. It is estimated that the rate of restenosis occurrence in patients who have undergone an angioplasty and stent procedure in randomized trials ranges between 30–40% [56,57]. Other studies, however, have reported incidence rates as high as 48.8% [58] or even 60% [5]. This natural variation in restenosis rates as described in the literature was recreated by the model on both the tissue and organ scales.

There were some innate assumptions in the model construction process that merit discussion. For instance, it was assumed that the majority of cells in the neointimal layer were SMCs and their proliferation and migration were the driving forces of the renarrowing of the lumen, under the influence and regulation of multiple other cells and cytokines. This assumption was supported by the literature [59], although there are other known factors in this process, such as extracellular matrix deposition and vessel remodeling (or persistent change in vessel size) [60]. This model clearly indicated that SMC proliferation and migration is the most important driving force in the development of restenosis, as extracellular matrix deposition and vessel remodeling were ignored in the model, but the model still could simulate the development of restenosis with high accuracy. The model's results do not signify that patients with higher SMC proliferation and migration will develop restenosis faster or more severely because of dynamic interactions among SMCs, other cells, and cytokines. From a clinical perspective, however, controlling SMC proliferation and migration may be a possible way to impede the development of restenosis. This is the therapeutic approach that drove the development of drug-eluting stents [59]. In that approach, the proliferation of SMCs and ECs is inhibited by the drug that coats on the drug-eluting stents. Unfortunately, such stents are not completely successful in improving patient outcomes because they are associated with other risks, such as late and very late thrombosis [61,62].

As described previously in the Materials and Methods section, the model can be dynamically manipulated in the model interface by editing the values for parameters such as the vessel diameter, number of struts, size of struts, length of stent, space of struts, number of stents and stent alignment. Such manipulation has have already been demonstrated in the validation simulations with three sets of input parameters. This type of simulations is used to simulate a group of patients in a similar situation. Therefore variations are observed in those simulations. In the future, the authors plan to integrate more patient-specific parameters into the model interface, such as platelets, leucocytes, and cytokines counts; the size of the targeted plaque; and vessel wall thickness. The updated model would then be able to produce more patient-specific results.

The motivation for not including plaque rupture and the corresponding intense inflammatory reactions in this model were explained at the beginning of the Materials and Methods section. In the future, the role of plaque rupture could be taken into account in an extended model. In such a model, anti-platelet and anti-inflammatory drugs, lipid, and interferon-γ would be introduced as agents in the model. The size and location of plaque are also important in this case and therefore would have to be taken into account in the model as well. The ruptured plaque releases a large number of inflammatory factors in a short period of time and triggers the activation of a large number of platelets that subsequently results in acute thrombosis [18]. Without proper control, both the strong inflammatory reaction and the acute thrombosis may lead to patient death. Therefore, simulating the consequences of plaque rupture is a critically important research question.

As mentioned in the Introduction section, the vast majority of patients, approximately 92%, who received the PCI procedures also underwent stent procedures simultaneously [3,63]. An important reason for this practice is that the elastic recoil right after balloon angioplasty can result in approximately 50% cross-sectional area loss on average [64]. Simultaneous stent placement is advantageous in that it can easily prevent elastic recoil from occurring. Conversely, implanting a stent also introduces further damage to the blood vessel. The model presented in this article was specifically created to simulate the response of the vessel to the concomitant angioplasty and stent procedures. However, since there are no similar models with a similar setting for the PCI procedure alone before this model, it can be problematic to determine the precise contributions from the stent in the development of in-stent restenosis. Accordingly, the result of this model cannot precisely identify the contributions of the stent to the lumen area loss when compared to the development of restenosis following a balloon angioplasty procedure. Therefore, even though the results obtained from the simulations in this model with varying stent parameters would be able to provide useful information for designing or testing different stents, a more accurate conclusion could be drawn after conducting simulations with a similar model where the consequence of angioplasty procedure alone is simulated. In the future, we plan to create an agent-based model to simulate the development of restenosis after only a balloon angioplasty procedure. The comparison between

the results from these two models should be able to further clarify the contribution of a stent to restenosis development.

As mentioned earlier in this section, the drugs that coat on drug-eluting stents inhibit the proliferation of all types of cells in the blood vessel and therefore inhibit the development of in-stent restenosis. However, patients with a drug-eluting stent have to undergo prolonged anti-platelet drug therapy because the damage to the endothelial cell lining and the media layer during the angioplasty and stent procedure can never be recovered, making platelet activation and subsequent thrombus formation a constant risk [65]. Because drug-eluting stents can effectively help patients to avoid in-stent restenosis and there are cheap anti-platelet drugs, for instance, aspirin [66], they have been widely used in recent years [67]. However, anti-platelet drugs can become a heavy burden for patients who do not respond well to the typical pharmaceuticals and patients who need to take multiple types of anti-platelet drugs to effectively avoid thrombosis [68,69].

In the future, we plan to create a model based on the setting of the current model that is capable of simulating the consequences of drug-eluting stent deployment. In that model, the proliferation and migration of SMC will not be so important while anti-platelet drugs will have an important role [70–73]. This drug-eluting stent model may be used to investigate the consequences of novel approaches and new technologies. For instance, the model would be helpful in investigating the possible results when the release of drug coated on the stent is delayed until the initial damage has been given time to heal. Such a controlled drug-eluting technology would be very promising because it would allow for inhibiting the proliferation of SMCs and ECs without the risk of late thrombosis. The model could provide critical information on the appropriate drug release timing to achieve this balance.

Conclusions

The developed agent-based model represents a simulation of the interplay between the major contributors in the development of restenosis in a human atherosclerotic blood vessel after an angioplasty and bare-metal stent deployment. The model simulated the body's response to the intervention and generated results consistent with serial imaging of human subjects across multiple studies. This model may serve as a tool to explore how different vessel cross-sections or stent arrangements may advance or reduce the development of restenosis in a blood vessel.

In the future, the authors will develop this model further to include more patient-specific physiological parameters and investigate the effects of plaque rupture. The authors will also create two parallel models, one for the angioplasty-only intervention and the other for the implantation of drug-eluting stents.

The model can be accessed at http://cpath.him.pitt.edu/stent/index.html.

Acknowledgments

We would like to thank the anonymous reviewers for their constructive comments, which significantly improved the final manuscript.

Author Contributions

Conceived and designed the experiments: LZ. Performed the experiments: AC. Analyzed the data: AC LZ. Contributed reagents/materials/analysis tools: AC LZ. Wrote the paper: AC LZ.

References

1. McCance KL, Huether SE (2009) Pathophysiology: The biologic basis for disease in adults and children. Maryland Heights, MO: Mosby. 1864 p.
2. Fitridge R, Thompson M (2007) Mechanisms of vascular disease: A textbook for vascular surgeons. Cambridge, UK: Cambridge University Press. 173–210.
3. Go AS, Mozaffarian D, Roger VL, Benjamin EJ, Berry JD, et al. (2014) Heart disease and stroke statistics–2014 update: a report from the american heart association. Circulation 129: e28–e292.
4. Stedman (2006) Stedman's Medical Dictionary. Philadelphia: Lippincott Wiliams & Wilkins.
5. Schillinger M, Minar E (2005) Restenosis after percutaneous angioplasty: the role of vascular inflammation. Vasc Health Risk Manag 1: 73–78.
6. Wasser K, Schnaudigel S, Wohlfahrt J, Psychogios MN, Knauth M, et al. (2011) Inflammation and in-stent restenosis: the role of serum markers and stent characteristics in carotid artery stenting. PLoS ONE 6: e22683.
7. Chen MS, John JM, Chew DP, Lee DS, Ellis SG, et al. (2006) Bare metal stent restenosis is not a benign clinical entity. Am Heart J 151: 1260–1264.
8. Muller DW, Ellis SG, Topol EJ (1992) Experimental models of coronary artery restenosis. J Am Coll Cardiol 19: 418–432.
9. Touchard AG, Schwartz RS (2006) Preclinical restenosis models: challenges and successes. Toxicol Pathol 34: 11–18.
10. Niazi M, Hussain M (2011) Agent-based computing from multi-agent systems to agent-based models: A visual survey. Springer Scientometrics 89: 479–499.
11. Wilensky U (1999) NetLogo. Center for Connected Learning and Computer-Based Modeling: Northwestern University, Evanston, IL.
12. Opal SM, DePalo VA (2000) Anti-inflammatory cytokines. Chest 117: 1162–1172.
13. Dinarello CA (2000) Proinflammatory cytokines. Chest 118: 503–508.
14. Thim T, Hagensen MK, Bentzon JF, Falk E (2008) From vulnerable plaque to atherothrombosis. J Intern Med 263: 506–516.
15. Meadows TA, Bhatt DL (2007) Clinical aspects of platelet inhibitors and thrombus formation. Circ Res 100: 1261–1275.
16. Waxman S, Freilich MI, Suter MJ, Shishkov M, Bilazarian S, et al. (2010) A case of lipid core plaque progression and rupture at the edge of a coronary stent: elucidating the mechanisms of drug-eluting stent failure. Circ Cardiovasc Interv 3: 193–196.
17. Kovanen PT, Mayranpaa M, Lindstedt KA (2005) Drug therapies to prevent coronary plaque rupture and erosion: present and future. Handb Exp Pharmacol: 745–776.
18. Drakopoulou M, Toutouzas K, Michelongona A, Tousoulis D, Stefanadis C (2011) Vulnerable plaque and inflammation: potential clinical strategies. Curr Pharm Des 17: 4190–4209.
19. Charo IF, Taub R (2011) Anti-inflammatory therapeutics for the treatment of atherosclerosis. Nat Rev Drug Discov 10: 365–376.
20. Karas SP, Gravanis MB, Santoian EC, Robinson KA, Anderberg KA, et al. (1992) Coronary intimal proliferation after balloon injury and stenting in swine: an animal model of restenosis. J Am Coll Cardiol 20: 467–474.
21. Rodero MP, Khosrotehrani K (2010) Skin wound healing modulation by macrophages. Int J Clin Exp Pathol 3: 643–653.
22. Kondo T, Ishida Y (2010) Molecular pathology of wound healing. Forensic Sci Int 203: 93–98.
23. Virmani R, Farb A (1999) Pathology of in-stent restenosis. Curr Opin Lipidol 10: 499–506.
24. Gawaz M, Langer H, May AE (2005) Platelets in inflammation and atherogenesis. J Clin Invest 115: 3378–3384.
25. Majesky MW, Lindner V, Twardzik DR, Schwartz SM, Reidy MA (1991) Production of transforming growth factor beta 1 during repair of arterial injury. J Clin Invest 88: 904–910.
26. Gordon S, Taylor PR (2005) Monocyte and macrophage heterogeneity. Nat Rev Immunol 5: 953–964.
27. Anderson JM, Rodriguez A, Chang DT (2008) Foreign body reaction to biomaterials. Semin Immunol 20: 86–100.
28. Ashcroft GS (1999) Bidirectional regulation of macrophage function by TGF-beta. Microbes Infect 1: 1275–1282.
29. Cerletti C, Tamburrelli C, Izzi B, Gianfagna F, de Gaetano G (2012) Platelet-leukocyte interactions in thrombosis. Thromb Res 129: 263–266.
30. Seye CI, Kong Q, Yu N, Gonzalez FA, Erb L, et al. (2007) P2 receptors in atherosclerosis and postangioplasty restenosis. Purinergic Signal 3: 153–162.
31. Stahl AL, Sartz L, Nelsson A, Bekassy ZD, Karpman D (2009) Shiga toxin and lipopolysaccharide induce platelet-leukocyte aggregates and tissue factor release, a thrombotic mechanism in hemolytic uremic syndrome. PLoS ONE 4: e6990.
32. Daigneault M, Preston JA, Marriott HM, Whyte MK, Dockrell DH (2010) The identification of markers of macrophage differentiation in PMA-stimulated THP-1 cells and monocyte-derived macrophages. PLoS ONE 5: e8668.
33. Berndt MC (2000) Platelets, thrombosis and the vessel wall. Amsterdam: Harwood Academic Publishers.
34. Monraats PS, Pires NM, Schepers A, Agema WR, Boesten LS, et al. (2005) Tumor necrosis factor-alpha plays an important role in restenosis development. FASEB J 19: 1998–2004.
35. Groschel K, Riecker A, Schulz JB, Ernemann U, Kastrup A (2005) Systematic review of early recurrent stenosis after carotid angioplasty and stenting. Stroke 36: 367–373.
36. Suwanabol PA, Kent KC, Liu B (2011) TGF-beta and restenosis revisited: a Smad link. J Surg Res 167: 287–297.
37. Rangamani P, Sirovich L (2007) Survival and apoptotic pathways initiated by TNF-alpha: modeling and predictions. Biotechnol Bioeng 97: 1216–1229.
38. Grainger DJ (2004) Transforming growth factor beta and atherosclerosis: so far, so good for the protective cytokine hypothesis. Arterioscler Thromb Vasc Biol 24: 399–404.
39. Tsai S, Hollenbeck ST, Ryer EJ, Edlin R, Yamanouchi D, et al. (2009) TGF-beta through Smad3 signaling stimulates vascular smooth muscle cell proliferation and neointimal formation. Am J Physiol Heart Circ Physiol 297: H540–549.
40. Welt FG, Rogers C (2002) Inflammation and restenosis in the stent era. Arterioscler Thromb Vasc Biol 22: 1769–1776.
41. Brown BN, Price IM, Toapanta FR, DeAlmeida DR, Wiley CA, et al. (2011) An agent-based model of inflammation and fibrosis following particulate exposure in the lung. Math Biosci 231: 186–196.
42. Li NY, Verdolini K, Clermont G, Mi Q, Rubinstein EN, et al. (2008) A patient-specific in silico model of inflammation and healing tested in acute vocal fold injury. PLoS ONE 3: e2789.
43. Alsheikh-Ali AA, Kitsios GD, Balk EM, Lau J, Ip S (2010) The vulnerable atherosclerotic plaque: scope of the literature. Ann Intern Med 153: 387–395.
44. Murphy BP, Savage P, McHugh PE, Quinn DF (2003) The stress-strain behavior of coronary stent struts is size dependent. Ann Biomed Eng 31: 686–691.
45. Kolodgie FD, Nakazawa G, Sangiorgi G, Ladich E, Burke AP, et al. (2007) Pathology of atherosclerosis and stenting. Neuroimaging Clin N Am 17: 285–301.
46. Stoeckel D, Bonsignore C, Duda S (2002) A survey of stent designs. Minim Invasive Ther Allied Technol 11: 137–147.
47. Botnar RM, Stuber M, Kissinger KV, Kim WY, Spuentrup E, et al. (2000) Noninvasive coronary vessel wall and plaque imaging with magnetic resonance imaging. Circulation 102: 2582–2587.
48. Blann AD, Wang JM, Wilson PB, Kumar S (1996) Serum levels of the TGF-beta receptor are increased in atherosclerosis. Atherosclerosis 120: 221–226.
49. Wildgruber M, Weiss W, Berger H, Wolf O, Eckstein HH, et al. (2007) Association of circulating transforming growth factor beta, tumor necrosis factor alpha and basic fibroblast growth factor with restenosis after transluminal angioplasty. Eur J Vasc Endovasc Surg 34: 35–43.
50. Kimura T, Nosaka H, Yokoi H, Iwabuchi M, Nobuyoshi M (1993) Serial angiographic follow-up after Palmaz-Schatz stent implantation: comparison with conventional balloon angioplasty. J Am Coll Cardiol 21: 1557–1563.
51. Hamid H, Coltart J (2007) 'Miracle stents'–a future without restenosis. McGill J Med 10: 105–111.
52. Chamie D, Costa JR Jr, Abizaid A, Feres F, Staico R, et al. (2010) Serial angiography and intravascular ultrasound: results of the SISC Registry (Stents In Small Coronaries). JACC Cardiovasc Interv 3: 191–202.
53. Hoffmann R, Mintz GS, Dussaillant GR, Popma JJ, Pichard AD, et al. (1996) Patterns and mechanisms of in-stent restenosis. A serial intravascular ultrasound study. Circulation 94: 1247–1254.
54. Pries AR, Reglin B, Secomb TW (2005) Remodeling of blood vessels: responses of diameter and wall thickness to hemodynamic and metabolic stimuli. Hypertension 46: 725–731.
55. Stefanescu RA, Shivakeshavan RG, Talathi SS (2012) Computational models of epilepsy. Seizure 21: 748–759.
56. Fischman DL, Leon MB, Baim DS, Schatz RA, Savage MP, et al. (1994) A randomized comparison of coronary-stent placement and balloon angioplasty in the treatment of coronary artery disease. N Engl J Med 331: 496–501.
57. Serruys PW, de Jaegere P, Kiemeneij F, Macaya C, Rutsch W, et al. (1994) A comparison of balloon-expandable-stent implantation with balloon angioplasty in patients with coronary artery disease. N Engl J Med 331: 489–495.
58. Mohan S, Dhall A (2010) A comparative study of restenosis rates in bare metal and drug-eluting stents. Int J Angiol 19: e66–72.
59. Costa MA, Simon DI (2005) Molecular basis of restenosis and drug-eluting stents. Circulation 111: 2257–2273.
60. Ward MR, Pasterkamp G, Yeung AC, Borst C (2000) Arterial remodeling. Mechanisms and clinical implications. Circulation 102: 1186–1191.
61. Otsuka F, Nakano M, Ladich E, Kolodgie FD, Virmani R (2012) Pathologic Etiologies of Late and Very Late Stent Thrombosis following First-Generation Drug-Eluting Stent Placement. Thrombosis 2012: 608593.

62. Zhang F, Qian J, Dong L, Ge J (2012) Super late stent thrombosis occurred at 8 years after drug-eluting stent implantation. Int J Cardiol 159: e53–55.

63. Auerbach D, Maeda J, Steiner C (2012) Hospital stays with cardiac stents, 2009. Rockville, MD: Agency for Healthcare Research and Quality.

64. King SB (2002) Restenosis following angioplasty. In: Waksman R, editor. Vascular Brachytherapy. 3rd ed. Armonk, NY: Futura Publishing Co., Inc. 3–11.

65. Chitkara K, Pujara K (2010) Drug-eluting Stents in Acute Coronary Syndrome: Is There a Risk of Stent Thrombosis with Second-Generation Stents? Eur J Cardiovasc Med 1: 20–24.

66. Homoncik M, Jilma B, Eichelberger B, Panzer S (2000) Inhibitory activity of aspirin on von Willebrand factor-induced platelet aggregation. Thromb Res 99: 461–466.

67. Roger VL, Go AS, Lloyd-Jones DM, Benjamin EJ, Berry JD, et al. (2012) Heart disease and stroke statistics–2012 update: a report from the American Heart Association. Circulation 125: e2–e220.

68. Poorhosseini HR, Hosseini SK, Davarpasand T, Lotfi Tokaldany M, Salarifar M, et al. (2012) Effectiveness of Two-Year versus One-Year Use of Dual Antiplatelet Therapy in Reducing the Risk of Very Late Stent Thrombosis after Drug-Eluting Stent Implantation. J Tehran Heart Cent 7: 47–52.

69. Lee KH, Ahn Y, Kim SS, Rhew SH, Jeong YW, et al. (2013) Comparison of Triple Anti-Platelet Therapy and Dual Anti-Platelet Therapy in Patients With Acute Myocardial Infarction Who Had No-Reflow Phenomenon During Percutaneous Coronary Intervention. Circ J 77: 2973–2981.

70. Friedman H, Mollon P, Lian J, Navaratnam P (2013) Clinical outcomes, health resource use, and cost in patients with early versus late dual or triple anti-platelet treatment for acute coronary syndrome. Am J Cardiovasc Drugs 13: 273–283.

71. Mulukutla SR, Marroquin OC, Vlachos HA, Selzer F, Toma C, et al. (2013) Benefit of long-term dual anti-platelet therapy in patients treated with drug-eluting stents: from the NHLBI dynamic registry. Am J Cardiol 111: 486–492.

72. Pappas C, Ntai K, Parissis JT, Anastasiou-Nana M (2013) Dual anti-platelet therapy in patients with G6PD deficiency after percutaneous coronary intervention. Int J Cardiol 165: 380–382.

73. Subban V, Kalidoss L, Sankardas MA (2012) Very late thrombosis of a paclitaxel-eluting stent after 72 months in a patient on dual anti-platelet therapy. Cardiovasc J Afr 23: e9–11.

74. Facoetti A, Mariotti L, Ballarini F, Bertolotti A, Nano R, et al. (2009) Experimental and theoretical analysis of cytokine release for the study of radiation-induced bystander effect. Int J Radiat Biol 85: 690–699.

75. DiMilla PA, Stone JA, Quinn JA, Albelda SM, Lauffenburger DA (1993) Maximal migration of human smooth muscle cells on fibronectin and type IV collagen occurs at an intermediate attachment strength. J Cell Biol 122: 729–737.

76. Sagnella SM, Kligman F, Anderson EH, King JE, Murugesan G, et al. (2004) Human microvascular endothelial cell growth and migration on biomimetic surfactant polymers. Biomaterials 25: 1249–1259.

77. Heikkila HM, Latti S, Leskinen MJ, Hakala JK, Kovanen PT, et al. (2008) Activated mast cells induce endothelial cell apoptosis by a combined action of chymase and tumor necrosis factor-alpha. Arterioscler Thromb Vasc Biol 28: 309–314.

78. Najean Y, Ardaillou N, Dresch C (1969) Platelet lifespan. Annu Rev Med 20: 47–62.

79. Noma H, Kato T, Fujita H, Kitagawa M, Yamano T, et al. (2009) Calpain inhibition induces activation of the distinct signalling pathways and cell migration in human monocytes. Immunology 128: e487–496.

80. Ferkol T, Perales JC, Mularo F, Hanson RW (1996) Receptor-mediated gene transfer into macrophages. Proc Natl Acad Sci USA 93: 101–105.

81. Heidenreich S (1999) Monocyte CD14: a multifunctional receptor engaged in apoptosis from both sides. J Leukoc Biol 65: 737–743.

82. Pillay J, den Braber I, Vrisekoop N, Kwast LM, de Boer RJ, et al. (2010) In vivo labeling with 2H2O reveals a human neutrophil lifespan of 5.4 days. Blood 116: 625–627.

20

Role of Far Infra-Red Therapy in Dialysis Arterio-Venous Fistula Maturation and Survival

Khalid Bashar[1]*, Donagh Healy[1], Leonard D. Browne[2], Elrasheid A. H. Kheirelseid[1], Michael T. Walsh[2], Mary Clarke – Moloney[1], Paul E. Burke[1], Eamon G. Kavanagh[1], Stewart Redmond Walsh[3]

1 Department of vascular surgery, University Hospital Limerick, Limerick, Ireland, 2 Centre for Applied Biomedical Engineering Research (CABER), Department of Mechanical, Aeronautical & Biomedical Engineering, Materials and Surface Science Institute, University of Limerick, Limerick, Ireland, 3 Department of surgery, National University of Ireland, Galway, Ireland

Abstract

Introduction: A well-functioning arteriovenous fistula (AVF) is the best modality for vascular access in patients with end-stage renal disease (ESRD) requiring haemodialysis (HD). However, AVFs' main disadvantage is the high rate of maturation failure, with approximately one third (20%–50%) not maturing into useful access. This review examine the use of Far-Infra Red therapy in an attempt to enhance both primary (unassisted) and secondary (assisted) patency rates for AVF in dialysis and pre-dialysis patients.

Method: We performed an online search for observational studies and randomised controlled trials (RCTs) that evaluated FIR in patients with AVF. Eligible studies compared FIR with control treatment and reported at least one outcome measure relating to access survival. Primary patency and secondary patency rates were the main outcomes of interest.

Results: Four RCTs (666 patients) were included. Unassisted patency assessed in 610 patients, and was significantly better among those who received FIR (228/311) compared to (185/299) controls (pooled risk ratio of 1.23 [1.12–1.35], p = 0.00001). In addition, the two studies which reported secondary patency rates showed significant difference in favour of FIR therapy-160/168 patients - compared to 140/163 controls (pooled risk ratio of 1.11 [1.04–1.19], p = 0.003).

Conclusion: FIR therapy may positively influence the complex process of AVF maturation improving both primary and secondary patency rates. However blinded RCTs performed by investigators with no commercial ties to FIR therapy technologies are needed.

Editor: Daniel Schneditz, Medical University of Graz, Austria

Funding: The authors have no support or funding to report.

Competing Interests: The authors have declared that no competing interests exist.

* Email: khalidbashar@rcsi.ie

Introduction

The number of patients with end stage renal disease (ESRD) requiring haemodialysis (HD) is steadily rising, a trend that is expected to continue [1]. Vascular access is a critical component in successful HD. A well-functioning arteriovenous fistula (AVF) is the best modality for HD vascular access [2–6]. AVF maturation is a complex process of remodelling. The newly formed fistula has to form a low resistance circuit capable of dilation to accommodate the increased blood flow required for HD. The AVF also has to be cannulated repeatedly with ease. The need for re-intervention to maintain patency should be minimal [2–4,6,7].

AVFs' main disadvantage is the high rate of maturation failure, with approximately one third (20%-50%) not maturing into useful access [8–10]. AVFs have higher primary failure rates to mature compared to grafts [8,11,12]. However they last longer, and with exclusion of fistulas that fail to mature primarily, the cumulative patency from formation to permanent failure is superior to grafts. AVFs also require fewer secondary interventions in the form of angioplasty, stenting or thrombectomy [8,13–16]. AVFs are associated with fewer complications compared to AVG and CVC in terms of infection, death, vascular access salvage procedures and hospitalizations [15,16]. Also, a mature AVF has a lower incidence of thrombosis and stenosis. This translates into prolonged patency rates and lower risk for infection [1,17–20].

Maturation of AVF depends on variable biomechanical forces. Remodelling of the arterial limb is characterised by vessel dilatation and outward hypertrophic remodelling of the intimal layer. Remodelling at the venous end can be accompanied by aggressive intimal thickening resulting in inward hypertrophic remodelling. Intimal hyperplasia (IH) is defined as the abnormal migration and proliferation of vascular smooth muscle cells provoked by injury, inflammation or stretch with associated

Table 1. Results of the study quality assessment.

Included study	Domain	Support for judgement	DH's judgement
Lai 2013 ESVS [37]	Random sequence generation	The method of generating the random sequence was not described.	Unclear
	Allocation concealment	No description of methods for maintaining allocation concealment.	Unclear
	Blinding of participants and personnel	Participants and personnel were not blinded. Dysfunctional access signs and other referral criteria could have a subjective component.	High risk of bias
	Blinding of outcome assessment	Outcome assessors were not blinded. Dysfunctional access signs and other referral criteria could have a subjective component.	High risk of bias
	Incomplete outcome data	Loss to follow up was minimal. Analysis was not by intention to treat. 9/59 control group patients crossed over to the intervention group potentially leading to bias in favour of the intervention	Unclear
	Selective reporting	No link to the protocol was given	Unclear
	Other sources of bias	None	Not available
Lin 2007 J Am Soc Neph [35]	Random sequence generation	A computerised minimisation algorithm was used	Low risk of bias
	Allocation concealment	Allocation sequence was kept by a study nurse who would not disclose allocations until time of intervention. Diagnosing malfunction in a fistula could have had a subjective element.	Unclear
	Blinding of participants and personnel	Participants and personnel were not blinded.	High risk of bias
	Blinding of outcome assessment	Outcome assessors were not blinded. Diagnosing malfunction in a fistula could have had a subjective element.	High risk of bias
	Incomplete outcome data	Loss to follow up was minimal and was similar between groups and was unlikely to influence results	Low risk of bias
	Selective reporting	Protocol was not available.	Unclear
	Other sources of bias	None	Not available
Lin 2013 AJKD [38]	Random sequence generation	A computer generated sequence was used	Low risk of bias
	Allocation concealment	Sealed opaque envelope were used to conceal allocation. There was no information in the manuscript or protocol on who had access to the envelopes and whether they were opened sequentially	Unclear
	Blinding of participants and personnel	No blinding. Diagnosing malfunction in a fistula could have had a subjective element.	High risk of bias
	Blinding of outcome assessment	Ultrasonographers were blinded however patients were not blinded. Diagnosing malfunction in a fistula could have had a subjective element.	High risk of bias
	Incomplete outcome data	Loss to follow up was similar between groups and unlikely to influence results	Low risk of bias
	Selective reporting	Link to protocol was provided (NCT01138254). Trial was not prospectively registered and there were several changes made including changes to outcomes.	High risk of bias
	Other sources of bias	None	Not available
Lin 2013 Neph Dial Transplant [36]	Random sequence generation	A computer generated sequence was used	Low risk of bias

Table 1. Cont.

Included study	Domain	Support for judgement	DH's judgement
	Allocation concealment	Sealed opaque envelope were used to conceal allocation. Two study nurses had access to the envelopes and there was no information in the manuscript or protocol on whether they were opened sequentially	Unclear
	Blinding of participants and personnel	No blinding. Diagnosing malfunction in a fistula could have had a subjective element.	High risk of bias
	Blinding of outcome assessment	No blinding. Diagnosing malfunction in a fistula could have had a subjective element.	High risk of bias
	Incomplete outcome data	Loss to follow up was similar between groups and unlikely to influence results	Low risk of bias.
	Selective reporting	All outcomes that were mentioned in the protocol were reported. The subgrouping based on polymorphisms of heme oxygenase-1 was not prespecified	Low risk of bias
	Other sources of bias	None	Not available

deposition of extracellular matrix in the intimal layer of the vein [21–23].

Far infra-red FIR therapy, which is a form of heat therapy, has been implicated in improvement of endothelial function and haemodynamics in coronary arteries, probably through up-regulating endothelial nitric oxide synthase (eNOS) expression in arterial endothelium leading to improved cardiac function in patients with chronic heart diseases [24]. Repeated leg hyperthermia using FIR has been shown to reduce oxidative stress in bed ridden type II diabetics [25].

FIR has also been reported to show encouraging results in phantom limb pain control [26], stimulation of the secretion of TGF-beta1 and activation of fibroblasts which may promote better wound healing independent of skin blood flow and skin temperature [27,28], reduction of both stress and fatigue levels of patients with end stage renal disease (ESRD) and stimulates the autonomic nervous system in those who are receiving regular haemodialysis (HD) [29].

This review was designed to examine the effect of FIR on AVF maturation using primary and secondary patency rates as the main outcomes of interest.

Methods

This systematic review and meta-analysis were conducted according to the Preferred Reporting Items for Systematic Review and Meta-Analysis (PRISMA) guidelines [30].

Eligibility Criteria

We included observational studies or randomised controlled trials (RCTs) that examined FIR therapy in patients with AVFs and ESRD. Eligible studies reported on AVF patency rates in FIR and non-FIR groups at one year or more following initiation of FIR therapy. Cases series and case reports were excluded. There was no restriction with regard to publication status or language.

Search strategy

A search of the literature for relevant studies was conducted in March 2014. We searched Medline without date restriction using

the free text "far infra-red". Additionally we used the strategy (["far infra-red" OR "far infrared" OR "post conditioning"] AND ["arteriovenous fistula" "dialysis" OR "end stage renal disease" OR "dialysis access" OR "access survival" OR "primary patency" OR "secondary patency" OR "fistula maturation]") to search CINAHL, EMBASE, the Cochrane library and Google Scholar. Bibliographies of included studies were searched for additional studies.

Abstracts of the relevant titles were subsequently obtained and evaluated for eligibility (KB, DH). Any remaining uncertainty was resolved by examination of the full article (KB, DH). Discussion with a third author (SRW) resolved discrepancies in cases of disagreement regarding eligibility.

The relevant outcomes for this review were primary patency – defined as unassisted AVF patency rates after at least 12 months of follow up - and secondary patency – defined as assisted patency rates after at least 12 months of follow up. The incidence of salvage procedures (endoluminal procedures or surgical procedures) for dysfunctional fistulas during follow up was a secondary outcome.

Data Collection

Data were extracted and checked for accuracy by two reviewers (KB, DH) independently and recorded on a Microsoft Excel spreadsheet. Any disagreements in extracting data were discussed between two reviewers (KB, DH), and if not settled this was resolved by consulting with a third reviewer (SRW). The following information regarding participant characteristics were recorded: age, sex, presence of co-morbidities, start of HD, primary and secondary patency rates, AVF salvage procedures, underlying cause of ESRD, definition of first AVF malfunction and overall access survival. The trials' inclusion and exclusion criteria were also recorded.

Quality assessment for risk of bias

The risk of bias for each study was assessed according to the criteria outlined in the in the Cochrane Handbook for Systematic Reviews of Interventions [31]. For each included study; the method used to perform random sequence generation, allocation concealment and blinding was described. The study was then

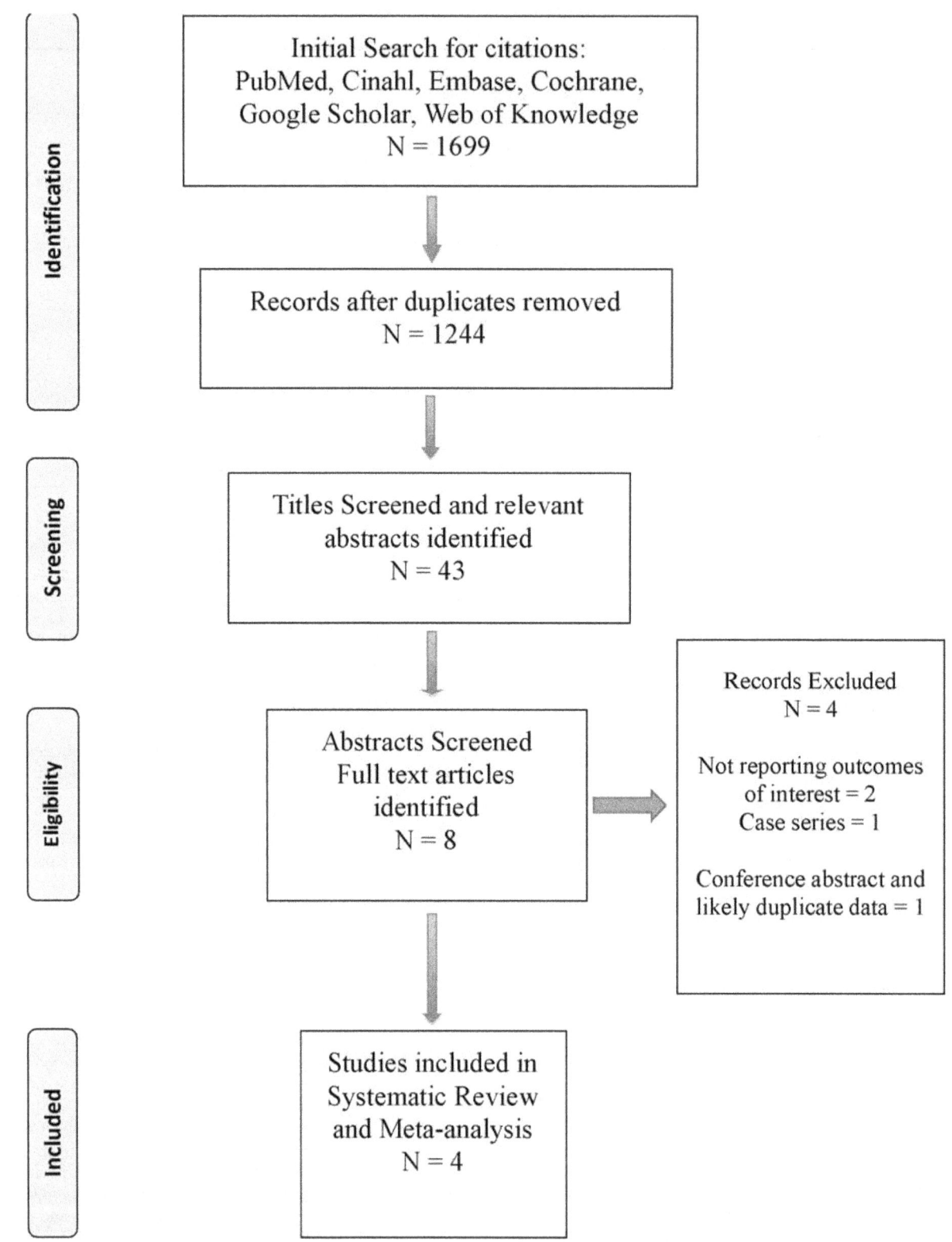

Figure 1. PRISMA 2009 Flow Diagram.

scrutinised for incomplete data outcomes, selective reporting and other potential sources of bias. Where possible, study protocols were obtained from trial registries to ascertain whether there was selective reporting within studies [Table 1].

Data analysis

Statistical analyses were performed using Review Manager version 5.2.8 [32]. Pooled risk ratios were calculated using the random effects model of DerSimonian and Laird [33]. For

Table 2. Inclusion & exclusion criteria and definition of AVF malfunction for included studies.

Study	Inclusion criteria	Exclusion criteria	Definition of AVF malfunction
Lin 2007 [35]	(1) Receiving 4 h of maintenance HD therapy three times weekly for at least 6 months at Taipei Veterans General Hospital, (2) Using a native AVF as the current vascular access for more than 6 months, without interventions within the last 3 months, and (3) Creation of AVF by cardiovascular surgeons in our hospital with the standardized surgical procedures of venous end-to-arterial side anastomosis in the upper extremity.	During the 1-yr follow-up, patients would be excluded from the study because of the following censoring criterion: (1) Renal transplantation, (2) Death with a functioning access, (3) Shifting to peritoneal dialysis, and (4) Loss of follow-up.	The need for any interventional procedure (surgery or angioplasty) to correct an occlusive or malfunctioning AVF that cannot sustain an extracorporeal blood flow >200 ml/min during HD after exclusion of the following stenosis-unrelated events: Infectious complication, progressive aneurysmal formation, or steal syndrome.
Lin 2013_AJKD [38]	(1) Aged 18–80 years, (2) Had CKD with estimated glomerular filtration rate (eGFR) of 5–20 mL/min/1.73 m^2, (3) Were not anticipated to receive dialysis or kidney transplantation within the next 3 months, and (4) Were undergoing AVF creation with venous end-to-arterial side anastomosis in the upper extremity.	(1) Those receiving an arteriovenous graft or cuffed tunnelled double-lumen catheter as the type of permanent vascular access, (2) Heart failure of New York Heart Association functional class III or IV, and (3) Episode of cardio- or cerebrovascular event or receiving intervention therapy within 3 months prior to screening.	The need for any interventional procedure (surgery or angioplasty) to correct an occlusive or malfunctioning fistula which could not sustain an extracorporeal blood flow >200 mL/min during HD after excluding the following stenosis-unrelated events, such as infectious complication, progressive aneurysmal formation or steal syndrome.
Lai_2013 [37]	(1) Received two or more PTA on the target lesions at upper extremities, with the last PTA successfully performed within the week before patient enrolment, and (2) After successful completion of at least 1 week of HD treatment, the patients with AVF or AVG were consecutively enrolled and randomly assigned to either a post-PTA FIR radiation group or a control group receiving the usual form radiation therapy at a 1:1 ratio.	(1) Received HD treatments other than three times a week, (2) Had previously received FIR radiation Therapy, (3) Received implantation of an endovascular stent, (4) Had multiple lesions that a single radiation field did not cover or the central lesion was considered too deep to be irradiated, (5) Missed FIR radiation treatments exceeding 10%, (6) Underwent renal transplantation, (7) Switched to peritoneal dialysis treatments, and (8) Had any severe disease with an estimated life expectancy of less than 1 year.	A significant lesion was defined as a lumen loss of 50% or more compared with adjacent normal vessel on angiography following dysfunctional diagnosis based on clinical signs suggestive of stenosis.
Lin_2013_NDT [36]	(1) Receiving 4 h of maintenance HD therapy three times weekly for at least 6 months at Taipei Veterans General Hospital, (2) Using a native AVF as the present vascular access for >6 months, without interventions within the last 3 months, and (3) Creation of AVF by cardiovascular surgeons in our hospital with the standardized surgical procedures of venous end-to-arterial side anastomosis in the upper extremity.	Received an AV graft as the first vascular access.	The need for any interventional procedure (surgery or angioplasty) to correct an occlusive or malfunctioning fistula which could not sustain an extracorporeal blood flow >200 mL/min during HD after excluding the following stenosis-unrelated events, such as infectious complication, progressive aneurysmal formation or steal syndrome.

continuous outcome variables the weighted mean difference (WMD) was calculated. The presence of statistical heterogeneity between studies was evaluated using the Cochran's Q statistic. P-values less than 5% were considered as statistically significant. Publication bias was assessed visually using a funnel plot, and additionally by comparing fixed and random effects modelling in a sensitivity analysis – this is a recognised method that can detect the influence of small-study effects [34].

Results

Study Selection

The results of the study selection process are summarized in the PRISMA flow diagram (Figure 1). The initial search yielded a total of 1669 citations, with 1244 citations remaining following removal of duplicates. The titles of these citations were screened with a total of 43 titles deemed potentially relevant. The abstracts of those titles were examined and eight full text articles were subsequently retrieved and examined. After assessing for eligibility

Table 3. Patients' Characteristics across included studies.

Study	Patients		Age		Gender M:F		Diabetes		Hypertension		Hx of AVF failure		Time on HD		Withdrawals
	FIR	Control	FIR	Control	FIR	Control	FIR	Control	FIR	Control	FIR	Control	FIR	Control	
Lin 2007 [35]	63/72	64/73	61.9±14.4	59.2±19.0	37:35	38:35	25	24	40	39	33	34	85.2±41.1	79.2±42.2	Creation of another vascular access because of the poor response to angioplasty: 1 patient receiving FIR therapy and four patients in control group. Patients were censored in case of: Renal transplantation ($n=3$), death with a functioning access ($n=5$), shifting to peritoneal dialysis ($n=4$) or loss of follow-up ($n=1$).
Lin 2013_AJKD [38]	60	62	63.2±18.5	63.0±14.4	32:28	35:27	28	23	18	20	-	-	Pre-dialysis	Pre-dialysis	Lost to F/U: FIR=1; Control=1. Shifting to PD: FIR=1; Control=1. Death e AVF: FIR=2; Control=3. Renal transplantation: FIR=1. New AVF (Infection): Control=1. D/C intervention: FIR=2; Control=1.
Lin 2013_NDT [36]	119/139	120/141	61.3±14.1	62.8±15.9	79:60	71:70	45	47	80	90	47	45	66.0±59.1	75.9±58.0	Underwent creation of another vascular access due to non-stenotic lesions: 3 patients receiving FIR therapy and 2 patients in the control group. Patients were censored in case of: Renal transplantation ($n=5$), death with a functioning access ($n=15$), shift to peritoneal dialysis ($n=5$) or loss of follow-up ($n=9$).
Lai 2013 [37]	69	50	62.7±10.9	63.1±12.5	32:37	24:26	42	28	48	38	All	All	50.4±42.0	58.8±56.4	Crossover patients: 9 from Control to FIR.

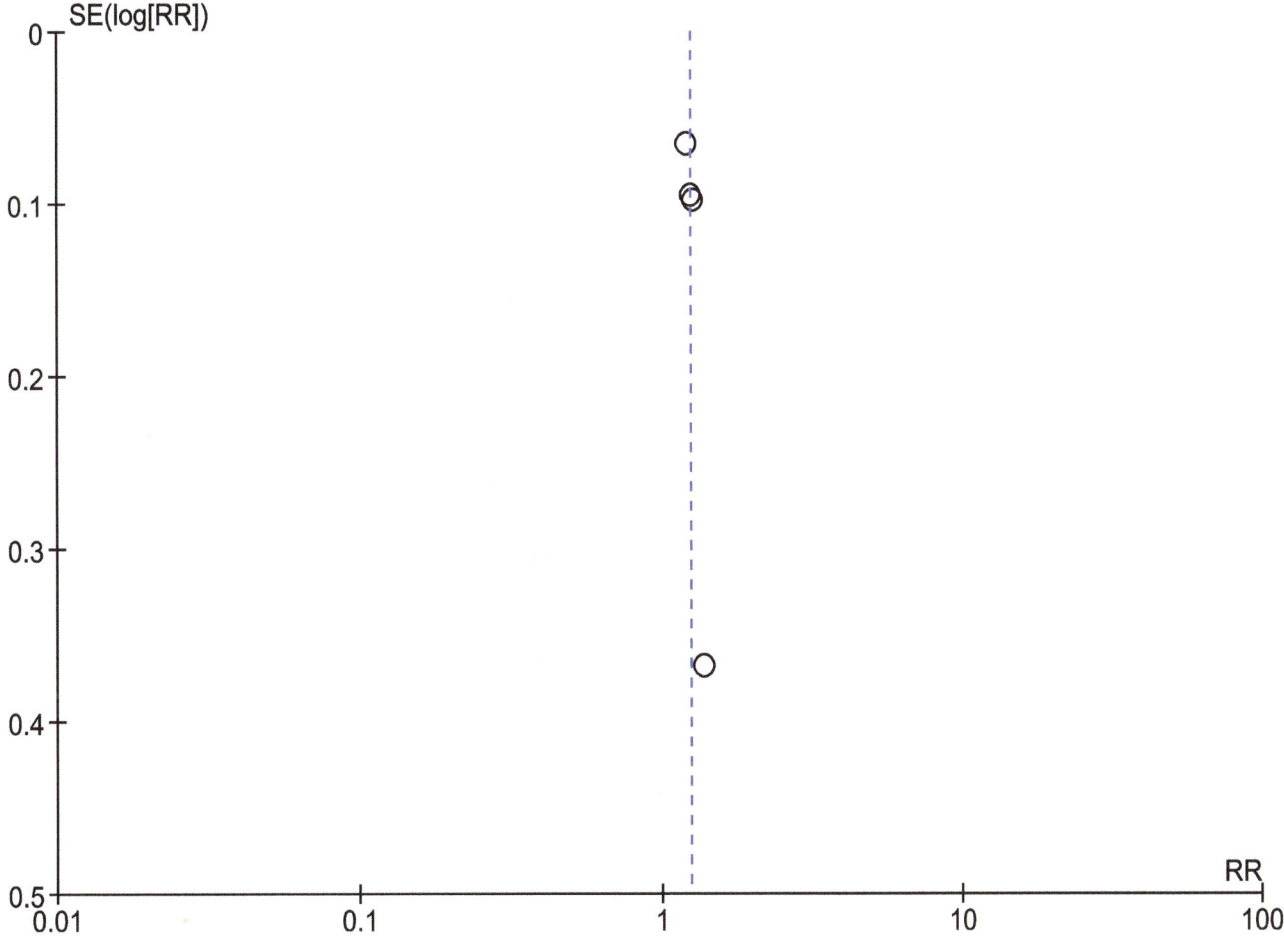

Figure 2. Forest Plot showing Primary AVFs patency at 12 months.

criteria, four RCT's were included in the review [35–38]. Three of those studies reported on patients with history of previous AVF who had been on HD prior to FIR therapy [35–37], while one study reported on patients with newly formed AVF not on HD [38]. We were not able to include another study by Lin et al [39] with a follow up of 3 months for primary patency rates as it was a conference abstract only, also we had concerns that the data in this study was used in another study by the same author [36] that has already been included in this review. Three studies were excluded from the final analysis after going through the full articles. Shipley et al followed their patients for six months in a case series of 20 patients – no control group - and reported maturation in 10 of those patients [40]. Two studies did not report on the outcomes of interest to the author of this systematic review [29,41].

Figure 3. Funnel plot for Primary AVFs patency at 12 months.

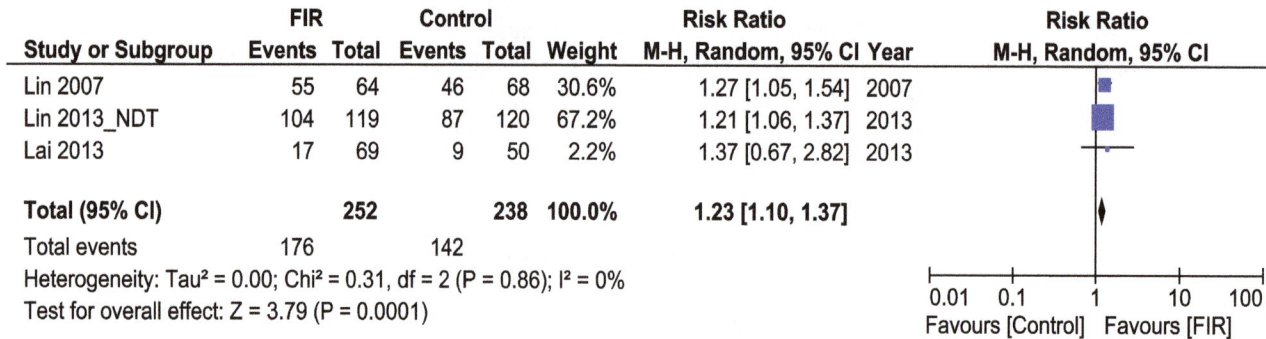

Figure 4. Forest Plot showing Primary AVFs patency at 12 months, Lin et al RCT on new AVFs excluded.

Characteristics of included studies

Far Infrared (FIR) technique. All studies included used the same technique for delivering of FIR therapy. WS TY101 FIR emitter (WS Far Infrared Medical Technology Co., Ltd., Taipei, Taiwan) was used in all studies which generates electromagnetic waves with wavelengths in the range between 5 and 25 (peak at 5–8.2 µm). The top radiator was set at a height of 20–30 cm above the surface of the AVF with the treatment time set at 40 min during HD three times per week.

Participants

The four studies included 666 patients, with 340 patients randomised to receive FIR therapy – median age 62.3±14.5 SD, while 326 were randomised to the control group – median age 62.0±14.5 SD. 348 patients were males–180 in FIR group and 168 in the control group, while females were 318, of those 160 received FIR therapy and 158 were controls.

Inclusion and exclusion criteria of studies are outlined in [Table 2], along with the definition of AVF malfunction for each of the included studies.

Apart from Lin et al who evaluated the effects of FIR in pre-dialysis patients with newly formed AVFs [38], the remaining RCTs included patients who already started HD. Mean time on HD in months for Lin et al [35] was 85.2±41.1 for FIR group and 79.2±42.2 for the control group, for Lai et al [37] FIR = 50.4±42 and control = 58.8±56.4 and for Lin et al in 2013 [36] FIR = 66.0±59.1 and control = 75.9±58.0. All patients in included trials received FIR therapy for 40 minutes per session three times a week for the duration of the study.

Lai et al studied patients with history of dysfunctional AVFs and repeated angioplasty. The mean life of the AVFs for their patients was 21.8±23.0 months for FIR group and 23.5±22.6 months for the controls [37]. 33 patients from 72 had history of AVF malfunction and 14 patients required surgical intervention, while 20 patients had a total of 49 angioplasty procedures in the FIR group compared to 34 patients from 73 with history of AVF malfunction, 13 of those required surgical intervention and 20 patients with total of 46 angioplasty procedures in the control group, in the RCT by Lin et al in 2007 [35]. Similarly, 47 patients had history of AVF malfunction with 12 patients requiring surgery from 139 and 35 patients underwent 79 angioplasty procedures in the FIR group, compared to 45 patients with history of malfunction, 13 patients of those required surgery and 32 patients underwent angioplasty as a salvage procedure in the control group in the study by Lin et al in 2013 [36]. All patients in both FIR and control groups had angioplasty procedures prior to recruitment in the study by Lai et al [37], while none of the patients included by Lin et al had a history of either surgical or angioplasty salvage procedures since they were all first time AVFs [38]. Lai et al had 9 of their patients who were initially randomised to the control group crossing over to the FIR group based on their request [37]. Clinical maturation was reported in 49 (81.7%) patients of 60 who received FIR therapy by Lin et all, compared to 37 (59.7%) from the 62 control subjects [38]. Sub –group analysis by age, gender and diagnosis of hypertension was not possible as this was not included in studies, and we did not have access to the raw data used by the authors. Other patients' characteristics are detailed in [Table 3].

Primary - unassisted - patency rates at 1 year

All of the 4 included studies (610 patients) reported on unassisted – primary – patency rate after 12 months of follow-up on the FIR therapy. 228/311 patients in FIR group had primarily patent AVFs at 12 months compared to 185/299 patients in the

Study or Subgroup	FIR Events	FIR Total	Control Events	Control Total	Weight	Risk Ratio M-H, Random, 95% CI	Risk Ratio M-H, Random, 95% CI
Lin 2013_AJKD	58	59	52	61	41.2%	1.15 [1.03, 1.29]	
Lin 2013_NDT	102	109	88	102	58.8%	1.08 [0.99, 1.19]	
Total (95% CI)		**168**		**163**	**100.0%**	**1.11 [1.04, 1.19]**	
Total events	160		140				

Heterogeneity: Tau² = 0.00; Chi² = 0.71, df = 1 (P = 0.40); I² = 0%
Test for overall effect: Z = 2.97 (P = 0.003)

0.01   0.1   1   10   100
Favours [Control]   Favours [FIR]

Figure 5. Forest plot showing assisted patency rates at 12 months.

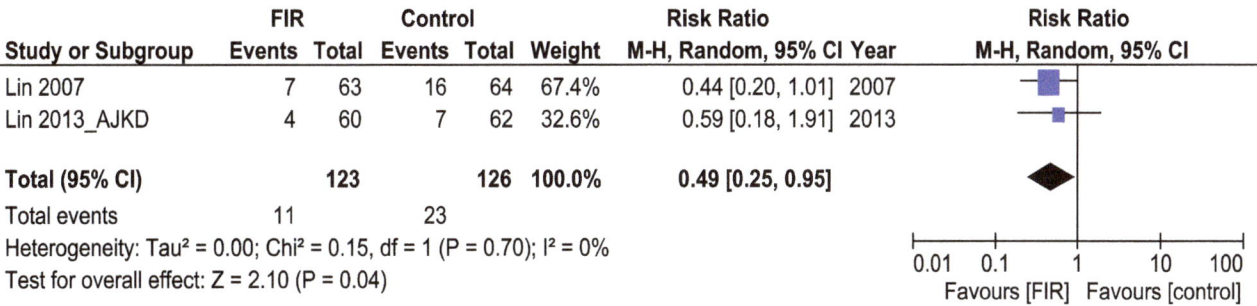

Figure 6. Forest plot showing surgical intervention for AVF malfunction.

control group. Pooled results showed significant difference between the two groups, with those who received FIR showing better primary patency rates compared to control (Pooled risk ratio = 1.23 [1.12, 1.35], 95% CI, p = 0.00001) [Figure 2]. There was no evidence of statistical heterogeneity (Cochran's Q = 0.33; degree of freedom (DF) = 3; p = 0.96; I^2 = 0%). The funnel plot did not suggest bias [Figure 3], and the result was unchanged when fixed effects modelling was used (pooled risk ratio1.24 [1.13–1.37], 95% CI, p<0.0001).

Excluding the RCT by Lin et al on newly formed AVFs in pre-dialysis patients [38] from the analysis for primary patency after 12 months, the remaining studies (490 patients) showed better results in the FIR group with 176/252 AVFs being patent at 12 months compared to 142/238 in the control group [35–37]. This was statistically significant (Pooled risk ratio = 1.23 [1.10, 1.37], 95% CI, p = 0.0001) [Figure 4]. There was no evidence of statistical heterogeneity (Cochran's Q = 0.31; degree of freedom (DF) = 2; p = 0.86; I^2 = 0%).

Secondary - assisted - patency rates

Data could be retrieved from 2 studies (331 patients) for analysis of assisted – secondary – patency rates at 12 months following salvage procedures [36,38]. 160/168 patients in the FIR group had patent AVFs following intervention for dysfunctional fistulas, compared to 140/163 patients in the control arm. Pooled results showed statistically significant difference favouring FIR therapy (Pooled risk ratio = 1.11 [1.04–1.19]; 95% CI, p = 0.003) [Figure 5]. There was no evidence of statistical heterogeneity (Cochran's Q = 0.71; degree of freedom (DF) = 1; p = 0.40; I^2 = 0%).

Intervention

Two studies [35,38] (249 patients) reported the need for intervention to salvage a dysfunctional AVF. Patients who received FIR therapy required less interventions, 11/123 patients compared to 23/126 patients in the control group. The difference was significant (Pooled risk ratio = 0.49 [0.25–0.985; 95% CI; p = 0.04] [Figure 6]. There was no evidence of statistical heterogeneity (Cochran's Q = 0.15; degree of freedom (DF) = 1; p = 0.70; I^2 = 0%).

Discussion

This review identified four studies (666 patients) which evaluated the use of FIR therapy to improve primary and secondary patency rates for AVFs in patients with ESRD. They all reported significant improvement in the outcome measures assessed in this review in favour of FIR therapy. Three of those studies (490 patients) were carried out on patients already started

HD sessions, and one study (122 patients) focused on pre-dialysis first time AVF maturation. All four trials following some form of randomisation, and the demographics of patients in included studies did not differ significantly. Pooled analysis showed that primary - unassisted - patency was significantly better in the FIR group (pooled risk ratio of 1.23 [1.12–1.35], p value of 0.0001). Secondary – assisted – patency was reported in two studies (279 patients) and was found to be significantly better in those who received FIR therapy (pooled risk ratio of 1.19 [1.07–1.31], p value of 0.0008).

Post-conditioning using Far Infra-Red therapy has been shown to increase the level of heme oxygenase-1 (HO-1) expression which protects against Ischaemia/reperfusion injury in study by Tu et al [42]. HO-1 is a known vasodilator and at the same time inhibits proliferation of vascular smooth muscle cells, platelet aggregation, and vasospasm leading to favourable conditions for maturation of AVFs. Also, Ikeda et al repeated thermal therapy was shown to up-regulate endothelial nitric oxide synthase expression in Syrian hamsters [24], a finding that was validated by Akasaki et al, who also reported increased angiogenesis via (eNOS) following repeated thermal therapy in mice with hindlimb ischemia. [43]. Kipshidze et al irradiated cultures of rabbit endothelial cells and smooth muscle cells with different doses of non-ablative infrared. They found that non-ablative infrared laser inhibited neointimal hyperplasia after coronary arteries angioplasty in cholesterol-fed rabbits for up to 60 days [44]. FIR therapy is still considered a novel treatment for AVF although the technique has been described since 2007 by Lin et al [35]. This review demonstrated a beneficial use of FIR therapy that improved both primary and secondary patency rates across all studies included. This statistically significant difference was consistent even when one excluded study for having only 3 months of follow-up was added to the sensitivity analysis [39]. Also, excluding the only RCT found by the authors on newly formed AVF did not alter the outcome of the pooled analysis in terms of significance.

FIR therapy was also shown to improve access flow (Qa). The study by Lin et al – which was one of the RCTs included in the review - showed that 40 min of FIR therapy in a single HD session could increase access flow of AVF by about 50 mL/min with a 1-year effect of improving Qa by up to 150 mL/min and increasing unassisted patency of AVF by about 18% in comparison with controls [35].

A serious limiting factor of this systematic review is that the four RCTs came from the same institution (Yang-Ming University in Taiwan), and three of the four were authored by the same two authors (Lin-cc and Yang-wc) [35,36,38]. Dr Lin-cc reported that he was receiving lecture fees from WS Far Infrared Medical Technology, the company that makes the infrared machines used in the studies raising the potential of bias.

Also, all the RCTs were performed in an unblinded fashion, which can impact outcomes as demonstrated by the fact that in one study nine patients opted to join the FIR group despite initially being allocated as controls. Blinding in clinical trials involving FIR therapy would involve additional costs in making machines that resemble the ones used to deliver FIR therapy. Those machines should be convincing to both staff and patients if effective double blinding is to be considered. However, blinding can be attempted by placing a screen between the FIR device and the patient. Also, double-blinding can be achieved by placing a box over the device and then creating simple mock devices that also appear as boxes. This review provides a thorough examination of published evidence supporting the use of FIR therapy to promote AVF access maturation in patients with ESRD in HD, and also for those who are likely to require dialysis in the near future. The meta-analysis showed overwhelming support for regular use of FIR therapy, however there were limitations that need to be considered. Finally, this review may serve to guide future advances in using repeated thermal therapy in postconditioning of AVFs.

Conclusion

Results from four RCTs suggest that regular use of FIR therapy in haemodialysis and pre-haemodialysis patients, in particular those with AVFs, can positively influence AVF function. However, more blinded randomised controlled, multicentre and international clinical trials are required. We also hope to see sub-group analysis in those studies, particularly by age (e.g. using 65 as cut-off), gender and diagnosis of hypertension.

Author Contributions

Conceived and designed the experiments: KB DH EK SRW MCM PB EK MW LB. Performed the experiments: KB DH EK SRW MCM PB EK MW LB. Analyzed the data: KB DH EK SRW MCM PB EK MW. Contributed reagents/materials/analysis tools: KB DH. Contributed to the writing of the manuscript: KB DH EK SRW MCM PB EK MW LB.

References

1. Frankel A (2006) Temporary access and central venous catheters. Eur J Vasc Endovasc Surg 31: 417–422.
2. NKF-KDOQI (2006) 2006 Updates Clinical Practice Guidelines and Recommendations.
3. Hoggard J, Saad T, Schon D, Vesely TM, Royer T (2008) Guidelines for venous access in patients with chronic kidney disease. A Position Statement from the American Society of Diagnostic and Interventional Nephrology, Clinical Practice Committee and the Association for Vascular Access. Semin Dial 21: 186–191.
4. Polkinghorne KR, Chin GK, Macginley RJ, Owen AR, Russell C, et al. (2013) KHA-CARI guideline: Vascular access - central venous catheters, arteriovenous fistulae and arteriovenous grafts. Nephrology (Carlton).
5. Stolic R (2013) Most important chronic complications of arteriovenous fistulas for hemodialysis. Med Princ Pract 22: 220–228.
6. McCann M, Einarsdottir H, Van Waeleghem JP, Murphy F, Sedgewick J (2008) Vascular access management 1: an overview. J Ren Care 34: 77–84.
7. Dixon BS (2006) Why don't fistulas mature? Kidney Int 70: 1413–1422.
8. Allon M, Robbin ML (2002) Increasing arteriovenous fistulas in hemodialysis patients: problems and solutions. Kidney Int 62: 1109–1124.
9. Rayner HC, Pisoni RL, Gillespie BW, Goodkin DA, Akiba T, et al. (2003) Creation, cannulation and survival of arteriovenous fistulae: data from the Dialysis Outcomes and Practice Patterns Study. Kidney Int 63: 323–330.
10. Lok CE, Oliver MJ, Su J, Bhola C, Hannigan N, et al. (2005) Arteriovenous fistula outcomes in the era of the elderly dialysis population. Kidney Int 67: 2462–2469.
11. Allon M, Lockhart ME, Lilly RZ, Gallichio MH, Young CJ, et al. (2001) Effect of preoperative sonographic mapping on vascular access outcomes in hemodialysis patients. Kidney Int 60: 2013–2020.
12. Oliver MJ, McCann RL, Indridason OS, Butterly DW, Schwab SJ (2001) Comparison of transposed brachiobasilic fistulas to upper arm grafts and brachiocephalic fistulas. Kidney Int 60: 1532–1539.
13. Allon M (2007) Current management of vascular access. Clin J Am Soc Nephrol 2: 786–800.
14. Dixon BS, Novak L, Fangman J (2002) Hemodialysis vascular access survival: upper-arm native arteriovenous fistula. Am J Kidney Dis 39: 92–101.
15. Ocak G, Rotmans JI, Vossen CY, Rosendaal FR, Krediet RT, et al. (2013) Type of arteriovenous vascular access and association with patency and mortality. BMC Nephrol 14: 79.
16. Polkinghorne KR, McDonald SP, Atkins RC, Kerr PG (2004) Vascular access and all-cause mortality: a propensity score analysis. J Am Soc Nephrol 15: 477–486.
17. Spergel LM, Ravani P, Roy-Chaudhury P, Asif A, Besarab A (2007) Surgical salvage of the autogenous arteriovenous fistula (AVF). J Nephrol 20: 388–398.
18. Brunori G, Bandera A, Valente F, Laudon A (2008) [Vascular access for dialysis in elderly: AVF versus permanent CVC]. G Ital Nefrol 25: 614–618.
19. McCann M, Einarsdottir H, Van Waeleghem JP, Murphy F, Sedgewick J (2010) Vascular access management III: central venous catheters. J Ren Care 36: 25–33.
20. Ma A, Shroff R, Hothi D, Lopez MM, Veligratli F, et al. (2013) A comparison of arteriovenous fistulas and central venous lines for long-term chronic haemodialysis. Pediatr Nephrol 28: 321–326.
21. Cox JL, Chiasson DA, Gotlieb AI (1991) Stranger in a strange land: the pathogenesis of saphenous vein graft stenosis with emphasis on structural and functional differences between veins and arteries. Prog Cardiovasc Dis 34: 45–68.
22. Davies MG, Hagen PO (1994) Pathobiology of intimal hyperplasia. Br J Surg 81: 1254–1269.
23. Newby AC, Zaltsman AB (2000) Molecular mechanisms in intimal hyperplasia. J Pathol 190: 300–309.
24. Ikeda Y, Biro S, Kamogawa Y, Yoshifuku S, Eto H, et al. (2001) Repeated thermal therapy upregulates arterial endothelial nitric oxide synthase expression in Syrian golden hamsters. Jpn Circ J 65: 434–438.
25. Kawaura A, Tanida N, Kamitani M, Akiyama J, Mizutani M, et al. (2010) The effect of leg hyperthermia using far infrared rays in bedridden subjects with type 2 diabetes mellitus. Acta Med Okayama 64: 143–147.
26. Huang CY, Yang RS, Kuo TS, Hsu KH (2009) Phantom limb pain treated by far infrared ray. Conf Proc IEEE Eng Med Biol Soc 2009: 1589–1591.
27. Toyokawa H, Matsui Y, Uhara J, Tsuchiya H, Teshima S, et al. (2003) Promotive effects of far-infrared ray on full-thickness skin wound healing in rats. Exp Biol Med (Maywood) 228: 724–729.
28. Capon A, Mordon S (2003) Can thermal lasers promote skin wound healing? Am J Clin Dermatol 4: 1–12.
29. Su LH, Wu KD, Lee LS, Wang H, Liu CF (2009) Effects of far infrared acupoint stimulation on autonomic activity and quality of life in hemodialysis patients. Am J Chin Med 37: 215–226.
30. Liberati A, Altman DG, Tetzlaff J, Mulrow C, Gotzsche PC, et al. (2009) The PRISMA statement for reporting systematic reviews and meta-analyses of studies that evaluate health care interventions: explanation and elaboration. PLoS Med 6: e1000100.
31. Higgins JP, Altman DG, Gotzsche PC, Juni P, Moher D, et al. (2011) The Cochrane Collaboration's tool for assessing risk of bias in randomised trials. BMJ 343: d5928.
32. The Nordic Cochrane Centre TCc (2012) Review Manager (RevMan) [Computer Program]. Version 5.2.
33. DerSimonian R, Laird NM (1983) Evaluating the Effect of Coaching on SAT Scores: A Meta-Analysis. Harvard Educational Review 53: 1–15.
34. Sterne JAC EM, Moher D (2011) Chapter 10: Addressing reporting biases. Higgins JPT, Green S (editors) Cochrane Handbook for Systematic Reviews of Intervention Version 5.1.0.
35. Lin CC, Chang CF, Lai MY, Chen TW, Lee PC, et al. (2007) Far-infrared therapy: a novel treatment to improve access blood flow and unassisted patency of arteriovenous fistula in hemodialysis patients. J Am Soc Nephrol 18: 985–992.
36. Lin CC, Chung MY, Yang WC, Lin SJ, Lee PC (2013) Length polymorphisms of heme oxygenase-1 determine the effect of far-infrared therapy on the function of arteriovenous fistula in hemodialysis patients: a novel physicogenomic study. Nephrol Dial Transplant 28: 1284–1293.
37. Lai CC, Fang HC, Mar GY, Liou JC, Tseng CJ, et al. (2013) Post-angioplasty far infrared radiation therapy improves 1-year angioplasty-free hemodialysis access patency of recurrent obstructive lesions. Eur J Vasc Endovasc Surg 46: 726–732.
38. Lin CC, Yang WC, Chen MC, Liu WS, Yang CY, et al. (2013) Effect of Far Infrared Therapy on Arteriovenous Fistula Maturation: An Open-Label Randomized Controlled Trial. Am J Kidney Dis.
39. W.-C LC-CY (2012) Far infrared therapy improves arteriovenous fistula maturation. Nephrology Dialysis Transplantation Conference: 50th ERA-EDTA Congress Istanbul Turkey Conference Start: 20120524 Conference End: 20120527.

40. Shipley T, Adam J, Sweeney D, Fenwick S, Mansy H, et al. (2012) Does far infrared therapy aid av fistula maturation and maintenance?. Nephrology Dialysis Transplantation Conference: 49th ERA-EDTA Congress Paris France Conference Start: 20120524 Conference End: 20120527 Conference Publication: (varpagings) 27 (ii261).

41. Lin CH, Lee LS, Su LH, Huang TC, Liu CF (2011) Thermal therapy in dialysis patients - a randomized trial. Am J Chin Med 39: 839–851.

42. Tu YP, Chen SC, Liu YH, Chen CF, Hour TC (2013) Postconditioning with far-infrared irradiation increases heme oxygenase-1 expression and protects against ischemia/reperfusion injury in rat testis. Life Sci 92: 35–41.

43. Akasaki Y, Miyata M, Eto H, Shirasawa T, Hamada N, et al. (2006) Repeated thermal therapy up-regulates endothelial nitric oxide synthase and augments angiogenesis in a mouse model of hindlimb ischemia. Circ J 70: 463–470.

44. Kipshidze N, Nikolaychik V, Muckerheidi M, Keelan MH, Chekanov V, et al. (2001) Effect of short pulsed nonablative infrared laser irradiation on vascular cells in vitro and neointimal hyperplasia in a rabbit balloon injury model. Circulation 104: 1850–1855.

21

Comparison of the Efficacy of Rosuvastatin versus Atorvastatin in Preventing Contrast Induced Nephropathy in Patient with Chronic Kidney Disease Undergoing Percutaneous Coronary Intervention

Yong Liu[1,9], Yuan-hui Liu[1,2,9], Ning Tan[1]*, Ji-yan Chen[1]*, Ying-ling Zhou[1], Li-wen Li[1], Chong-yang Duan[3], Ping-Yan Chen[3], Jian-fang Luo[1], Hua-long Li[1], Wei-Guo[1]

1 Department of Cardiology, Guangdong Cardiovascular Institute, Guangdong General Hospital, Guangdong Academy of Medical Sciences, Guangzhou, Guangdong, China, 2 Southern medical university, Guangzhou, Guangdong, China, 3 Department of Biostatistics, School of Public Health and Tropical Medicine, Southern Medical University, Guangzhou, China

Abstract

Objectives: We prospectively compared the preventive effects of rosuvastatin and atorvastatin on contrast-induced nephropathy (CIN) in patients with chronic kidney disease (CKD) undergoing percutaneous coronary intervention (PCI).

Methods: We enrolled 1078 consecutive patients with CKD undergoing elective PCI. Patients in Group 1 (n = 273) received rosuvastatin (10 mg), and those in group 2 (n = 805) received atorvastatin (20 mg). The primary end-point was the development of CIN, defined as an absolute increase in serum creatinine ≥0.5 mg/dL, or an increase ≥25% from baseline within 48–72 h after contrast medium exposure.

Results: CIN was observed in 58 (5.4%) patients. The incidence of CIN was similar in patients pretreated with either rosuvastatin or atorvastatin (5.9% vs. 5.2%, p = 0.684). The same results were also observed when using other definitions of CIN. Clinical and procedural characteristics did not show significant differences between the two groups (p>0.05). Additionally, there were no significant inter-group differences with respect to in-hospital mortality rates (0.4% vs. 1.5%, p = 0.141), or other in-hospital complications. Multivariate logistic regression analysis revealed that rosuvastatin and atorvastatin demonstrated similar efficacies for preventing CIN, after adjusting for potential confounding risk factors (odds ratio = 1.17, 95% confidence interval, 0.62–2.20, p = 0.623). A Kaplan–Meier survival analysis showed that patients taking either rosuvastatin or atorvastatin had similar incidences of all-cause mortality (9.4% vs. 7.1%, respectively; p = 0.290) and major adverse cardiovascular events (29.32% vs. 23.14%, respectively; p = 0.135) during follow-up.

Conclusions: Rosuvastatin and atorvastatin have similar efficacies for preventing CIN in patients with CKD undergoing PCI.

Editor: Garyfalia Drossopoulou, National Centre for Scientific Research "Demokritos", Greece

Funding: This study was supported by grant from the National Natural Science Foundation of China (grant no. 81270286). The funders had no role in the study design, data collection and analysis, decision to publish, or preparation of the manuscript; the work was not funded by any industry sponsors.

Competing Interests: The authors have declared that no competing interests exist.

* Email: tanning100@126.com (NT); cgy01973@126.com (JYC)

9 These authors contributed equally to this work.

Introduction

Contrast-induced nephropathy (CIN) is an important and well-known complication in patients undergoing percutaneous coronary intervention (PCI). CIN also causes prolonged in-hospital stays and excess health care costs, and represents a powerful predictor of short and long term adverse outcomes [1,2,3]. CIN occurs even more frequently in patients with chronic kidney disease (CKD), with a reported incidence as high as 20–26.6% [3,4]. However, other than periprocedural hydration with normal saline, limiting the amount of contrast medium (CM), and using iso- or low-osmolar CM, few strategies are effective for preventing CIN.

Statins belong to a drug class that has pleiotropic effects on the vasculature and improves endothelial function, probably by increasing nitric oxide synthetase bioavailability and decreasing oxidative stress [5,6,7]. These properties counteract specific pathophysiologic mechanisms that promote the development of CIN [2,8]. In recent years, increasing evidence has supported the preventive effect of atorvastatin on CIN development in patients undergoing PCI [9,10]. Additionally, two large randomized control trials (RCTs) demonstrated that rosuvastatin significantly reduced the risk of CIN and improved short term clinical outcomes [11,12]. However, not all statins (especially, rosuvastatin and atorvastatin) are equivalent; they vary in several properties, including low-density lipoprotein (LDL) cholesterol lowering potency, lipophilicity, renoprotection, anti-inflammatory effects, and their effects on myocardial function [13,14]. Whether these differences significantly influence their effect on preventing CIN remains unknown. Recently, Kaya et al. (ROSA-CIN trial) conducted a study including 198 ST-segment elevation myocardial infarction (STEMI) patients undergoing primary PCI to determine if rosuvastatin and atorvastatin had similar efficacies for preventing CIN [15]. However, the number of enrolled patients was too small to draw definite conclusions; additional large trials are required to confirm their similarity. Therefore, we performed a prospective study to compare the preventive effects of rosuvastatin and atorvastatin on CIN in patients with CKD undergoing PCI.

Patients and Methods

Patient population

We prospectively enrolled consecutive CKD patients undergoing PCI at Guangdong Cardiovascular Institute, Guangdong General Hospital, China, between March 2010 and September 2012. The inclusion criteria included: patients with an estimated glomerular filtration rate (eGFR) of 30–90 mL/min/1.73 m^2 (CKD stages II and III), and patients pretreated with either atorvastatin (20 mg) or rosuvastatin (10 mg), at equivalent standard doses [16]. Statin pretreatment was defined as taking a statin 2–3 days before CM exposure and 2–3 days after the procedure. Patients were excluded if they had undergone chronic statin therapy (>14 days); had been treated with simvastatin or other statins; had a history of heart failure (defined as NYHA III/IV or Killip class II–IV), pregnancy, CM allergy, CM exposure during the previous 7 days; or had been treated with potentially nephroprotective (e.g., N-acetylcysteine or theophylline) or nephrotoxic (e.g., steroids, non-steroidal anti-inflammatory drugs, aminoglycosides, amphotericin B) drugs [17]. We also excluded patients with CKD stages 0, IV or V; hepatic insufficiency; or who had undergone renal transplantation or dialysis.

This study protocol was approved by the Guangdong General Hospital ethics committee and the study conformed to the Declaration of Helsinki. Written informed consent was obtained from all patients before the procedure.

Biochemical investigations

Serum creatinine (SCr) levels were measured upon admission and within 48–72 h after CM exposure. Blood urea nitrogen (BUN), creatine kinase MB, fasting glucose, electrolytes, fasting lipid profiles, albumin, and other standard clinical parameters were measured in the morning before the procedure. The eGFR was evaluated using the 4-variable Modification of Diet in Renal Disease equation based on Chinese patients [18]. Left ventricular function was echocardiographically evaluated in each patient within a 24-h period before the PCI.

PCI and medications

PCI was performed by experienced interventional cardiologists according to standard clinical practice using standard techniques. Nonionic, low-osmolar CM was used in all patients (either Iopamiron or Ultravist, both at 370 mg I/mL). Normal saline (0.9%) at a rate of 1 mL/kg/h (0.5 mL/kg/h if the patient's left ventricular ejection fraction (LVEF) was <40%) was administered intravenously 3–12 h before and 6–12 h after CM exposure. Antiplatelet agents (aspirin/clopidogrel), β-adrenergic blocking agents, statins, diuretics, angiotensin-converting enzyme inhibitors, and inotropic drugs were used at the attending cardiologist's discretion, according to clinical protocols derived from interventional guidelines.

Clinical outcomes

Follow-up events were carefully monitored and recorded by trained nurses through office visits and telephone interviews conducted, at 1, 6, 12, and 24 months after cardiac catherization.

The primary end-point was CIN development, defined as an absolute increase in SCr ≥0.5 mg/dL or a relative increase ≥25% from baseline, within 48–72 h after CM exposure. Additional end points included: CIN, as defined by other criteria [17], and major in-hospital or long-term adverse clinical events (MACEs), including all-cause mortality, non-fatal myocardial infarction, target vessel revascularization, CIN requiring renal replacement therapy, and stroke.

The other CIN definitions included: an absolute increase in SCr of ≥0.5 mg/dL within 48–72 h (CIN2); an absolute increase in SCr of ≥0.3 mg/dL within 48 h (CIN3); a SCr increase of ≥50% (1.5 fold from baseline) within 48 h (CIN4); and CIN5 (CIN3 or CIN4) [17].

Statistical analysis

SAS version 9.2 (SAS Institute, Cary, NC, USA) was used for all analyses. Continuous variables are described as means ± SD or medians, and categorical variables as absolute values (percentages). Comparisons of between-groups differences were performed using Student's t-test or the Wilcoxon rank sum test (if not normally distributed) for continuous variables and a chi-square or Fisher's exact test for categorical variables. Logistic regression analysis was performed using CIN as the dependent variable. Variables that were statistically significant according to a univariate analysis, were included in the final multivariate model to identify CIN predictors. Cumulative event curves for both groups of patients were created using the Kaplan-Meier survival method and compared using the log-rank test. All statistical tests were 2-tailed and statistical significance was inferred if P<0.05.

Results

Baseline characteristics between patients pretreated with atorvastatin and rosuvastatin

A total of 1078 consecutive CKD patients, pretreated with atorvastatin or rosuvastatin were analyzed (mean age, 65.2±10.1 years; mean eGFR, 69.8±14.0 mL/min/1.73 m^2; mean Mehran score, 4.3±3.2). Clinical and procedural characteristics were not significantly different between the two groups. In particular, the proportions of patients with diabetes mellitus (DM, P = 0.091), age ≥75 years (P = 0.200), or anemia (P = 0.187) were similar in both groups. The baseline SCr (P = 0.495) and eGFR (P = 0. 704) levels were also similar between the two groups, as were the mean LVEF (rosuvastatin 59.96±11.18% vs. atorvastatin 59.05±11.77%, P = 0.291), CM volumes used (rosuvastatin 133.36±67.75 mL vs. atorvastatin 132.37±70.13 mL, P = 0.838), and Mehran risk scores (rosuvastatin 4.06±2.86 vs. atorvastatin 4.42±3.31, P = 0.095). (Table 1).

Preventive effect of statins on CIN and in hospital outcomes

Overall, CIN was observed in 58 patients (5.4%). Compared with patients without CIN, patients with CIN had a significantly higher rate of in-hospital mortality (10.34% vs. 0.69%, P<0.001),

Table 1. Baseline clinical characteristics of study participants.

Variables	Rosuvastatin (n = 273)	Atorvastatin (n = 805)	P
Demographics			
Age, (y)	65.28±9.89	65.79±10.28	0.425
Age>75 y, (%)	36(13.2%)	126(15.7%)	0.443
Females (%)	57(20.9%)	187(23.2%)	0.423
Weight (kg)	65.58±10.18	65.17±10.24	0.409
SBP (mmHg)	133.07±21.64	131.01±20.44	0.158
DBP (mmHg)	76.64±11.44	75.31±11.23	0.093
Heart rate (bpm)	74.33±12.32	72.94±12.15	0.105
Medical history, n (%)			
Smokers	108(39.6%)	301(37.4%)	0.523
Hypertension	176(64.5%)	506(62.9%)	0.633
Diabetes	56(20.5%)	206(25.6%)	0.091
Dyslipidemia	41(15.0%)	112(13.9%)	0.651
Prior MI	31(11.4%)	100(12.4%)	0.641
Prior CABG	4(1.5%)	8(1.0%)	0.521
Laboratory findings			
Baseline SCr (μmol/L)	99.29±24.77	98.17±23.07	0.495
Baseline-eGFR DDEeGFR (mL/min/1.73 m^2)	69.49±14.83	69.86±13.73	0.704
Log-NT-pro-BNP (pg/mL)	5.59±1.76	5.66±1.68	0.573
hs-CRP (mg/L)	12.02±21.96	10.10±19.77	0.281
LVEF, %	59.96±11.18	59.05±11.77	0.291
Total cholesterol (mmol/L)	4.23±1.08	4.29±1.94	0.660
Triglyceride (mmol/L)	1.44±0.89	1.79±8.17	0.329
LDL (mmol/L)	2.53±0.94	2.48±0.86	0.548
HbA1c, %	6.53±1.53	6.49±1.20	0.679
HG, g/L	132.21±14.77	132.57±16.54	0.733
Anemia, n (%)	86(31.5%)	289(35.9%)	0.187
Serum albumin, g/L	34.76±3.95	35.47±4.29	0.018
Uric acid, μmol/L	374.81±103.30	389.95±108.719	0.074
Medication, n (%)			
ACEI/ARB	242(88.6%)	729(90.6%)	0.361
β-bloker	237(86.8%)	720(89.4%)	0.235
Calcium channel blocker	70(25.6%)	163(20.2%)	0.061
Diuretics	27(9.9%)	101(12.5%)	0.241
Procedural characteristic			
Contrast volume (mL)	133.36±67.75	132.37±70.13	0.838
Contrast exposure time (min) (min)	73.37±43.97	71.96±47.34	0.669
Number of diseased vessels (n)	2.14±1.05	2.03±1.12	0.156
Number of stents (n)	1.68±1.20	1.60±1.19	0.387
Contrast volume/eGFR ratio	2.07±1.28	2.01±1.22	0.467
Mehran score	4.06±2.86	4.42±3.31	0.095

Abbreviations: SBP: systolic blood pressure; DBP: diastolic blood pressure. MI: myocardial infarction; CABG: coronary artery bypass grafting; SCr: serum creatinine; eGFR: estimated glomerular filtration rate; NT-pro-BNP: N-Terminal Pro-B-Type natriuretic peptide; hs-CRP: high sensitivity C reactive protein; LVEF: left ventricular ejection fraction; LDL: low density lipoprotein; HbA1c: hemoglobin A1c; HG: hemoglobin: ACEI/ARB: angiotensin-converting enzyme inhibitor/angiotensin receptor blocker; Mehran score: model to define contrast-induced nephropathy (CIN) by Mehran et al. Anemia was defined using World Health Organization criteria: baseline hematocrit value <39% for men and <36% for women.

and other in hospital complications, such as the requirement for renal replacement therapy (3.4% vs. 0.4%, P = 0.002) and the use of intra-aortic balloon pump (IABP; 10.34% vs. 1.18%, P<0.001). (Figure 1).

The incidences of CIN were similar between patients pretreated with either rosuvastatin or atorvastatin (5.9% vs. 5.2%, P = 0.684); similar results were also obtained using the alternate CIN definitions. In addition, there were no significant differences

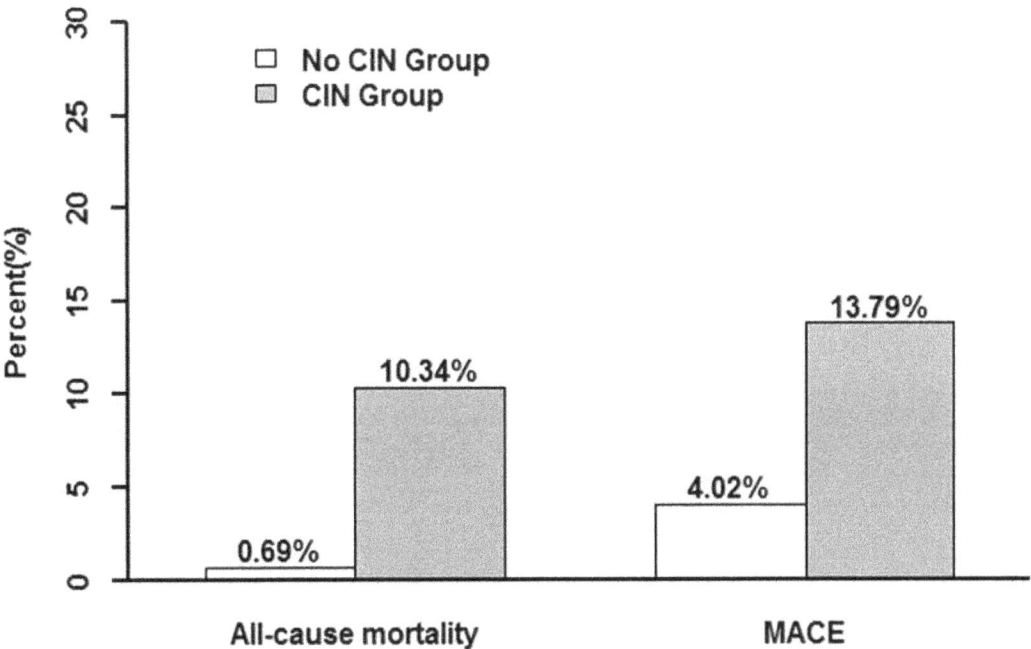

Figure 1. Multivariate logistic analysis associating contrast-induced nephropathy with various risk indicators.

between the two groups with regard to the rate of in-hospital mortality (0.4% vs. 1.5%, P = 0.141). However, patients treated with rosuvastatin had a lower incidence of in-hospital MACEs than those treated with atorvastatin (1.8% vs. 5.5%, P = 0.013) (Table2).

Multivariate logistic regression analysis revealed that pretreatment with rosuvastatin had a similar effect as atorvastatin pretreatment regarding the development of CIN in patients undergoing PCI (odds ratio [OR] = 1.17, 95% confidence interval [CI], 0.62–2.20, P = 0.623), even after adjusting for potential confounding risk factors (age >75 years, eGFR ≤60 mL/min/1.73 m², DM, anemia, CM >100 mL, IABP, LVEF<40%, primary PCI). Age >75 years (P = 0.029), IABP (P = 0.023), and primary PCI (P = 0.007) were other independent predictors of CIN in this population. (Figure 2).

Clinical outcomes during follow-up

The median follow-up period was 2.51±0.86 years (inter quartile range, 1.80–3.27 years) and was continued for all patients who survived to discharge.

To determine the relationship between the accumulated risk of adverse events and rosuvastatin or atorvastatin pretreatment, a Kaplan–Meier survival analysis was performed. Patients pretreated either rosuvastatin or atorvastatin demonstrated a similar incidence of all-cause mortality (7.76% vs. 5.36%, P = 0.193) or MACEs (26.48% vs. 21.28%, P = 0.243), as illustrated in Figure 3. In addition, patients who developed CIN had a higher rate of all-cause mortality than those who did not (cumulative rate of mortality, 22.73% vs. 5.07%, P<0.001). A similar result was found for MACEs. (43.18% vs. 21.50%, P = 0.002). (Figure 4).

Table 2. In-hospital events in patients treated with rosuvastatin or atorvastatin.

Variables	Rosuvastatin (n = 273)	Atorvastatin (n = 805)	P
CIN1	16 (5.9%)	42 (5.2%)	0.684
CIN2	5 (1.8%)	13 (1.6%)	0.809
CIN3	10 (3.7%)	33 (4.1%)	0.750
CIN4	2 (0.7%)	10 (1.2%)	0.488
CIN5	10 (3.7%)	33 (4.1%)	0.750
Death	1 (0.4%)	12 (1.5%)	0.141
Renal replacement therapy	1 (0.4%)	5 (0.6%)	0.625
Hypotension	3 (1.1%)	16 (2.0%)	0.335
IABP	3 (1.1%)	15 (1.9%)	0.394
Acute heart failure	2 (0.7%)	11 (1.4%)	0.407
Cerebrovascular accident	0 (0.0%)	3 (0.4%)	0.312

Abbreviations: CIN: contrast induced nephropathy; IABP: intra-aortic ballon pump.

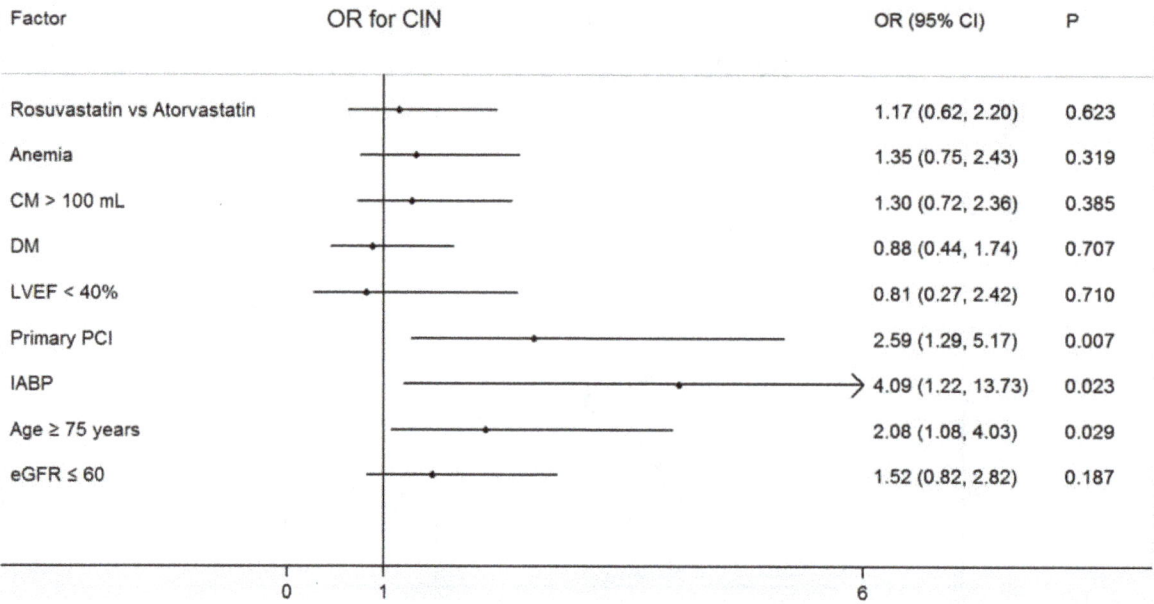

Factor	OR for CIN	OR (95% CI)	P
Rosuvastatin vs Atorvastatin		1.17 (0.62, 2.20)	0.623
Anemia		1.35 (0.75, 2.43)	0.319
CM > 100 mL		1.30 (0.72, 2.36)	0.385
DM		0.88 (0.44, 1.74)	0.707
LVEF < 40%		0.81 (0.27, 2.42)	0.710
Primary PCI		2.59 (1.29, 5.17)	0.007
IABP		4.09 (1.22, 13.73)	0.023
Age ≥ 75 years		2.08 (1.08, 4.03)	0.029
eGFR ≤ 60		1.52 (0.82, 2.82)	0.187

Figure 2. The prevalence of in-hospital all-cause mortality or major adverse cardiovascular events in patients with or without contrast-induced nephropathy.

Discussion

The present study may be the first to demonstrate that pretreatments with either rosuvastatin or atorvastatin have similar efficacies for preventing CIN in patients with CKD undergoing PCI.

The prevention of CIN is an important concern because it affects patient morbidity and mortality, especially in CKD patients [3,4]. In the current study, we found that the incidence of CIN was 5.4%, in agreement with previous studies [3]. Similar to previous studies, we found that patients developing CIN had a higher risk of poor in-hospital and long-term clinical outcomes. Because, few strategies have been demonstrated to be effective for preventing CIN [17]. The development of new strategies to decrease CIN occurrence, especially for high-risk CKD patients is urgently needed. This has led to an increased interest in the preventive

effects of statins (especially, atorvastatin and rosuvastatin) on CIN development in patients undergoing PCI.

However, conflicting results have been published. Kandula et al [19] reported an observational study (239 patients with statins, 114 without statins), that showed statin treatment was not associated with CIN prevention, after adjusting for the propensity of receiving statins (OR = 1.6, 95% CI: 0.86–3.22, P = 0.12). In contrast, another study based on a database of 29,409 patients undergoing emergent and non-emergent PCI [20], reported that patients using statins had a lower risk of CIN than did those not using statins (4.4% vs. 5.9%, P<0.001). Similar results were demonstrated by Hoshi et al [21]. Other than these observational studies, many RCTs have been conducted to address this topic. Toso et al [22] performed a prospective RCT, including 304 patients, to investigate the efficacy of short-term high dose atorvastatin on preventing CIN development in patients with

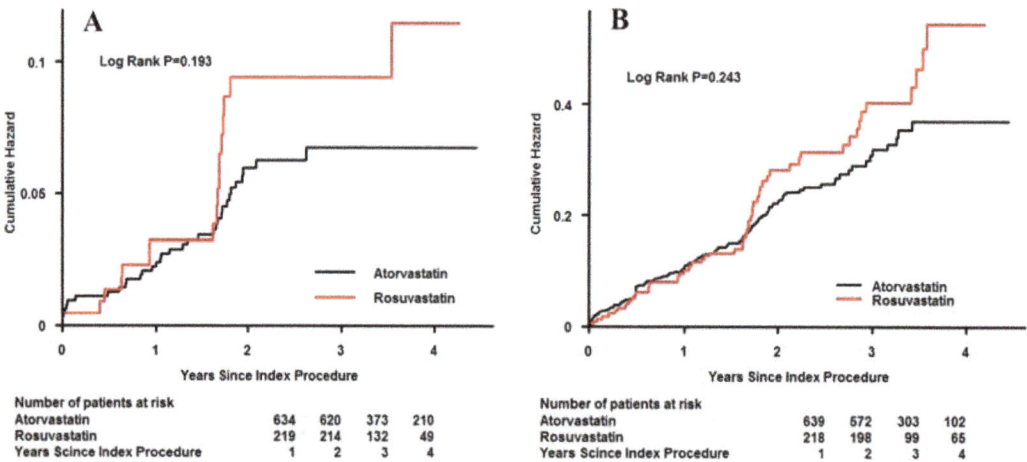

Figure 3. Cumulative rate of follow-up all-cause mortality (A) or major adverse cardiovascular events (B) in patients initially treated with rosuvastatin or atorvastatin.

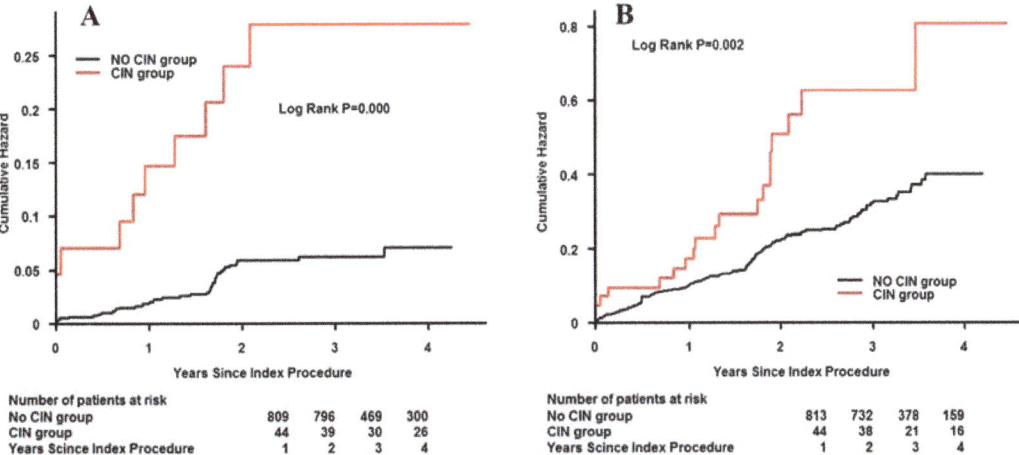

Figure 4. Cumulative rate of follow-up all-cause mortality (A) or major adverse cardiovascular events (B) in patients with or without contrast-induced nephropathy.

CKD undergoing PCI. The results showed that short-term high doses of atorvastatin, administered periprocedurally, did not decrease CIN occurrence in patients with pre-existing CKD. However, another group [10] enrolled 410 patients with CKD in an RCT and demonstrated that a single high dose of atorvastatin administered within a 24 h period before CM exposure, was effective at reducing the CIN rate. Similar findings have been reported from subsequent RCTs [9,21,23]. A previous meta-analysis of 7 RCTs, with a total of 1399 patients (693 patients receiving high-dose statins, 706 receiving low-dose or no statins) revealed that atorvastatin was beneficial for preventing of CIN [24], which is in agreement with our recent meta-analysis [25].

Two large RCTs recently demonstrated that rosuvastatin pretreatment, upon admission, could reduce CIN occurrence in patients undergoing PCI. Leoncini et al [11] reported that acute coronary syndrome patients, without ST-segment elevation, who were treated with rosuvastatin (40 mg on-admission, followed by 20 mg/day) experienced less CIN than patients not receiving rosuvastatin. Similarly, in patients with type 2 DM and CKD, another group showed that rosuvastatin significantly reduced the risk of CIN after CM exposure [12]. Accordingly, although guideline committees have not recommended this CIN-prevention strategy, researchers are increasingly considering statins as an effective drug for preventing CIN, based on the existing evidence.

Although the mechanism of statins in CIN prevention remains unknown, the following mechanisms may play important roles. In addition to their intended impact on blood cholesterol levels, statins are also known to have pleiotropic effects. Previous studies showed that statins treatment could prevent renal tubular cell apoptosis and increase survival signaling pathways [10]. However, the direct toxic effects of CM on renal cells, leading cell necrosis or apoptosis, are thought to contribute to the CIN pathogenesis. Preventing CM-induced renal cell apoptosis seems to play an important role in the statins' effects on CIN [10]. In addition, endothelial dysfunction, another major contributor to CIN progression, is caused by a nitric oxide (NO) and endothelin-1 imbalance, after CM exposure. Statins may help correct this imbalance by increasing NO production and reducing endothelin-1 synthesis [26]. Furthermore, C-reactive protein (CRP), as a marker of systemic inflammation, is also associated with CIN, and patients with high periprocedural CRP levels are at high risk for developing CIN [9,27,28]. Recent studies have demonstrated that the preventive effect of statins on CIN development parallels a

significant decrease in post-procedural CRP levels [12]. Thus, statins may reduce inflammation by inhibiting pro-inflammatory mediator synthesis [29], and may have a reno-protective effect during CM exposure by attenuating inflammatory responses.

Different statins (e.g., atorvastatin and rosuvastatin) vary in their LDL-lowering potency, lipophilicity, reno-protection, and anti-inflammatory effects [13,14]. However, whether the difference (hydrophilic and lipophilic) between statins influences their ability to reduce CIN risk is unclear. Rosuvastatin, a hydrophilic statin, has acute pleiotropic effects, and has been demonstrated to reduce LDL more aggressively, without increasing complications, and improve patient prognosis better than the other statins [30]; it also, exerts a beneficial reno-protective effect in patients with renal dysfunction [31]. Additionally, rosuvastatin has a longer plasma half-life and stronger anti-inflammatory effects than atorvastatin [32,33]. Because patients with CKD have significantly higher mean CRP levels [34], rosuvastatin may be more effective in these patients. Furthermore, Thiago et al demonstrated that rosuvastatin performed better than atorvastatin or simvastatin, in an experimental murine model of cigarette smoke-induced acute lung inflammation, because of better attenuation of both inflammation and oxidative stress parameters [35]. A recent meta-analysis reported that rosuvastatin might also increase apolipoprotein A-I levels at all doses more than atorvastatin [36]; apolipoprotein A-I can stabilize lipoprotein structure and has anti-inflammatory and antioxidant properties [37]. Based on these difference between rosuvastatin and atorvastatin, we hypothesized that rosuvastatin would differ from atorvastatin with respect to their abilities to prevent CIN.

To date, large studies investigating the CIN-risk reduction differences between rosuvastatin and atorvastatin have not been reported. One recent study, including 192 patients (94 taking rosuvastatin, 98 taking atorvastatin), compared the effects of different statins on CIN in STEMI patients treated with primary PCI; both statins had similar efficacies for preventing CIN. The study also suggested that the incidence of Killip class ≥ 2 patients ranged from 91.8–94.7% [15]. Therefore, increased of SCr in those patients may be the result of hemodynamic compromise due to acute impairment of cardiac pump function after extended myocardial infarction, rather than the direct effect of CM exposure [38]. However, in our study, the patients had relatively stable hemodynamic status because patients with a history of heart failure (NYHA $\geq$ III and Killip $\geq$ II) were excluded. Thus, CM administration may play a major role and the reduced risk of CIN may be a true reflection of the statins' effects. In our study, patients receiving rosuvastatin displayed higher levels of hs-CRP than did those treated with atorvastatin, suggesting that these patients would be more likely to develop CIN, based on the previous evidence [27,28]. However, our findings demonstrated that the incidence of CIN in rosuvastatin-treated patients was similar to that in atorvastatin- treated patients; the patients were relatively well balanced with respect to their baseline clinical and angiography characteristics. Although we did not demonstrate that rosuvastatin was superior to atorvastatin for preventing CIN, the results may not be surprising considering that different factors are involved in CIN development and that different patho-physiological mechanisms coexist.

The present study also demonstrated the patients pretreated with rosuvastatin or atorvastatin had similar risks of all-cause mortality and MACEs. In addition, we demonstrated that age > 75 years, IABP use, and primary PCI were independent risk factors of CIN, but not an eGFR $\leq$60 mL/min/1.73 m^2. However, Ando et al have demonstrated that eGFR as a continuous variable was a risk factor for CIN in STEMI patients treated with primary PCI [39]. This might be related to the different patient populations included in the two studies.

Limitations

There are several limitations to this study. First, this was a prospective, observational study conducted at a single center. Therefore, causality cannot be ascribed. Second, our study

population was limited to CKD (stage II and III) patients, so the results may not extend to patients with other stage of CKD or those without CKD. Third, due to variations in the timing of measurements, we may have missed the post-procedural SCr peak. Furthermore, we did not use cystatin C which is a more sensitive biomarker and increases faster than SCr after CIN. Thus, the true incidence of CIN may have been underestimated. Fourth, SCr levels were not systematically measured during the follow-up period. Fifth, in consideration of previous studies revealed that high-dose atorvastatin (40 or 80 mg) pretreatment was more effective than low-dose (20 mg) or no statin therapy [24], we did not investigate the protective efficacies of different doses in our study.

Conclusions

Our study demonstrated that rosuvastatin pretreatment exerts an effect similar to atorvastatin in preventing CIN in high risk patients with CKD undergoing PCI. Thus, future head to head studies are required to compare hydrophilic and lipophilic statins to determine if they reduce CIN risks differently.

Author Contributions

Conceived and designed the experiments: YL YHL NT JYC. Performed the experiments: YL YHL YLZ LWL JFL HLL WG. Analyzed the data: YL YHL CYD PYC. Contributed to the writing of the manuscript: YHL YL. Contributed to revising manuscript critically for important intellectual content: NT JYC.

References

1. Wi J, Ko YG, Kim JS, Kim BK, Choi D, et al. (2011) Impact of contrast-induced acute kidney injury with transient or persistent renal dysfunction on long-term outcomes of patients with acute myocardial infarction undergoing percutaneous coronary intervention. Heart 97: 1753–1757.

2. Seeliger E, Sendeski M, Rihal CS, Persson PB (2012) Contrast-induced kidney injury: mechanisms, risk factors, and prevention. Eur Heart J 33: 2007–2015.

3. Tsai TT, Patel UD, Chang TI, Kennedy KF, Masoudi FA, et al. (2014) Contemporary Incidence, Predictors, and Outcomes of Acute Kidney Injury in Patients Undergoing Percutaneous Coronary Interventions: Insights From the NCDR Cath-PCI Registry. JACC Cardiovasc Interv 7: 1–9.

4. Dangas G, Iakovou I, Nikolsky E, Aymong ED, Mintz GS, et al. (2005) Contrast-induced nephropathy after percutaneous coronary interventions in relation to chronic kidney disease and hemodynamic variables. Am J Cardiol 95: 13–19.

5. Wassmann S, Faul A, Hennen B, Scheller B, Bohm M, et al. (2003) Rapid effect of 3-hydroxy-3-methylglutaryl coenzyme a reductase inhibition on coronary endothelial function. Circ Res 93: e98–e103.

6. Ongini E, Impagnatiello F, Bonazzi A, Guzzetta M, Govoni M, et al. (2004) Nitric oxide (NO)-releasing statin derivatives, a class of drugs showing enhanced antiproliferative and antiinflammatory properties. Proc Natl Acad Sci U S A 101: 8497–8502.

7. Luvai A, Mbagaya W, Hall AS, Barth JH (2012) Rosuvastatin: a review of the pharmacology and clinical effectiveness in cardiovascular disease. Clin Med Insights Cardiol 6: 17–33.

8. Wong PC, Li Z, Guo J, Zhang A (2012) Pathophysiology of contrast-induced nephropathy. Int J Cardiol 158: 186–192.

9. Patti G, Ricottini E, Nusca A, Colonna G, Pasceri V, et al. (2011) Short-term, high-dose Atorvastatin pretreatment to prevent contrast-induced nephropathy in patients with acute coronary syndromes undergoing percutaneous coronary intervention (from the ARMYDA-CIN [atorvastatin for reduction of myocardial damage during angioplasty–contrast-induced nephropathy] trial. Am J Cardiol 108: 1–7.

10. Quintavalle C, Fiore D, De Micco F, Visconti G, Focaccio A, et al. (2012) Impact of a high loading dose of atorvastatin on contrast-induced acute kidney injury. Circulation 126: 3008–3016.

11. Leoncini M, Toso A, Maioli M, Tropeano F, Villani S, et al. (2014) Early high-dose rosuvastatin for contrast-induced nephropathy prevention in acute coronary syndrome: Results from the PRATO-ACS Study (Protective Effect of Rosuvastatin and Antiplatelet Therapy On contrast-induced acute kidney injury and myocardial damage in patients with Acute Coronary Syndrome). J Am Coll Cardiol 63: 71–79.

12. Han Y, Zhu G, Han L, Hou F, Huang W, et al. (2014) Short-term rosuvastatin therapy for prevention of contrast-induced acute kidney injury in patients with diabetes and chronic kidney disease. J Am Coll Cardiol 63: 62–70.

13. Toth PP (2014) An update on the benefits and risks of rosuvastatin therapy. Postgrad Med 126: 7–17.

14. DiNicolantonio JJ, Lavie CJ, Serebruany VL, O'Keefe JH (2013) Statin wars: the heavyweight match–atorvastatin versus rosuvastatin for the treatment of atherosclerosis, heart failure, and chronic kidney disease. Postgrad Med 125: 7–16.

15. Kaya A, Kurt M, Tanboga IH, Isik T, Ekinci M, et al. (2013) Rosuvastatin versus atorvastatin to prevent contrast induced nephropathy in patients undergoing primary percutaneous coronary intervention (ROSA-cIN trial). Acta Cardiol 68: 489–494.

16. Jones PH, Davidson MH, Stein EA, Bays HE, McKenney JM, et al. (2003) Comparison of the efficacy and safety of rosuvastatin versus atorvastatin, simvastatin, and pravastatin across doses (STELLAR* Trial). Am J Cardiol 92: 152–160.

17. Stacul F, van der Molen AJ, Reimer P, Webb JA, Thomsen HS, et al. (2011) Contrast induced nephropathy: updated ESUR Contrast Media Safety Committee guidelines. Eur Radiol 21: 2527–2541.

18. Ma YC, Zuo L, Chen JH, Luo Q, Yu XQ, et al. (2006) Modified glomerular filtration rate estimating equation for Chinese patients with chronic kidney disease. J Am Soc Nephrol 17: 2937–2944.

19. Kandula P, Shah R, Singh N, Markwell SJ, Bhensdadia N, et al. (2010) Statins for prevention of contrast-induced nephropathy in patients undergoing non-emergent percutaneous coronary intervention. Nephrology (Carlton) 15: 165–170.

20. Khanal S, Attallah N, Smith DE, Kline-Rogers E, Share D, et al. (2005) Statin therapy reduces contrast-induced nephropathy: an analysis of contemporary percutaneous interventions. Am J Med 118: 843–849.

21. Hoshi T, Sato A, Kakefuda Y, Harunari T, Watabe H, et al. (2014) Preventive effect of statin pretreatment on contrast-induced acute kidney injury in patients undergoing coronary angioplasty: Propensity score analysis from a multicenter registry. Int J Cardiol 171: 243–249.

22. Toso A, Maioli M, Leoncini M, Gallopin M, Tedeschi D, et al. (2010) Usefulness of atorvastatin (80 mg) in prevention of contrast-induced nephropathy in patients with chronic renal disease. Am J Cardiol 105: 288–292.

23. Li W, Fu X, Wang Y, Li X, Yang Z, et al. (2012) Beneficial effects of high-dose atorvastatin pretreatment on renal function in patients with acute ST-segment elevation myocardial infarction undergoing emergency percutaneous coronary intervention. Cardiology 122: 195–202.

24. Li Y, Liu Y, Fu L, Mei C, Dai B (2012) Efficacy of short-term high-dose statin in preventing contrast-induced nephropathy: a meta-analysis of seven randomized controlled trials. PLoS One 7: e34450.

25. Liu YH, Liu Y, Duan CY, Tan N, Chen JY, et al. (2014) Statins for the Prevention of Contrast-Induced Nephropathy After Coronary Angiography/ Percutaneous Interventions: A Meta-analysis of Randomized Controlled Trials.

Journal ofCardiovascular Pharmacology and Therapeutics. pii: 1074248414549462. [Epub ahead of print].

26. Almuti K, Rimawi R, Spevack D, Ostfeld RJ (2006) Effects of statins beyond lipid lowering: potential for clinical benefits. Int J Cardiol 109: 7–15.

27. Liu YH, Liu Y, Tan N, Chen JY, Chen J, et al. (2014) Predictive value of GRACE risk scores for contrast-induced acute kidney injury in patients with ST-segment elevation myocardial infarction before undergoing primary percutaneous coronary intervention. Int Urol Nephrol 46: 417–426.

28. Liu Y, Tan N, Zhou YL, Chen YY, Chen JY, et al. (2012) High-sensitivity C-reactive protein predicts contrast-induced nephropathy after primary percutaneous coronary intervention. J Nephrol 25: 332–340.

29. Tawfik MK, Ghattas MH, Abo-Elmatty DM, Abdel-Aziz NA (2010) Atorvastatin restores the balance between pro-inflammatory and anti-inflammatory mediators in rats with acute myocardial infarction. Eur Rev Med Pharmacol Sci 14: 499–506.

30. Betteridge DJ, Gibson JM, Sager PT (2007) Comparison of effectiveness of rosuvastatin versus atorvastatin on the achievement of combined C-reactive protein (<2 mg/L) and low-density lipoprotein cholesterol (<70 mg/dl) targets in patients with type 2 diabetes mellitus (from the ANDROMEDA study). Am J Cardiol 100: 1245–1248.

31. Ridker PM, MacFadyen J, Cressman M, Glynn RJ (2010) Efficacy of rosuvastatin among men and women with moderate chronic kidney disease and elevated high-sensitivity C-reactive protein: a secondary analysis from the JUPITER (Justification for the Use of Statins in Prevention-an Intervention Trial Evaluating Rosuvastatin) trial. J Am Coll Cardiol 55: 1266–1273.

32. Qu HY, Xiao YW, Jiang GH, Wang ZY, Zhang Y, et al. (2009) Effect of atorvastatin versus rosuvastatin on levels of serum lipids, inflammatory markers and adiponectin in patients with hypercholesterolemia. Pharm Res 26: 958–964.

33. Herregods MC, Daubresse JC, Michel G, Lamotte M, Vissers E, et al. (2008) Discovery Belux: comparison of rosuvastatin with atorvastatin in hypercholesterolaemia. Acta Cardiol 63: 493–499.

34. Fox ER, Benjamin EJ, Sarpong DF, Nagarajarao H, Taylor JK, et al. (2010) The relation of C-reactive protein to chronic kidney disease in African Americans: the Jackson Heart Study. BMC Nephrol 11: 1.

35. Ferreira TS, Lanzetti M, Barroso MV, Rueff-Barroso CR, Benjamim CF, et al. (2014) Oxidative Stress and Inflammation Are Differentially Affected by Atorvastatin, Pravastatin, Rosuvastatin, and Simvastatin on Lungs from Mice Exposed to Cigarette Smoke. Inflammation.

36. Takagi H, Umemoto T (2014) A meta-analysis of randomized head-to-head trials for effects of rosuvastatin versus atorvastatin on apolipoprotein profiles. Am J Cardiol 113: 292–301.

37. Walldius G, Jungner I (2004) Apolipoprotein B and apolipoprotein A-I: risk indicators of coronary heart disease and targets for lipid-modifying therapy. J Intern Med 255: 188–205.

38. Goldberg A, Hammerman H, Petcherski S, Zdorovyak A, Yalonetsky S, et al. (2005) Inhospital and 1-year mortality of patients who develop worsening renal function following acute ST-elevation myocardial infarction. Am Heart J 150: 330–337.

39. Ando G, Morabito G, de Gregorio C, Trio O, Saporito F, et al. (2013) Age, glomerular filtration rate, ejection fraction, and the AGEF score predict contrast-induced nephropathy in patients with acute myocardial infarction undergoing primary percutaneous coronary intervention. Catheter Cardiovasc Interv 82: 878–885.

22

Mapping Intravascular Ultrasound Controversies in Interventional Cardiology Practice

David Maresca[1]*, Samantha Adams[2], Bruno Maresca[3], Antonius F. W. van der Steen[1,4,5]

1 Department of Biomedical Engineering, Erasmus University Medical Centre, Rotterdam, the Netherlands, **2** Tilburg Institute for Law, Technology and Society, Tilburg University, Tilburg, the Netherlands, **3** Centre de recherche pour l'étude et l'observation des conditions de vie, Paris, France, **4** Interuniversity Cardiology Institute of the Netherlands, Utrecht, the Netherlands, **5** Imaging Science and Technology, Delft University of Technology, Delft, the Netherlands

Abstract

Intravascular ultrasound is a catheter-based imaging modality that was developed to investigate the condition of coronary arteries and assess the vulnerability of coronary atherosclerotic plaques in particular. Since its introduction in the clinic 20 years ago, use of intravascular ultrasound innovation has been relatively limited. Intravascular ultrasound remains a niche technology; its clinical practice did not vastly expand, except in Japan, where intravascular ultrasound is an appraised tool for guiding percutaneous coronary interventions. In this qualitative research study, we follow scholarship on the sociology of innovation in exploring both the current adoption practices and perspectives on the future of intravascular ultrasound. We conducted a survey of biomedical experts with experience in the technology, the practice, and the commercialization of intravascular ultrasound. The collected information enabled us to map intravascular ultrasound controversies as well as to outline the dynamics of the international network of experts that generates intravascular ultrasound innovations and uses intravascular ultrasound technologies. While the technology is praised for its capacity to measure coronary atherosclerotic plaque morphology and is steadily used in clinical research, the lack of demonstrated benefits of intravascular ultrasound guided coronary interventions emerges as the strongest factor that prevents its expansion. Furthermore, most of the controversies identified were external to intravascular ultrasound technology itself, meaning that decision making at the industrial, financial and regulatory levels are likely to determine the future of intravascular ultrasound. In light of opinions from the responding experts', a wider adoption of intravascular ultrasound as a stand-alone imaging modality seems rather uncertain, but the appeal for this technology may be renewed by improving image quality and through combination with complementary imaging modalities.

Editor: Wang Zhan, University of Maryland, College Park, United States of America

Funding: Funding of the Dutch Technology Foundation STW. The funders had no role in study design, data collection and analysis, decision to publish, or preparation of the manuscript.

Competing Interests: The authors have declared that no competing interests exist.

* E-mail: david.maresca@espci.fr

Introduction

Tremendous advances occurred during the last 40 years in the field of medical imaging of the heart and the coronary vasculature, triggered by the increasing need to reduce acute myocardial infarctions. The intravascular imaging route led to the development of X-ray angiography in the 1960's, balloon angioplasty and related techniques in the late 1970's and early 1980's. Meanwhile, in the early 1970's, academic research programs focused on developing two-dimensional real-time ultrasound imaging of the heart, transferring in particular knowledge from underwater acoustics to medicine [1]. This noninvasive route led to echocardiography, an imaging modality acclaimed for its radiation free nature but lacking the resolution to image the coronary vasculature.

The need for a technique able to provide high resolution images of diseased coronary artery wall structures, referred to as vulnerable plaques [2] and primarily responsible for myocardial infarctions, arose in the early 1990's when false-negative coronary angiography cases became evident [3]. Intravascular ultrasound (IVUS) is a catheter-based echocardiography modality that was patented in 1972 [4] and further developed to investigate the status of the coronary artery wall. The tip of an IVUS catheter incorporates a single piezoelectric transducer (40 to 60 MHz frequency range) or a circular array of transducers (20 MHz) to generate circular cross sectional images of the arterial wall, perpendicular to the longitudinal artery axis. Single transducer IVUS images are acquired by mechanically rotating the transducer over 360 degrees, whereas in circular array IVUS the ultrasound beam is steered electronically. The resolution of IVUS images is of the order of 100 µm in the axial direction, 300 µm in the lateral direction [5], and IVUS imaging depth typically ranges from 5 to 10 mm. IVUS technology has played an important role in the standardization of balloon angioplasty and stent treatments. Before intervention, IVUS can provide the artery lumen diameter, the plaque morphology and burden [6] thanks to the delineation of the external elastic membrane, and can be used to select optimal stent dimensions. Post intervention, IVUS is also useful to control stent apposition and possible complications. In addition, IVUS technology proved to be very useful in cardiovascular research. Since plaque progression and regression can be accurately measured with IVUS, the efficacy of new cardiovascular therapies on plaque volume can be quantified. IVUS also serves as gold standard for the evaluation of new intravascular modalities. Next to the estimation of plaque burden, the most valued IVUS function is calcium detection. Unfortunately, predicting the risk for future acute cardiovascular events requires knowledge of plaque composition [7], which is not provided by conventional IVUS. Several IVUS signal processing techniques have been developed at an academic level to augment IVUS capabilities in detecting and characterizing coronary artery plaques at risk [8,9] but failed to reach clinical practice so far.

Looking back, the realization of IVUS is undoubtedly a technical success. Twenty years after its introduction in the clinic in the early 1990's, IVUS technology continues to bring scientific insight into the pathophysiology of the coronary artery disease and helps guiding percutaneous coronary interventions. To date, the noninvasive imaging techniques capable of identifying coronary artery wall lesions are magnetic resonance imaging (MRI) and multi-slice computed tomography (MSCT), but their resolution remains inferior to *in situ* catheter techniques. Minimally invasive imaging techniques include coronary angiography, angioscopy, IVUS, intravascular optical coherence tomography (OCT), the combination of near infrared reflectance spectroscopy (NIRS) with IVUS [10]. OCT in particular has emerged as a rival for IVUS by generating more superficial but higher resolution images of the arterial wall.

Surprisingly, IVUS innovation appears relatively limited since its introduction in the clinic, especially in terms of image quality. Significant academic innovations such as IVUS flow [11,12], IVUS palpography [8,13], harmonic IVUS [14,15] and contrast-enhanced IVUS [9,16] were to date not taken up by industry. Furthermore, IVUS remains a niche technology, whose clinical practice did not vastly expand nor disappear. IVUS reimbursement varies considerably worldwide which reveals a contrasted adoption of IVUS. In Japan, IVUS is reimbursed separately since 1994, even for diagnostic use. In the United States, IVUS is not reimbursed but procedure codes leave enough room for IVUS utilization where necessary. In the rest of the world, there is no separate reimbursement for IVUS. IVUS market penetration worldwide follows accordingly.

Following scholarship in sociology of innovations, we were interested in understanding both the reasons for current adoption practices and prospects for further adoption or development of the technology in the future. As part of this, we sought to outline issues related to the technology, which are often referred to as 'controversies' [17], meaning that they can still be disputed, negotiated, etc. and practice, whereby the end result is still unknown. Understanding the various issues at stake for the respondents is important because how these further develop in practice can shape the future of the technology. To identify these issues, we took a qualitative approach. This approach combined a survey of experts currently generating innovations and/or using IVUS technologies with a social network analysis of their interactions.

Materials and Methods

To outline the dynamics of the network of experts that generates IVUS innovations and uses IVUS technologies, we conducted a survey of biomedical experts with experience in the technology and practice of IVUS. To that end, we selected a deliberative sample of potential respondents: a representative group of 49 experts dealing with the question of IVUS innovation or adjacent fields. Potential respondents were identified through publications in the field and confirmed through an expert check (Professor van der Steen, head of the Biomedical Engineering Department of the Thorax Centre, Erasmus University Medical Center, the Nether-

lands). Identified experts comprised interventional cardiologists, academic and corporate engineers, corporate leaders and public and private funders. For ethical considerations, the questionnaire data were collected under the agreement that data sourcing was kept anonymous. Questionnaire answers were pooled, randomized and analyzed anonymously. Participants were aware that their responses would be used in this study and that their company names may be included.

Survey design

We developed a questionnaire [18] with a combination of open and closed questions on IVUS innovation and refined it through face-to-face interviews with three experts. After revision, the questionnaire was issued to all other experts. The questionnaire started with two open questions about coronary atherosclerosis diagnostic in humans: "*What is the best method available to diagnose human coronary atherosclerosis?*" and "*What would be an ideal technique to diagnose coronary arteries?*". The first question permitted to review the coronary diagnostic tools that are currently appraised. The second question aimed at highlighting the limitations of existing diagnostic tools and identifying future diagnostic solutions with strong potential in the respondents' opinion. The questionnaire continued with questions focused on IVUS. To characterize the homogeneity of the respondents, we asked them to rate (from 0 - not so much, to 10 - extensive) their technical, clinical and market knowledge representation of IVUS. We collected their opinions on the advantages and disadvantages of IVUS. Next came two central questions: the room IVUS technology has left for improvement (to be rated from 0 - no room, to 10 - lots of room), and the likelihood of the existence of IVUS 20 years from now (to be rated from 0 – uncertain, to 10 - certain). These questions were inserted to quantify the future perspective of IVUS technology in the respondents' opinion. Next, we asked what the reimbursement procedure was for new medical devices in the respondent's country of residence before to specifically address the status of IVUS reimbursement. Then, we asked what were the prevailing factors that could explain the continuous but limited clinical utilization of IVUS in the respondents' opinion. Interventional cardiologists were specifically asked how IVUS helps them complete the regular tasks of their job. All these questions were inserted to collect material explaining the current adoption of IVUS. The last part contained of questions on the additional factors likely to impact IVUS innovation (e.g. educational efforts in IVUS, role of patents, and competition between experts in the IVUS market). Finally, we provided room for further comments related to IVUS technology that the respondents might want to share.

Network analysis

In the second part of the questionnaire, we asked the respondents to indicate the frequency and nature of their interaction with other identified experts. We analyzed the level of interaction among our deliberative sample of respondents using the social network analysis software UCINET (Harvard University, Boston, USA) [19]. A clique analysis was performed, assembling groups of four members or more who declared symmetric interactions [20]. Subsequently, we proceeded to a hierarchical cluster analysis of the respondents' adjacency in the network: an algorithm ordered the respondents hierarchically based on their level of similarity (amount of clique memberships shared by pairs of experts) and their proximity in the network. We displayed the result as a hierarchical clustering tree diagram using UCINET (see Figure 1). Having registered the bonds between experts, which informs on the professional network architecture, as well as the respondents' opinions on IVUS technology, we could map IVUS controversies and discuss their implications for the future of IVUS with respect to the position of the respondents in the network. It is important to realize that the individuals who contributed to this study represent a part of a bigger professional network, which is a limitation of this study. However, we postulate that the group of respondents that was surveyed is representative of the hierarchies and opinions present in the community of experts that generates IVUS innovations and uses IVUS technologies.

Description of the respondents

With the initial list of potential respondents, 38 international institutions were represented (20 American, 9 Dutch, 3 Canadian, 2 Japanese, 2 French, 1 German, and 1 South Korean). The list comprised the following types of respondents:

- Fifteen corporate leaders, encompassing IVUS companies (Boston Scientific, Volcano, Terumo, Infraredx, Silicon Valley Medical Instruments and Colibri Technologies), a company fostering competing intravascular technologies, two general medical ultrasound companies, and a clinical research organization with experience in interventional cardiology.

- Fourteen cardiologists conducting clinical research involving IVUS or practicing IVUS-guided percutaneous coronary interventions (PCI). The group identified comprised key opinion

leaders as well as international cardiologists in activity performing IVUS related research.

- Ten engineers involved with IVUS innovation or related fields. This included two academic engineers who filed constitutive IVUS inventions, four academic engineers currently in activity as well as four corporate engineers.

- Ten funders involved with IVUS innovation or related fields. Six were public funders and four private funders. Public funders represented public research organizations, public technology foundations. Private funders encompassed private technology foundations and investment firms.

Of the initial 49 experts, 23 returned a completed questionnaire. We analyzed the responses by first reassigning them into pertinent categories. Among cardiologists (8 respondents), a distinction was made between opinion-leading cardiologists (3 respondents) and academic IVUS users (5 respondents), based on internal knowledge of the field of IVUS and top authors tracking on a biomedical experts platform. Among corporate leaders (6 respondents), a distinction was made between IVUS companies (4 respondents) and related field companies (2 respondents). Public and Private funders were merged in a single group because of the limited contributions (2 respondents). Finally, engineers (7 respondents) were divided into academic (5 respondents) or corporate engineers (2 respondents).

For figure and citation purposes, we labeled IVUS corporate leaders as *IVUS Corp Leader*, corporate leaders in adjacent fields as

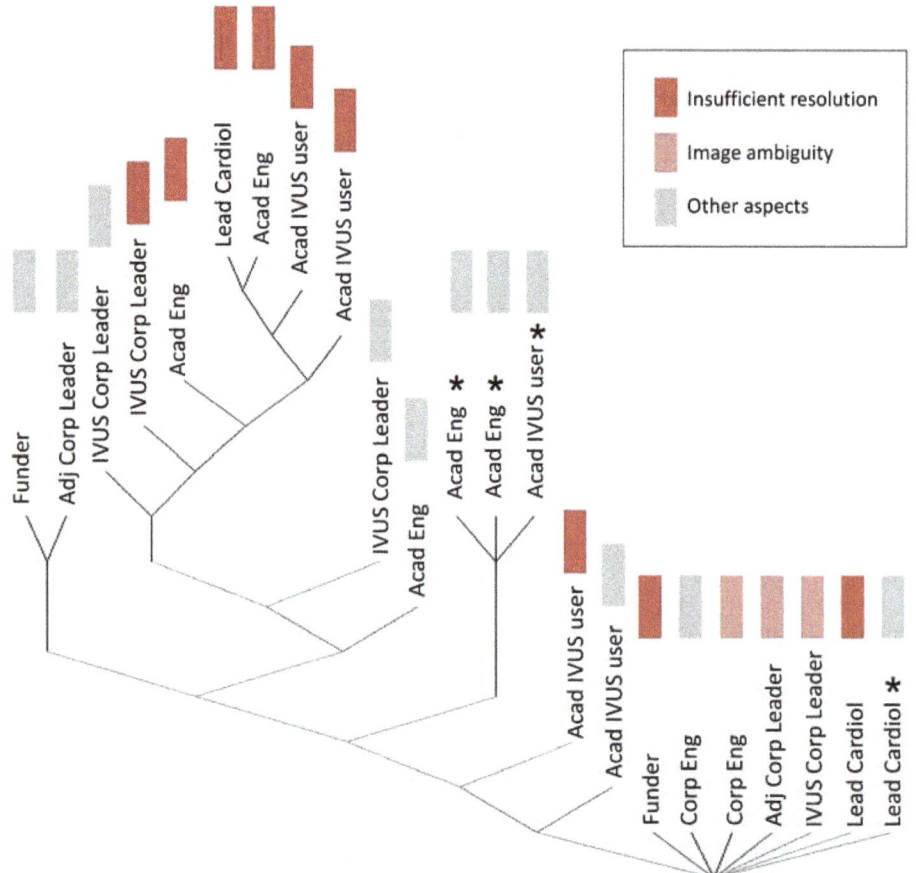

Figure 1. Respondents' perception of intravascular ultrasound resolution. Early experts are indicated with a star. Experts that were the least central in the network, who declared a limited level of interaction with other members, appear at the bottom of the diagram. The diagram can be subdivided as follows: a base of peripheral experts that are the least central in the network, a middle group, including early IVUS experts, with an intermediate centrality level, and finally the leading group of the network gathering the most central experts.

Adj Corp Leader, opinion leading cardiologists as *Lead Cardiol*, academic IVUS users as *Acad IVUS Users*, academic engineers as *Acad Eng*, corporate engineers as *Corp Eng* and funders as *Funder*.

Results

Self-characterization of the respondents

Overall, respondents demonstrated a homogeneously high technical knowledge (total average of 8.1) and clinical knowledge (total average of 7.6) of IVUS, indicating that we successfully surveyed experts involved at the technical and medical interface of IVUS. The technical knowledge was well aligned among all categories of experts. Engineers reported a deficit in clinical knowledge (average of 6.0), below cardiologists and corporate leaders, indicating that they do not perceive themselves as medical specialists. Respondents' market knowledge appeared to be more widespread (total average of 7.0), above average for opinion-leading cardiologists and corporate leaders and below average for academic IVUS users. The experts' knowledge representation of IVUS reimbursement policies worldwide was the lowest (total average of 5.0). IVUS corporate leaders and corporate leaders of related fields were above average while corporate engineers and funders were below. Cardiologists and academic engineers were average. Corporate leaders naturally appeared to be more focused than the rest on the non-technical factors that governing the development of medical technologies.

Historical context of IVUS introduction

Twenty years elapsed between the registration of the first IVUS patent in 1972 [4] and its transfer to clinical research in the early 1990's [21,22], when the technology caught the attention of interventional cardiologists willing to visualize coronary artery wall lesions. This was clear, for example, in this response from a European respondent:

"As the big worry for cardiac echography was to see through the ribs, the idea of a phased array catheter was suggested. But in the meantime, the external linear array proved to be successful. People could see the heart and babies. Since the noninvasive approach worked, people forgot about the phased array catheter until the early nineties, when the need for a high resolution technique able to characterize coronary artery lesions emerged." *(Acad Eng)*

The introduction of IVUS as a high tech medical device followed a classical path. It first started as an academic engineering project aiming at developing intracardiac echocardiography in real time. IVUS technology eventually found light as a high resolution tool to characterize coronary artery lesions, as a result of the academic collaboration of cardiologists and engineers. This was clear, for example, in this response about the advantages of IVUS from Canadian respondent:

"It [IVUS] has good penetration through blood and soft tissue, enabling estimation of vessel dimension, vessel remodeling, and plaque burden with high sensitivity and specificity in identifying coronary calcifications". *(Acad Eng)*

The second phase of IVUS introduction was its adoption by industry. The industrial development and aim given to IVUS was largely shaped by Boston Scientific. This is evident, for example, in this response from the US:

"In the first 10 years, Mansfield/Boston Scientific and CVIS were alone; then BSC bought CVIS and merged their platform." *(IVUS Corp Leader)*

As Boston scientific is primarily a stent manufacturer, IVUS holds an adjacent technology position within the company portfolio. IVUS was positioned as a percutaneous coronary intervention (PCI) guidance tool, allowing for peri-interventional planning and assessment of complications. This role is clear, for example, in the response of an interventional cardiologist who explains how IVUS helps him complete the regular tasks of his job:

"IVUS-guided PCI:

1. PRE: Plaque assessment, luminal diameters, stent length sizing.
2. INTRA: Stent apposition, re-entry in dissected planes, ante/retrograde chronic total occlusion (CTO).
3. POST: thrombus, edge prolapse, dissection, etc." *(Lead Cardiol)*

This tells us that the use of IVUS evolved from a research diagnostic tool to a PCI intervention guidance tool. It raises the question of the role for intracoronary imaging technologies. To date, IVUS technology is perceived as well aligned within the product portfolio of IVUS companies. This was reported in this response from the US:

"All companies try to create a coronary artery imaging platform. For Boston Scientific and Terumo, IVUS is an adjacent market. For Volcano, Infraredx, it is a central market." *(Funder)*

The third stage of the introduction of IVUS is its reimbursement via public health policy. Overall, the reimbursement process for a new medical device consists in the following: evidence-based medicine must prove benefits in using the technology. Subsequently, randomized clinical trials are to be conducted to determine whether the technology leads to an improved effectiveness in terms of patient outcome as well as a superior cost-effectiveness than the standard of care. The reality of IVUS reimbursement appears contrasted. In the US, the situation was reported as follows:

"There is no separate reimbursement for IVUS and it must be bundled into the existing Diagnosis-related group (DRG) for the specific coronary intervention. A separate set of cost-effectiveness and clinical utility data would be required to create stand-alone IVUS reimbursement" *(IVUS Corp Leader)*

This indicates that IVUS only partially fulfills the usual requirements for the reimbursement of a new device in the United States. Most notably, it appears that the technology has failed to demonstrate clinical utility. Yet, several respondents pointed at the clear dissymmetry in the reimbursement of IVUS that exists worldwide. This was clear, for example, in this response from the US:

"Separate reimbursement exists in Japan, where IVUS penetration is widely viewed as the deepest in any part of the world. This is not circumstantial. The second highest major market penetration is in the US, where it is not reimbursed separately but in which specific procedure codes do leave enough room for IVUS utilization where necessary. The lowest penetration exists in EU and Asia/Latin America markets where per-procedure economics are tightest and no separate reimbursement exists. Thus, while there is undoubtedly strong clinical belief in the utility of IVUS, there is an undeniable correlation between where that clinical belief manifests and where the economic policies are most accommodating." *(IVUS Corp Leader)*

Japan's separate reimbursement of IVUS is unique worldwide and seems to be the result of a stronger belief in the utility of IVUS interventional cardiology practice. Nonetheless, the status of IVUS reimbursement is a strong indicator of a contrasted acceptance of the technology and reveals that IVUS must be engaged into a set of controversies.

Open debates surrounding IVUS technology

By reviewing the contributors' answers, we identified six controversies revolving around IVUS technology; a controversy being defined as a debate surrounding a technique, for which the outcome has not yet been determined [17,23]. The controversies identified are reported in Table 1.

- The first controversy concerns the invasive nature of IVUS. It opposes experts who perceive invasiveness as a limitation, e.g. by preventing the screening of asymptomatic patients, to experts who relativize the minimal invasiveness of IVUS in light of the interventional nature of their job.

- The second controversy identified concerns the resolution of IVUS imaging. It opposes experts who perceive IVUS resolution as insufficient to detect important features of atherosclerotic

plaques (e.g. thrombi, thin cap fibroatheroma, plaque composition) and/or consider IVUS images as difficult to interpret, to experts who praise the sufficient clarity of IVUS whose resolution provides well validated quantitative measurements of atherosclerotic plaques (e.g. size and shape of coronary lesions, residual lumen, calcium detection, clear images of stent struts).

- The third controversy concerns the practicability of IVUS as a diagnostic tool. It opposes experts who consider that IVUS is an expensive and late diagnostic solution (restricted to patients who already need an intervention) which is tedious to analyze, to experts who praise the local knowledge of the plaque provided by IVUS and therefore its prognostic value, as well as the fact that IVUS is relatively quick to use.

- The fourth controversy concerns the utility of IVUS as a percutaneous coronary intervention (PCI) guidance tool. It opposes experts considering that IVUS has a limited impact on clinical decision making and failed to prove clinical benefits in terms of PCI treatment outcome, to experts who consider that IVUS improves safety overall by resolving ambiguous anatomy on angiograms (for example at the left main coronary artery), permits the adequate selection of stent landing zones and stent size, and allows for the evaluation of post-intervention complications.

- The fifth controversy concerns the impact of IVUS reimbursement on IVUS utilization worldwide. It opposes experts who consider that IVUS current reimbursement leaves enough room for an appropriate use and that expansion is primarily limited by the lack of demonstrated IVUS benefits, to experts who consider that a separate reimbursement of IVUS, even for diagnostic use, would favor its development as observed in Japan.

- The sixth controversy concerned the means invested in the education of IVUS experts. In light of the absence of clearly

Table 1. Ongoing IVUS controversies conveyed by the respondents.

Controversy	Positive responses	Negative responses
Invasiveness of IVUS	"Minimally invasive"; "The technique is invasive but I am an interventional cardiologist. IVUS takes 30 seconds"	"IVUS is very invasive to find the site of interest"; "A major disadvantage is that IVUS is invasive"
Resolution of IVUS	"High resolution and similarity to pathology"; "It has good penetration through blood and soft tissue, enabling estimation of vessel dimension, vessel remodeling, and plaque burden with high sensitivity and specificity in identifying coronary calcifications"	"Unacceptably poor resolution"; "Resolution is not enough for some particular purpose (Thin Cap Fibroatheroma)"
Usefulness of IVUS as diagnostic tool	"In order to understand the local problem, a catheter is the best"; "Large investigation range in combination with pull-back"; "Relatively quick, you can see obstruction, size and shape of the lesion (morphology)"; "Well validated quantitative measurements, many related outcome evidence by IVUS measurements (example, minimum stent area to predict future revascularization), easy to learn/use"; "Resolves ambiguous anatomy on angiogram, especially at left main"	"Intra-coronary imaging is too invasive and too late to use"; "most information not needed in daily practice unless complication"; "Lack of clarity of the images (I think I know what I'm looking at but not entirely sure) and the difficulty of acquiring those images"; "A catheter does not provide a complete view of the vascular tree"
Usefulness of IVUS as PCI guidance tool	"Inadequacy of angiography to guide clinical decision making in complex anatomy"; "Clinical trials have shown that the use of IVUS is reasonable during PCI for several indications. The medical literature continues to demonstrate limitation of angiographic-only guidance for PCI"	"Clinical impact on decision making is limited"; "There is no large clinical trial to show the benefit of using IVUS"; "Absence of evidence based medicine guidelines/Competition with FFR&OCT"
Impact of IVUS reimbursement on IVUS innovation	"Separate reimbursement exists in Japan, where IVUS penetration is widely viewed as the deepest in any part of the world. This is not circumstantial"; "Japan has reimbursement even for diagnostic IVUS. If not, the usage will decrease to half of now"	"Reimbursable for appropriate use"; "I think the biggest limit is the lack of investment in academic research"; "It affects the clinical use. Institutions like the Thoraxcenter simply supply the difference, but in peripheral hospitals the clinical use is affected. The IVUS innovation is an academic/industrial process and is financed by other means"
Educational efforts in IVUS	"A focused educational program is needed for realizing the potential of this technique"	"Today it's a niche technology, teaching efforts questionable given poor penetration"

demonstrated clinical benefits in using IVUS, some experts consider that enough educational efforts are consented (live cases at conferences, publications, experts visits), while others consider that because IVUS technology is not exploited at its full potential, a global educational effort is required (e.g. exposure of cardiologists in training, creation of a certification program, online consulting systems).

It is interesting to note that only one of the six controversies identified - the ongoing debate on IVUS resolution - was intrinsic to the technology itself. All others appeared as peripheral debates surrounding IVUS practice and questioning aspects of interventional cardiology practice in general. Nonetheless, the amount of controversies identified is not negligible and raises the question of the future of IVUS, especially since the field of intracoronary imaging has become more competitive with the introduction of OCT. In particular, the role of intravascular imaging seems to be questioned: is the goal to mimic histology, to perform prognostic imaging and/or to provide procedure guidance?

Mapping IVUS controversies

In order to analyze controversies by taking into account the social network dynamics, we projected the respondents' opinions on the UCINET tree diagram (Methods section). In Figure 1, we projected the opinions of the respondents who mentioned "resolution" when answering to the question of the disadvantages of IVUS. By doing so, we mapped the ongoing debate on the resolution of IVUS imaging (identified earlier as the only one intrinsic to the technology of IVUS). It appeared that the six most central experts in the network perceive IVUS resolution as insufficient. Interestingly, the figure reveals that none of the historic experts (marked with a star in the figure) cited resolution as a disadvantage of IVUS. From their perspective, IVUS was introduced as a high resolution technique, filling a void in interventional cardiology. Figure 1 displays therefore the evolution of the debate on resolution since the introduction of IVUS. We know that IVUS image quality did not drastically change since its introduction. Still it changed from high to low at the advent of OCT. A clear change in understanding of what "high resolution" means is observed, independent from the developmental path of IVUS technology: it indicates a mutual shaping between technology and society.

Future perspective for IVUS technology

When looking at the distribution of the answers of the respondents to the two central questions (the room for improvement left for IVUS technology and the perspective of existence in 20 years), we observed a singular double-peak distribution (Figure 2).

This result clearly indicates that two populations coexist in the IVUS network surveyed, one optimistic and one pessimistic about the technology perspective. We rearranged the responses into two categories, the positive opinions (values above 6) and the negative opinions (values below 6). Academic engineers were the most optimistic when rating the room for improvement that IVUS technology has (average of 7.8), which is natural considering that they are professionally invested in IVUS innovation. Academic IVUS users were optimistic as well (7.3) followed by IVUS corporate leaders (6.8). On the contrary, corporate engineers appeared pessimistic (4.5) while other corporate leaders were the most pessimistic (1.5). Logically, it appears that the judgment on the room for improvement of IVUS is directly dependent on the degree of investment the experts have in IVUS: engineers and corporate leaders involved with other intravascular technologies were negative about the innovation potential that IVUS has left.

Results were projected on the tree diagram in Figure 3, showing that historic experts emerge as the principal subgroup sharing a positive opinion about the room for innovation left for IVUS technology. Note that most central experts, who are currently professional active, conveyed a rather negative opinion.

Concerning the existence of IVUS in 20 years, the optimistic group gathered academic IVUS users (7.1), academic engineers (6.6) and IVUS corporate leaders (6.5). The pessimistic group was made of the opinion-leading cardiologists (4.3), other corporate leaders (4.0) and funders (3.3). Engineers and IVUS corporate leaders were convinced of the future of the technology. Conversely, opinion-leading cardiologists and funders were skeptical about the future of IVUS. Again, historic experts shared an optimistic vision of the future of IVUS as for the previous question. Central experts in the network appeared more balanced. Experts with a low centrality (potentially less tied to IVUS) were rather pessimistic.

When the answers to both questions are coupled, it appears that academic engineers, academic IVUS users and IVUS corporate leaders share a globally optimistic view, whereas opinion-leading cardiologists, other corporate leaders and funders shared a globally pessimistic view. Therefore, a major conclusion is that opinion-leading cardiologists and funders, who orientate innovation due to their position, disclosed a pessimistic opinion of the existence of IVUS technology 20 years from now. Their regard on the future of the technology was clearly exposed, for example, in this response from the US:

"In my opinion, the use of IVUS only makes sense as part of conventional angioplasty. If it were incorporated as part of the procedure, then there would not be a need for a second invasive procedure. However, the fact that IVUS is invasive may limit its capability for growth, especially if non-invasive MRI and CT coronary diagnostic imaging capabilities reach the point that they become more attractive, competitive diagnostic procedures. This may be possible in the near future, and might decrease the need for invasive diagnostic procedures like IVUS.

A more important consideration would be the results of comparative effectiveness studies of IVUS, compared to conventional angioplasty. If it could be proved that IVUS increased longevity or decreased complications, this would contribute toward making this procedure more attractive to practitioners" (Funder)

Discussion

This study demonstrates that the development and positioning of IVUS, in the high-tech environment of interventional cardiology adjunctive devices, is shaped by co-developing controversies surrounding the technology. We questioned why IVUS neither expanded nor disappeared since its introduction 40 years ago. The capacity of IVUS to estimate total coronary plaque burden was almost unanimously reported by the respondents and appears as the principal advantage of IVUS. IVUS is the only clinical tool capable of measuring plaque burden in vivo [24] and was shown to be a predictor of major adverse cardiovascular events [6]. For this reason, the technology is praised in cardiovascular research since it allows for longitudinal studies of atherosclerosis progression. IVUS can also rely on an extensive publication database and has become the gold standard to compare to when introducing a new intravascular imaging technology. Therefore, one possible

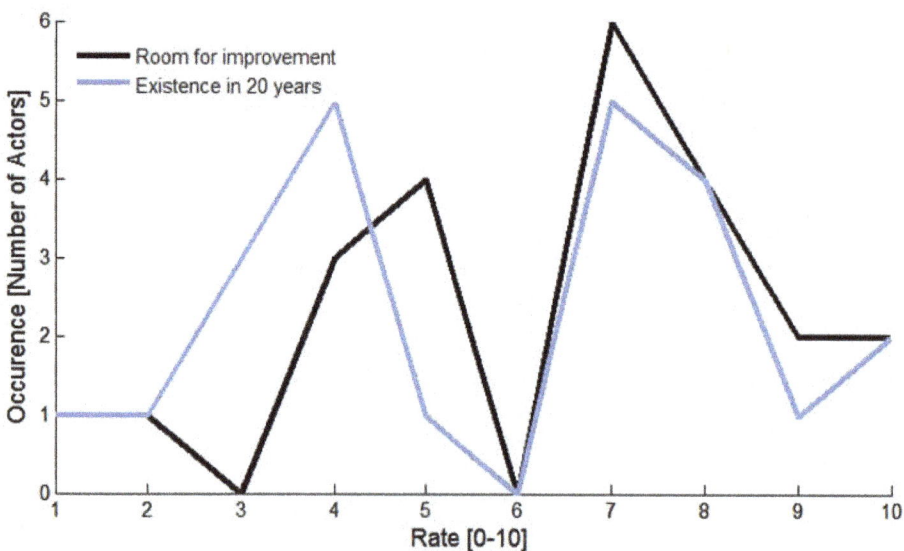

Figure 2. Future perspective of intravascular ultrasound according to the respondents.

explanation is that it is the utilization of IVUS in cardiovascular research that kept the technology running in academic medical centers.

On the other hand, the absence of good reimbursement was clearly reported as directly limiting the clinical use of IVUS (or would affect its use in the case of Japan). But respondents from the United States, Europe and Japan alike also reported that the

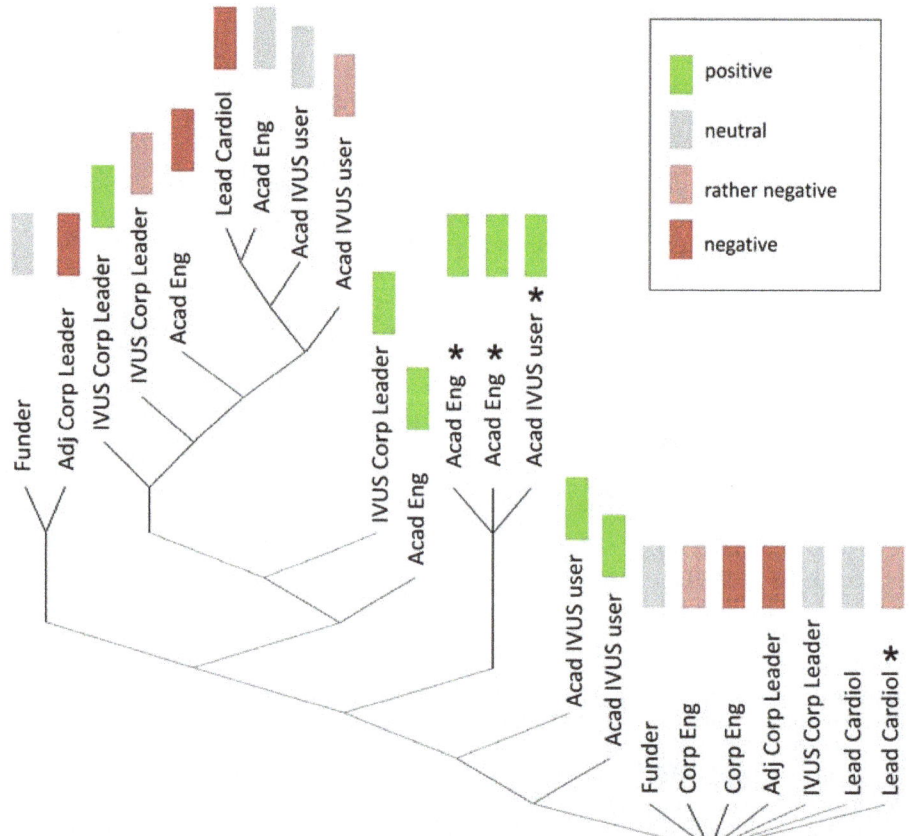

Figure 3. Room for innovation in intravascular ultrasound according to the respondents. Early experts are indicated with a star. Least central experts in the network appear at the bottom of the diagram and most central experts at the top.

creation of stand-alone reimbursement for a medical device requires cost-effectiveness and clinical utility data. Therefore, we can pose the question whether it is the lack of demonstrated medical evidence in favor of IVUS technology that prevented the creation of a stand-alone IVUS reimbursement, with the exception of Japan where the technology was reimbursed in 1994.

The case of IVUS reimbursement in Japan can be explained by two converging factors. First, an early interest for IVUS technology (in 1993 IVUS was used in Japanese hospitals for clinical research), which was originally offering both the highest resolution available in interventional cardiology and validated quantitative and outcome related measurements (e.g. "minimum stent area to predict future vascularization"). Second, a reimbursement accreditation procedure for approving a new medical device that is "not inferior to existing alternatives but does not have to be superior in every aspect". Other countries adopted a wait-and-see stance, as a stand-alone IVUS reimbursement requires a set of "cost-effectiveness and clinical utility data". Penetration of IVUS is the lowest in Europe, Latin America and Asia where reimbursement policies are the least accommodating. It is the combination of a strong belief in the clinical utility of IVUS and an accommodating economic policy that fosters the use of the technology. A Japanese respondent reported that if IVUS was not reimbursed in Japan, its use would be halved compared to now. Ulucanlar et al. [25] recently argued that 'technology identities' e.g. their novelty, effectiveness, utility, risks and requirements are socially constructed and shape technology adoption. Here we show in the case in the particular case of IVUS that the 'identity' of a given technology can vary geographically.

Several other lessons relevant for both the future of IVUS and the introduction of new intracoronary imaging techniques can be learned from this sociological study of IVUS innovation. We observed that the only controversy intrinsic to IVUS technology was the debate on IVUS resolution. It is important to analyze at the architecture of the network of IVUS experts surveyed when evaluating the implications of this controversy. The tree diagram (Figure 1) can be subdivided in three groups: a base of peripheral experts that are the least central in the network, a middle group of early IVUS experts with an intermediate centrality level and finally, the leading group of the network gathering the most central experts. Experts at the top of the diagram are likely to be in close collaboration and/or competition with each other and to be the most deeply involved with IVUS or adjacent technologies. Furthermore, their point of view is dominant because of their central position in the network. But they are also likely to have the highest interest in promoting a given imaging modality. Since the six most central experts in this survey are all indicating that IVUS resolution is insufficient, we can assume that improvements are mandatory for the future of the technology. Note that a significant enhancement in IVUS image quality could be achieved by improving IVUS lateral resolution, currently three times worse than axial resolution [5]. This strategy was investigated academically by Chandrana et al. [15] but did not materialize industrially to date.

Interestingly, we observed that the middle group of early experts who were involved with the introduction of IVUS pointed at other IVUS limitations than resolution. Certainly because, from their perspective, IVUS filled a void in the interventional cardiology space and entered as the highest resolution modality. On the contrary, peripheral experts are likely to be involved to a lesser extent with IVUS and potentially give a more positive judgment of the advantages and disadvantages of IVUS technology. This observation is in line with the concept of "certainty trough"

developed by Donald A. MacKenzie [26], which states that knowledge producers from a peripheral discipline attribute less uncertainty to technology from another discipline than those involved directly in knowledge production. More than resolution, it is the ambiguity of IVUS images that the respondents incriminate, telling us that understanding IVUS images requires expertise. Whether a higher resolution will solve image interpretation issues is not clear. Despite its microscopic resolution, OCT is still in a phase of standardization, proven benefits have not been demonstrated yet and the technology is not exempt of artifacts, which makes OCT image interpretation an expert's task as well.

Several respondents stressed the need for focused educational programs in order to fully realize the potential of intracoronary imaging techniques. They criticized the lack of exposure of medical doctors to these techniques at resident stage. Educational efforts in IVUS were considered as "hobbyist" by an early European practitioner. And the relevance of educational efforts was questioned by others given the poor penetration of IVUS. When characterizing themselves, engineers declared a deficit in clinical knowledge of IVUS compared to other groups, whereas technical knowledge was homogeneously high among experts. A more extensive education of engineers to the reality of IVUS clinical procedures and catheter laboratory workflow might prove to be critical for the successful introduction of future intracoronary imaging modalities. Complementarily, educating interventional cardiologists further in the physics of intravascular imaging could improve patient treatment, by helping them to recognize image artifacts and hence secure their diagnosis. It is likely that a more substantial knowledge overlap between interventional cardiologists, biomedical engineers, industry leaders and investors would accelerate IVUS innovation. The evolution of cardiac interventions based on new medical technology was shown to be progressing along co-evolving pathways: advances in scientific understanding indeed, but more important improvements of the ability to develop and use medical technologies as well as learning in medical practice [27].

Most central experts in the network had a skeptical perception of the potential for innovation that IVUS technology has left (Figure 3). This can be understood from a historical perspective as the field of IVUS faced a relative lack of IVUS innovation in the past 20 year. 40 MHz IVUS was reported as early as 1991 in scientific literature [20,21] and remains the standard product of major IVUS companies today; image quality in IVUS did not experience major breakthroughs in 20 years. Several respondents criticized the lack of competition in the IVUS market, which potentially stifles innovation. These respondents also called for the creation of new start-ups to re-energize clinical translation. IVUS companies happened to sit on innovation in some cases therefore limiting the dissemination of new technological developments. It was reported that patents have played a role, but that most of them are now obsolete. Academic engineers were the only ones that appeared clearly positive about the potential left for IVUS innovation (Figure 2), probably because they envision potential refinements in IVUS technology.

Given that five of the six identified controversies are external to IVUS technology, we can hypothesize that decision making at the industrial, financial and regulatory levels will orientate predominantly future innovations in intracoronary imaging. As reported earlier, a major conclusion is that opinion-leading cardiologists and funders, who shape innovation to a large extent, disclosed a pessimistic opinion of the existence of IVUS technology 20 years from now. In general, minimally invasive imaging modalities are logically not perceived as adequate for the early screening of coronary atherosclerosis in asymptomatic patients. First, because the information they provide is local (as opposed to a full view of the coronary anatomy e.g. angiography/MRI/CT) and second because of their invasive character. Therefore, wide adoption of intravascular imaging will depend on added benefits for cardiac patients requiring intervention. If a medical consensus advocates the identification of flow limiting lesions, then the combination of fractional flow reserve (FFR) and angiography is sufficient [28]. If medical guidelines state that the assessment of plaque vulnerability is critical, then intravascular imaging techniques will play a role as prognostic tools. In any case, next generation IVUS technologies as well as new intravascular technologies will compete with OCT in terms of image quality and guidance of stent apposition, and with the combination of angiography and FFR in terms of clinical decision making.

Conclusion

To date, IVUS remains valuable as it is the only clinical tool capable of imaging plaque burden *in vivo* and because it is grounded in extensive scientific literature. Mapping IVUS controversies revealed that the appeal of intravascular ultrasound may be renewed by improving (lateral) image resolution and/or through combination with other imaging modalities. An integrated IVUS-OCT catheter, providing OCT resolution and IVUS penetration simultaneously, was recently evaluated *in vivo* [29]. This technical solution has the merit to solve the issue of IVUS resolution. Other combined modalities were mentioned such as NIRS-IVUS [30] and intravascular photoacoustics [31]. These may provide an enhanced characterization of the arterial wall but will still need to act on IVUS image quality. In all cases

miniaturization and integration of independent modalities will weigh on cost-effectiveness.

The successful translation of future intravascular imaging technologies in interventional cardiology practice will require a rapid demonstration of clinical utility, which is a necessary condition for an efficient reimbursement; otherwise, hospitals cannot afford to use it. Finally, this must be coupled on a willingness of care practitioners to gain experience in a range of quickly developing technologies [32] in order to improve patient care. Unless, of course, in the advent of preventive medicine, the amount of percutaneous coronary interventions decreases drastically.

The future of IVUS as a stand-alone modality appears uncertain due to a lack of demonstrated benefits of the technology in terms of patient outcomes. Moreover, its use in cardiovascular research is likely to erode with the emergence of newer intravascular imaging techniques. As time passes, competition among adjunctive interventional cardiology devices increases, whereby the chance that IVUS will reach stand-alone reimbursement decreases.

Acknowledgments

We warmly thank all the respondents for their time and answers, their valuable contributions made this study possible.

Author Contributions

Conceived and designed the experiments: DM SA BM AvdS. Performed the experiments: DM. Analyzed the data: DM SA BM AvdS. Contributed reagents/materials/analysis tools: DM SA BM AvdS. Wrote the paper: DM SA BM AvdS.

References

1. Yoxen E (1987) Seeing with sound: a study of the development of medical images. The social construction of technological systems: New directions in the sociology and history of technology. Boston: MIT Press. 281 p.
2. Muller JE, Tofler GH, Stone PH (1989) Circadian variation and triggers of onset of acute cardiovascular disease. Circulation 79: 733–743
3. Glagov S, Weisenberg E, Zarins CK (1987) Compensatory enlargement of human atherosclerotic coronary arteries. N Engl J Med 316: 1371–1375.
4. Bom N, Lancee CT (1972) Apparatus for ultrasonically examining a hollow organ. UK Patent no.1402192.
5. Maresca D, Jansen K, Renaud G, van Soest G, Li X, et al. (2012) Intravascular ultrasound chirp imaging. Appl Phys Lett 100: 043703.
6. Stone GW, Maehara A, Lansky AJ, De Bruyne B, Cristea E, et al. (2011) A prospective natural-history study of coronary atherosclerosis. N Engl J Med 364: 226–235.
7. Davies MJ (1996) Stability and instability: Two faces of coronary atherosclerosis: The Paul Dudley White lecture 1995. Circulation 94: 2013–2020.
8. Céspedes EI, De Korte CL, Van Der Steen AFW (2000) Intraluminal ultrasonic palpation: assessment of local and cross-sectional tissue stiffness. Ultrasound Med Biol 26: 385–396.
9. Goertz DE, Frijlink ME, Tempel D, Van Damme LCA, Krams R, et al. (2006) Contrast harmonic intravascular ultrasound: A feasibility study for vasa vasorum imaging. Invest Radiol 41: 631–638.
10. Jansen K, van Soest G, van der Steen AFW (2012) Photoacoustic imaging of coronary arteries: Current status and potential clinical applications. Coronary atherosclerosis: current management and treatment. London: Informa Healthcare. 166 p.
11. Li W, Van Der Steen AFW, Lancée CT, Céspedes I, Bom N (1998) Blood flow imaging and volume flow quantitation with intravascular ultrasound. Ultrasound Med Biol 24: 203–214.
12. Carlier SG, Li W, Ignacio Céspedes E, Van der Steen AFW, Hamburger JN, et al. (1998) Simultaneous morphological and functional assessment of a renal artery stent intervention with intravascular ultrasound. Circulation 97: 2575–2576.
13. Schaar JA, De Korte CL, Mastik F, Strijder C, Pasterkamp G, et al. (2003) Characterizing Vulnerable Plaque Features with Intravascular Elastography. Circulation 108: 2636–2641.
14. Frijlink ME, Goertz DE, Van Damme LCA, Krams R, Van Der Steen AFW (2006) Intravascular ultrasound tissue harmonic imaging in vivo. IEEE Trans Ultrason Ferroelectr Freq Control 53: 1844–1851.
15. Chandrana C, Kharin N, Vince GD, Roy S, Fleischman AJ (2010) Demonstration of second-harmonic IVUS feasibility with focused broadband miniature transducers. IEEE Trans Ultrason Ferroelectr Freq Control 57: 1077–1085.
16. Maresca D, Skachkov I, Renaud G, Jansen K, van Soest G, et al. (2014) Imaging Microvasculature with Contrast-Enhanced Ultraharmonic Ultrasound. Ultrasound Med Biol. In press
17. Callon M (1987) Society in the Making: The Study of Technology as a Tool for Sociological Analysis. The social construction of technological systems: New directions in the sociology and history of technology. Boston: MIT Press. 83 p.
18. Tsai W (2001) Knowledge transfer in intraorganizational networks: Effects of network position and absorptive capacity on business unit innovation and performance. Acad Manag J 44: 996–1004.
19. Borgatti SP, Everett MG, Freeman LC (2002) Ucinet for Windows: Software for Social Network Analysis. Harvard, MA: Analytic Technologies.
20. Luce RD, Perry AD (1949) A method of matrix analysis of group structure. Psychometrika 14: 95–116.
21. Nissen SE, Gurley JC, Grines CL, Booth DC, McClure R, et al. (1991) Intravascular ultrasound assessment of lumen size and wall morphology in normal subjects and patients with coronary artery disease. Circulation 84: 1087–1099.
22. Gussenhoven EJ, Frietman PA V, The SHK, Van Suylen RJ, Van Egmond FC, et al. (1991) Assessment of medial thinning in atherosclerosis by intravascular ultrasound. Am J Cardiol 68: 1625–1632.
23. Venturini T (2010) Diving in magma: How to explore controversies with actor-network theory. Public Underst Sci 19: 258–273.
24. Kubo T, Akasaka T (2012) What is the optimal imaging tool for coronary atherosclerosis? Coronary atherosclerosis: current management and treatment. London: Informa Healthcare. 250 p.
25. Ulucanlar S, Faulkner A, Peirce S, Elwyn G (2013) Technology identity: The role of sociotechnical representations in the adoption of medical devices. Soc Sci Med 98: 95–105.
26. MacKenzie DA (1993) Inventing accuracy: A historical sociology of nuclear missile guidance. Boston: MIT press.
27. Morlacchi P, Nelson RR (2011) How medical practice evolves: Learning to treat failing hearts with an implantable device. Res Policy 40: 511–525.
28. Tonino PAL, De Bruyne B, Pijls NHJ, Siebert U, Ikeno F, et al. (2009) Fractional flow reserve versus angiography for guiding percutaneous coronary intervention. N Engl J Med 360: 213–224.

29. Li J, Li X, Mohar D, Raney A, Jing J, et al. (2014) Integrated IVUS-OCT for Real-Time Imaging of Coronary Atherosclerosis. JACC Cardiovasc Imaging 7: 101–103.

30. Madder RD, Goldstein JA, Madden SP, Puri R, Wolski K, et al. (2013) Detection by Near-Infrared Spectroscopy of Large Lipid Core Plaques at Culprit Sites in Patients With Acute ST-Segment Elevation Myocardial Infarction. JACC Cardiovasc Interv 6: 838–846.

31. Jansen K, van Soest G, van der Steen AFW (2014) Intravascular Photoacoustic Imaging: A New Tool for Vulnerable Plaque Identification. Ultrasound Med Biol. In Press.

32. Rosenberg L, Schlich T (2012) Twenty-first Century Surgery: Have we Entered Uncharted Waters? *Bull Am Coll Surg* 97: 6–11.

23

Association between Tissue Characteristics of Coronary Plaque and Distal Embolization after Coronary Intervention in Acute Coronary Syndrome Patients: Insights from a Meta-Analysis of Virtual Histology-Intravascular Ultrasound Studies

Song Ding[◊], Longwei Xu[◊], Fan Yang, Lingcong Kong, Yichao Zhao, Lingchen Gao, Wei Wang, Rende Xu, Heng Ge, Meng Jiang, Jun Pu*, Ben He*

From Department of Cardiology, Ren Ji Hospital, School of Medicine, Shanghai Jiao Tong University, Shanghai, China

Abstract

Background and Objectives: The predictive value of plaque characteristics assessed by virtual histology-intravascular ultrasound (VH-IVUS) including fibrous tissue (FT), fibrofatty (FF), necrotic core (NC) and dense calcium (DC) in identifying distal embolization after percutaneous coronary intervention (PCI) is still controversial. We performed a systematic review and meta-analysis to summarize the association of pre-PCI plaque composition and post-PCI distal embolization in acute coronary syndrome patients.

Methods: Studies were identified in PubMed, OVID, EMBASE, the Cochrane Library, the Current Controlled Trials Register, reviews, and reference lists of relevant articles. A meta-analysis using both fixed and random effects models with assessment of study heterogeneity and publication bias was performed.

Results: Of the 388 articles screened, 10 studies with a total of 872 subjects (199 with distal embolization and 673 with normal flow) met the eligibility of our study. Compared with normal flow groups, significant higher absolute volume of NC [weighted mean differences (WMD): 5.79 mm^3, 95% CI: 3.02 to 8.55 mm^3; $p<0.001$] and DC (WMD: 2.55 mm^3, 95% CI: 0.22 to 4.88 mm^3; $p=0.03$) were found in acute coronary syndrome patients with distal embolization. Further subgroup analysis demonstrated that the predictive value of tissue characteristics in determining distal embolization was correlated to clinical scenario of the patients, definition of distal embolization, and whether the percutaneous aspiration thrombectomy was applied.

Conclusion: Our study that pooled current evidence showed that plaque components were closely related to the distal embolization after PCI, especially the absolute volume of NC and DC, supporting further studies with larger sample size and high-methodological quality.

Editor: Claudio Moretti, S.G.Battista Hospital, Italy

Funding: This work was supported by the National Natural Science Foundation of China (81330006, 81170192, 81270282, 81070176, and 81400261), International Cooperation Program of Shanghai Committee of Science and Technology (12410708300), Shanghai Leading Medical Talents Program and Shanghai Leading Talents Program (LJ10007), Program for New Century Excellent Talents in University from Ministry of Education of China (NCET-12-0352), Shanghai Shuguang Program (12SG22), Key Basic Research Program of Shanghai Committee of Science and Technology (14JC1404500), and Shanghai Jiao Tong University Science and Technology Foundation (Grant No. YZ1005). The funders had no role in study design, data collection and analysis, decision to publish, or preparation of the manuscript.

Competing Interests: The authors have declared that no competing interests exist.

* Email: pujun310@hotmail.com (JP); heben1025@hotmail.com (BH)

◊ These authors contributed equally to this work.

Introduction

Rationale

Distal embolization (DE) is a common complication after percutaneous coronary intervention (PCI), particularly in the setting of acute coronary syndrome (ACS) or vein graft intervention, which may result in microvascular obstruction and no-reflow phenomenon [1,2]. This undesirable side effect of PCI has been confirmed to be associated with increased post-procedural myocardial infarction, in-hospital mortality, and long-term adverse events [3–5]. However, there is no effective strategy for prediction and prevention of DE, which is an important issue for interventional cardiology.

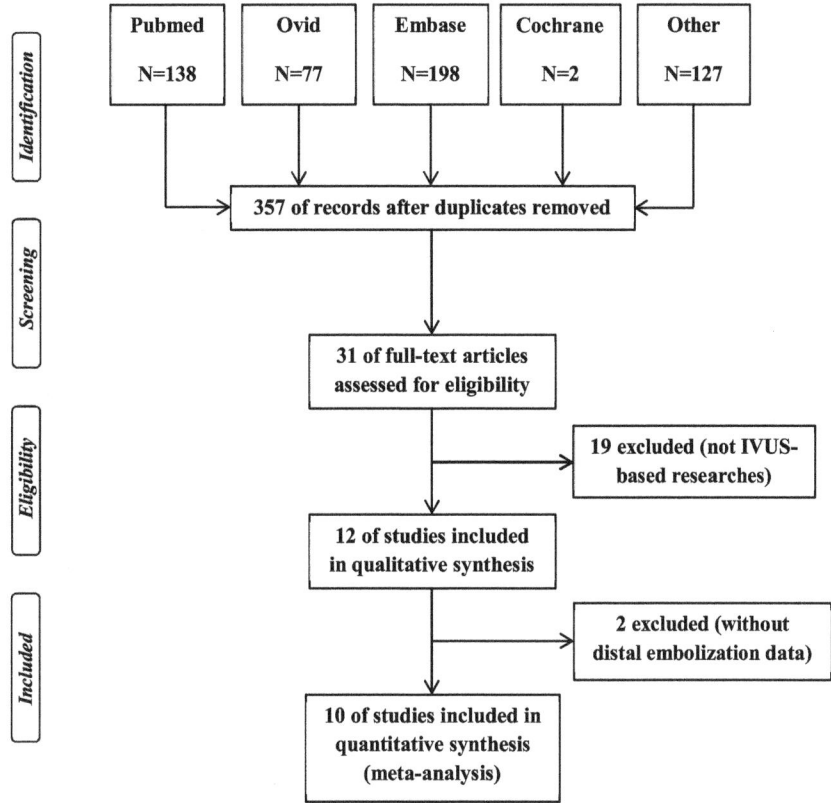

Figure 1. Process of study selection.

Although several studies using grayscale intravascular ultrasound (IVUS) have indicated that plaque characteristics identified by pre-interventional IVUS (i.e., a large plaque burden, a lipid-pool-like image, and positive remodeling) maybe associated with the angiographic no-reflow phenomenon in ACS patients [6–10], gray-scale IVUS is dependent on the simple interpretation of acoustic reflections and of limited value for identifying specific plaque components [11]. Recently, some new methods able to assess both plaque morphology and tissue characteristics, such as virtual histology-IVUS (VH-IVUS), have become clinically available. VH-IVUS is based on spectral and amplitude analysis of IVUS backscattered radiofrequency that allows for characterization of in-vivo atherosclerotic plaque into four types: fibrous (FT), fibrofatty (FF), necrotic core (NC), and dense calcium (DC) [12–23]. However, whether pre-PCI plaque characteristics of culprit lesion assessed by VH-IVUS could predict post-PCI angiographic DE, and which plaque components are associated with no-reflow phenomenon remain debated. We therefore performed a systematic review that pooled current evidence to investigate the relationship between pre-PCI plaque composition characteristics assessed by VH-IVUS and post-PCI DE phenomenon in ACS patients.

Methods

Search strategy

PubMed, Ovid, EMBASE, and the Cochrane Library databases were searched in their entirety from January 2002 to April 2013. Complex search strategies were formulated using the following MESH terms and text words: intravascular ultrasound, virtual

histology, IVUS, VH-IVUS, plaque component, plaque composition, plaque characteristic, no reflow, DE, microembolization, and obstruction. In order to identify any studies missed by the literature searches, we had searched reference lists of all eligible studies and relevant review articles. In addition, we searched from published and ongoing trials in clinical trial registries (Clinical-Trials.gov, Controlled-trials.com and the WHO International Clinical Trials Registry Platform). Searches were not restricted by language, time published, or publication status. Duplicate reports were eliminated (Appendix S1).

Study selection

We included studies when the following criteria were met:(1) Plaque characteristics were assessed by VH-IVUS; (2) VH-IVUS was performed before coronary intervention in ACS patients; and (3) DE was defined according to angiographic evidence or clinical relevancy. Studies without normal flow (NF) group were excluded from our analysis.

Data extraction

Two reviewers (D. S. and P. J.) assessed the eligibility of studies using a standardized form developed for this purpose in duplicate and independently. Disagreements were adjudicated by resolved by consensus. Data extraction was completed by the same observers using a standardized data extraction form developed for this study. The following information was extracted from each study: sample size, mean age, gender distribution, risk factors, clinical scenario, definition of DE, and the volume (mm³)and percentage of each tissue component of plaque (including FT, FF, NC, and DC). Several studies met our inclusion criteria but were

Table 1. Basical characteristics of studies included in meta-analysis (Normal flow vs. distal embolization).

Study	Study interval	Location	Sample size (n)	Design	Clinical scenario	PAT	Definition of distal embolization
Bae 2008	NR	Daejeon, South Korea	45/12	RSC	AMI	Yes	TIMI flow grade ≤2
Higashikuni 2008	2005.6-2006.4	Tokyo, Japan	40/9	RSC	ACS (AMI and UA)	Yes	Decrease of at least 1 grade in TIMI
Hong 2009	NR	Washington DC, United States	42/38	RSC	UA	No	cTnI elevation >3X the ULN
Hong 2011	2006.2-2008.1	Gwangju, South Korea	166/24	RSC	ACS (STEMI, NSTEMI and UA)	No	TIMI flow grade ≤2
Kawaguchi 2007	2005.8-2006.12	Gunma, Japan	60/11	PSC	AMI (STEMI)	Yes	ST-segment re-elevation
Nakamura 2007	2006.1-2006.3	Saitama, Japan	42/8	PSC	AMI (STEMI)	Yes	Decrease in TIMI flow grade
Ohshima 2009	2007.1-2007.12	Ehime, Japan	24/20	PSC	AMI (STEMI)	Yes	TIMI flow grade ≤2
Ohshima 2011	NR	Ehime, Japan	19/34	RSC	AMI (STEMI)	Yes	TIMI flow grade ≤2
Shin 2011	NR	Ulsan, South Korea	90/22	RSC	UA	No	CK-MB elevation >1X the ULN
Zhao 2013	2010.9-2011.11	Zhengzhou, China	145/21	RSC	UA	Yes	TIMI flow grade ≤2

ACS, acute coronary injury; AMI, acute myocardial infarction; NR, not reported; NSTEMI, non ST-segment elevation myocardial infarction; PAT, percutaneous aspiration thrombectomy; PSC, prospective single center; RSC, retrospective single center; STEMI, ST-segment elevation myocardial infarction; ULN, upper limit of normal.

Table 2. Clinical characteristics of studies included in meta-analysis (Normal flow vs. distal embolization).

Study	Mean age (years)	Males (%)	Comorbidities			Pre-PCI use of Aspirin (%)	Use of Statins	Use of GP IIb/IIIa inhibitor	Use of Statins	Use of distal protectiondevices
			HT (%)	DM (%)	HL (%)					
Bae 2008	56.2/67.5	82.2/66.7	40.0/33.3	13.3/33.3	31.1/25.0	100/100	NR	0/0	NR	No
Higashikuni 2008	66.6/60.6	92.5/77.8	70.0/55.6	30.0/55.6	65.0/8	30.0/44.4	22.5/22.2	0/0	22.5/22.2	No
Hong 2009	65/63	47.6/76.3	64.3/73.7	23.8/31.6	NR	92.9/86.8	NR	14.3/10.5	NR	No
Hong 2011	60.5/60.1	65.7/58.3	52.4/70.8	19.3/25	NR	NR	NR	23.5/29.2	NR	NR
Kawaguchi 2007	NR	NR	68.3/81.8	41.7/9.1	45.0/81.8	NR	NR	0/0	NR	No
Nakamura 2007	65.3/58.5	85.7/87.5	42.9/25.0	23.8/37.5	61.9/62.5	100/100	NR	0/0	NR	No
Ohshima 2009	66.0/74.0	83.3/65.0	58.3/75.0	54.2/60.0	62.5/45.0	100/100	NR	NR	NR	No
Ohshima 2011	73/67	68.4/85.3	78.9/70.6	26.3/38.2	47.4/61.8	100/100	NR	NR	NR	No
Shin 2011	61.4/65.5	61.1/50.0	51.1/72.7	32.2/22.7	53.3/63.6	100/100	21.1/27.3	0/0	21.1/27.3	No
Zhao 2013	51/49	66.2/66.6	59.3/61.9	26.9/47.6	NR	100/100	98.6/95.2	NR	98.6/95.2	No

DM, diabetes mellitus; HT, hypertension; HL, hyperlipidaemia; NR, not reported;

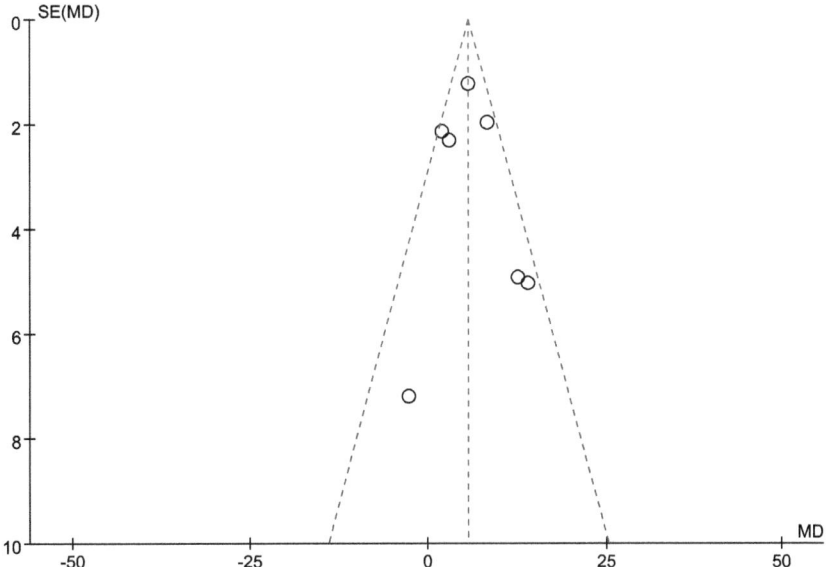

Figure 2. Funnel plot for necrotic core volume outcome data of involved studies.

missing data vital to our analysis; in these cases, we contacted the authors to obtain raw data whenever possible.

Statistical analysis

Statistical analysis in this study was carried out using RevMan software version 5.2 (The Cochrane Collaboration). Results were summarized as weighted mean differences (WMD) with their associated 95% confidence intervals (CI) using both fixed and random effects models, the latter was more conservative where heterogeneity beyond that expected by chance alone was encountered. In addition, the odds ratio (OR) was calculated for baseline comorbidities. Heterogeneity between studies was analyzed by the Q statistic and the I^2 statistic. A p value of the Q statistic <0.1 was defined as an indicator of heterogeneity, and an I^2 <50% indicated that the magnitude of the heterogeneity might not be significant. Funnel plots were plotted to investigate possible small study effects/publication bias by using Revman 5.2. Planned subgroup analyses were conducted based on the clinical scenario, definition of DE, and whether percutaneous aspiration thrombectomy was applied.

Quality assessment

Methodological quality was assessed independently by 2 reviewers (D. S. and P. J.) using the Newcastle-Ottawa Scale.

Results

Search result

After initial literature search, we identified 388 potential studies, of which 357 studies were excluded based on the title and abstracts, because they were unrelated papers, reviews, editorials, letters, case reports or animal studies. The remaining 31 articles were considered of interest and examined in full-text. Of these, 19 studies those were not IVUS-based were excluded. Of the remainder, 2 studies without DE data were excluded [12,13]. Therefore, 10 observational studies were included in our final meta-analysis [14–23]. Figure 1 shows the study selection process.

Characteristics of included studies

Table 1 and 2 summarize the main features of the included studies. A total of 872 patients (199 patients in DE group and 673 patients in NF group) were enrolled in the 10 studies, and the sample sizes were 44–190 in each study. Among the included studies, 5 studies involved AMI patients [14,18–21] (4 of them only involved STEMI patients), 3 studies enrolled unstable angina (UA) patients [16,22,23], and the remaining 2 studies involved ACS (including both AMI and UA) patients [15,17]. Percutaneous aspiration thrombectomy was performed before IVUS examinations in 7 studies [14,15,18–21,23]. There were no significant differences between DE and NF groups in age and gender of patients. Moreover, there was no significant difference in the incidence of hypertension (OR: 1.36, 95% CI: 0.95 to 1.95, $p = 0.10$), diabetes (OR: 1.36, 95% CI: 0.94 to 1.96, $p = 0.10$) and hyperlipidaemia (OR: 1.44, 95% CI: 0.89 to 2.31, $p = 0.13$) between the two groups. A Funnel plot for NC volume outcome data was used to assess any potential small study effects or publication bias (Figure 2). The Funnel plot was roughly symmetrical as to the mean-effect size line.

Moreover, we evaluated the quality of primary studies using the Newcastle–Ottawa Scale, a validated technique for assessing the quality of observational and non randomized studies. As shown in Table 3, all observational studies were intermediate to low intermediate bias risk as assessed by the Newcastle-Ottawa Scale for quality assessment risk evaluation of adequacy of selection, comparability of study groups, and assessment of outcome or exposure.

Relationship between coronary plaque characteristics and DE

As shown in Table 4, Figure 3 and 4, the absolute volume and percentage of four different plaque compositions through the entire culprit lesion were assessed. Compared with NF group, the overall pooled results with random-effects analysis showed DE group had significant higher absolute volume of NC (WMD: 5.79 mm³, 95% CI: 3.02 to 8.55 mm³; $p<0.001$) and DC (WMD:

Table 3. Newcastle-Ottawa Scale of bias risk for the involved studies.

Study	Adequacy of selection			Comparability	Outcomes assessment		
	Representativeness of the exposed cohort	Selection of the non-exposed cohort	Ascertainment of exposure		Assessment of Outcomes	Follow-up period long enough for outcome to occur	Adequacy of follow-up period among cohorts
Bae 2008	**	**	***	***	**	**	**
Higashikuni 2008	**	**	***	***	***	**	**
Hong 2009	**	**	**	***	**	**	**
Hong 2011	**	**	***	***	**	**	**
Kawaguchi 2007	**	**	**	**	**	**	**
Nakamura 2007	**	**	***	***	***	**	**
Ohshima 2009	**	**	***	***	**	**	**
Ohshima 2011	**	**	***	***	***	**	**
Shin 2011	**	**	**	**	**	**	**
Zhao 2013	**	**	***	**	**	**	**

Asterisks are the star rating as per the Newcastle-Ottawa Scale; ** and *** indicate highest rating for these categories.

2.55 mm^3, 95% CI: 0.22 to 4.88 mm^3; $p = 0.03$). The difference between the two groups was not statistically significant with respect to percentage of NC (WMD: 4.35%, 95% CI: -1.44% to 10.15%; $p = 0.14$) and DC (WMD: 0.81%, 95% CI: -1.20% to 2.82%; $p = 0.43$). In addition, there were no significant differences in absolute volume and percentage of FT and FF at the entire culprit lesions between the two groups. Substantial statistical heterogeneity was detected in all of the comparisons among these trials, except for the absolute volume of FT ($I^2 = 0$%).

Subgroup analysis

Planned subgroup analyses were conducted based on the different clinical scenario, definition of DE, and whether percutaneous aspiration thrombectomy was applied (Table 5 and 6). Subgroup analysis by different clinical scenario showed that patients with DE had significantly higher absolute volume and percentage of NC (WMD: 6.61 mm^3, 95% CI: 4.11 to 9.12 mm^3; p<0.001 and WMD: 8.64%, 95% CI: 5.29% to 11.99%; p< 0.001) in subgroup of UA patients.

In order to assess the impact of the definition of DE in determining DE on our analyses, subgroup analysis by angiographic or clinical relevance definition was performed. The results showed that there was significantly higher absolute volume of NC (WMD: 7.13 mm3, 95% CI: 4.40 to 9.87 mm3; p = 0.04) in subgroup of DE in clinical relevance definition.

In order to investigate whether percutaneous aspiration thrombectomy would affect the outcomes, trials were divided into two subgroups according to whether thrombectomy was applied. The results showed that in the subgroup without thrombectomy, patients with DE had significantly higher absolute volume and percentage of NC (WMD: 7.47 mm3, 95% CI: 4.25 to 10.69 mm3; p<0.001 and WMD: -7.45%, 95% CI: 4.38% to 10.53%; p<0.001), and significantly lower absolute volume of FF (WMD: -7.38 mm3, 95% CI: -9.86 to -4.90 mm3; p<0.001).

Discussion

The present meta-analysis that pooled all currently available published data indicated that, among four phenotypes of coronary plaque composition assessed by VH-IVUS, absolute volume of NC components was closely related to the DE after PCI in ACS patients. Besides, absolute volume of DC component might also be related to the DE after PCI. Further subgroup analysis revealed that the predictive value of VH-IVUS plaque characteristics in determining DE was correlated to the clinical scenario of the patients, the definition of DE, and whether percutaneous aspiration thrombectomy was applied.

Two recent review/meta-analyses [24,25] that investigated the relationship between plaque characteristics and DE after PCI have also reported that the extent of NC was larger in patients with DE. The meta-analysis by Jang et al. [24] evaluated the effect of plaque characteristics on embolization after PCI by grayscale-IVUS and VH-IVUS, and found that the morphologic characteristics of plaque derived from grayscale-IVUS (i.e.,eccentric plaque, ruptured plaque, and attenuated plaque) and the NC component derived from VH-IVUS are closely related to the DE phenomenon after PCI. The systematic review by Claessen et al. [25] summarized the published data on the use of plaque composition assessment by VH-IVUS to predict the occurrence of DE, and found that the NC component was associated with DE in all but 2 of the 11 reviewed studies. In the present study, we performed a systematic review that pooled all the currently available published data investigating the relationship between pre-PCI plaque composition characteristics assessed by VH-IVUS and post-PCI

Table 4. Composition of plaque by VH-IVUS.

Study		Absolute volume (mm³)				Percentage (%)			
		FT	FF	DC	NC	FT	FF	DC	NC
Bae 2008	Reflow	83.8 (66.8)	18.0 (18.6)	12.7 (13.9)	28.8 (26.0)	NR	NR	NR	NR
	No reflow	119.6 (61.7)	36.7 (25.5)	9.3 (8.9)	26.1 (21.0)	NR	NR	NR	NR
Higashikuni 2008	Reflow	NR	NR	NR	NR	68.3 (10.2)	15.5 (7.1)	4.8 (3.6)	11.7 (7.9)
	No reflow	NR	NR	NR	NR	59.6 (11.2)	12.0 (9.7)	4.7 (3.3)	22.1 (9.3)
Hong 2009	Reflow	33.9(14.2)	16.9(11.6)	3.2(3.0)	7.9(4.4)	55.0(11.6)	27.5(13.0)	4.8(3.4)	12.8(8.4)
	No reflow	38.4(19.0)	13.1(9.9)	3.8(3.0)	13.6(6.4)	55.7(13.1)	19.0(9.3)	5.5(3.9)	19.8(10.4)
Hong 2011	Reflow	77 (75.4)	20 (25.4)	10 (11.5)	16 (16.9)	61 (9.9)	16 (9.9)	9 (6.8)	14 (8.0)
	No reflow	76 (50.0)	15 (18.5)	19 (20.0)	30 (23.8)	55 (14.0)	9 (6.1)	14 (8.0)	22 (11.0)
Kawaguchi 2007	Reflow	68.2 (35.3)	13.2 (11.4)	9.6 (13.9)	20.4 (19.2)	NR	NR	NR	NR
	No reflow	67.1 (30.7)	9.8 (10.4)	12.2 (8.6)	32.9 (14.1)	NR	NR	NR	NR
Nakamura 2007	Reflow	NR	NR	NR	NR	67.0 (1.5)	17.0 (1.1)	4.8 (0.6)	11.2 (1.2)
	No reflow	NR	NR	NR	NR	68.3 (2.1)	23.1 (3.5)	2.6 (0.6)	6.3 (1.0)
Ohshima 2009	Reflow	56.6 (21.8)	8.6 (5.2)	6.5 (5.3)	12.0 (7.4)	67.8 (10.2)	10.1 (3.9)	7.8 (5.2)	14.3 (6.7)
	No reflow	56.2 (32.6)	14.2 (11.4)	10.3 (7.6)	14.1 (6.7)	57.5 (10.7)	14.5 (9.6)	11.8 (8.9)	15.8 (7.4)
Ohshima 2011	Reflow	57.0 (33.3)	14.7 (11.5)	9.3 (6.0)	13.7 (6.7)	57.5 (11.0)	14.8 (9.7)	11.3 (9.0)	15.8 (7.6)
	No reflow	67.5 (29.7)	15.0 (11.7)	11.0 (8.8)	16.8 (10.0)	61.2 (10.8)	13.4 (8.1)	10.2 (7.2)	15.3 (6.0)
Shin 2011	Reflow	NR	NR	3.9 (3.7)	8.8 (5.8)	NR	NR	NR	NR
	No reflow	NR	NR	9.1 (5.8)	17.2 (8.8)	NR	NR	NR	NR
Zhao 2013	Reflow	NR	NR	NR	NR	59.24 (6.72)	17.90 (3.21)	8.36 (3.13)	14.50 (5.48)
	No reflow	NR	NR	NR	NR	50.26 (8.72)	15.29 (2.83)	9.53 (2.99)	24.92 (10.04)

Data are presented as mean (SD)
FT, fibrous tissue; FF, fibrofatty; NC, necrotic core; DC, dense calcium.

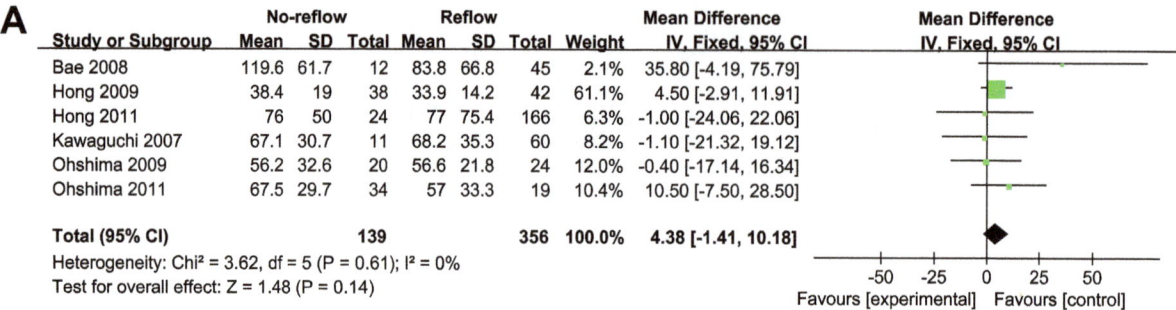

Figure 3. Absolute volume comparison of four different plaque compositions through the entire culprit lesion between the normal flow group and the distal embolization group. (A) Absolute fibrous volume comparison; (B) Absolute fibrofatty volume comparison; (C) Absolute dense calcium volume comparison; (D) Absolute necrotic core volume comparison;

DE phenomenon in ACS patients, and we updated the meta-analysis by adding two VH-IVUS studies [22,23] that did not include in the previous meta-analysis by Jang et al. [24]. We found that absolute volume of NC component, but not percentage of NC component, was closely related to the DE after PCI in ACS patients, confirming the findings of previous review/meta-analyses. In addition, our analysis that pooled all current evidence found

that besides NC volume, absolute DC volume was also closely related to the DE phenomenon after PCI. There is some evidence which indicated that DC might be related to DE. For example, pathologic studies revealed that coronary calcification is related to the total plaque burden, NC component, plaque erosion or rupture that is responsible for coronary thrombosis [26–29]. In addition, some studies have also reported that coronary calcium

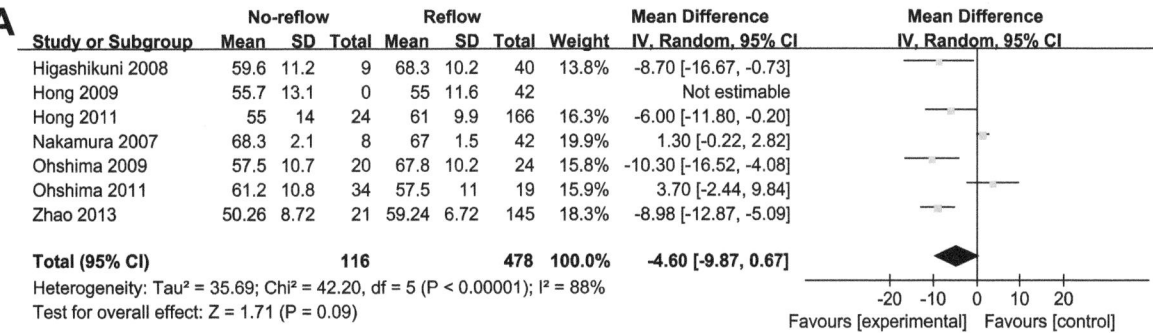

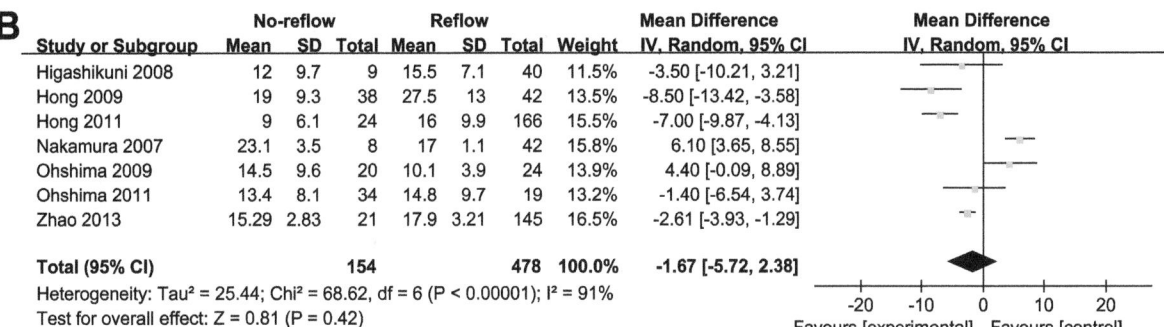

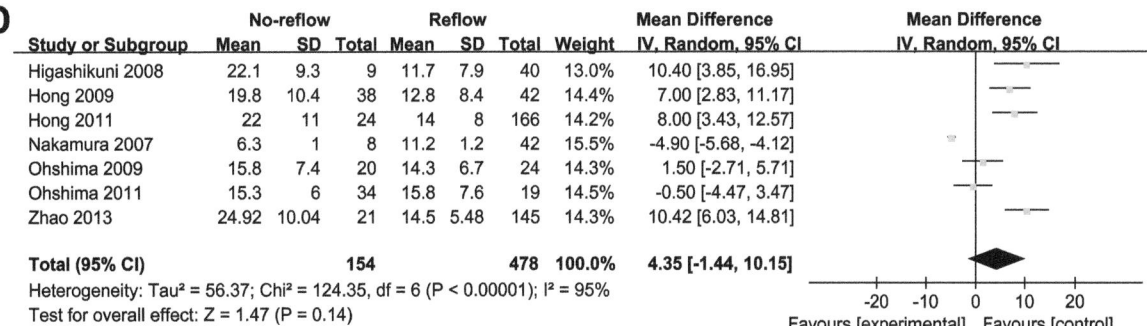

Figure 4. Percentage comparison of four different plaque compositions through the entire culprit lesion between the normal flow group and the distal embolization group. (A) Fibrous percentage comparison; (B) Fibrofatty percentage comparison; (C) Dense calcium percentage comparison; (D) Necrotic core percentage comparison.

was associated with coronary event including myocardial infarction or death in symptomatic/asymptomatic persons [30–33].

In our analysis, we noted a considerable degree of heterogeneity among the included trials. Thus, we performed further subgroup analyses and tried to appraise the possible sources of differences and heterogeneity among trials. Our results suggested that the

clinical scenario of the patients, the definition of DE and the use of thrombectomy may influence the correlation between tissue characteristics of coronary plaque and DE. When analyzed in the context of clinical scenario, increased absolute volume of NC was found in DE group in studies including UA patients, but not in those including AMI patients. This phenomenon might be

Table 5. Subgroup analyses of the association of the absolute volume of plaque components with the onset of distal embolization.

Subgroup	FT WMD (95% CI, mm³)	p	FF WMD (95% CI, mm³)	p	DC WMD (95% CI, mm³)	p	NC WMD (95% CI, mm³)	p
Clinical scenario								
AMI	5.21 (−4.93, 15.35)	0.31	3.17 (−3.25, 9.59)	0.33	1.81 (−0.81, 4.44)	0.18	3.56 (−0.37, 7.50)	0.08
Unstable angina	4.50 (−2.91, 11.91)	0.23	−3.80 (−8.51, 0.91)	0.11	2.77 (−1.73, 7.27)	0.23	6.61 (4.11, 9.12)	<0.001
Definition of distal embolization								
Angiographic evidence	5.62 (−4.83, 16.07)	0.29	3.11 (−3.77, 10.00)	0.38	2.44 (−1.34, 6.22)	0.21	3.88 (−0.62, 8.38)	0.09
Clinical relevancy	3.84 (−3.12, 10.80)	0.28	−3.67 (−7.54, 0.20)	0.06	2.71 (−0.88, 6.29)	0.14	7.13 (4.40, 9.87)	<0.001
Thrombectomy								
With thrombectomy	−4.36 (−10.42, 1.71)	0.16	0.80 (−3.89, 5.49)	0.74	0.06 (−2.17, 2.30)	0.96	3.56 (−0.37, 7.50)	0.08
Without thrombectomy	−2.57 (−9.14, 3.99)	0.44	−7.38 (−9.86, −4.90)	<0.001	2.59 (−1.60, 6.77)	0.23	7.47 (4.25, 10.69)	<0.001

FT, fibrous tissue; FF, fibrofatty; NC, necrotic core; DC, dense calcium; WMD, weighted mean differences; AMI, acute myocardial infarction.

Table 6. Subgroup analyses of the association of the percentage of plaque components with the onset of distal embolization.

Subgroup	FT WMD (95% CI, %)	p	FF WMD (95% CI, %)	p	DC WMD (95% CI, %)	p	NC WMD (95% CI, %)	p
Clinical scenario								
AMI	−1.48 (−8.40, 5.44)	0.68	3.49 (−0.68, 7.66)	0.10	−0.18 (−3.89, 3.53)	0.92	−1.67 (−6.04, 2.70)	0.45
Unstable angina	−4.34 (−13.81, 5.14)	0.37	−5.06 (−10.75, 0.63)	0.08	0.97 (−0.07, 2.02)	0.07	8.64 (5.29, 11.99)	<0.001
Definition of distal embolization								
Angiographic evidence	−4.60 (−9.87, 0.67)	0.09	−0.61 (−4.91, 3.70)	0.78	0.87 (−1.49, 3.24)	0.47	3.91 (−2.30, 10.11)	0.22
Clinical relevancy	0.70 (−4.75, 6.15)	0.80	−8.50 (−13.42, −3.58)	<0.001	0.70 (−0.91, 2.31)	0.39	7.00 (2.83, 11.17)	0.001
Thrombectomy								
With thrombectomy	5.21 (−4.93, 15.35)	0.31	3.17 (−3.25, 9.59)	0.33	1.81 (−0.81, 4.44)	0.18	3.07 (−3.45, 9.59)	0.36
Without thrombectomy	3.98 (−3.07, 11.04)	0.27	−4.09 (−8.19, 0.01)	0.05	3.85 (−0.46, 8.17)	0.08	7.45 (4.38, 10.53)	<0.001

FT, fibrous tissue; FF, fibrofatty; NC, necrotic core; DC, dense calcium; WMD, weighted mean differences; AMI, acute myocardial infarction.

explained by the rupture and migration of NC plaque in AMI patients. In addition, VH-IVUS is limited to detecting thrombus (in fact, thrombus appears as either fibrotic or fibrofatty plaque depending on the age of the thrombus) [34]. Moreover, large amount of NC may have migrated into the distal coronary bed before or during primary PCI in AMI patients [14]. An unexpected finding in our analysis was that no association was found between plaque components and DE in the subgroup of angiographically defined DE. Although angiography has been commonly used as a gold standard for assessing DE, TIMI flow grade is a subjective method to assess epicardial blood flow. As suggested by published literatures, the qualitative nature of TIMI grade renders it somewhat dependent on the technical skill of the observer, and significant differences were found in inter-observer variabilities among different reports, particularly for TIMI 2 grade (Kappa value was 0.4963 for inter-observer variability), which may introduce selection bias in the enrollment of the participants [35,36].

In addition, our results indicated that pre-stent percutaneous aspiration thrombectomy may also be a important factor in determining the predictive value of VH-IVUS-derived plaque characteristics.

Study limitations

Several important limitations of our study should be taken into account, in order to place our findings in the proper context. Firstly, as mentioned above, there was considerable heterogeneity in patient characteristics, use of pre-stent thrombectomy, and definitions of DE among the included trials. Secondly, although the consensus document recommends measurement of the absolute and relative components of each plaque at the minimum

lumen site and over the whole lesion, these measurements were not usually reported uniformly in the individual studies involved in our study. Thirdly, although our pooled analysis found that besides NC volume, absolute DC volume was also closely related to the DE phenomenon after PCI, more evidence should be obtained to confirm this finding because only two of the studies included in our meta-analysis reported statistically significant association between DC component and post-PCI DE. Finally, all of the involved trials were non-randomized studies and of small sample sizes, which might have brought some bias. Therefore further studies with larger sample size and high-methodological quality are needed.

Acknowledgments

The authors gratefully acknowledge the authors of the original studies.

Author Contributions

Conceived and designed the experiments: SD LX RX JP BH. Performed the experiments: SD LX RX JP BH. Analyzed the data: SD LX FY LK YZ LG WW RX. Contributed reagents/materials/analysis tools: SD LX HG MJ JP BH. Wrote the paper: SD LX RX LK JP BH.

References

1. Morishima I, Sone T, Okumura K, Tsuboi H, Kondo J, et al. (2000) Angiographic no-reflow phenomenon as a predictor of adverse long-term outcome in patients treated with percutaneous transluminal coronary angioplasty for first acute myocardial infarction. J Am Coll Cardiol 36: 1202–1209.
2. Grines CL, Cox DA, Stone GW, Garcia E, Mattos LA, et al. (1999) Coronary angioplasty with or without stent implantation for acute myocardial infarction. Stent Primary Angioplasty in Myocardial Infarction Study Group. N Engl J Med 341: 1949–1956.
3. Pu J, Shan P, Ding S, Qiao Z, Jiang L, et al. (2011) Gender differences in epicardial and tissue-level reperfusion in patients undergoing primary angioplasty for acute myocardial infarction. Atherosclerosis 215: 203–208.
4. Cura FA, L'Allier PL, Kapadia SR, Houghtaling PL, Dipaola LM, et al. (2001) Predictors and prognosis of suboptimal coronary blood flow after primary coronary angioplasty in patients with acute myocardial infarction. Am J Cardiol 88: 124–128.
5. Ding S, Pu J, Qiao ZQ, Shan P, Song W, et al. (2010) TIMI myocardial perfusion frame count: a new method to assess myocardial perfusion and its predictive value for short-term prognosis. Catheter Cardiovasc Interv 75: 722–732.
6. Iijima R, Shinji H, Ikeda N, Itaya H, Makino K, et al. (2006) Comparison of coronary arterial finding by intravascular ultrasound in patients with "transient no-reflow" versus "reflow" during percutaneous coronary intervention in acute coronary syndrome. Am J Cardiol 97: 29–33.
7. Ohshima K, Ikeda S, Kadota H, Yamane K, Izumi N, et al. (2013) Impact of culprit plaque volume and composition on myocardial microcirculation following primary angioplasty in patients with ST-segment elevation myocardial infarction: virtual histology intravascular ultrasound analysis. Int J Cardiol 167: 1000–1005.
8. Kusama I, Hibi K, Kosuge M, Nozawa N, Ozaki H, et al. (2007) Impact of plaque rupture on infarct size in ST-segment elevation anterior acute myocardial infarction. J Am Coll Cardiol 50: 1230–1237.
9. Tanaka A, Kawarabayashi T, Nishibori Y, Sano T, Nishida Y, et al. (2002) No-reflow phenomenon and lesion morphology in patients with acute myocardial infarction. Circulation 105: 2148–2152.
10. Katayama T, Kubo N, Takagi Y, Funayama H, Ikeda N, et al. (2006) Relation of atherothrombosis burden and volume detected by intravascular ultrasound to angiographic no-reflow phenomenon during stent implantation in patients with acute myocardial infarction. Am J Cardiol 97: 301–304.
11. Pu J, Mintz GS, Brilakis ES, Banerjee S, Abdel-Karim AR, et al. (2012) In vivo characterization of coronary plaques: novel findings from comparing greyscale

and virtual histology intravascular ultrasound and near-infrared spectroscopy. Eur Heart J 33: 372–383.
12. Bose D, von Birgelen C, Zhou XY, Schmermund A, Philipp S, et al. (2008) Impact of atherosclerotic plaque composition on coronary microembolization during percutaneous coronary interventions. Basic Res Cardiol 103: 587–597.
13. Yamada R, Okura H, Kume T, Neishi Y, Kawamoto T, et al. (2010) Target lesion thin-cap fibroatheroma defined by virtual histology intravascular ultrasound affects microvascular injury during percutaneous coronary intervention in patients with angina pectoris. Circ J 74: 1658–1662.
14. Bae JH, Kwon TG, Hyun DW, Rihal CS, Lerman A (2008) Predictors of slow flow during primary percutaneous coronary intervention: an intravascular ultrasound-virtual histology study. Heart 94: 1559–1564.
15. Higashikuni Y, Tanabe K, Tanimoto S, Aoki J, Yamamoto H, et al. (2008) Impact of culprit plaque composition on the no-reflow phenomenon in patients with acute coronary syndrome: an intravascular ultrasound radiofrequency analysis. Circ J 72: 1235–1241.
16. Hong YJ, Mintz GS, Kim SW, Lee SY, Okabe T, et al. (2009) Impact of plaque composition on cardiac troponin elevation after percutaneous coronary intervention: an ultrasound analysis. JACC Cardiovasc Imaging 2: 458–468.
17. Hong YJ, Jeong MH, Choi YH, Ko JS, Lee MG, et al. (2011) Impact of plaque components on no-reflow phenomenon after stent deployment in patients with acute coronary syndrome: a virtual histology-intravascular ultrasound analysis. Eur Heart J 32: 2059–2066.
18. Kawaguchi R, Oshima S, Jingu M, Tsurugaya H, Toyama T, et al. (2007) Usefulness of virtual histology intravascular ultrasound to predict distal embolization for ST-segment elevation myocardial infarction. J Am Coll Cardiol 50: 1641–1646.
19. Nakamura T, Kubo N, Ako J, Momomura S (2007) Angiographic no-reflow phenomenon and plaque characteristics by virtual histology intravascular ultrasound in patients with acute myocardial infarction. J Interv Cardiol 20: 335–339.
20. Ohshima K, Ikeda S, Watanabe K, Yamane K, Izumi N, et al. (2009) Relationship between plaque composition and no-reflow phenomenon following primary angioplasty in patients with ST-segment elevation myocardial infarction—analysis with virtual histology intravascular ultrasound. J Cardiol 54: 205–213.
21. Ohshima K, Ikeda S, Kadota H, Yamane K, Izumi N, et al. (2011) Cavity volume of ruptured plaque is an independent predictor for angiographic no-reflow phenomenon during primary angioplasty in patients with ST-segment elevation myocardial infarction. J Cardiol 57: 36–43.

22. Shin ES, Garcia-Garcia HM, Garg S, Park J, Kim SJ, et al. (2011) The assessment of Shin's method for the prediction of creatinine kinase-MB elevation after percutaneous coronary intervention: an intravascular ultrasound study. Int J Cardiovasc Imaging 27: 883–892.

23. Zhao XY, Wang XF, Li L, Zhang JY, Du YY, et al. (2013) Plaque characteristics and serum pregnancy-associated plasma protein A levels predict the no-reflow phenomenon after percutaneous coronary intervention. J Int Med Res 41: 307–316.

24. Jang JS, Jin HY, Seo JS, Yang TH, Kim DK, et al. (2013) Meta-analysis of plaque composition by intravascular ultrasound and its relation to distal embolization after percutaneous coronary intervention. Am J Cardiol 111: 968–972.

25. Claessen BE, Maehara A, Fahy M, Xu K, Stone GW, et al. (2012) Plaque composition by intravascular ultrasound and distal embolization after percutaneous coronary intervention. JACC Cardiovasc Imaging 5: S111–118.

26. Taylor AJ, Burke AP, O'Malley PG, Farb A, Malcom GT, et al. (2000) A comparison of the Framingham risk index, coronary artery calcification, and culprit plaque morphology in sudden cardiac death. Circulation 101: 1243–1248.

27. Pu J, Mintz GS, Biro S, Lee JB, Sum ST, et al. (2014) Insights into echo-attenuated plaques, echolucent plaques, and plaques with spotty calcification: novel findings from comparisons among intravascular ultrasound, near-infrared spectroscopy, and pathological histology in 2,294 human coronary artery segments. J Am Coll Cardiol 63: 2220–2233.

28. Schmermund A, Schwartz RS, Adamzik M, Sangiorgi G, Pfeifer EA, et al. (2001) Coronary atherosclerosis in unheralded sudden coronary death under age 50: histo-pathologic comparison with 'healthy' subjects dying out of hospital. Atherosclerosis 155: 499–508.

29. Virmani R, Kolodgie FD, Burke AP, Farb A, Schwartz SM (2000) Lessons from sudden coronary death: a comprehensive morphological classification scheme for atherosclerotic lesions. Arterioscler Thromb Vasc Biol 20: 1262–1275.

30. Keelan PC, Bielak LF, Ashai K, Jamjoum LS, Denktas AE, et al. (2001) Long-term prognostic value of coronary calcification detected by electron-beam computed tomography in patients undergoing coronary angiography. Circulation 104: 412–417.

31. Shaw LJ, Raggi P, Schisterman E, Berman DS, Callister TQ (2003) Prognostic value of cardiac risk factors and coronary artery calcium screening for all-cause mortality. Radiology 228: 826–833.

32. Detrano R, Hsiai T, Wang S, Puentes G, Fallavollita J, et al. (1996) Prognostic value of coronary calcification and angiographic stenoses in patients undergoing coronary angiography. J Am Coll Cardiol 27: 285–290.

33. Raggi P, Cooil B, Shaw LJ, Aboulhson J, Takasu J, et al. (2003) Progression of coronary calcium on serial electron beam tomographic scanning is greater in patients with future myocardial infarction. Am J Cardiol 92: 827–829.

34. Maehara A, Mintz GS, Weissman NJ. (2009) Advances in intravascular imaging. Circ Cardiovasc Interv 2: 482–490.

35. Steigen TK, Claudio C, Abbott D, Schulzer M, Burton J, et al. (2008) Angiographic core laboratory reproducibility analyses: implications for planning clinical trials using coronary angiography and left ventriculography end-points. Int J Cardiovasc Imaging 24: 453–462.

36. Gibson CM, Cannon CP, Daley WL, Dodge JT, Jr., Alexander B, Jr., et al. (1996) TIMI frame count: a quantitative method of assessing coronary artery flow. Circulation 93: 879–888.

Permissions

The contributors of this book come from diverse backgrounds, making this book a truly international effort. This book will bring forth new frontiers with its revolutionizing research information and detailed analysis of the nascent developments around the world.

We would like to thank all the contributing authors for lending their expertise to make the book truly unique. They have played a crucial role in the development of this book. Without their invaluable contributions this book wouldn't have been possible. They have made vital efforts to compile up to date information on the varied aspects of this subject to make this book a valuable addition to the collection of many professionals and students.

This book was conceptualized with the vision of imparting up-to-date information and advanced data in this field. To ensure the same, a matchless editorial board was set up. Every individual on the board went through rigorous rounds of assessment to prove their worth. After which they invested a large part of their time researching and compiling the most relevant data for our readers.

The editorial board has been involved in producing this book since its inception. They have spent rigorous hours researching and exploring the diverse topics which have resulted in the successful publishing of this book. They have passed on their knowledge of decades through this book. To expedite this challenging task, the publisher supported the team at every step. A small team of assistant editors was also appointed to further simplify the editing procedure and attain best results for the readers.

Apart from the editorial board, the designing team has also invested a significant amount of their time in understanding the subject and creating the most relevant covers. They scrutinized every image to scout for the most suitable representation of the subject and create an appropriate cover for the book.

The publishing team has been an ardent support to the editorial, designing and production team. Their endless efforts to recruit the best for this project, has resulted in the accomplishment of this book. They are a veteran in the field of academics and their pool of knowledge is as vast as their experience in printing. Their expertise and guidance has proved useful at every step. Their uncompromising quality standards have made this book an exceptional effort. Their encouragement from time to time has been an inspiration for everyone.

The publisher and the editorial board hope that this book will prove to be a valuable piece of knowledge for researchers, students, practitioners and scholars across the globe.

List of Contributors

Thibaut Caruba
Pharmacie, Hôpital Européen Georges Pompidou, APHP, Paris, France

Sandrine Katsahian
URC Hô pital Henri Mondor, APHP, Cré teil, France
Equipe 22, Centre de Recherche des Cordeliers, UMRS 762 INSERM, Paris, France

Catherine Schramm and Anaïs Charles Nelson
URC Hô pital Henri Mondor, APHP, Créteil, France

Pierre Durieux
Equipe 22, Centre de Recherche des Cordeliers, UMRS 762 INSERM, Paris, France
Département de Santé Publique et Informatique, Hôpital Européen Georges Pompidou, APHP, Paris

Dominique Bégué
Facultéde Pharmacie, Université RenéDescartes, Paris, France

Yves Juilliére
Cardiologie, Institut Lorrain du Coeur et des Vaisseaux Louis Mathieu, Nancy, France

Olivier Dubourg
Cardiologie, Hôpital Ambroise Paré, APHP, Boulogne Billancourt, France Universitéde Versailles-Saint Quentin, Montigny-Le-Bretonneux, France

Nicolas Danchin
Cardiologie, Hôpital Européen Georges Pompidou, APHP, Paris, France, 10 Facultéde Médecine, Université René Descartes, Paris, France

Brigitte Sabatier
Pharmacie, Hôpital Européen Georges Pompidou, APHP, Paris, France
Equipe 22, Centre de Recherche des Cordeliers, UMRS 762 INSERM, Paris, France

Weiwei Wu
Department of Vascular Surgery, Peking Union Medical College Hospital, Chinese Academy of Medical Science, Beijing, China
Department of Vascular Surgery, Beijing Tsinghua Changgung Hospital, Beijing Tsinghua University, Beijing, China

Surong Hua, Yongjun Li, Wei Ye, Bao Liu, Xiaojun Song, Yuehong Zheng and Changwei Liu
Department of Vascular Surgery, Peking Union Medical College Hospital, Chinese Academy of Medical Science, Beijing, China

Yangguang Yin and Xiaohui Zhao
Cardiovascular Disease Research Center, Xinqiao Hospital, Third Military Medical University, Chongqing, China

Yao Zhang
The Evidence Based Medicine and Clinic Epidemiology Center, Third Military Medical University, Chongqing, China

Jolanta M. Siller-Matula, Irene M. Lang, Thomas Neunteufl and Gerald Maurer
Department of Cardiology, Medical University of Vienna, Vienna, Austria

Marek Kozinski and Jacek Kubica
Department of Cardiology and Internal Medicine, Collegium Medicum of the Nicolaus Copernicus University, Bydgoszcz, Poland

Katarzyna Linkowska and Tomasz Grzybowski
Institute of Molecular and Forensic Genetics, Collegium Medicum of the Nicolaus Copernicus University, Bydgoszcz, Poland

Bernd Jilma
Department of Clinical Pharmacology, Medical University of Vienna, Vienna, Austria

Chih-Cheng Wu
Cardiovascular center, National Taiwan University Hospital, Hsinchu Branch, Hsinchu, Taiwan
School of Medicine, National Taiwan University, Taipei, Taiwan
School of Medicine, National Yang-Ming University, Taipei, Taiwan

Po-Hsun Huang
Division of Cardiology, Taipei Veterans General Hospital, Taipei, Taiwan
Department of Medicine, National Yang-Ming University, Taipei, Taiwan

Institute of Clinical Medicine, National Yang-Ming University, Taipei Taiwan
School of Medicine, National Yang-Ming University, Taipei, Taiwan Cardiovascular Research Center, National Yang-Ming University, Taipei, Taiwan

Chao-Lun Lai
Cardiovascular center, National Taiwan University Hospital, Hsinchu Branch, Hsinchu, Taiwan
School of Medicine, National Taiwan University, Taipei, Taiwan

Hsin-Bang Leu
Healthcare and Management Center, Taipei Veterans General
Hospital, Taipei, Taiwan
Cardiovascular center, National Taiwan University Hospital, Hsinchu Branch, Hsinchu, Taiwan
Cardiovascular Research Center, National Yang-Ming University, Taipei, Taiwan

Jaw-Wen Chen
Division of Cardiology, Taipei Veterans General Hospital, Taipei, Taiwan
Department of Medical Research and Education, Taipei Veterans General Hospital, Taipei, Taiwan
Cardiovascular Research Center, National Yang-Ming University, Taipei, Taiwan
Institute and Department of Pharmacology, National Yang-Ming University, Taipei, Taiwan

Shing-Jong Lin
Division of Cardiology, Taipei Veterans General Hospital, Taipei, Taiwan
Department of Medical Research and Education, Taipei Veterans General Hospital, Taipei, Taiwan
Department of Medicine, National Yang-Ming University, Taipei, Taiwan
Institute of Clinical Medicine, National Yang-Ming University, Taipei, Taiwan
School of Medicine, National Yang-Ming University, Taipei, Taiwan
Cardiovascular Research Center, National Yang-Ming University, Taipei, Taiwan

Liwen Ye, Qingwei Chen, Guiqion Li, Wei Deng and Dazhi Ke
Department of Geriatrics Cardiology, the Second Affiliated Hospital of Chongqing Medical University, Chongqing, China

Minming Zheng
Chongqing Ophthalmology Research Center for the Senile, the Second Affiliated Hospital of Chongqing Medical University, Chongqing, China
Department of Ophthalmology, the Second Affiliated Hospital of Chongqing Medical University, Chongqing, China

Truls Råmunddal, Christian Dworeck, Oskar Angerås, Jacob Odenstedt, Dan Ioanes, Göran Matejka, Per Albertsson and Elmir Omerovic
Department of Cardiology, Sahlgrenska University Hospital, Gothenburg, Sweden

Loes Hoebers and ose P. S. Henriques
Department of Cardiology, Academic Medical Center, Amsterdam, The Netherlands

GÖran Olivecrona and Jan Harnek
Department of Coronary Heart Disease, Skåne University Hospital, Scania, Sweden

Ulf Jensen, Mikael Aasa and Risto Jussila
Department of Cardiology, Stockholm South General Hospital, Stockholm, Sweden

Stefan James and Bo Lagerqvist
Department of Medical Sciences, Uppsala University, Uppsala, Sweden

Raffaele Piccolo, Gennaro Galasso, Ernesto Capuano, Stefania De Luca, Giovanni Esposito and Bruno Trimarco
Department of Advanced Biomedical Sciences, Federico II University, Naples, Italy

Federico Piscione
Department of Medicine and Surgery, University of Salerno, Salerno, Italy

Pier Woudstra, Peter Damman, Wichert J. Kuijt, Wouter J. Kikkert, Maik J. Grundeken, Peter M. van Brussel , Karel T. Koch, JoséP. S. Henriques, Jan J. Piek, Jan G. P. Tijssen and Robbert J. de Winter
Heart Center, Academic Medical Center – University of Amsterdam, Amsterdam, The Netherlands

An K. Stroobants, Jan P. van Straalen and Johan C. Fischer
Department of Clinical Chemistry, Academic Medical Center – University of Amsterdam, Amsterdam, The Netherlands

Joo Myung Lee, Jonghanne Park, Ki-Hyun Jeon, Ji-hyun Jung, Sang Eun Lee, Jung-Kyu Han, Han-Mo Yang, Kyung Woo Park, Hyun-Jae Kang and Bon-Kwon Koo
Department of Internal Medicine and Cardiovascular Center, Seoul National University Hospital, Seoul, Korea

Hack-Lyoung Kim
Cardiovascular Center, Seoul National University, Boramae Medical Center, Seoul, Korea

Sang-Ho Jo
Division of Cardiology, Department of Internal Medicine, Hallym University Sacred Heart Hospital, Anyang-si, Gyeonggi-do, Korea

Hyo-Soo Kim
Department of Internal Medicine and Cardiovascular Center, Seoul National University Hospital, Seoul, Korea
Department of Molecular Medicine and Biopharmaceutical Sciences, Graduate School of Convergence Science and Technology, Seoul National University, Seoul, Korea

Alexandra R. Lucas, Erbin Dai, Liying Liu, Hao Chen and Sriram Ambadapadi
Division of Cardiovascular Medicine, Departments of Medicine and Molecular Genetics & Microbiology, College of Medicine, University of Florida, Gainesville, Florida, United States of America

Raj K. Verma, Sheela Kesavalu, Mercedes Rivera, Irina Velsko and Sasanka Chukkapalli
Department of Periodontology, College of Dentistry, University of Florida, Gainesville, Florida, United States of America

Lakshmyya Kesavalu
Department of Periodontology, College of Dentistry, University of Florida, Gainesville, Florida, United States of America Department of Oral
Biology, College of Dentistry, University of Florida, Gainesville, Florida, United States of America

Xiao-Lin Li, Jian-Jun Li, Yuan-Lin Guo, Cheng-Gang Zhu, Rui-Xia Xu, Sha Li, Ping Qing, Na-Qiong Wu, Li- Xin Jiang, Bo Xu and Run-Lin Gao
Division of Dyslipidemia, State Key Laboratory of Cardiovascular Disease, Fu Wai Hospital, National Center for Cardiovascular Diseases, Chinese Academy of Medical Sciences and Peking Union Medical College, XiCheng District, Beijing, China

Wei-Chieh Lee, Tzu-Hsien Tsai, Yung-Lung Chen, Cheng-Hsu Yang, Shyh-Ming Chen, Chien-Jen Chen, Cheng-Jei Lin, Cheng-I Cheng and Chi-Ling Hang
Division of Cardiology, Department of Internal Medicine, Kaohsiung Chang Gung Memorial Hospital and Chang Gung University College of Medicine, Kaohsiung, Taiwan

Chiung-Jen Wu
Center for Translational Research in Biomedical Sciences, Kaohsiung Chang Gung Memorial Hospital and Chang Gung University College of Medicine, Kaohsiung, Taiwan

Hon-Kan Yip
Institute of Shock Wave Medicine and Tissue Engineering, Kaohsiung Chang Gung Memorial Hospital and Chang Gung University College of Medicine, Kaohsiung, Taiwan

Ching-Hui Huang
Division of Cardiology, Department of Internal Medicine, Changhua Christian Hospital, Changhua, Taiwan
Department of Biological Science and Technology, National Chiao Tung University, Hsinchu, Taiwan

Chia-Chu Chang
Division of Nephrology, Department of Internal Medicine, Changhua Christian Hospital, Changhua, Taiwan
School of Medicine, Chung Shan Medical University, Taichung, Taiwan

Chen-Ling Kuo and Ching-Shan Huang
Vascular and Genomic Research Center, Changhua Christian Hospital, Changhua, Taiwan

Tzai-Wen Chiu and Chih-Sheng Lin
Department of Biological Science and Technology, National Chiao Tung University, Hsinchu, Taiwan

Chin-San Liu
Vascular and Genomic Research Center, Changhua Christian Hospital, Changhua, Taiwan
Department of Neurology, Changhua Christian Hospital, Changhua, Taiwan
Graduate Institute of Integrative Medicine, China Medical University, Taichung, Taiwan

Song-Bai Deng, Jing Wang, Ling Wu, Xiao-Dong Jing, Yu-Ling Yan, Jian-Lin Du, Ya-Jie Liu and Qiang She
Department of Cardiology, The Second Affiliated Hospital of Chongqing Medical University, Chongqing, China

Jun Xiao
Department of Cardiology, The Medical Emergency Center of Chongqing, Chongqing, China

Hai-Mu Yao, De-Liang Shen, You-You Du, Jin-Ying Zhang, Ling Li and Luo-Sha Zhao
Department of Cardiology, the First Affiliated Hospital of Zhengzhou University, Zhengzhou, P. R. China

Tong-Wen Sun, Xiao-Juan Zhang and You-Dong Wan
Department of Integrated ICU, the First Affiliated Hospital of Zhengzhou University, Zhengzhou, P. R. China

Pei-Chuan Li and Ming-Jyh Sheu
School of Pharmacy, China Medical University, Taichung, Taiwan

Chun-Hsu Pan
College of Pharmacy, Taipei Medical University, Taipei, Taiwan

Chin-Ching Wu
Department of Public Health, China Medical University, Taichung, Taiwan

Wei-Fen Ma
School of Nursing, China Medical University, Taichung, Taiwan

Chieh-Hsi Wu
School of Pharmacy, China Medical University, Taichung, Taiwan
College of Pharmacy, Taipei Medical University, Taipei, Taiwan
Department of Biological Science and Technology, China Medical
University, Taichung, Taiwan

Bo Kyung Koo
Department of Internal Medicine, Seoul National University College of Medicine, Seoul, Republic of Korea
Department of Internal Medicine, Boramae Medical Center, Seoul, Republic of Korea

Chang-Hoon Lee
Department of Internal Medicine, Seoul National University College of Medicine, Seoul, Republic of Korea

Bo Ram Yang
Division of Clinical Epidemiology, Medical Research Collaborating Center, Seoul National University College of Medicine, Seoul, Republic of Korea
Department of Preventive Medicine, Seoul National University College of Medicine, Seoul, Republic of Korea

Seung-sik Hwang
Department of Social and Preventive Medicine, Inha University School of Medicine, Incheon, Republic of Korea

Nam-Kyong Choi
Division of Clinical Epidemiology, Medical Research Collaborating Center, Seoul National University College of Medicine, Seoul, Republic of Korea
Institute of Environmental Medicine, Seoul National University Medical Research Center, Seoul, Republic of Korea

Antonia E. Curtin
Department of Bioengineering, University of Pittsburgh, Pittsburgh, Pennsylvania, United States of America

Leming Zhou
Department of Bioengineering, University of Pittsburgh, Pittsburgh, Pennsylvania, United States of America
Department of Health Information Management, University of Pittsburgh, Pittsburgh, Pennsylvania, United States of America

Khalid Bashar, Donagh Healy, Elrasheid A. H. Kheirelseid, Mary Clarke – Moloney, Paul E. Burke and Eamon G. Kavanagh
Department of vascular surgery, University Hospital Limerick, Limerick, Ireland

Leonard D. Browne and Michael T. Walsh
Centre for Applied Biomedical Engineering Research (CABER), Department of Mechanical, Aeronautical & Biomedical Engineering, Materials and Surface Science Institute, University of Limerick, Limerick, Ireland

Stewart Redmond Walsh
Department of surgery, National University of Ireland, Galway, Ireland

Yong Liu, Ning Tan, Ji-yan Chen, Ying-ling Zhou, Li-wen Li, Jian-fang Luo, Hua-long Li and Wei-Guo
Department of Cardiology, Guangdong Cardiovascular Institute, Guangdong General Hospital, Guangdong Academy of Medical Sciences, Guangzhou, Guangdong, China

Yuan-hui Liu
Department of Cardiology, Guangdong Cardiovascular Institute, Guangdong General Hospital, Guangdong Academy of Medical Sciences, Guangzhou, Guangdong, China Southern medical university, Guangzhou, Guangdong, China

Chong-yang Duan and Ping-Yan Chen
Department of Biostatistics, School of Public Health and Tropical Medicine, Southern Medical University, Guangzhou, China

David Maresca
Department of Biomedical Engineering, Erasmus University Medical Centre, Rotterdam, the Netherlands

Samantha Adams
Tilburg Institute for Law, Technology and Society, Tilburg
University, Tilburg, the Netherlands

Bruno Maresca
Centre de recherche pour l'e´tude et l'observation des conditions de vie, Paris, France

Antonius F. W. van der Steen
Department of Biomedical Engineering, Erasmus University Medical Centre, Rotterdam, the Netherlands
Interuniversity Cardiology Institute of the Netherlands, Utrecht, the Netherlands, Imaging Science and Technology, Delft University of Technology, Delft, the Netherlands
Imaging Science and Technology, Delft University of Technology, Delft, the Netherlands

Song Ding, Longwei Xu, Fan Yang, Lingcong Kong, Yichao Zhao, Lingchen Gao, Wei Wang, Rende Xu, Heng Ge, Meng Jiang and Jun Pu, Ben He
From Department of Cardiology, Ren Ji Hospital, School of Medicine, Shanghai Jiao Tong University, Shanghai, China

Index